Controversies in Neurocritical Care

Prasanna Udupi Bidkar
Mathangi Krishnakumar
Editors

Controversies in Neurocritical Care

BYWORD BOOKS™

Springer

Editors
Prasanna Udupi Bidkar
Division of Neuroanaesthesiology and Neurocritical Care, Department of Anesthesiology and Critical Care
Jawaharlal Institute of Postgraduate Medical Education and Research (JIPMER)
Puducherry, Pondicherry, India

Mathangi Krishnakumar
Surgical and Neuro Intensive Care Unit, Department of Anaesthesia
St John's Medical College Hospital
Bangalore, Karnataka, India

ISBN 978-981-95-4418-9 ISBN 978-981-95-4419-6 (eBook)
https://doi.org/10.1007/978-981-95-4419-6

Jointly published with Byword Books
Co-publishing partnership between Byword Books Private Limited and Springer Nature Singapore Pte Ltd.
The registered company address is 152 Beach Road, #21-01/04 Gateway East, Singapore, 189721, Singapore

This Springer imprint is published by the registered company Springer Nature Singapore Pte Ltd.
The registered company address is: 152 Beach Road, #21-01/04 Gateway East, Singapore 189721, Singapore

To the mentors, pioneers, and relentless thinkers in Neurocritical Care—who questioned dogma, embraced debate, and made progress possible through intellectual courage.

To the patients who trusted us in their most vulnerable moments, and to the families who stood by them—this book is a testament to the courage it takes to face the uncertainty in Neurocritical Care.

Foreword 1

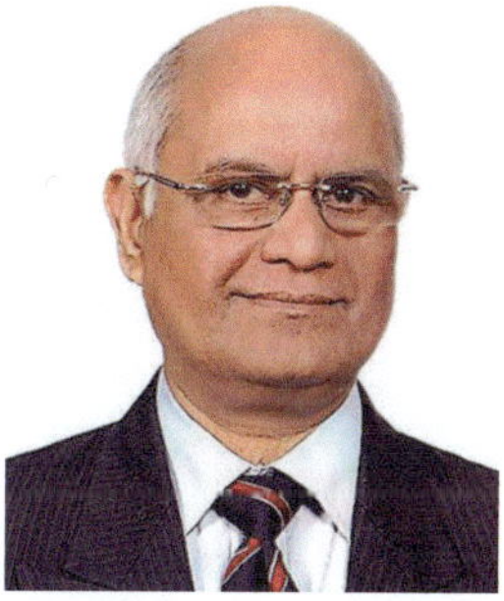

Neurocritical care has grown remarkably since its inception as a postoperative neurosurgical intensive care way back in 1923. Advances in technology, better understanding of the pathophysiology of neurocritical illnesses, and improved hemodynamic and neuro monitoring are major contributing factors for its phenomenal growth. The utilization of neurocritical care units has been associated with sharp decline in mortality rates, decrease in ICU and hospital stay, and improved functional outcome. Independent departments of neurocritical care have been established both in public sector and corporate hospitals in India to provide best possible care to critically ill neurological patients.

To keep pace with the advancements and growth of neurocritical care, it is prudent to have reading materials, books, and journals to guide the caregivers and neurocritical care fellows. Dr. Prasanna Bidkar, who was my DM Neuroanaesthesiology and Neurocritical care student, along with Dr. Mathangi Krishnakumar, a dynamic and very active neurointensivist, has taken the lead in publishing the book entitled *Controversies in Neurocritical Care*. We generally tend to extrapolate Western literature to our Indian context which may not be quite correct. Genetic predisposition and racial and environmental factors with resource crunch may seriously affect the incidence and outcome. This book can fill the void. The book has 24 chapters covering all controversial topics of neurocritical care. Renowned teachers and researchers of neurocritical care from reputed centers of India have contributed to these chapters.

I am confident that this book will be of immense help not only to the students of neurocritical care but will be a great referral book for all neuroscientists. I congratulate Dr. Prasanna and Dr. Mathangi for this commendable effort.

Emeritus Consultant
Neuroanaesthesiology and Neurocritical Care
Fortis Memorial Research Institute
Gurugram, India

Hari Hara Dash

Foreword 2

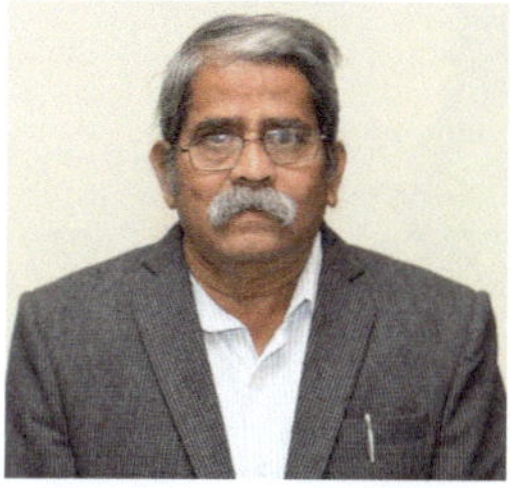

Neurocritical care is full of controversies because brain is a complex organ and pathology of brain is full of dilemmas. These controversies pose problems for the clinicians managing patients in neurocritical care. A lot of research is going on into resolving these ambiguities, but the problems still remain. In this book Prof. Bidkar and Dr. Mathangi have made an attempt to bring out the various controversies involved in the management of neurocritical care patients. They are not suggesting definite solutions for all these problems, but they are bringing about clarity in understanding these issues so that management of neurocritical care patients becomes more rational.

Controversies exist regarding the management of hemodynamics in various critical care situations, anticoagulation in cerebral venous thrombosis and thromboprophylaxis postoperatively. Dilemmas exist in the use of antiepileptics in refractory status epilepticus. There are no clear-cut guidelines on ventilatory strategy in patients with brain injury and sedation practices in neurocritical care unit. A lot of literature has accumulated on neuroprotective strategies in brain-injured patients with no clarity on what the ideal technique is in each clinical situation. There are difficulties regarding brain death certification and end-of-life care.

All the above controversies and many others have been addressed by the authors in this book. To the extent possible, they provided evidence-based approaches to these problems. But on a lot of issues there is no concrete evidence one way or the other.

They still remain the focus of future research. Until concrete answers are found out for these issues, clinical practices should be based on pragmatic approaches with best interest of the patient in mind.

Retired Senior Professor of Neuroanaesthesia and Neurocritical Care
National Institute of Mental Health and Neurosciences (NIMHANS)
Bangalore, India

G. S. Umamaheswara Rao

Preface

Neurocritical care is a science of vigilance—where decisions are measured in milliseconds, outcomes often hang in balance, and certainty is a luxury few can afford. In this field, controversy is not an anomaly but a companion; it is the by-product of progress, the residue of unanswered questions, and the spark that fuels clinical innovation.

Controversies in Neurocritical Care was conceived as a response to the real-world dilemmas faced by neurointensivists, anesthesiologists, neurologists, neurosurgeons, and critical care practitioners. The practice of neurocritical care in our context is as dynamic as it is diverse, influenced by resource availability, institutional culture, patient heterogeneity, and evolving evidence—often from faraway systems that may not mirror our own. Against this backdrop, we recognized the need for a textbook that does not offer prescriptive formulas but encourages thoughtful engagement with complexity.

Each chapter dissects a core controversy, balancing available evidence with pragmatic insight, and encourages the reader to think beyond protocol-driven care. From the management of traumatic brain injury to ethical considerations in end-of-life care, we have attempted to curate a dialogue rather than deliver a decree.

This is a book that acknowledges the imperfect nature of medical science, especially in critically ill neurological patients, and invites readers to embrace uncertainty—not passively, but with curiosity and clinical acumen.

Our contributors, drawn from academic institutions across India, have been unafraid to question dogma, examine conflicting data, and present balanced perspectives. The aim is not to create consensus, but to sharpen clinical judgment and promote academic discourse.

With gratitude to our mentors, colleagues, and learners—whose questions were often the genesis of these chapters—we offer this book as both a reference and a conversation.

If this book provokes reflection, challenges assumptions, or even sparks a spirited corridor debate—we will consider our mission accomplished.

Puducherry, Pondicherry, India — Prasanna Udupi Bidkar
Bangalore, Karnataka, India — Mathangi Krishnakumar

Contents

About the Editors

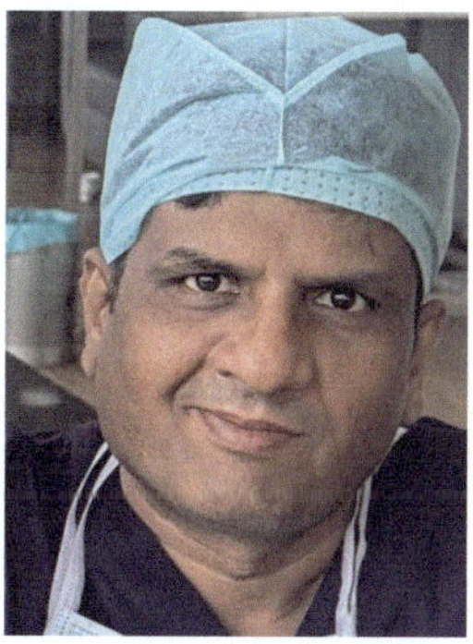

Prasanna Bidkar, MD,DNB,DM(Neuroanaesthesia), MBA is a Professor and Head of Division of Neuroanaesthesiology and Neurocritical Care at the Jawaharlal Institute of Postgraduate Medical Education and Research (JIPMER), Pondicherry, India. He has more than 20 years of experience in the field of Neuroanaesthesiology and Neurocritical care. He has more than 100 publications and has delivered 250 invited guest lectures. He has authored 2 books on Acute Neuro Care and Manual of airway management and 35 book chapters in various books on neurosciences. He is recipient of many awards and has been part of multiple Internationally funded (PHRI Canada) multicenter trials. He is the founder member and first treasurer of Neurocritical Care Society of Inda (NCSI) and course chairman for DM – Neuroanesthesiology and Neurocritical care at JIPMER, Pondicherry.

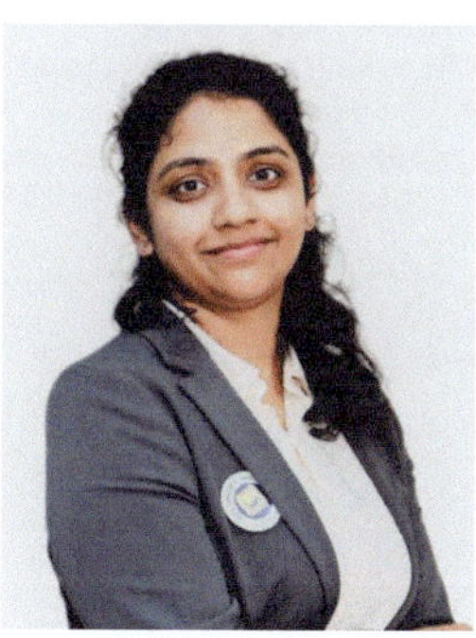

Mathangi Krishnakumar, MD, DM, PDF (Neurocritical Care) is an alumni of Armed Forces Medical College (AFMC) Pune and has completed her DM Neuroanesthesiology and Neurocritical care from NIMHANS, Bangalore. Currently she is working as Associate Professor in the neurosurgical and general intensive care at the St John's Medical College Hospital, Bengaluru, India. She has received multiple appreciation awards published several publications, authored book chapters, and has been a regular faculty in various national conferences. She has organized many CME, workshops and national conference.

Traumatic Brain Injury

1

Keshav Goyal, Suman Sokhal, and Varun Chelani

Abstract

Traumatic brain injury presents a myriad of challenges in both its acute management and long-term care. The continuously evolving research behind traumatic brain injury (TBI) has generated new evidence over the years and created controversies with existing beliefs. The chapter tries to throw light on some of the important practical issues encompassing prehospital, emergency, and intensive care management of TBI patients.

Keywords

Traumatic brain injury (TBI) · Intracranial pressure (ICP) monitoring · Cerebral perfusion pressure (CPP) · Decompressive craniectomy · Multimodal neuromonitoring

1.1 Introduction

Current treatment of traumatic brain injury (TBI) patients is mostly dependent on the Brain Trauma Foundation (BTF) guidelines and institutional protocols. One-size-fits-all is not possible, given the heterogeneity in TBI pathology and other patient-related factors. Within this complex landscape of TBI, several controversies persist, stirring debate among clinicians and researchers. This section will deal with a few common controversies and delve into the related recent evidence to guide the management of TBI patients.

K. Goyal (✉) · S. Sokhal · V. Chelani
Department of Neuroanaesthesiology & Critical Care, All India Institute of Medical Sciences, New Delhi, Delhi, India

P. U. Bidkar, M. Krishnakumar (eds.), *Controversies in Neurocritical Care*, https://doi.org/10.1007/978-981-95-4419-6_1

The common topics of controversy discussed are:

1. TBI management in specialized neurocritical care units
2. Prehospital intubation by paramedics
3. Need for individualization of thresholds
4. Tranexamic acid in TBI
5. Cerebrospinal fluid (CSF) diversion procedures
6. Mannitol vs. hypertonic saline
7. Anti-seizure prophylaxis
8. Primary or secondary decompression
9. Hypothermia in TBI
10. Neuromonitoring in TBI

1.1.1 TBI Management in Neurocritical Care Units

Q: Should TBI be managed in specialised Neuro ICU?

Neurocritical care units (NCUs) are specialized intensive care units dedicated to managing critically ill patients with neurological and neurosurgical conditions. NCUs offer a multidisciplinary team of neurointensivists, neurosurgeons, neurologists, and critical care nurses with advanced monitoring techniques such as intracranial pressure monitoring (ICP), cerebral oxygenation monitoring, and electroencephalography (EEG), enabling early detection of complications and implementation of targeted interventions to optimize patient outcomes.

Evidence:

- An extensive observational study (1989–2003) from England and Wales concluded that TBI patients treated in neurosurgical centers were associated with a 26% decrease in mortality and a 2.15 times decrease in the odds of death if matched with a non-neurosurgical facility [1].
- The "*Point of View*" paper by Smith et al. delineated aspects for improved outcomes at NCUs as protocolized care, improved control of brain and systemic physiology by neurointensivists, multimodal monitoring, and rapid access to interventions [2].
- In 2013, the Risk Adjustment in Neurocritical care (RAIN) study confirmed better outcomes in neuroscience-associated critical care units. The RAIN study found that treatment in NCUs is more cost-effective than combined neuro and general ICU care due to high mean-lifetime quality-adjusted life-years (QALYs) [3].
- According to the findings of a recent review and meta-analysis, neurocritical care services offer better mortality rates and functional outcomes for adults with brain injury. Patients in neurocritical care units have a 17% lower relative risk of dying or having an unfavorable functional outcome when compared to patients in conventional ICUs [4].

- The evidence provides the basis for the National Institute for Clinical Excellence (NICE 2023), which advises that all patients with sTBI should be transferred to NCUs independent of the requirement for neurosurgery. If it is not possible to transfer patients who do not require neurosurgery, continue to liaise with neurosciences over clinical management [5].
- Monteiro et al. compared the neuro ICU management backed by multimodal neuro monitoring to general intensive care unit management after acute brain injury. They concluded that patients managed at NCUs had an odds ratio of 0.228, i.e., a lower risk of poor outcome. Neurocritical care management was associated with better outcomes at various time points at intensive care unit discharge, at 28 days, at 3 months, and at 6 months after trauma [6].

  The probable reasons for better outcomes in NCUs may be: [7]

  1. Brain-centered care and a more experienced multidisciplinary team can identify signs of neurological decline as soon as possible
  2. Strictly following guidelines to prevent secondary brain injury
  3. Optimal and effective use of multimodal brain monitoring techniques
  4. Physiotherapy and neurorehabilitation centers
  5. Better communication and focus

Conclusion:

The benefits of managing TBI in NCUs outweigh the drawbacks; emphasize the importance of managing patients at NCUs, especially for sTBI. However, access to specialized NCUs and transfer time should be considered. Resource constraints, including bed availability and staffing shortages, can strain NCUs' capacity to accommodate all TBI patients, and good communication with neuro intensivists may help in better patient management.

1.1.2 Prehospital Intubation by Paramedics

Q. Yes or No?

Post-trauma patients with sTBI are susceptible to clogging of the airway and hypoxia. Endotracheal intubation (ETI) performed by paramedics is a common practice in many emergency medical services (EMS) systems to secure the airway, prevent hypoxemia, and decrease secondary brain injury. On the other hand, ETI performed by inexperienced paramedics may even compromise the airway and ventilation, lead to iatrogenic injuries and transport delays, and thus contribute to exacerbating secondary brain injury and adverse outcomes.

Evidence:

- Davis and colleagues demonstrated that intubation leads to increased deaths if attempted by less efficient EMS providers [8]. Choffat's prospective trial concluded that prehospital intubation improves outcomes for patients with sTBI and an injury severity score (ISS) ≥ 25; however, all intubations in this study were performed by trained medical personnel [9].

- The Excellence in Prehospital Injury Care (EPIC) study conducted in the USA followed the implementation of the prehospital TBI guidelines wherein clinical protocols suggested supplementation of high-flow oxygen to all TBI cases if needed, bag-mask ventilation using airway maneuvers and airway adjuncts, and ETI to be performed only if an experienced advanced life support (ALS) provider is available. This implementation of guidelines was independently associated with improvement in survival among patients with sTBI and in the severe, prehospital intubated group [10].
- Data from CENTER-TBI ($n = 4509$) concluded that prehospital intubation had improved recovery after chest and abdominal injuries (extracranial injury), whereas in-hospital intubation improved the outcome of head injury patients and associated Glasgow Coma Scale (GCS) scores of ≤10. The possible reasons for poor outcomes in prehospital intubation in TBI patients were a post-intubation rise in ICP, use of sedatives, and associated hypotension and hyperventilation in intubated patients [11].
- Bossers et al. conducted an analysis using a Dutch nationwide trauma registry and concluded that the impact of prehospital intubation on mortality may vary based on the EMS clinician's experience. Therefore, it is advisable to involve prehospital personnel who are highly skilled in intubation whenever it is deemed necessary [12].

Conclusion: Endotracheal intubation, before reaching the hospital in patients with sTBI, is advantageous only if done by qualified experts in concordance with established recommendations; otherwise, the airway can be managed with bag-mask ventilation by paramedics. If the transport time is longer, then the senior physician should ideally be a part of the EMS team, or at least the paramedical staff should be well-trained for intubation.

1.1.3 Need for Individualization of Thresholds?

Q. What should the systolic blood pressure (SBP) threshold be in TBI?

If cerebral autoregulation is disturbed after TBI, maintaining a stable systolic blood pressure (SBP) becomes decisive to prevent both insufficient and excessive cerebral blood flow. So, the SBP threshold is crucial in critically ill patients with a head injury.

Evidence:

- Berry et al. conducted a retrospective analysis ($N = 15{,}733$) on adult trauma patients to find out the optimal threshold of SBP in predefined age categories (15–49 years, 50–69 years, and ≥ 70 years). Lower mortality was seen when 100–110 mm Hg was the threshold [13]. To reduce deaths and to improve functional outcome, the Brain Trauma Foundation (BTF) guidelines advocated for maintaining SBP at ≥100 mm Hg and ≥ 110 mm Hg for patients aged 50–69 years and for 15–49 or ≥ 70 years, respectively [14].

- Spaite et al. studied prehospital hypotension cutoff points for mortality in moderate-to-severe TBI in patients aged >10 years. After analyzing the data, they concluded that there was a linear relationship between the lowest value of prehospital SBP and the probability of mortality, but they were unable to find any identifiable threshold between 40 and 119 mm Hg. They mentioned that 90 mm Hg as a physiological cutoff point may be incorrect. The adjusted mortality characteristic showed three different features: (1) chances of death decrease gradually between 40 and 125 mm Hg, (2) remain low from 130 to 180 mm Hg, and (3) then increase rapidly above 180 mm Hg [15].
- A recent study based on 1,54,725 adult patients with isolated TBI showed that systolic blood pressure (SBP) under 110 mm Hg should be considered as the cutoff for hypotension in adult patients aged 50–69. The risk of in-hospital mortality decreases as SBP increases, leveling off at 110 mm Hg [16].

Conclusion: In sTBI, systolic blood pressure must be maintained at ≥100–110 mm Hg. Similarly, very high SBP (>180 mm Hg) should be controlled in previously normotensive patients. Still, these numbers are just a guide, there is a need for an individualized approach based on various patient factors, including cerebral autoregulation.

Q. What should the cerebral perfusion pressure (CPP) and ICP thresholds be in TBI?

The BTF guidelines suggest treating ICP above 22 mm Hg to reduce mortality rates both in the hospital and within 2 weeks post-injury for sTBI patients. Additionally, they recommend maintaining a CPP of 60–70 mm Hg to ensure survival and to achieve favorable outcomes [14]. However, an ideal CPP target is needed due to the variability in cerebral autoregulation across individuals and the evolving nature of injury. This makes a one-size-fits-all approach impractical.

Evidence:

- Sorrentino and colleagues determined critical threshold values for cerebral perfusion pressure (CPP), intracranial pressure (ICP), and the pressure-reactivity index (PRx) and found that 22 mm Hg for ICP and 70 mm Hg for CPP were the optimal thresholds for adults for both reducing mortality and improving neurological outcome. For patients with impaired regulation (PRx ≥0.05), those with CPP <70 had significantly poorer outcomes [17].
- Lazaridis et al. suggested that the pressure-reactivity index (PRx) can be used to individualize the ICP threshold by plotting the connection between ICP and PRx [18].
- Donnelly et al. investigated a CPP autoregulation range and concluded that a plausible alternative to the fixed CPP (60–70 mm Hg) was individualized autoregulation-guided CPP management in sTBI patients [19].

- Tas et al. in the COGiTATE study assessed the practicability and safety of cerebral autoregulation-guided CPP (CPPopt) in head-injured patients who require ICP monitoring. They concluded that tailoring one's care by aiming for a variable, optimal CPP is achievable and safe in TBI patients [20].
- Beqiri et al., in their CENTER-TBI sub-study analysis, studied the lower edge of CPP in TBI patients. They concluded that if CPP was below the lower limit of reactivity, then it increased the risk of mortality within the first week after injury [21].
- Brasil et al.'s survey of global experienced professionals managing severe head injury patients across low-middle-income countries (LMICs) and high-income countries (HICs) concluded that skilled clinicians have a tendency to individualize ICP management. Waveform analysis of ICP, added to noninvasive techniques, potentially enhances individualized patient care, especially in LMICs [22].

Conclusion: Cerebral autoregulation should be assessed using multimodal monitoring. Individualized CPP and ICP thresholds shall be the way forward to meet the unique needs of TBI patients for better outcomes. ICP is not only a number, but waveforms should also be assessed.

1.1.4 Tranexamic Acid in TBI

Q. Yes or no? If yes, then what should be the timing? Dose? In which patients?

In TBI patients, the incidence of coagulation dysfunction is as high as 60%. It is mainly initiated by endogenous plasminogen activator, causing excessive fibrinolysis, hematoma expansion, cerebral edema, and raised ICP. Tranexamic acid (TXA), an antifibrinolytic agent, blocks the lysine binding sites on plasminogen molecules and inhibits the conversion of plasminogen to plasmin, thereby reducing fibrinolysis and stabilizing blood clots [23]. But its administration is also associated with complications like seizures, thromboembolism, hypotension, anaphylaxis, etc.

Evidence:

- Initial enthusiasm for TXA in TBI was seen in the CRASH-2 trial, which found that the early intravenous dosing of TXA (loading followed by infusion) within 3 h of injury significantly reduced mortality in bleeding trauma patients. As isolated TBI was not an inclusion criterion, this prompted further investigation, specifically into the TBI scenario [23].
- CRASH-3, a large-scale randomized controlled trial (RCT) conducted on over 12,000 isolated TBI patients, concluded that, TXA administration within 3 h of head injury starting with a dose of 1 g over 10 min followed by an infusion of 1 g over 8 h significantly reduced head injury-related deaths in mild-to-moderate TBI patients, though it did not improve overall survival or outcomes in severe TBI [24].

- Rowell et al. executed a study to determine whether TXA initiated in the out-of-hospital setting improves neurologic outcome in patients with moderate or severe TBI when administered within 2 h of injury. They found that, in comparison with placebo, TXA did not significantly improve 6-month neurologic outcome or progression of intracranial hematoma [25].
- A systematic review by Lawati et al. concluded that in acute TBI, TXA neither increases side effects nor affects outcome, but it could potentially reduce the growth of a hematoma as seen in follow-up imaging [26].
- While another systematic review in acute TBI patients, by Song et al., concluded that TXA administration reduced both hematoma progression and mortality, the incidence of neurosurgery and pulmonary embolism remained comparable to those observed with the placebo [27].

Conclusion: Current evidence is inconclusive in warranting routine administration of TXA in all patients, but it may be useful in mild-to-moderate TBI patients. Though bleeding multi-trauma patients should receive it early (<3 h of injury), otherwise administration of TXA should be individualized as per patient profile in TBI.

1.1.5 CSF Diversion Procedures

Q. Yes or No?

CSF diversion (External Ventricular Drain or Lumbar Drain) is considered a tier I approach for intracranial hypertension management in TBI. But it is associated with risks and complications like hemorrhage, infection, catheter malposition, over drainage, and cerebrospinal fluid leaks.

Evidence:

- BTF guidelines suggest that when the initial GCS score is <6, CSF drainage should be used to lower ICP in patients during the first 12 h after the injury [14]. It is based on a retrospective study by Griesdale et al. that demonstrated a statistically insignificant trend for lower mortality with CSF drainage (EVD) in patients with a GCS score < 6 but increased mortality during hospital stay and 28 days post-injury in patients with a GCS score ≥ 6 [28].
- A retrospective trial by Akbib et al. concluded that during the first 4 min of opening the external ventricular drain (EVD), intracranial pressure (ICP) decreased by 5.7 ± 0.6 mm Hg, cerebral perfusion pressure (CPP) increased by 4.1 ± 1.2 mm Hg, and brain tissue oxygenation ($PbtO_2$) increased by 1.15 ± 0.26 mm Hg. Hence, they concluded that ICP, CPP, and $PbtO_2$ improved with CSF drainage of EVD when the opening pressure is above 25 mm Hg [29].
- Recent research on comparative effectiveness challenged the role of CSF diversion in 1000 children with sTBI. Despite decreased ICP in the children, no relation was found between CSF diversion procedures and improved outcomes at 6 months [30].

Q. Continuous or intermittent drainage? What is the optimal timing?

There is a difference in opinion regarding the continuous monitoring of ICP and only intermittently draining CSF or continuous drainage of CSF with intermittent ICP measurements. Otherwise, the intraparenchymal fiberoptic catheter may be used for ICP measurements along with EVD for continuous drainage.

Evidence:

- Nwachuku et al., in their retrospective study, examined the effects of continuous versus intermittent cerebrospinal fluid (CSF) drainage on intracranial pressure (ICP) in sTBI adults and concluded that open EVD with continuous CSF drainage led to better control of intracranial pressure (ICP) during the management [31]. However, continuous drainage may lead to ventricular collapse and EVD obstruction [32].
- Chau et al. published a systematic review on the optimal timing of external ventricular drainage after sTBI and highlighted the lack of high-quality research on this topic [33].
- Recently, Taylor and colleagues investigated whether early EVD insertion (within 24 h of injury) may result in better 6-month functional outcomes in patients with moderate-to-severe TBI compared with EVD insertion >24 h after injury [34].

Conclusion: CSF diversion procedures may decrease ICP and increase CPP in TBI patients, but their role in functional outcomes is still inconclusive. If CSF diversion is used, the early and continuous CSF drainage can result in better overall ICP control. Still, the risk-benefit ratio should be considered before the procedure.

1.1.6 Mannitol Versus Hypertonic Saline

Q. Which hyperosmotic agent is preferred in TBI: mannitol or hypertonic saline?

Mannitol and hypertonic saline (HTS) are the most often used hyperosmotic agents for the management of intracranial hypertension in TBI patients [35]. Hypertonic saline is used in 3.0–23.4% concentrations.

Evidence:

- Miyoshi et al. carried out a meta-analysis to find the effects of HTS versus mannitol in TBI patients in prehospital, casualty, and ICU settings. No significant difference in mortality was seen using either of the agents for controlling raised ICP [36].
- Alternative systematic review and meta-analysis also concluded that both agents can effectively decrease ICP. Onset time was similar in both, but 3% HTS reduced ICP more easily and was sustained for longer. The duration of mannitol action is affected by the infusion rate due to rapid renal elimination. Serious side

effects like acute renal insufficiency and rebound cerebral edema are more common with mannitol [37].
- Han et al. concluded that 30–60 min after administration in patients with TBI, HTS caused a greater fall in ICP and increased CPP in comparison with mannitol [38].
- Post-hoc analysis of osmotherapy in the erythropoietin trial in TBI concluded that an increase in acute kidney injury was seen in the early (within 2 days) use of mannitol [39].
- Roquilly et al. compared the continuous infusion of 20% hypertonic saline, plus standard care, and standard care alone for 6-month neurological outcomes in moderate-to-severe head injury patients continuous hyperosmolar therapy for traumatic brain injury (COBI Trial). Both groups were comparable, and 20% HTS did not show any significant benefit [40].
- Bernhardt et al. conducted a meta-analysis, including RCTs beyond the year 2000, in which they compared HTS vs. other ICP-lowering treatments in patients with TBI across all age groups. They found that there was no significant difference in the length of hospital or ICU stay, neurological function, mortality, or uncontrolled ICP. Though serum sodium levels were comparatively higher in patients receiving HTS [41].

Conclusion:

Either of the agents can be used to decrease ICP with equal efficacy in adult TBI, with a slight sustained effect with HTS. HTS is preferred over mannitol in patients with acute renal failure and hemodynamically unstable patients (the osmotic diuretic effect of mannitol further decreases BP and CPP). HTS should be used cautiously in patients with impaired cardiac function, as volume overload may precipitate congestive cardiac failure and pulmonary edema. Serum electrolytes should be monitored with both agents, especially sodium and chloride levels, when using HTS. HTS can be given as a bolus or continuous infusion; formulations and infusion rates vary by institution, and no practice protocols exist.

1.1.7 Anti-seizure Prophylaxis in TBI

Seizures are a common complication following TBI. On EEG recordings, post-traumatic seizures (PTS) may be 12% and subclinical seizures may be approximately as high as 20–25%. Early PTS occurs within the first week after injury, while late seizures may happen weeks to years post-injury and are, often associated with the development of post-traumatic epilepsy (PTE). Some studies have compared the safety and efficacy of Phenytoin (PHT) with Levetiracetam (LEV), as Levetiracetam does not require therapeutic level monitoring, has predicted metabolism, no protein binding, and a minimal adverse event profile. Anti-seizure prophylaxis in patients with TBI is a widely debated topic within neurocritical care, primarily due to varying evidence about its efficacy and the potential for adverse effects from prolonged anti-seizure medication use.

Q. Yes Or No? If yes, then how long? Which drug?

Evidence:

- Tamkin et al. conducted an RCT to assess the impact of Phenytoin on early and late PTS. Phenytoin significantly decreased the incidence of early PTS without modifying the incidence of late PTS and mortality despite having adequate therapeutic levels of Phenytoin on the day of their first late seizure [42].
- Based on the above and other RCTs, the BTF currently recommends administering prophylactic anti-epileptic drugs (AEDs) for the first 7 days to decrease the incidence of early post-traumatic seizures in severe TBI [14].
- The long-term use of anti-seizure drugs is associated with a worse rehabilitation outcome assessed with the GCS score and the functional independence measure (FIM) [43].
- A 21-day prophylactic Phenytoin therapy was also compared with a 7-day Phenytoin therapy in TBI patients, but the 21-day therapy was not found to be effective and was also associated with more adverse side effects [44].
- A prospective, randomized, and single-centered trial comparing LEV versus PHT in patients with sTBI concluded that LEV showed lower disability and higher glasgow outcome scale (GOS) at 6 months after injury. Patients in the LEV group experienced fewer instances of gastrointestinal issues [45].
- Wang et al. led a systematic review and network meta-analysis comparing the efficacy of anticonvulsant drugs given prophylactically following TBI. They concluded that, though there is currently no strong evidence, AEDs are superior to placebo in preventing early post-traumatic seizure [46].
- A recent meta-analysis comparing the effects of LEV and PHT on seizures in TBI patients concluded that both drugs are comparable in reducing the incidence of PTS, but patients treated with LEV had a significantly shorter duration of ICU stay and a lower incidence of drug-related adverse effects [47].

Conclusion: AEDs should be considered for the first 7 days after TBI to prevent early PTS. After 7 days, the evidence does not support a benefit in reducing late PTS, but AEDs are associated with increased side effects and poor rehabilitation. LEV may be used as an alternative to PHT for seizure prophylaxis, possibly with fewer drug-related adverse effects.

1.1.8 Primary and Secondary Decompression

Primary decompression involves early surgical intervention shortly after the injury at the time of hematoma evacuation (emergency), while secondary decompression occurs as a delayed procedure to treat refractory ICP, resistant to maximal management (ultimate).

Q. Primary Decompressive Craniectomy (DC) or Craniotomy?

Acute extradural hematoma (AEDH) is less likely to be associated with intraparenchymal brain injury, so craniotomy is usually done. However, acute subdural hematoma (ASDH) is usually complicated by intraparenchymal lesions and cerebral edema. There is no concrete evidence to support osteoplastic craniotomy or primary DC in patients with these lesions, and it is a matter of controversy to date.

Evidence:

- Phen et al., in a systematic review and meta-analysis, found that patients who need primary DC already have a worse clinical status and consequently poorer postoperative outcome compared to craniotomy [48]. Similar results were observed in elderly patients with TBI in a retrospective cohort [49]. On the other hand, a recent retrospective study concluded better functional outcomes in patients with ASDH undergoing primary DC compared with craniotomy among adult patients with an initial GCS score > 4 [50].
- The current RESCUE-ASDH trial (multicenter randomized controlled trial) in patients with traumatic ASDH comparing craniotomy with primary DC found that disability and quality-of-life outcomes were similar between the two approaches at 12 months. In the craniotomy group, additional surgery was required in a higher proportion, but they had lower wound complications as compared to the craniectomy group [51].
- Essen et al. analyzed data from a CENTER-TBI study to compare 6-month functional outcomes in patients undergoing primary DC versus craniotomy. The authors concluded that primary decompressive craniectomy (DC) did not lead to improved functional outcomes as compared to craniotomy. The authors cautioned against the use of primary DC [52].
- The prospective randomized evaluation of decompressive ipsilateral craniectomy for traumatic acute epidural hematoma (PREDICT-AEDH) trial is currently ongoing and awaiting results as it will help in decision-making to improve patient outcome in AEDH patients with associated brain swelling in clinical practice [53].

Conclusion: There is no superiority of primary DC over craniotomy in patients with ASDH; hence, the decision should be individualized and restricted to patients who are salvageable with significant intraoperative brain swelling.

Q. What is the current status of secondary decompressive craniectomy?

Evidence:

- Research regarding secondary DC has been published in decompressive craniectomy (DECRA) and RESCUEicp trials. The DECRA trial by Cooper et al. investigated the outcomes of early decompressive craniectomy in severe TBI patients and found a reduction in mortality rates but increased rates of severe disability compared to standard care [54]. RESCUEicp concluded that patients with TBI and associated refractory intracranial hypertension and secondary DC led to lower mortality but more chances of these patients remaining in a vegetative state at 6 months as compared to conservative care [55].

- Kolias et al., in conducting a secondary analysis of the RESCUEicp trial, concluded that even at 24 months, patients with decompressive craniectomy for refractory ICP had a sustained reduction in mortality and were more likely to improve over time versus patients in the medical group [56].
- Zhang et al., in their meta-analysis, found that when compared to control groups, DC reduced mortality (31%) among patients with TBI [57].

Conclusion: Secondary DC can be used as a tier 3 therapy to reduce ICP and mortality, but with poor functional outcomes, and the majority of patients remain vegetative. The family should be involved in the discussion regarding practical outcomes before considering DC in TBI patients.

1.1.9 Hypothermia in TBI

Q. Yes or No? Optimal timing?

Hypothermia, the deliberate reduction of body temperature, has garnered attention as a potential neuroprotective strategy in TBI management. However, the efficacy, optimal timing, and safety of hypothermia remain subjects of controversy in clinical practice.

Evidence:

- The Eurotherm3235 trial by Andrews et al. enrolled 387 sTBI patients with ICP > 20 mm Hg even after Stage 1 treatments. They were divided into standard care or hypothermia (32–35 °C for at least 48 h) plus the standard care group. The trial was prematurely terminated due to safety concerns, as the outcome was worse in the therapeutic hypothermia group than in the standard care alone group. Serious adverse events such as cardiac arrhythmias, hyperkalemia, pneumonia, and acute respiratory distress syndrome (ARDS) were more common in the hypothermia group than in the standard care group [58].
- Prophylactic hypothermia trial to lessen traumatic brain injury—a randomized clinical trial (POLAR-RCT) found no neurologic outcome benefits after using early prophylactic hypothermia (in both the out-of-hospital and emergency department (ED) settings with a target temperature of 33 °C ± 0.5 °C for at least 72 h) for patients with sTBI [59].
- Hui et al., in their trial on sTBI, studied the safety and efficacy of long-term (5 days) mild hypothermia (34–35 °C) with refractory intracranial hypertension (LTH-1) and concluded that, in comparison with normothermia, there was no significant improvement in the neurological outcome at 6 months [60].

- The recent systematic reviews and meta-analyses concluded that in TBI patients, therapeutic hypothermia does not show any benefit over normothermia in terms of mortality and functional outcome [61].

Conclusion:

The current data do not find any evidence to support hypothermia in the management of TBI patients in terms of mortality or functional outcome; rather, it is associated with more complications. Early prophylactic hypothermia has no role in TBI patients. There is strong evidence that the use of therapeutic hypothermia lowers ICP; however, reduced ICP does not necessarily lead to improved outcomes. It can be considered as tier III therapy to reduce ICP, considering and discussing the risk-benefit with the family of the patient.

1.1.10 Neuromonitoring in TBI

Neuromonitoring techniques in the management of TBI are offering potential improvements in patient outcomes through precise measurements of brain function and physiology. Important neuromonitoring techniques include cerebral hemodynamics (ICP, CPP, and TCD), cerebral oxygenation ($SjvO_2$, near-infrared spectroscopy (NIRS), and $PbtO_2$), cerebral metabolism (microdialysis), and cerebral functional monitoring (EEG, etc.). Despite theoretical advantages, the question of whether multimodality neuromonitoring should be the standard of care remains controversial.

Q. Yes or No?
Q. Does it change the outcome?
Q. Choice of neuromonitoring?

Evidences:

- The landmark BEST TRIP trial in TBI, conducted in Bolivia and Ecuador, challenged ICP monitoring and showed that ICP monitoring, as compared to clinical examination and imaging, did not lead to any outcome difference [62].
- Multiple large observational studies (>10,000 patients) with moderate-quality evidence found that treatment guided by information from the ICP monitor was associated with a decrease in 2-week post-injury mortality and in-hospital stay [63, 64].
- A recent meta-analysis in TBI patients by Perdomo et al. concluded that there is no evidence that ICP monitoring reduces mortality [65].
- A systematic review on continuous near-infrared spectroscopy (NIRS) monitoring in adults with TBI found that NIRS measurements reflect changes in intracranial pressure, brain tissue oxygen tension ($PbtO_2$), and cerebrovascular reactivity indices. Though these were low-quality, contradictory data, they highlight the

need for more prospective studies [66]. Recent data do not suggest NIRS as an adequate substitute for $PbtO_2$ monitoring in moderate-to-severe TBI [67].
- The BOOST II trial studied the role of multimodal ICP and $PbtO_2$ monitoring in reducing brain tissue hypoxia. They found a trend toward lower mortality and more favorable outcomes than ICP-only treatment [68]. The trial led to the initiation of (BOOST-3): a multicenter, randomized, and blinded-endpoint trial to compare $PbtO_2$ and ICP monitoring versus ICP alone on functional outcome at 180 (±30) days in patients with severe TBI [69].
- The similarly planned OXY-TC trial done in France concluded that combined ICP and $PbtO_2$ monitoring, poor neurological outcomes, and mortality at 6 months in sTBI patients were not reduced [70].
- The brain oxygen neuroprotection with normobaric and augmented oxygenation (BONANZA) trial will also conclude whether the strategy guided by $PbtO_2$ affects long-term neurological and functional outcomes in patients with sTBI [71].

Conclusion: Management based on the combination of clinical, radiological, and data from multimodality monitoring will result in better outcomes in TBI patients. ICP monitoring is the standard of care in many centers, and moving away may be detrimental. ICP is not only the number but also the waveform that should be assessed for the management of TBI patients. Results of the BOOST-3 and BONANZA trials will guide the usefulness of a combination of ICP and $PbtO_2$ monitoring.

1.2 Conclusion

While the controversies in TBI management are challenging, they also fuel a dynamic field that is continuously evolving. As we move forward, clinical practice and research must be informed by a robust evidence base, interdisciplinary collaboration, and a commitment to patient-centered care. As RCTs, especially in TBI, are technically demanding, time-consuming, and not feasible ethically, comparative effectiveness research (CENTER-TBI, ADAPT) may be the way forward to answer the controversies.

1.2.1 Landmark Trials

1. CRASH 3 trial [24]: A randomized, placebo-controlled trial of 12,737 adults with TBI. On comparing the TXA vs. placebo groups in patients treated within 3 h of injury, the risk of head injury-related death was 18.5% versus 19.8%, respectively. This mortality benefit was seen in mild-to-moderate TBI but not in severe TBI patients [24].
2. BOOST-3 trial [69]: It was conducted to determine if there is any evidence of clinical efficacy of PbtO2 monitoring compared to treatment based on ICP monitoring alone. Patients with severe TBI requiring placement of ICP monitors

within 6 h of injury will be enrolled. They will be randomized into either of the treatment protocols based on ICP monitoring alone or the combination of ICP and PbtO2 monitoring. The primary outcome will be the Glasgow Outcome Scale-Extended (GOS-E) measured at 6 months post-injury. Other secondary outcomes include assessment of functional, cognitive, and behavioral outcomes at 6 months; safety; survival to discharge; shortened time to follow commands; and reduction of total brain hypoxia exposure [69].

3. COGiTATE trial [20]: This research investigated the practical use as well as the risks associated with using cerebral autoregulation to guide the CPP management of patients who experienced TBI, whose ICP needed to be monitored (TBIicp patients). The CPPopt-guided therapy: assessment of target effectiveness (COGiTATE) parallel two-arm feasibility trial took place in four tertiary centers. For every patient enrolled in the study, the BTF guideline-recommended range or the individualized CA-guided CPP targets were used to randomize the participants into two groups. No significant differences between groups were noted for TIL or other safety endpoints. In summary, we conclude that an individual and dynamic CA-guided target CPP is definitely feasible and safe in TBIicp patients [20].

References

1. Patel HC, Bouamra O, Woodford M, King AT, Yates DW, Lecky FE. Trauma audit and research network. Trends in head injury outcome from 1989 to 2003 and the effect of neurosurgical care: an observational study. Lancet. 2005;366(9496):1538–44.
2. Teig M, Smith M. Where should patients with severe traumatic brain injury be managed? All patient should be managed in a neurocritical care unit. J Neurosurg Anesthesiol. 2010 Oct;22(4):357–9.
3. Harrison DA, Prabhu G, Grieve R, Harvey SE, Sadique MZ, Gomes M, et al. Risk adjustment in Neurocritical care (RAIN)—prospective validation of risk prediction models for adult patients with acute traumatic brain injury to use to evaluate the optimum location and comparative costs of neurocritical care: a cohort study. Health Technol Assess. 2013;17(23):1–350.
4. Pham X, Ray J, Neto AS, Laing J, Perucca P, Kwan P, O'Brien TJ, Udy AA. Association of neurocritical care services with mortality and functional outcomes for adults with brain injury: a systematic review and meta-analysis. JAMA Neurol. 2022;79(10):1049–58.
5. NICE. Head injury: assessment and early management. London: National Institute for Health and Care Excellence (NICE); 2023.
6. Monteiro E, Ferreira A, Mendes ER, Silva SRE, Maia I, Dias CC, et al. Neurocritical care management supported by multimodal brain monitoring after acute brain injury. Crit Care Sci. 2023;35(2):196–202.
7. Tweedie I. Neuro-critical care versus general critical care for neurological injury: beneficial evidence. J Neuroanaesthesiol Crit Care. 2016;3:62–5.
8. Davis DP, Koprowicz KM, Newgard CD, Daya M, Bulger EM, Stiell I, Nichol G, Stephens S, Dreyer J, Minei J, Kerby JD. The relationship between out-of-hospital airway management and outcome among trauma patients with Glasgow coma scale scores of 8 or less. Prehosp Emerg Care. 2011;15(2):184–92.
9. Choffat C, Delhumeau C, Fournier N, Schoettker P. Effect of pre-hospital intubation in patients with severe traumatic brain injury on outcome: a prospective cohort study. J Clin Med. 2019;8(4):470.

10. Spaite DW, Bobrow BJ, Keim SM, Barnhart B, Chikani V, Gaither JB, et al. Association of Statewide Implementation of the prehospital traumatic brain injury treatment guidelines with patient survival following traumatic brain injury: the excellence in prehospital injury care (EPIC) study. JAMA Surg. 2019;154(7):e191152.
11. Gravesteijn B, et al. CENTER-TBI collaborators. Tracheal intubation in traumatic brain injury: a multicentre prospective observational study. Br J Anaesth. 2020;125(4):505–17.
12. Bossers SM, Verheul R, van Zwet EW, Bloemers FW, Giannakopoulos GF, Loer SA, et al. Prehospital intubation of patients with severe traumatic brain injury: a Dutch Nationwide trauma registry analysis. Prehosp Emerg Care. 2023;27(5):662–8.
13. Berry C, Ley EJ, Bukur M, et al. Redefining hypotension in traumatic brain injury. Injury. 2012;43(11):1833–7.
14. Carney N, Totten AM, O'Reilly C, Ullman JS, Hawryluk GW, Bell MJ, et al. Guidelines for the management of severe traumatic brain injury. Fourth Edition Neurosurg. 2017;80(1):6–15.
15. Spaite DW, Hu C, Bobrow BJ, Chikani V, Sherrill D, Barnhart B, Gaither JB, Denninghoff KR, Viscusi C, Mullins T, Adelson PD. Mortality and prehospital blood pressure in patients with major traumatic brain injury: implications for the hypotension threshold. JAMA Surg. 2017;152(4):360–8.
16. Gaitanidis A, Breen KA, Maurer LR, Saillant NN, Kaafarani HMA, Velmahos GC, Mendoza AE. Systolic blood pressure <110 mm hg as a threshold of hypotension in patients with isolated traumatic brain injuries. J Neurotrauma. 2021;38(7):879–85.
17. Sorrentino E, Diedler J, Kasprowicz M, et al. Critical thresholds for cerebrovascular reactivity after traumatic brain injury. Neurocrit Care. 2012;16(2):258–66.
18. Lazaridis C, DeSantis SM, Smielewski P, Menon DK, Hutchinson P, Pickard JD, Czosnyka M. Patient-specific thresholds of intracranial pressure in severe traumatic brain injury. J Neurosurg. 2014;120(4):893–900.
19. Donnelly J, Czosnyka M, Adams H, Robba C, Steiner LA, Cardim D, Cabella B, Liu X, Ercole A, Hutchinson PJ, Menon DK, Aries MJH, Smielewski P. Individualizing thresholds of cerebral perfusion pressure using estimated limits of autoregulation. Crit Care Med. 2017;45(9):1464–71.
20. Tas J, Beqiri E, van Kaam RC, Czosnyka M, Donnelly J, Haeren RH, et al. Targeting autoregulation-guided cerebral perfusion pressure after traumatic brain injury (COGiTATE): a feasibility randomized controlled clinical trial. J Neurotrauma. 2021;38(20):2790–800.
21. CENTER-TBI HR ICU participants and investigators. The lower limit of reactivity as a potential individualised cerebral perfusion pressure target in traumatic brain injury: a CENTER-TBI high-resolution sub-study analysis. Crit Care. 2023;27(1):194.
22. Brasil S, Godoy DA, Videtta W, Rubiano AM, Solla D, Taccone FS et al. A comprehensive perspective on intracranial pressure monitoring and individualized management in neurocritical care: results of a survey with global experts. Neurocrit Care. 2024.
23. CRASH-2 trial collaborators; effects of tranexamic acid on death, vascular occlusive events, and blood transfusion in trauma patients with significant haemorrhage (CRASH-2): a randomised, placebo-controlled trial. Lancet. 2010;376(9734):23–32.
24. CRASH-3 trial collaborators. Effects of tranexamic acid on death, disability, vascular occlusive events and other morbidities in patients with acute traumatic brain injury (CRASH-3): a randomised, placebo-controlled trial. Lancet. 2019;394(10210):1713–23.
25. Rowell SE, Meier EN, McKnight B, Kannas D, May S, Sheehan K, et al. Effect of out-of-hospital Tranexamic acid vs placebo on 6-month functional neurologic outcomes in patients with moderate or severe traumatic brain injury. JAMA. 2020;324(10):961–74.
26. Lawati KA, Sharif S, Maqbali SA, Rimawi HA, Petrosoniak A, Belley-Cote EP, et al. Efficacy and safety of tranexamic acid in acute traumatic brain injury: a systematic review and meta-analysis of randomized-controlled trials. Intensive Care Med. 2021;47(1):14–27.
27. Song JX, Wu JX, Zhong H, Chen W, Zheng JC. Therapeutic efficacy of tranexamic acid on traumatic brain injury: a systematic review and meta-analysis. Scand J Trauma Resusc Emerg Med. 2024;32(1):18.

28. Griesdale DE, McEwen J, Kurth T, Chittock DR. External ventricular drains and mortality in patients with severe traumatic brain injury. Can J Neurol Sci. 2010;37(1):43–88.
29. Akbik OS, Krasberg M, Nemoto EM, Yonas H. Effect of cerebrospinal fluid drainage on brain tissue oxygenation in traumatic brain injury. J Neurotrauma. 2017;34(22):3153–7.
30. Puccio Bell MJ, Rosario BL, Kochanek PM, Adelson PD, Morris KP, Au AK, et al. Approaches and decisions for acute Pediatric TBI (ADAPT) investigators. Comparative effectiveness of diversion of cerebrospinal fluid for children with severe traumatic brain injury. JAMA Netw Open. 2022;5(7):e2220969. https://doi.org/10.1001/jamanetworkopen.2022.20969.
31. Nwachuku EL, Puccio AM, Fetzick A, Scruggs B, Chang YF, Shutter LA, et al. Intermittent versus continuous cerebrospinal fluid drainage management in adult severe traumatic brain injury: assessment of intracranial pressure burden. Neurocrit Care. 2014;20(1):49–53.
32. Chau CYC, Craven CL, Rubiano AM, Adams H, Tülü S, Czosnyka M, Servadei F, Ercole A, Hutchinson PJ, Kolias AG. The evolution of the role of external ventricular drainage in traumatic brain injury. J Clin Med. 2019;8(9):1422.
33. Chau CYC, Mediratta S, McKie MA, Gregson B, Tulu S, Ercole A, Solla DJF, Paiva WS, Hutchinson PJ, Kolias AG. Optimal timing of external ventricular drainage after severe traumatic brain injury: a systematic review. J Clin Med. 2020;9(6):1996.
34. Taylor JD, Bailey M, Cooper DJ, French C, Menon DK, Nichol AD, et al. Association between early external ventricular drain insertion and functional outcomes 6 months following moderate-to-severe traumatic brain injury. J Neurotrauma. 2024;41(11–12):1364–74.
35. De Vivo P, Del Gaudio A, Ciritella P, Puopolo M, Chiarotti F, Mastronardi E. Hypertonic saline solution: a safe alternative to mannitol 18% in neurosurgery. Minerva Anestesiol. 2001;67(9):603–11.
36. Miyoshi Y, Kondo Y, Suzuki H, Fukuda T, Yasuda H, Yokobori S. Neuroresuscitation task force and the guidelines editorial committee. Effects of hypertonic saline versus mannitol in patients with traumatic brain injury in prehospital, emergency department, and intensive care unit settings: a systematic review and meta-analysis. J Intensive Care. 2020;12(8):61.
37. Shi J, Tan L, Ye J, Hu L. Hypertonic saline and mannitol in patients with traumatic brain injury: a systematic and meta-analysis. Medicine (Baltimore). 2020;99(35):e21655.
38. Han C, Yang F, Guo S, Zhang J. Hypertonic saline compared to mannitol for the management of elevated intracranial pressure in traumatic brain injury: a meta-analysis. Front Surg. 2022;7(8):765784.
39. Skrifvars MB, Bailey M, Moore E, Mårtensson J, French C, Presneill J, et al. Erythropoietin in traumatic brain injury (EPO-TBI) investigators and the Australian and New Zealand Intensive Care Society (ANZICS) clinical trials group. A post hoc analysis of osmotherapy use in the erythropoietin in traumatic brain injury study-associations with acute kidney injury and mortality. Crit Care Med. 2021;49(4):e394–403.
40. Roquilly A, Moyer JD, Huet O, Lasocki S, Cohen B, Dahyot-Fizelier C, et al. Effect of continuous infusion of hypertonic saline vs standard care on 6-month neurological outcomes in patients with traumatic brain injury: the COBI randomized clinical trial. JAMA. 2021;325(20):2056–66.
41. Bernhardt K, McClune W, Rowland MJ, Shah A. Hypertonic saline versus other intracranial-pressure-lowering agents for patients with acute traumatic brain injury: a systematic review and meta-analysis. Neurocrit Care. 2024;40(2):769–84.
42. Temkin NR, Dikmen SS, Wilensky AJ, Keihm J, Chabal S, Winn HR. A randomized, double-blind study of phenytoin for the prevention of post-traumatic seizures. N Engl J Med. 1990;323(8):497–502.
43. Pingue V, Mele C, Nardone A. Post-traumatic seizures and antiepileptic therapy as predictors of the functional outcome in patients with traumatic brain injury. Sci Rep. 2021;11(1):4708.
44. Kumar S, Bharti AK, Prasad RS, Kumari S, Singh A, Yadav G. Efficacy of phenytoin for 7 days versus 21 days as prophylactic anticonvulsant in traumatic brain injury patients – a comparative study. J Family Med Prim Care. 2022;11(8):4805–10.
45. Szaflarski JP, Sangha KS, Lindsell CJ, Shutter LA. Prospective, randomized, single-blinded comparative trial of intravenous levetiracetam versus phenytoin for seizure prophylaxis. Neurocrit Care. 2010;12(2):165–72.

46. Wang BC, Chiu HY, Luh HT, Lin CJ, Hsieh SH, Chen TJ, Wu CR, Chen PY. Comparative efficacy of prophylactic anticonvulsant drugs following traumatic brain injury: a systematic review and network meta-analysis of randomized controlled trials. PLoS One. 2022;17(3):e0265932.
47. Karamian A, Farzaneh H, Taheri M, Seifi A. Effectiveness of Levetiracetam versus phenytoin in preventing seizure in traumatic brain injury patients: a systematic review and meta-analysis. Clin Neurol Neurosurg. 2024;240:108251.
48. Phan K, Moore JM, Griessenauer C, Dmytriw AA, Scherman DB, Sheik-Ali S, et al. Craniotomy versus Decompressive Craniectomy for acute subdural hematoma: systematic review and meta-analysis. World Neurosurg. 2017;101:677–85.
49. Kinoshita T, Yoshiya K, Fujimoto Y, Kajikawa R, Kiguchi T, Hara M, et al. Decompressive Craniectomy in conjunction with evacuation of intracranial Hemorrhagic lesions is associated with worse outcomes in elderly patients with traumatic brain injury: a propensity score analysis. World Neurosurg. 2016;89:187–92.
50. Abouhashem S, Eldawoody H. Functional outcome after primary decompressive craniectomy for acute subdural hematoma in severe traumatic brain injury. Turk Neurosurg. 2022;32:211–20.
51. Hutchinson PJ, Adams H, Mohan M, Devi BI, Uff C, Hasan S, et al. British neurosurgical trainee research collaborative, NIHR Global Health research group on acquired brain and spine injury, and RESCUE-ASDH trial collaborators; RESCUE-ASDH trial collaborators. Decompressive Craniectomy versus craniotomy for acute subdural hematoma. N Engl J Med. 2023;388(24):2219–29.
52. van Essen TA, van Erp IAM, Lingsma HF, Pisică D, Yue JK, Singh RD, et al. CENTER-TBI investigators and participants. Comparative effectiveness of decompressive craniectomy versus craniotomy for traumatic acute subdural hematoma (CENTER-TBI): an observational cohort study. EClinicalMedicine. 2023;63:102161.
53. Yang C, Huang X, Feng J, Xie L, Hui J, Li W, et al. Prospective randomized evaluation of Decompressive ipsilateral Craniectomy for traumatic acute epidural hematoma (PREDICT-AEDH): study protocol for a randomized controlled trial. Trials. 2021;22(1):421.
54. Cooper DJ, Rosenfeld JV, Murray L, Arabi YM, Davies AR, D'Urso P, et al. DECRA trial investigators; Australian and New Zealand Intensive Care Society clinical trials group. Decompressive craniectomy in diffuse traumatic brain injury. N Engl J Med. 2011;364(16):1493–502.
55. Hutchison PJ, Corteen E, Czosnyka M, Kolias AG, Timofeev IS, Timothy J, et al. Decompressive craniectomy in traumatic brain injury: the randomized multicenter RESCUEicp study. Acta Neurochir Suppl. 2006;96:17–20.
56. Kolias AG, Adams H, Timofeev IS, Corteen EA, Hossain I, Czosnyka M, et al. RESCUEicp trial collaborators. Evaluation of outcomes among patients with traumatic intracranial hypertension treated with Decompressive Craniectomy vs standard medical care at 24 months: a secondary analysis of the RESCUEicp randomized clinical trial. JAMA Neurol. 2022;79(7):664–71.
57. Zhang Q, Li Y, Chang X. Role of decompressive craniectomy in the management of traumatic brain injury-a meta-analysis of randomized controlled trials. Ann Indian Acad Neurol. 2023;26(6):966–74.
58. Andrews PJ, Sinclair HL, Rodriguez A, et al. Hypothermia for intracranial hypertension after traumatic brain injury. N Engl J Med. 2015;373(25):2403–12.
59. Cooper DJ, Nichol AD, Bailey M, Bernard S, Cameron PA, Pili-Floury S, et al. Effect of early sustained prophylactic hypothermia on neurologic outcomes among patients with severe traumatic brain injury: the POLAR randomized clinical trial. JAMA. 2018;320(21):2211–20.
60. Hui J, Feng J, Tu Y, Zhang W, Zhong C, Liu M, et al. LTH-1 trial collaborators. Safety and efficacy of long-term mild hypothermia for severe traumatic brain injury with refractory intracranial hypertension (LTH-1): a multicenter randomized controlled trial. EClinicalMedicine. 2021;32:100732.

61. Martyniuk A, Hart S, Lannon M, Mastrolonardo A, Kabbani A, Hafeez DA, et al. Therapeutic hypothermia compared with Normothermia in adults with traumatic brain injury; functional outcome, mortality, and adverse effects: a systematic review and meta-analysis. Neurocrit Care. 2024.
62. Chesnut RM, Temkin N, Carney N, Dikmen S, Rondina C, Videtta W, et al. Global Neurotrauma research group. A trial of intracranial-pressure monitoring in traumatic brain injury. N Engl J Med. 2012;367(26):2471–81.
63. Alali AS, Fowler RA, Mainprize TG, et al. Intracranial pressure monitoring in severe traumatic brain injury: results from the American College of Surgeons trauma quality improvement program. J Neurotrauma. 2013;30(20):1737–46.
64. Talving P, Karamanos E, Teixeira PG, et al. Intracranial pressure monitoring in severe head injury: compliance with brain trauma foundation guidelines and effect on outcomes: a prospective study. J Neurosurg. 2013;119(5):1248–54.
65. Florez-Perdomo WA, Mishra R, Moscote-Salar LR, Cincu R, Maurya VP, et al. Intracranial pressure monitoring in patients with traumatic brain injury: an umbrella review of systematic review and meta-analysis. J Neurointensive Care. 2024;7(1):18–28.
66. Mathieu F, Khellaf A, Ku JC, Donnelly J, Thelin EP, Zeiler FA. Continuous near-infrared spectroscopy monitoring in adult traumatic brain injury: a systematic review. J Neurosurg Anesthesiol. 2020;32(4):288–99.
67. Gomez A, Griesdale D, Froese L, Yang E, Thelin EP, Raj R, et al. Temporal statistical relationship between regional cerebral oxygen saturation (rSO_2) and brain tissue oxygen tension ($PbtO_2$) in moderate-to-severe traumatic brain injury: a Canadian high resolution-TBI (CAHR-TBI) cohort study. Bioengineering (Basel). 2023;10(10):1124.
68. Okonkwo DO, Shutter LA, Moore C, Temkin NR, Puccio AM, Madden CJ, et al. Brain oxygen optimization in severe traumatic brain injury phase-II: a phase II randomized trial. Crit Care Med. 2017;45(11):1907–14.
69. Bernard F, Barsan W, Diaz-Arrastia R, Merck LH, Yeatts S, Shutter LA. Brain oxygen optimization in severe traumatic brain injury (BOOST-3): a multicentre, randomised, blinded-endpoint, comparative effectiveness study of brain tissue oxygen and intracranial pressure monitoring versus intracranial pressure alone. BMJ Open. 2022;12(3):e060188.
70. Payen JF, Launey Y, Chabanne R, Gay S, Francony G, Gergele L, et al. OXY-TC trial collaborators. Intracranial pressure monitoring with and without brain tissue oxygen pressure monitoring for severe traumatic brain injury in France (OXY-TC): an open-label, randomised controlled superiority trial. Lancet Neurol. 2023;22(11):1005–14.
71. BONANZA – ANZICS [Internet]. Available from: https://www.anzics.com.au/current-active-endorsed-research/bonanza/.

Controversies in the Neurocritical Care Management of Aneurysmal Subarachnoid Hemorrhage

2

Amiya Kumar Barik and Kiran Jangra

Abstract

Critical care management of a patient with aneurysmal subarachnoid hemorrhage (aSAH) is quite challenging because it involves not only the brain but also the other major organ systems of the body. The secondary effects of a ruptured aneurysm are life-threatening and are difficult to treat. The existing evidence on the neurocritical care management of aSAH is not very clear and gives rise to many controversies. This chapter focuses on the major controversies, including timing of aneurysm repair; coiling versus clipping as a modality for aneurysm repair; use of antifibrinolytic therapy in acute aSAH; blood pressure goals before aneurysm treatment; vasospasm and delayed cerebral ischemia (DCI) prevention and treatment strategies; and pressure vs flow augmentation. The existing literature supports early aneurysm repair as soon as feasible. Coiling is favored in the posterior circulation, and clipping is preferred in a large hematoma. For good-grade and anterior circulation, both techniques are equally good, but coiling may have a better functional outcome at 1 year but not at 5 years. For blister aneurysms, flow diverters appear to be an appealing choice. Routine use of antifibrinolytics is not recommended; prophylactic blood pressure augmentation is not recommended, while for the treatment of DCI, hemodynamic augmentation needs to be individualized.

Keywords

Aneurysmal subarachnoid hemorrhage (ASAH)Vasospasm · Delayed cerebral ischemia (DCI) · Coiling vs. clipping · Hemodynamic augmentation

A. K. Barik · K. Jangra (✉)
PGIMER, Chandigarh, Punjab, India

P. U. Bidkar, M. Krishnakumar (eds.), *Controversies in Neurocritical Care*,
https://doi.org/10.1007/978-981-95-4419-6_2

2.1 Introduction

Subarachnoid hemorrhage (SAH) is the abnormal presence of blood between the arachnoid membrane and the pia mater in the brain, which can be traumatic or nontraumatic. Intracranial aneurysm rupture is the most common cause of nontraumatic SAH, known as aneurysmal subarachnoid hemorrhage (aSAH) [1]. The incidence of aSAH is approximately 6.1 per 100,000 person-years, and the prevalence is almost 8.09 million cases worldwide, the highest being in Japan and Finland [2, 3]. The major risk factors associated with aSAH are hypertension, cigarette smoking, alcohol, and drug abuse; female sex, age 35–60 years, and ≥ intracranial aneurysm in first-degree relatives [4].

The intensive care management of aSAH requires a multidisciplinary approach. The goal of management is to prevent rebleeding, which is best achieved either by endovascular coiling or by clipping of the aneurysm. In due course, prevention and management of various complications, such as DCI, vasospasm, cerebral edema, hydrocephalus, raised intracranial pressure, and seizures, become important aspects of neurocritical care in these patients. Although various guidelines were formulated in the past for the meticulous management of aSAH, there are a few gray areas where consensus may vary among various institutions. This chapter focuses on commonly encountered controversies in the management of patients with aSAH. The main controversies that will be discussed in this chapter are listed in Table 2.1.

Table 2.1 Various controversies in the management of aSAH

1.	Timings of aneurysm repair
2.	Coiling vs. clipping as a modality for aneurysm repair
3.	Use of antifibrinolytic therapy in acute aSAH
4.	Blood pressure goals before aneurysm treatment
5.	Vasospasm prevention and treatment strategies
6.	Pressure vs. flow augmentation

aSAH aneurysmal subarachnoid hemorrhage, *DCI* delayed cerebral ischemia

2.2 Timings of Aneurysm Repair

Rebleeding is one of the most feared complications following aSAH, and securing the aneurysm either with clipping or coiling is the most effective way to prevent it. However, the timing of aneurysm surgery has been the topic of debate for a long time. Earlier, the patients were mostly operated on during the late phase (2 or 3 weeks after the hemorrhage). In the early phase (initial 2 weeks), the brain parenchyma is inflamed and swollen due to the inflammation incited by the bleed. It might result in poor operative conditions and a high risk of complications [5–7]. The patients were not usually operated on during the period of maximum risk of vasospasm (4–10th day after SAH) due to the increased risk of delayed cerebral ischemia (DCI).

Later on, a Cochrane review on the timing of surgery after aSAH, with only one randomized clinical trial, found that early surgery (days 0–3) had the best outcome, and intermediate surgery (days 4–7) was the worst [8, 9]. A systematic review that included ten observational studies, along with this trial, observed that both early (days 0–3) and intermediate (days 4–7) surgeries produced better outcomes than late surgery [10]. However, delaying treatment beyond 7–10 days (the typical delayed cerebral ischemia phase) is not recommended. These studies changed the protocol for the timing of surgeries in many places; thereafter, more and more studies came up confirming the results [10–13].

The timing of ruptured aneurysm repair in good-grade aSAH have not been studied directly. Only one small trial of 159 patients demonstrated that early surgery (0–3 days from SAH) resulted in lower death and dependence at 3 months compared to intermediate surgery (4–7 days) or late surgery ($\geq$8 days) in the pre-coiling era [14]. Subsequently, a meta-analysis of various retrospective and prospective observational studies and randomized trials (International Subarachnoid Aneurysm Trial (ISAT)), including both clipping and coiling within 24, 48, or 72 h from SAH, reported the outcome benefits of early treatment (<24 h) in patients with aSAH, including high-grade SAH [9, 10, 12, 14, 15].

2.2.1 Current Recommendations [16]

The aneurysm should be repaired as soon as feasible after aSAH to reduce the risk of rebleeding and to facilitate treatment of DCI. Preferably, the definitive treatment of the aneurysm should not be delayed past the period of DCI.

2.2.2 Knowledge Gaps

Though early treatment of the aneurysm is recommended, the exact time frame of treatment has not been defined, and various time frames have been used in the literature. There are sparse data regarding the patients' quality of life and neurocognitive outcomes after surgery within 6 h (ultra-early) of the onset of symptoms and emergency surgery/intervention (24/7), including nighttime. In such situations, suboptimal logistic conditions and surgery on unoptimized patients have the potential for detrimental outcomes.

2.3 Coiling Versus Clipping

The goal of initial management of the aSAH is to completely obliterate the sac of the aneurysm [17, 18]. Whenever complete obliteration is not possible, it can be partially occluded (mainly at the ruptured site), and the definitive repair can be carried out within 1–3 months, depending on the patient's condition [13].

Mainly, aneurysms are obliterated using two techniques: clipping and coiling. For clipping the neck of the aneurysm, after craniotomy, the surgical clip is applied at the neck of the aneurysm so that it is isolated from the cerebral circulation [19]. Endovascular coiling is performed under C-arm guidance, where the detachable coils are inserted into the sac through a microcatheter. This reduces the blood flow of the aneurysmal sac, resulting in subsequent obliteration of the aneurysm by thrombus formation [20].

A patient-centric decision by the expert team (neurosurgeon and neurointerventionist) is desirable in selecting the suitable treatment option, coiling versus clipping [21]. Among the patients with large (>50 cm^3) intracerebral hematoma (ICH) after aneurysm rupture, evacuation of the hematoma followed by clipping is a reasonable choice [22]. However, in the case of smaller ICH (<30 cm^3), coiling can be performed without clot evacuation [22–24].

The prospective randomized trial has reported significantly better clinical outcomes with coiling in posterior circulation aneurysms than clipping [20, 25, 26]. Endovascular coiling is preferred for elderly patients (>70 years), posterior circulation, and ruptured aneurysms, which carry a high surgical risk for general anesthesia. However, the late clinical trials failed to show the benefit of coiling over clipping in patients >70 years old [27–29]. The ISAT study favored clipping among young (< 40 years) patients, with less benefit of coiling in those <50 [27]. They observed that in patients >65 years, coiling was superior in internal carotid and posterior communicating artery aneurysms, but clipping was superior for ruptured middle cerebral artery (MCA) aneurysms.

Similarly, middle and anterior cerebral aneurysms with associated intraparenchymal hematoma are approached surgically for clipping. In the case of very large and more complex aneurysms, these two modalities can be combined for better results. The endovascular treatment was revolutionized by the discovery of the Guglielmi platinum detachable coils. Other treatment options to obliterate the aneurysmal sac that can be useful are stent-assisted coiling, balloon-assisted coiling, flow diverters, and embolic agents. Stent-assisted coiling and flow diverters are preferred for more complex aneurysms but are associated with a higher risk of complications compared to clipping and primary coiling [30, 31]. Performing a ventriculostomy and initiating an antiplatelet drug before the endovascular procedure can reduce the risk of ventriculostomy-related hemorrhage [31]. Novel flow diverters are new rays of hope in the field of endovascular treatment, considering their lower complication rates.

2.3.1 Recommendations

The collective data showed significantly favorable data for death or dependency at 1 year with coiling, but not at 5 years. However, there was a higher incidence of rebleeding and seizures in patients who underwent coiling [20, 27, 32]. Therefore, the treatment option needs to be individualized, considering the patient's condition (aneurysm size, shape, and location; patient's health on admission, and preexisting systemic illness). Pertaining to the high thrombogenicity of stent-assisted coiling and flow diverters, dual antiplatelet therapy is necessary, which increases the risk of hemorrhagic complications, especially in acute SAH.

2.3.2 Knowledge Gap

Studies comparing clipping and coiling for outcomes like quality of life (QOL) and neurocognitive function are needed. Clipping is usually favored for ruptured anterior circulation aneurysms, including internal carotid artery (ICA) bifurcation, ACOM, and MCA aneurysms, but the supporting data are quite limited. The long-term outcomes data are limited for the use of emerging novel endovascular techniques and flow diverters.

2.4 Use of Antifibrinolytic Therapy in Acute aSAH

The only effective way of reducing rebleeding is by obliteration of the aneurysm as early as possible [33, 34]. The use of antifibrinolytic therapy may decrease the rebleeding risk in the acute phase, but the trials were inconsistent, and the functional outcomes were not improved [35, 36]. Ultra-early tranexamic acid after subarachnoid hemorrhage (ULTRA) is a high-quality randomized trial that evaluated early tranexamic acid administration among aSAH patients. It failed to show its beneficial role in reducing the risk of bleeding and improving functional outcomes [37].

2.4.1 Recommendations

The routine use of antifibrinolytics is not recommended. However, for patients who are already on anticoagulants, emergency reversal is strongly recommended.

2.4.2 Knowledge Gaps

The role of antifibrinolytics may still be there in situations where definitive treatment of the ruptured aneurysm is delayed due to logistical or medical issues.

2.5 Blood Pressure (BP) Goals Before Aneurysm Treatment

The role of early control of hypertension on the risk of rebleeding is also inconsistent [34, 38, 39]. However, severe hypertension at the time of presentation should be treated, and sudden fluctuations in blood pressure should be avoided [40]. Although the target BP is still dubious, a meta-analysis carried out to evaluate the factors responsible for early rebleeding states that systolic BP more than 160 mm Hg was associated with an increased risk of bleeding compared to BP less than 140 mm Hg [40, 41]. Gradual reduction of BP is recommended if it is more than 180–200 mm Hg. Avoiding an mean arterial pressure (MAP) below 65 mm Hg and closely monitoring neurological status are recommended during blood pressure reduction.

2.5.1 Recommendations

Current evidence is insufficient to recommend any specific BP targets. However, a few factors like BP at presentation, history of hypertension, renal insufficiency, signs of brain swelling, and hydrocephalus need to be considered before targeting BP [42].

2.5.2 Knowledge Gaps

Future research should be directed to determine the optimal BP before aneurysm obliteration. Still, it is not clear whether the therapeutic targets should be systolic BP, mean arterial pressure, or the proportional reduction in BP. The technique of blood pressure lowering without compromising cerebral perfusion pressure in the absence of intracranial pressure (ICP) monitoring is still not known.

2.6 Vasospasm Prevention and Treatment Strategies

Cerebral vasospasm is the narrowing of the cerebral arteries. It is one of the most common complications encountered following aSAH. Its incidence varies from 30% to 50% and is the leading cause of morbidity and mortality [43]. It is mostly evident between the 4th and 14th day and resolves spontaneously after the 21st day following aSAH [43]. The risk factors for vasospasm are the age of the patient, size, and location of the aneurysm; clinical grade and severity of SAH; presence of intracerebral or intraventricular hemorrhage, and acute hydrocephalus. Although the pathogenesis of cerebral vasospasm is unclear, the breakdown of blood products and calcium-dependent and -independent cerebral vasoconstriction is thought to be a possible cause. The breakdown of blood products causes smooth muscle contraction and endothelial damage, leading to cerebral vasospasm and may give rise to DCI [43].

DCI is defined as the occurrence of a focal neurological deficit or a decrease of at least 2 points on the glasgow coma scale (GCS) lasting for at least 1 h without any other causes. The diagnosis of DCI is a challenge for clinicians; along with serial neurological examinations, other modalities, such as transcranial Doppler (TCD), CT angiography (CTA), CT perfusion (CTP), and electroencephalogram (EEG), can be helpful [44].

2.6.1 Treatment of Cerebral Vasospasm and DCI Following aSAH

Managing DCI can be challenging for clinicians following aSAH. The presence of angiographic evidence of vasospasm is a major predictor of morbidity and mortality. Although the mechanism of development of DCI is incompletely understood, a few mechanisms that are thought to contribute to it are cortical spreading depolarization, failure of autoregulation, blood–brain barrier disruption, and microthrombosis. Therefore, preventive measures and treatments are targeted at these possible mechanisms [45].

Preventive measures of DCI can focus on managing systemic or local medications and interventions.

2.6.2 Systemic Medications

The US FDA approved *nimodipine* (a dihydropyridine calcium channel-blocker) for the management of vasospasm following aSAH. It is the therapeutic agent of choice. It is administered at an oral dose of 60 mg six times per day for 21 days. It is found to be beneficial in the prevention of DCI and in improving functional status. However, the ideal time for starting nimodipine is still debatable. It can be given via intravenous or intra-arterial routes, but the data are not adequate to recommend any specific route of administration [46]. In case of hypotension occurring following nimodipine infusion, it should not be stopped; instead, hypotension should be managed using the available medical interventions.

Clazosentan, an endothelin receptor antagonist, was studied in three major trials (CONSCIOUS-1, −2, and −3) to treat vasospasm-related morbidity and mortality in patients with aSAH. In CONSCIOUS-1, 15 mg/h of clazosentan was reported to be beneficial in a dose-dependent manner for moderate-to-severe angiographic vasospasm [47]. However, in the CONSCIOUS-2 trial, a dose of 5 mg/h failed to show any improvement in morbidity, incidence of new-onset cerebral ischemia, or mortality in patients undergoing aneurysmal clipping [48]. Thus, considering its findings, the CONSCIOUS-3 trial involving aSAH patients undergoing endovascular coiling was stopped prematurely [49].

Other medications considered for the management of the systemic vasospasm include *magnesium, cilostazol, fasudil, omega-3 fatty acids, erythropoiesis-stimulating hormone erythropoietin (EPO), statins, and anti-inflammatory drugs. Magnesium* is a physiological antagonist of calcium that causes vascular smooth muscle relaxation, resulting in vasodilatation. Few trials were carried out using magnesium among aSAH patients, but they failed to show any significant beneficial effect. One trial demonstrated that a serum magnesium concentration of 2.0–2.5 mmol/liter might reduce ischemia on CT, but without any long-term benefit [50]. Similarly, a trial using intravenous magnesium (Intravenous Magnesium Sulfate for Aneurysmal Subarachnoid Hemorrhage (IMASH)) also failed to show significant improvement in aSAH [51]. MESH-2 (The Magnesium Sulfate For Aneurysmal Subarachnoid Hemorrhage) trial was carried out using 64 mmol of magnesium, but without any evidence of a beneficial role on the outcome measured by the modified Rankin Scale (mRS) at 3 months [52].*Cilostazol* is a selective phosphodiesterase-3 inhibitor. It has an antithrombotic and antiplatelet effect. Studies show conflicting evidence among patients with aSAH. A study showed improved clinical outcomes when used at a dose of 100 mg twice daily orally for 14 days [53]. Another study showed a decreased incidence of symptomatic and angiographic vasospasm without any significant benefit on the 6-month outcome [54]. Following non-approval of nimodipine in Japan, a Rho-kinase inhibitor named *fasudil* first came into the picture for the management of vasospasm [55, 56]. A study comparing fasudil (30 mg IV bolus daily) with nimodipine found a comparable effect on the vasospasm, whereas fasudil had a better outcome after 1 month of follow-up [57]. *Eicosapentaenoic acid* is an omega-3 fatty acid having cardio and cerebrovascular-protective effects [58]. It has antiplatelet and vasodilatory effects, which make it a potential drug for the treatment of cerebral vasospasm following aSAH [59]. However, its effect on long-term follow-up is still questionable [60]. *Erythropoietin (EPO),* an erythropoiesis-stimulating hormone that can be used at a dose of 30,000 IU consecutively for 3 days, has shown a significant improvement in brain tissue oxygen tension among patients with cerebral vasospasm [61]. This effect could be due to the anti-inflammatory effect and the restoration of autoregulation by the EPO. The *Simvastatin* in Aneurysmal Subarachnoid Hemorrhage (STASH) study using a statin did not show any significant beneficial role in symptomatic vasospasm or long-term follow-up [62]. Other drugs that have shown promising results for vasospasm and need to be explored in the future are unfractionated heparin postoperatively (8 U/kg/h), methylprednisolone, and intrathecal medications for clearing heme-degradation products such as haptoglobin, deferoxamine, and vitamin D [63, 64]. Neural ganglia blocks, such as stellate ganglion block, are used to treat symptomatic vasospasm. However, their impact on DCI requires high-quality research.

2.6.3 For Topical or Mechanical Therapy for DCI

A topical or mechanical approach to prevent DCI bypasses the systemic side effects of the various drugs and focuses on the area affected by the vasospasm. Among the various available routes, the intraventricular route by the preexisting external ventricular drain is preferred. In a retrospective trial, *nicardipine* was used among patients with clinical vasospasm at a dose of 4 mg, 8–12 hourly intraventricularly, leading to a significant reduction in mean cerebral blood flow (CBF) velocities in the MCA and ACA [65].

Alongside, drugs can be locally applied to the vasospasm site after surgical exposure. Four mg of nicardipine can be applied as a pellet implantation, which releases the drug slowly for almost 2 weeks [66]. Few studies have evaluated the role of nicardipine implants after surgical clipping, and found them to be effective in preventing the development of DCI, cerebral infarct, and 1-year outcomes measured by mRS [67]. Other methods to prevent local DCI are drainage of the interventricular blood by using a lumbar cerebrospinal fluid (CSF) drain and a cisternal drain. An randomized controlled trial (RCT) showed a lower incidence of vasospasm and a better 10-day outcome following the application of the lumbar drain; however, the effect was weaned off at 6 months [68]. The application of drugs like *papaverine and urokinase* is also tried locally, but of limited benefit [69, 70]. Even though *papaverine* is a historically effective vasodilator, it is usually avoided due to its neurotoxicity [71]. Intra-arterial infusions in combination with angioplasty targeted to different levels of the cerebral vasculature allow access of vasodilators to the entire vasculature in diffuse spasm [72].

2.7 Treatment Strategies for DCI

2.7.1 Induced Hypertension

Induced hypertension can be effective in treating DCI. However, a hypertension induction in the management of aneurysmal subarachnoid hemorrhage with secondary ischemia (HIMALAIA) study compared the role of induced hypertension vs. no hypertension in the DCI among aSAH patients. However, it was prematurely halted and failed to show any supporting evidence [73].

2.7.2 Intraventricular Nicardipine

It can be a potential treatment option for DCI. A retrospective study evaluated the role of intraventricular nicardipine on TCD-diagnosed vasospasm. It showed positive results in its role, but without any significant difference in the clinical outcome.

2.7.3 Neuroradiological Treatments

Interventional neuroradiological procedures are effective in cases where the vasospasm is refractory to medical management. Transluminal balloon angioplasty (TBA) and intra-arterial spasmolysis (IAS) are the available treatment options. Although there is no consensus regarding the two treatment strategies, the TBA has a long-lasting effect and can treat proximal vasospasm, whereas the IAS has a transient effect and treats distal vasospasm [74, 75]. The drugs used for spasmolysis are nimodipine, papaverine, fasudil, and colforsin. A trial compared prolonged intra-arterial nimodipine infusion with no interventional procedure and found a better 6-month outcome in the nimodipine group [76]. In another trial, similar outcomes were noted among patients treated with endovascular therapy and induced hypertension [77].

2.8 Pressure Versus Flow Augmentation

2.8.1 Evidence for Blood Pressure Augmentation for Increasing Cerebral Blood Flow

The evidence for hemodynamic augmentation is very sparse, and various guidelines make different recommendations. Most of the guidelines are consistent in maintaining euvolemia, but the choice of ionotrope or vasopressor remains a controversial topic [78]. The neurocritical care guidelines state that in the absence of high-quality data regarding or against BP or cardiac output augmentation for the prevention and treatment of DCI, the use of hemodynamic augmentation techniques should be judicious and individualized [79]. The American Heart Association (AHA)/ American Society of Anesthesiologists (ASA) guidelines recommend that it may be reasonable to elevate SBP to slow down the progression and reduce the severity of DCI following aSAH [80]. In these recommendations, there was a single randomized controlled trial that aimed to enroll 240 patients but was prematurely discontinued after recruiting 21 patients in the induced hypertension arm and 20 patients in the no hypertension arm, in view of the lack of effect on cerebral perfusion and slow recruitment [81]. Hence, these guidelines mainly draw their conclusion from the observational data of large, multicenter studies reporting an improvement in approximately 80% of symptomatic patients after induced hypertension [82]. A pilot study evaluating 35 patients by Rondeau et al. compared norepinephrine-induced BP augmentation and dobutamine-induced cardiac index augmentation and observed no difference in angiographic vasospasm with the two techniques [83]. An observational (prospective and retrospective) study by Lakhal et al. compared a combined technique of intravenous milrinone and induced hypertension with hypertension alone for treating cerebral vasospasm [84]. They observed that 29% of patients showed poor tolerance to IV milrinone, but it was associated with better long-term neurological and radiological outcomes and a lower incidence of angioplasty.

2.8.2 Evidence for Cardiac Output Augmentation for Increasing Cerebral Blood Flow

Later, flow-directed studies were carried out targeting the blood flow in cerebral vessels. Figure 2.1 depicts a complex hypothesis that explains how augmenting cardiac output increases cerebral blood flow irrespective of blood pressure. One such study was conducted by Mutoh et al., where early-goal-directed therapy (EGDT)

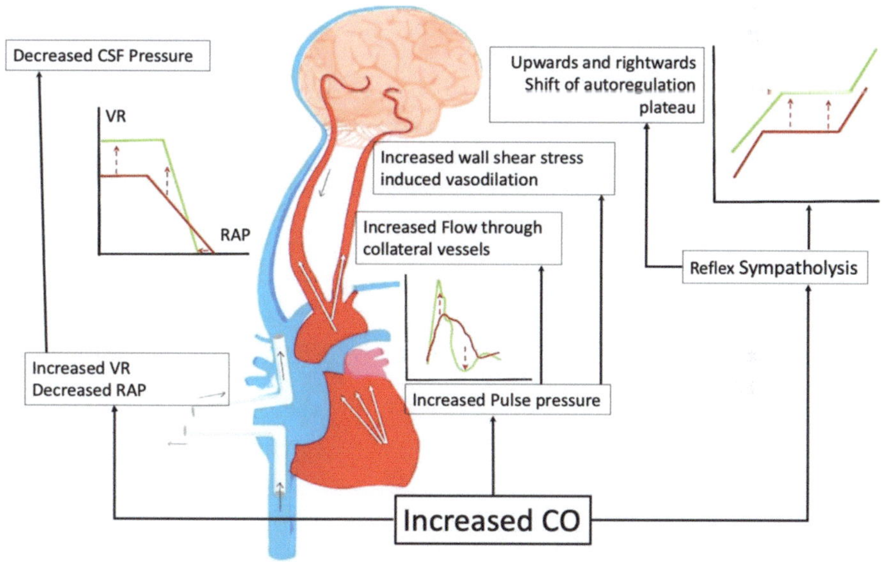

Fig. 2.1 Diagrammatic representation of the mechanism of cerebral blood flow augmentation by an increase in cardiac output. An increase in cardiac output increases the pulsatility of the flow through baroreceptors, which leads to sympatholysis, resulting in the pressure-autoregulation plateau shift toward the right and upward. Pulsatile flow may increase collateral flow in the cerebral vascular tree and induce vasodilation through increases in oscillatory wall shear stress. Increased cardiac output reduces right atrial pressure, which is transmitted to the cerebral venous system. Thus, intracranial pressure is reduced through a decrease in cerebrospinal fluid production, thereby increasing cerebral blood flow. In the graphs, the red traces represent the baseline relationship, the green traces show the state after the cardiac output is independently increased, and the dotted red arrows show the differences between baseline and high cardiac output states. ABP arterial blood pressure, CBF cerebral blood flow, CO cardiac output, CPP cerebral perfusion pressure, CSF cerebrospinal fluid, RAP right atrial pressure, VR venous return

using preload volume and cardiac output was compared with standard treatment (fluid balance or central venous pressure) [85]. The EGDT group received dobutamine or milrinone during GCI to achieve a global end-diastolic volume index (GEDI) of 800–900 ml/m^2 and a cardiac index of 4 L/min/m^2 or clinical improvement. Even though the incidence of DCI was unchanged for the whole group, the subgroups of patients with poor-grade aSAH also showed a lower incidence of DCI in the EGDT group. The patients with coexisting cardiopulmonary complications and poor-grade aSAH also showed a higher proportion of favorable functional outcomes at 3 months in the EGDT group [85]. Similarly, other studies also found a lower rate of DCI in the goal-directed therapy group [39, 41, 85, 86].

2.8.3 Recommendations

To date, large multicenter randomized controlled trials are not available, so the optimal hemodynamic targets are still undetermined.

2.9 Conclusion

To conclude, we have summarized the recommendations of two major guidelines, AHA/ASA and Neurocritical Care Society (NCS), in Table 2.2. Both guidelines agree with each other in almost all recommendations, except for a few points that may not be discussed in both guidelines.

Table 2.2 Summary of the recommendations from the recent guideline

S. no.	Topic	AHA/ASA guidelines [80]	NCS guidelines [79]
1.	Blood pressure (BP) targets for the prevention of rebleeding of ruptured aneurysm	Although it is *reasonable* to treat severe hypertension on presentation, there is insufficient evidence to recommend a particular BP target. Sudden, profound reduction of BP should be avoided	Lack of evidence to recommend a specific blood pressure reduction goal does not necessarily imply that *blood pressure reduction is not helpful* before aneurysm treatment
2.	Antifibrinolytics for the prevention of rebleeding of ruptured aneurysm	The routine use of antifibrinolytic therapy is *not recommended* because of a lack of benefit	*Recommend against* the administration of antifibrinolytic therapy to prevent rebleeding of ruptured aneurysms in patients with aSAH (strong recommendation, high-moderate quality of evidence)

(continued)

Table 2.2 (continued)

S. no.	Topic	AHA/ASA guidelines [80]	NCS guidelines [79]
3.	Calcium channel blockers prophylaxis	In patients with aSAH, *early initiation of enteral nimodipine is beneficial* in preventing DCI and improving functional outcomes	*Recommend the administration of oral nimodipine* in patients with aSAH to reduce DCI and cerebral infarction, and to improve functional outcome (strong recommendation, moderate quality of evidence) We *recommend against the administration of intravenous nicardipine* For the prevention of DCI because of increased risk of adverse effects (strong recommendation, moderate quality of evidence) There is insufficient evidence to recommend for or against the administration of calcium channel blockers other than nicardipine by intravenous or intraventricular routes
4.	Endothelin antagonists	Not discussed	*Recommend against endothelin receptor antagonist* administration Because of lack of benefit on mortality and functional outcomes and an increased risk of adverse events (strong recommendation—high quality of evidence)
5.	Statins	In patients with aSAH, routine use of statin therapy to improve outcomes is not recommended	*Recommend against starting* statin treatment to reduce DCI or improve functional outcomes in aSAH because of lack of benefit (strong recommendation, high-quality evidence)
6.	Magnesium/ therapeutic hypermagnesemia	In patients with aSAH, routine use of intravenous magnesium to improve neurological outcomes is not recommended	*Recommend against the use of targeted hypermagnesemia* to improve outcomes in aSAH due to lack of benefit (strong recommendation, moderate-quality evidence)
7.	Hemodynamic management—blood pressure and cardiac output augmentation	For patients with aSAH at risk of DCI, *prophylactic hemodynamic augmentation should not be performed* to reduce iatrogenic patient harm SBP elevation may reduce the progression and severity of DCI in vasospasm No reccomendation for pressure versus flow augmentation	There are insufficient quality data to recommend for or against blood pressure or cardiac output augmentation for the prevention and treatment of DCI. Due to the associated risks, use of *these interventions should be judicious and tailored to the patient's individual hemodynamic profile*

AHA American Heart Association, *ASA* American Society of Anesthesiologists, *aSAH* aneurysmal subarachnoid hemorrhage, *DCI* delayed cerebral ischemia, *NCS* neurocritical care society

References

1. Toth G, Cerejo R. Intracranial aneurysms: review of current science and management. Vasc Med. 2018;23(3):276–88.
2. Etminan N, Chang HS, Hackenberg K, de Rooij NK, Vergouwen MDI, Rinkel GJE, et al. Worldwide incidence of aneurysmal subarachnoid hemorrhage according to region, time period, blood pressure, and smoking prevalence in the population: a systematic review and meta-analysis. JAMA Neurol. 2019;76:588–97.
3. Tsao CW, Aday AW, Almarzooq ZI, Anderson CAM, Arora P, Avery CL, et al. On behalf of the American Heart Association Council on epidemiology and prevention statistics committee and stroke statistics subcommittee. Heart disease and stroke statistics—2023 update: a report from the American Heart Association. Circulation. 2023;147:e93–e621.
4. Juvela S, Porras M, Poussa K. Natural history of unruptured intracranial aneurysms: probability of and risk factors for aneurysm rupture. J Neurosurg. 2000;93(3):379–87.
5. Kassell NF, Drake CG. Timing of aneurysm surgery. Neurosurgery. 19821;10:514–9.
6. Adams CB, Loach AB, O'laoire SA. Intracranial aneurysms: analysis of results of microneurosurgery. BMJ. 1976;11:607–9.
7. Bohm E, Hugosson R. Experiences of surgical treatment of 400 consecutive ruptured cerebral arterial aneurysms. Acta Neurochir. 1978;40:33–43.
8. Whitfield PC, Kirkpatrick PJ. Timing of surgery for aneurysmal subarachnoid haemorrhage. Cochrane Database Syst Rev. 2001;2:CD001697.
9. Ohman J, Heiskanen O. Timing of operation for ruptured supratentorial aneurysms: a prospective randomized study. J Neurosurg. 1989;70:55–60.
10. de Gans K, Nieuwkamp DJ, Rinkel GJ, Algra A. Timing of aneurysm surgery in subarachnoid hemorrhage: a systematic review of the literature. Neurosurgery. 2002;50:336–40.
11. Rawal S, Alcaide-Leon P, Macdonald RL, Rinkel GJ, Victor JC, Krings T, et al. Meta-analysis of timing of endovascular aneurysm treatment in subarachnoid haemorrhage: inconsistent results of early treatment within 1 day. J Neurol Neurosurg Psychiatry. 2017;88:241–8.
12. Oudshoorn SC, Rinkel GJ, Molyneux AJ, Kerr RS, Dorhout Mees SM, Backes D, et al. Aneurysm treatment <24 versus 24- 72 h after subarachnoid hemorrhage. Neurocrit Care. 2014;21:4–13.
13. Campi A, Ramzi N, Molyneux AJ, Summers PE, Kerr RS, Sneade M, et al. Retreatment of ruptured cerebral aneurysms in patients randomized by coiling or clipping in the International Subarachnoid Aneurysm Trial (ISAT). Stroke. 2007;38:1538–44.
14. Wong GK, Boet R, Ng SC, Chan M, Gin T, Zee B, Poon WS. Ultra-early (within 24 hours) aneurysm treatment after subarachnoid hemorrhage. World Neurosurg. 2012;77:311–5.
15. Zhao B, Rabinstein A, Murad MH, Lanzino G, Panni P, Brinjikji W. Surgical and endovascular treatment of poor-grade aneurysmal subarachnoid hemorrhage: a systematic review and meta-analysis. J Neurosurg Sci. 2017;61:403–15.
16. Hoh BL, Ko NU, Amin-Hanjani S, Chou SHY, Cruz-Flores S, Dangayach NS, Derdeyn CP. Guideline for the management of patients with aneurysmal subarachnoid hemorrhage: a guideline from the American Heart Association/American Stroke Association. Stroke. 2023;54(7):e314–70.
17. Munich SA, Cress MC, Rangel-Castilla L, Sonig A, Ogilvy CS, Lanzino G, et al. Neck remnants and the risk of aneurysm rupture after endovascular treatment with coiling or stent-assisted coiling: much ado about nothing? Neurosurgery. 2019;84:421–7.
18. Pierot L, Barbe C, Herbreteau D, Gauvrit JY, Januel AC, Bala F, et al. Rebleeding and bleeding in the year following intracranial aneurysm coiling: analysis of a large prospective multi- center cohort of 1140 patients: analysis of recanalization after endovascular treatment of intracranial aneurysm (ARETA) study. J Neurointerv Surg. 2020;12:1219–25.
19. Brisman JL, Song JK, Newell DW. Cerebral aneurysms. N Engl J Med. 2006;355(9):928–39.

20. Lindgren A, Vergouwen MD, van der Schaaf I, Algra A, Wermer M, Clarke MJ, et al. Endovascular coiling versus neurosurgical clipping for people with aneurysmal subarachnoid haemorrhage. Cochrane Database Syst Rev. 2018;8(8):CD003085.
21. McDougall CG, Spetzler RF, Zabramski JM, Partovi S, Hills NK, Nakaji P, et al. The Barrow ruptured aneurysm trial. J Neurosurg. 2012;116:135–44.
22. Guresir E, Beck J, Vatter H, Setzer M, Gerlach R, Seifert V, et al. Subarachnoid hemorrhage and intracerebral hematoma: incidence, prognostic factors, and outcome. Neurosurgery. 2008;63:1088–93.
23. de los Reyes K, Patel A, Bederson JB, Frontera JA. Management of sub-arachnoid hemorrhage with intracerebral hematoma: clipping and clot evacuation versus coil embolization followed by clot evacuation. J Neurointerv Surg. 2013;5:99–103.
24. Niemann DB, Wills AD, Maartens NF, Kerr RS, Byrne JV, Molyneux AJ. Treatment of intracerebral hematomas caused by aneurysm rupture: coil placement followed by clot evacuation. J Neurosurg. 2003;99:843–7.
25. Spetzler RF, McDougall CG, Albuquerque FC, Zabramski JM, Hills NK, Partovi S, et al. The Barrow ruptured aneurysm trial: 3-year results. J Neurosurg. 2013;119:46–157.
26. Spetzler RF, McDougall CG, Zabramski JM, Albuquerque FC, Hills NK, Russin JJ, et al. The Barrow ruptured aneurysm trial: 6-year results. J Neurosurg. 2015;123:609–17.
27. Molyneux AJ, Kerr RS, Yu LM, Clarke M, Sneade M, Yarnold JA, et al. International subarachnoid aneurysm trial (ISAT) collaborative group. International subarachnoid aneurysm trial (ISAT) of neurosurgical clipping versus endovascular coiling in 2143 patients with ruptured intracranial aneurysms: a randomised comparison of effects on survival, dependency, seizures, rebleeding, subgroups, and aneurysm occlusion. Lancet. 2005;366:809–17.
28. Ido K, Kurogi R, Kurogi A, Nishimura K, Arimura K, Nishimura A, et al. J-ASPECT Study Collaborators. Effect of treatment modality and cerebral vasospasm agent on patient outcomes after aneurysmal subarachnoid hemorrhage in the elderly aged 75 years and older. PLoS One. 2020;15:e0230953.
29. Ohkuma H, Shimamura N, Naraoka M, Katagai T. Aneurysmal subarachnoid hemorrhage in the elderly over age 75: a systematic review. Neurol Med Chir (Tokyo). 2017;57:575–83.
30. Giorgianni A, Agosti E, Molinaro S, Terrana AV, Vizzari FA, Nativo L, et al. Flow diversion for acutely ruptured intracranial aneurysms treatment: a retrospective study and literature review. J Stroke Cerebrovasc Dis. 2022;31:106284.
31. Cagnazzo F, Di Carlo DT, Petrella G, Perrini P. Ventriculostomy-related hemorrhage in patients on antiplatelet therapy for endovascular treatment of acutely ruptured intracranial aneurysms: a meta-analysis. Neurosurg Rev. 2020;43:397–406.
32. Molyneux AJ, Birks J, Clarke A, Sneade M, Kerr RS. The durability of endovascular coiling versus neurosurgical clipping of ruptured cerebral aneurysms: 18-year follow-up of the UK cohort of the international subarachnoid aneurysm trial (ISAT). Lancet. 2015;385:691–7.
33. Kassell NF, Torner JC, Jane JA, Haley EC Jr, Adams HP. The international cooperative study on the timing of aneurysm surgery, part 2: surgical results. J Neurosurg. 1990;73:37–47.
34. Wijdicks EF, Vermeulen M, Murray GD, Hijdra A, van Gijn J. The effects of treating hypertension following aneurysmal subarachnoid hemorrhage. Clin Neurol Neurosurg. 1990;92:111–7.
35. Shi M, Yang C, Chen ZH, Xiao LF, Zhao WY. Efficacy and safety of tranexamic acid in aneurysmal subarachnoid hemorrhage: a systematic review and meta-analysis of randomized controlled trials. Front Surg. 2021;8:790149.
36. Baharoglu MI, Germans MR, Rinkel GJ, Algra A, Vermeulen M, van Gijn J, et al. Antifibrinolytic therapy for aneurysmal subarachnoid haemorrhage. Cochrane Database Syst Rev. 2013;2013:Cd001245.
37. Post R, Germans MR, Tjerkstra MA, Vergouwen MDI, Jellema K, Koot RW, et al. ULTRA Investigators. Ultra-early tranexamic acid after subarachnoid haemorrhage (ULTRA): a randomised controlled trial. Lancet. 2021;397:112–8.
38. Ohkuma H, Tsurutani H, Suzuki S. Incidence and significance of early aneurysmal rebleeding before neurosurgical or neurological management. Stroke. 2001;32:1176–80.

39. Calviere L, Gathier CS, Rafiq M, Koopman I, Rousseau V, Raposo N, et al. Rebleeding after aneurysmal subarachnoid hemorrhage in two centers using different blood pressure management strategies. Front Neurol. 2022;13:836268.
40. Ascanio LC, Enriquez-Marulanda A, Maragkos GA, Salem MM, Alturki AY, Ravindran K, et al. Effect of blood pressure variability during the acute period of subarachnoid hemorrhage on functional outcomes. Neurosurgery. 2020;87:779–87.
41. Tang C, Zhang TS, Zhou LF. Risk factors for rebleeding of aneurysmal subarachnoid hemorrhage: a meta-analysis. PLoS One. 2014;9:e99536.
42. Steiner T, Juvela S, Unterberg A, Jung C, Forsting M, Rinkel G. European stroke organization guidelines for the management of intracranial aneurysms and subarachnoid haemorrhage. Cerebrovasc Dis. 2013;35:93–112.
43. Harders AG, Gilsbach JM. Time course of blood velocity changes related to vasospasm in the circle of Willis measured by transcranial Doppler ultrasound. J Neurosurg. 1987;66:718–28.
44. Hoh BL, Cheung AC, Rabinov JD, Pryor JC, Carter BS, Ogilvy CS. Results of a prospective protocol of computed tomographic angiography in place of catheter angiography as the only diagnostic and pretreatment planning study for cerebral aneurysms by a combined neurovascular team. Neurosurgery. 2004;54:1329–40.
45. Abdulazim A, Heilig M, Rinkel G, Etminan N. Diagnosis of delayed cerebral ischemia in patients with aneurysmal subarachnoid Hemorrhage and triggers for intervention. Neurocrit Care. 2023;39(2):311–9.
46. Veldeman M, Höllig A, Clusmann H, Stevanovic A, Rossaint R, Coburn M. Delayed cerebral ischaemia prevention and treatment after aneurysmal subarachnoid haemorrhage: a systematic review. Br J Anaesth. 2016;117(1):17–40.
47. Macdonald RL, Kassell NF, Mayer S, Ruefenacht D, Schmiedek P, Weidauer S, et al. Clazosentan to over-come neurological ischemia and infarction occurring after subarachnoid hemorrhage (CONSCIOUS-1): randomized, double-blind, placebo-controlled phase 2 dose-finding trial. Stroke. 2008;39:3015–21.
48. Macdonald RL, Higashida RT, Keller E, Mayer SA, Molyneux A, Raabe A, et al. Clazosentan, an endothelin receptor antagonist, in patients with aneurysmal subarachnoid haemorrhage undergoing surgical clipping: a randomised, double-blind, placebo-controlled phase 3 trial (CONSCIOUS-2). Lancet Neurol. 2011;10:618–25.
49. Macdonald RL, Higashida RT, Keller E, Mayer SA, Molyneux A, Raabe A, et al. Randomized trial of clazosentan in patients with aneurysmal subarachnoid hemorrhage undergoing endovascular coiling. Stroke. 2012;43:1463–9.
50. Westermaier T, Stetter C, Vince GH, Pham M, Tejon JP, Eriskat J, et al. Prophylactic intravenous magnesium sulfate for treatment of aneurysmal subarachnoid hemorrhage: a randomized, placebo-controlled, clinical study. Crit Care Med. 2010;38:1284–90.
51. Wong GK, Poon WS, Chan MT, Boet R, Gin T, Ng SC, et al. Intravenous magnesium sulphate for aneurysmal subarachnoid hemorrhage (IMASH): a randomized, double-blinded, placebo-controlled, multicenter phase III trial. Stroke. 2010;41:921–6.
52. Dorhout Mees SM, Algra A, Vandertop WP, van Kooten F, Kuijsten HA, Boiten J, et al. Magnesium for aneurysmal subarachnoid haemorrhage (MASH-2): a randomised placebo-controlled trial. Lancet. 2012;380:44–9.
53. Suzuki S, Sayama T, Nakamura T, Nishimura H, Ohta M, Inoue T, et al. Cilostazol improves outcome after subarachnoid hemorrhage: a preliminary report. Cerebrovasc Dis. 2011;32:89–93.
54. Senbokuya N, Kinouchi H, Kanemaru K, Ohashi Y, Fukamachi A, Yagi S, et al. Effects of cilostazol on cerebral vasospasm after aneurysmal subarachnoid hemorrhage: a multicenter prospective, randomized, openlabel blinded end point trial. J Neurosurg. 2013;118:121–30.
55. Shibuya M, Suzuki Y, Sugita K, Saito I, Sasaki T, Takakura K, et al. Effect of AT877 on cerebral vasospasm after aneurysmal subarachnoid hemorrhage. Results of a prospective placebo-controlled double-blind trial. J Neurosurg. 1992;76:571–7.

56. Committee for Guidelines for Management of Aneurysmal Subarachnoid Hemorrhage, Japanese Society on Surgery for Cerebral Stroke. Evidence-based guidelines for the management of aneurysmal subarachnoid hemorrhage. English edition. Neurol Med Chir (Tokyo). 2012;52(6):355–429.
57. Zhao J, Zhou D, Guo J, Ren Z, Zhou L, Wang S, et al. Efficacy and safety of fasudil in patients with subarachnoid hemorrhage: final results of a randomized trial of fasudil versus nimodipine. Neurol Med Chir (Tokyo). 2011;51:679–83.
58. De Caterina R. N-3 fatty acids in cardiovascular disease. N Engl J Med. 2011;364:2439–50.
59. Tanaka K, Ishikawa Y, Yokoyama M, Origasa H, Matsuzaki M, Saito Y, et al. Reduction in the recurrence of stroke by eicosapentaenoic acid for hypercholesterolemic patients: subanalysis of the JELIS trial. Stroke. 2008;39:2052–8.
60. Yoneda H, Shirao S, Nakagawara J, Ogasawara K, Tominaga T, Suzuki M. A prospective, multicenter, randomized study of the efficacy of eicosapentaenoic acid for cerebral vasospasm: the EVAS study. World Neurosurg. 2014;81:309–15.
61. Helbok R, Shaker E, Beer R, Chemelli A, Sojer M, Sohm F, et al. High dose erythropoietin increases brain tissue oxygen tension in severe vasospasm after subarachnoid hemorrhage. BMC Neurol. 2012;12:32.
62. Kirkpatrick PJ, Turner CL, Smith C, Hutchinson PJ, Murray GD. Simvastatin in aneurysmal subarachnoid haemorrhage (STASH): a multicentre randomised phase 3 trial. Lancet Neurol. 2014;13:666–75.
63. Simard JM, Aldrich EF, Schreibman D, James RF, Polifka A, Beaty N. Low-dose intravenous heparin infusion in patients with aneurysmal subarachnoid hemorrhage: a preliminary assessment. J Neurosurg. 2013;119:1611–9.
64. Gomis P, Graftieaux JP, Sercombe R, Hettler D, Scherpereel B, Rousseaux P. Randomized, double-blind, placebo-controlled, pilot trial of high-dose methylprednisolone in aneurysmal subarachnoid hemorrhage. J Neurosurg. 2010;112:681–8.
65. Webb A, Kolenda J, Martin K, Wright W, Samuels O. The effect of intraventricular administration of nicardipine on mean cerebral blood flow velocity measured by transcranial Doppler in the treatment of vasospasm following aneurysmal subarachnoid hemorrhage. Neurocrit Care. 2010;12:159–64.
66. Kasuya H. Clinical trial of nicardipine prolonged-release implants for preventing cerebral vasospasm: multicenter cooperative study in Tokyo. Acta Neurochir Suppl. 2011;110:165–7.
67. Schneider UC, Dreher S, Hoffmann KT, Schmiedek P, Kasuya H, Vajkoczy P. The use of nicardipine prolonged release implants (NPRI) in microsurgical clipping after aneurysmal subarachnoid haemorrhage: comparison with endovascular treatment. Acta Neurochir. 2011;153:2119–25.
68. Al-Tamimi YZ, Bhargava D, Feltbower RG, Hall G, Goddard AJ, Quinn AC, Ross SA. Lumbar drainage of cerebrospinal fluid after aneurysmal subarachnoid hemorrhage: a prospective, randomized, controlled trial (LUMAS). Stroke. 2012;43(3):677–82.
69. Litrico S, Almairac F, Gaberel T, et al. Intraventricular fibrinolysis for severe aneurysmal intraventricular hemorrhage: a randomized controlled trial and meta-analysis. Neurosurg Rev. 2013;36:523–30.
70. Etminan N, Beseoglu K, Eicker SO, Turowski B, Steiger HJ, Hanggi D. Prospective, randomized, open-label phase II trial on concomitant intraventricular fibrinolysis and low frequency rotation after severe subarachnoid hemorrhage. Stroke. 2013;44:2162–8.
71. Smith WS, Dowd CF, Johnston SC, et al. Neurotoxicity of intra-arterial papaverine preserved with chlorobutanol used for the treatment of cerebral vasospasm after aneurysmal subarachnoid hemorrhage. Stroke. 2004;35:2518–22.
72. Cooke D, Seiler D, Hallam D, Kim L, Jarvik JG, Sekhar L, Ghodke B. Does treatment modality affect vasospasm distribution in aneurysmal subarachnoid hemorrhage: differential use of intra-arterial interventions for cerebral vasospasm in surgical clipping and endovascular coiling populations. J Neurointerv Surg. 2010;2:139–44.
73. Gathier CS, van den Bergh WM, Slooter AJ. HIMALAIA (hypertension induction in the management of aneurysmal subarachnoid hemorrhage with secondary ischaemia): a ran-

domized single-blind controlled trial of induced hypertension vs. no induced hypertension in the treatment of delayed cerebral ischemia after subarachnoid hemorrhage. Int J Stroke. 2014;9:375–80.
74. Bulsara KR, Günel M, Amin-Hanjani S, Chen PR, Connolly ES, Friedlander RM. Results of a national cerebrovascular neurosurgery survey on the management of cerebral vasospasm/ delayed cerebral ischemia. J Neurointerv Surg. 2015;7:408–11.
75. Hollingworth M, Chen PR, Goddard AJ, Coulthard A, Söderman M, Bulsara KR. Results of an international survey on the investigation and endovascular management of cerebral vasospasm and delayed cerebral ischemia. World Neurosurg. 2015;83:1120–6.e1.
76. Bele S, Proescholdt MA, Hochreiter A, Schuierer G, Scheitzach J, Wendl C, et al. Continuous intraarterial nimodipine infusion in patients with severe refractory cerebral vasospasm after aneurysmal subarachnoid hemorrhage: a feasibility study and outcome results. Acta Neurochir. 2015;157:2041–50.
77. Mortimer AM, Steinfort B, Faulder K, Bradford C, Finfer S, Assaad N, et al. The detrimental clinical impact of severe angiographic vasospasm may be diminished by maximal medical therapy and intensive endovascular treatment. J Neurointerv Surg. 2015;7:881–7.
78. Deem S, Diringer M, Livesay S, Treggiari MM. Hemodynamic management in the prevention and treatment of delayed cerebral ischemia after aneurysmal subarachnoid hemorrhage. Neurocrit Care. 2023;39(1):81–90.
79. Treggiari MM, Rabinstein AA, Busl KM, Caylor MM, Citerio G, Deem S, et al. Guidelines for the neurocritical care management of aneurysmal subarachnoid hemorrhage. Neurocrit Care. 2023;39(1):1–28.
80. Hoh BL, Ko NU, Amin-Hanjani S, Hsiang-Yi Chou S, Cruz-Flores S, Dangayach NS, et al. 2023 guideline for the management of patients with aneurysmal subarachnoid hemorrhage: a guideline from the American Heart Association/American Stroke Association. Stroke. 2023;54(7):e314–70.
81. Gathier CS, van den Bergh WM, van der Jagt M, Ver-weij BH, Dankbaar JW, Müller MC, et al. HIMALAIA study group. Induced hypertension for delayed cerebral ischemia after aneurysmal subarachnoid hemorrhage: a randomized clinical trial. Stroke. 2018;49:76–83.
82. Haegens NM, Gathier CS, Horn J, Coert BA, Verbaan D, van den Bergh WM. Induced hypertension in preventing cerebral infarction in delayed cerebral ischemia after subarachnoid hemorrhage. Stroke. 2018;49:2630–6.
83. Rondeau N, Cinotti R, Rozec B, Roquilly A, Floch H, Groleau N, et al. Dobutamine-induced high cardiac index did not prevent vasospasm in subarachnoid hemorrhage patients: a randomized controlled pilot study. Neurocrit Care. 2012;17:183–90.
84. Lakhal K, Hivert A, Alexandre PL, Fresco M, Robert-Edan V, Rodie-Talbere PA, et al. Intravenous milrinone for cerebral vasospasm in subarachnoid hemorrhage: the MILRISPASM controlled before-after study. Neurocrit Care. 2021;35:669–79.
85. Mutoh T, Kazumata K, Terasaka S, Taki Y, Suzuki A, Ishikawa T. Early intensive versus minimally invasive approach to postoperative hemodynamic management after subarachnoid hemorrhage. Stroke. 2014;45:1280–4.
86. Anetsberger A, Gempt J, Blobner M, Ringel F, Bogdanski R, Heim M, et al. Impact of goal-directed therapy on delayed ischemia after aneurysmal subarachnoid hemorrhage: randomized controlled trial. Stroke. 2020;51:2287–96.

Controversies in the Management of Acute Ischemic Stroke

3

Ponniah Vanamoorthy, Sindhu Priya, and Mathangi Krishnakumar

Abstract

Acute ischemic stroke (AIS) represents a critical neurological emergency requiring timely diagnosis and evidence-based intervention. Despite advancements in reperfusion strategies and imaging techniques, the management of AIS remains fraught with controversies. This chapter explores key areas of debate, including the choice and timing of neuroimaging, thrombolytic therapy beyond the traditional 4.5-h window, eligibility in elderly patients and those with comorbidities, use of tenecteplase versus alteplase, and thrombolysis in patients on direct oral anticoagulants. Additional areas of contention include rescue therapies following failed thrombectomy, optimal blood pressure targets post-intervention, and the role of dual antiplatelet therapy and genetic resistance. The chapter also evaluates diagnostic approaches to patent foramen ovale and examines evolving strategies in neuroprotection and anesthesia during endovascular therapy. Through a critical appraisal of current evidence and clinical guidelines, this chapter highlights the need for individualized treatment strategies and further research to resolve ongoing dilemmas in AIS management.

Keywords

Acute ischemic stroke · Thrombolysis · Endovascular therapy · Neuroprotection Blood pressure management

P. Vanamoorthy (✉) · S. Priya
Neuro Anaesthesia & Critical Care, Kauvery Hospital, Chennai, Tamil Nadu, India

M. Krishnakumar
Surgical and Neuro Intensive care unit, Department of Anaesthesia, St John's Medical College Hospital, Bengaluru, Karnataka, India

P. U. Bidkar, M. Krishnakumar (eds.), *Controversies in Neurocritical Care*,
https://doi.org/10.1007/978-981-95-4419-6_3

3.1 Introduction

Acute ischemic stroke (AIS) necessitates prompt and precise management to minimize neurologic damage and improve patient outcomes. However, the management of AIS is fraught with controversies, primarily due to the complexities of the condition and the evolving nature of medical research. This document explores some of the key controversies in AIS management.

3.2 Imaging

In the treatment of acute ischemic stroke, time is of the essence, and the treatment decision can be made only after brain imaging. Computed tomography (CT) scans are the preferred initial imaging of choice in most institutes, but now there is a shift in practice, and many centers have begun to use MRI (magnetic resonance imaging) as the first imaging modality.

Non-contrast CT, computed tomography angiography (CTA), and computed tomography perfusion (CTP) are essential components of imaging protocols for ischemic "code-stroke" evaluations [1]. Studies have shown that the total scan duration for CT/CTA is about 7 min, and CT/CTA/CTP is around 10 min. In centers using MRI as the primary diagnostic tool, standardized stroke MRI protocols take about 10 min [2].

Diffusion-weighted imaging (DWI) is currently the most effective sequence for detecting brain infarction earlier than CT or other MR sequences. It has high sensitivity (88–100%), specificity (95–100%), and accuracy (95%) in identifying ischemic core within minutes of onset [1]. MRI also gives more precise localization of the ischemic lesion, more accurate detection of stroke mimics, likely better quantification of the ischemic core, and the capability to estimate the delay from stroke onset in patients with unknown onset [3].

Due to the lower time of acquisition of MRI images with diffusion, many centers are adopting MRI as the first neuroimaging modality (Table 3.1).

Table 3.1 Advantages and disadvantages of imaging modalitites

CT	MRI
Scan time short for non-contrast CT scan	The minimum sequences take 13 min. Efforts are being made to shorten the time to 6 min
Short scan time makes patient cooperation easier	Sedation may be required for the patient
Can be done safely in patients with pacemakers, metallic foreign body, aneurysm clips, implantable devices, and hemodynamically unstable patients	Needs to be done with caution (but recently many of the medical devices are MR compatible or MR conditional)
Easily available	Not all centers are equipped with MRI scan machines
Lesser diagnostic capability for early stroke	More diagnostic capability and rule out stroke mimics

3.3 Thrombolytic Therapy

3.3.1 Timing of Administration

Reperfusion strategies with intravenous thrombolysis (IVT) are the standard established treatment of care for patients with AIS who present within a 5-h window period from the onset of stroke symptoms. A recent meta-analysis found that administration of a thrombolytic agent in select patients (with known time of onset and perfusion mismatch on CT or MRI) who present between 4.5 and 9 h after symptom onset had improved functional outcomes compared with placebo [4].

A similar study on IVT for ischemic stroke beyond 4.5 h without mechanical thrombectomy showed good functional outcomes compared to standard medical care, despite higher odds of spontaneous intracerebral hemorrhage and a nonsignificant increase in mortality [5].

With the advent of advanced neuroimaging and widespread stroke awareness programs, the traditional 4.5-h time frame can be modified to improve functional outcomes.

3.4 Thrombolysis in Patients Taking Direct Oral Anticoagulants (DOACs)

1. Intravenous thrombolytics should not routinely be administered to patients on DOACs who present with acute ischemic stroke. In comprehensive stroke centers with access to specialized tests for DOAC levels and reversal agents, thrombolysis could be considered. Decisions should be individualized in consultation with thrombosis specialists, patients, and their families.
2. The benefits and risks of administering IV thrombolysis to a patient treated with a combination of antiplatelet and low-dose DOAC (e.g., COMPASS trial protocol) remain unclear. Treatment may be considered in consultation with a stroke expert.

3.5 Eligibility Criteria

The criteria for selecting patients for thrombolytic therapy also spark debate. Age, stroke severity, and comorbidities influence eligibility. While some argue for broader inclusion to maximize therapeutic benefits, others warn of increased adverse effects.

Age: Elderly patients (>80 years) represent one-third of all strokes. Historical age restrictions were based on underrepresentation in trials. However, the IST-3 and SITS-UTMOST trials demonstrated the safe use of alteplase in those over 80 years. The european stroke organisation (ESO) and AHA/ASA now no longer specify an upper age limit, promoting broader access to thrombolysis [6].

3.5.1 Minor Stroke and Wake-Up Stroke

These cases pose challenges in assessing functional impairment and risk-benefit balance of thrombolysis. Ongoing studies are examining optimal thresholds for treatment decisions.

3.5.2 Tenecteplase for Thrombolysis

Tenecteplase is a genetically modified tPA with greater fibrin specificity and a longer half-life than alteplase. It offers ease of administration as a bolus, reducing the risk of medication error, transfer delays, and dose interruption. The TRACE-2 and ATTEST-2 trials concluded that 0.25 mg/kg of tenecteplase was not inferior to alteplase for stroke thrombolysis [7, 8].

ESO guidelines strongly recommend tenecteplase (0.25 mg/kg) as an alternative to alteplase (0.9 mg/kg) for patients with AIS within 4.5 h of onset [9, 10]. National guidelines in the UK and Ireland also support this approach.

The EXTEND-IA TNK Part 2 trial compared tenecteplase doses of 0.25 vs. 0.4 mg/kg and found no significant differences in reperfusion or functional outcomes [11]. The NOR-TEST 2 trial reported safety concerns with the 0.4 mg/kg dose, supporting the lower dose in clinical practice.

3.6 Contraindications for Thrombolysis

Unruptured Aneurysm: Advanced neuroimaging often detects incidental aneurysms. Despite historical concerns, recent literature supports the safety of thrombolysis in such patients, with similar rates of symptomatic intracranial hemorrhage [12, 13].

Poor Pre-Stroke mRS: AHA/ASA guidelines do not consider preexisting disability (mRS >2) an absolute contraindication for thrombolysis. ESO guidelines recommend treatment for all eligible patients within 4.5 h, regardless of premorbid status, although the evidence quality is low. Meta-analyses have shown that patients with disability (mRS 3–5) had better outcomes with IVT compared to no treatment, without increased risks [14].

3.7 Choice of Thrombolytic Agent: Tenecteplase Versus Alteplase

Numerous trials have evaluated tenecteplase as a potential replacement for alteplase. Results consistently show non-inferiority in efficacy, and some suggest better recanalization and lower intracerebral hemorrhage (ICH) risk. As a result, many centers have adopted tenecteplase at 0.25 mg/kg (max 25 mg) as an alternative to alteplase 0.9 mg/kg [7–11].

3.8 Rescue Therapy After a Failed Mechanical Thrombectomy

Despite successful recanalization, re-occlusion occurs in 10–30% of patients after mechanical thrombectomy, often due to underlying atherosclerosis exacerbated by instrumentation. Unsuccessful recanalization is an independent predictor of mortality [15].

Medical management options include antithrombotics such as aspirin, clopidogrel, heparin, ticagrelor, and intravenous tirofiban. Rescue stenting is also being increasingly explored as a strategy to improve outcomes [16].

There is currently no consensus on the optimal antiplatelet or anticoagulation regimen in this setting, and practice varies widely between institutions. Tirofiban, a glycoprotein IIb/IIIa receptor antagonist, has been highlighted for its endogenous thrombolytic effects and short half-life, making it a feasible adjunct in the acute setting [17].

Studies suggest that intravenous tirofiban, when administered after failed thrombectomy, improves recanalization rates without increasing the risk of symptomatic intracerebral hemorrhage [18]. Rescue stenting in these patients has been associated with better 90-day functional outcomes, although the quality of evidence remains low [19, 20].

3.9 Endovascular Therapy (EVT)

3.9.1 Patient Selection

Endovascular therapy is now standard for large-vessel occlusion strokes. However, selection criteria remain controversial. Some advocate broadening inclusion criteria to include patients with minor strokes, while others recommend stringent imaging and clinical selection to reduce unnecessary risks.

Key trials such as MR CLEAN, EXTEND-IA, SWIFT PRIME, and REVASCAT excluded patients with blood pressures >185/110 mmHg, while endovascular treatment for small core and anterior circulation proximal occlusion with emphasis on minimizing CT to recanalization times (ESCAPE trial) allowed broader inclusion [21].

Current Canadian guidelines recommend that all eligible patients should receive IV thrombolysis even if they are candidates for EVT [strong recommendation; high quality of evidence].

3.9.2 Stroke with Patent Foramen Ovale (PFO)

PFO is a common congenital intracardiac shunt that can facilitate paradoxical embolism, contributing to cryptogenic stroke. Detection techniques include:

- *Transthoracic Echocardiography (TTE)*: Noninvasive and accessible, but lower sensitivity (~46%).

- *Transesophageal Echocardiography (TEE)*: Gold standard with ~90% sensitivity and >95% specificity.
- *Transcranial Doppler (TCD)*: Noninvasive, sensitive (~96%), and useful at bedside, but may yield false positives from extracardiac shunts [22–24].

TCD has been shown to outperform TTE in detecting right-to-left shunts (RLS) and complements TEE for detailed anatomical evaluation. Both TEE and TCD are essential in guiding secondary prevention strategies in cryptogenic strokes associated with PFO [25, 26] (Table 3.2).

Table 3.2 Monitoring in patent foramen ovale

Monitor	Transthoracic echocardiography	Trans esophageal echocardiography	Transcranial doppler
Advantages	Noninvasive, easy to use, relatively low cost, reproducible, comfortable for patients; it provides visualization of cardiac structures and helps in diagnosing coexisting septal aneurysm and other cardiac pathologies; performed in normal respiration and Valsalva manuever to maximize the sensitivity and specificity for detection of RLS. Preferred initial diagnostic modality	2D and 3D TEE offers significant anatomic details	Noninvasive (compared with TEE), cost-effective, valid, and easily reproducible bedside procedure, patient comfort, rapid and semiquantitative assessment of shunt size, and has an ability to identify extracardiac and intracardiac shunting; studies can be performed in normal respiration and Valsalva maneuver to maximize the sensitivity and specificity for detection of RLS; no sedation needed.
Disadvantages	Poor image quality, least sensitive, detects only one-half the instances of PFOs found either on TEE or TCD. Sensitivity can be increased by following protocols, including injections of agitated saline with Valsalva manuvre.	TEE is a semi-invasive procedure, sedation may be required, which may hinder patient's cooperation for Valsalva maneuver, patient needs to be nil-per-oral; procedure-related complications–Esophageal injury, bleeding. Challenging to do in patients with altered mental status and coagulopathy	It does not provide additional information on other structural cardiac lesions and aortic-arch atherosclerosis; an absent temporal window, especially in older females, results in poor insonation because TCD images the cerebral vessels particularly the middle cerebral artery, the RLS may occur due to other malformations such as an arteriovenous fistula (AVF), or venous air embolism, which would lead to a false-positive diagnosis of a PFO

(continued)

Table 3.2 (continued)

Monitor	Transthoracic echocardiography	Trans esophageal echocardiography	Transcranial doppler
	TTE has a sensitivity of 46%, specificity of 98%	TEE has a sensitivity of ~90% and a specificity >95% as compared to tissue confirmatory diagnosis on autopsy	Transcranial Doppler (TCD) is very sensitive (96%) and specific (92%)

3.10 Antithrombotic Therapy

3.10.1 Dual Versus Single Antiplatelet Therapy (DAPT Versus SAPT)

Dual antiplatelet therapy (DAPT) with aspirin and clopidogrel for 21 days is recommended in minor strokes and transient ischemic attack (TIA). However, resistance to these agents due to genetic polymorphisms, especially CYP2C19, affects clinical outcomes [27, 28].

The acute stroke or transient ischemic attack treated with ticagrelor and aspirin for prevention of stroke and death (THALES trial) demonstrated that aspirin-ticagrelor reduced the 30-day risk of disabling stroke or death compared to aspirin alone, albeit with increased bleeding [29].

A network meta-analysis comparing aspirin+clopidogrel vs. aspirin+ticagrelor found both combinations superior to aspirin alone, with no significant difference between the combinations themselves [30].

Point-of-care tests such as VerifyNow and thromboelastography (TEG) platelet mapping can help identify non-responders and guide individualized therapy [31, 32].

3.10.2 Anticoagulation in Cardioembolic Stroke

In patients with atrial fibrillation and other cardioembolic sources, anticoagulation is standard. However, the timing of initiation post-stroke is debated. Early initiation reduces recurrence but increases hemorrhagic risk. Guidelines vary, and clinical judgment based on imaging, infarct size, and bleeding risk is essential.

3.11 Management of Blood Pressure

3.11.1 Acute Phase Management

Blood pressure (BP) management in AIS remains a major area of debate. Elevated BP is common and may support perfusion of the ischemic penumbra. However, excessive BP may also increase the risk of hemorrhagic transformation, especially after thrombolysis or thrombectomy.

Current guidelines recommend:

- *Before IV thrombolysis:* BP should be <185/110 mm Hg
- *After IV thrombolysis:* Maintain BP <180/105 mm Hg for the first 24 h [33–35]

Trials such as the stroke acute management with urgent risk-factor assessment and improvement (registry/trial program in Japan) (*SAMURAI) rt-PA Registry* and *Transl Stroke Res 2016* show that BP variability is associated with worse outcomes, including symptomatic intracranial hemorrhage [33, 34].

In endovascular therapy (EVT) trials such as *MR CLEAN*, *REVASCAT*, and *SWIFT PRIME*, patients with BP >185/110 mmHg were excluded. Hence, this value is often used as a threshold in current EVT protocols [21].

However, recent trials exploring tighter BP control have yielded mixed results:

- *BP-TARGET*: No clear benefit from intensive BP lowering post-EVT.
- *ENCHANTED2/MT*: Showed worse outcomes with intensive BP lowering (<120 mmHg), especially in populations with intracranial atherosclerosis [36].

Ongoing trials (BEST-II, OPTIMAL_BP, and CRISIS I) aim to clarify ideal BP targets based on the degree of reperfusion and vascular status.

Key Consideration: In patients with successful recanalization (TICI 2b-3), SBP 120–140 mm Hg may be optimal. In unsuccessful reperfusion (TICI 0–2a) or poor collaterals, higher targets (140–180 mm Hg) may be appropriate.

3.11.2 Induced Hypertension (iHTN)

Induced hypertension is being evaluated as a strategy to augment cerebral perfusion in patients with acute ischemic stroke who show signs of neurological deterioration or have hypoperfusion syndromes.

The *SETIN-HYPERTENSION trial* evaluated phenylephrine-induced BP elevation in non-cardioembolic strokes. It demonstrated safety and possible efficacy, especially when initiated within 3 h of early neurological deterioration (END) [37].

Mechanistically, iHTN enhances perfusion via improved cerebral perfusion pressure and collateral circulation, particularly in large-vessel occlusions or small-vessel occlusions with progressive thrombosis.

3.11.3 Anesthesia for Endovascular Therapy

Sedation versus general anesthesia (GA) during EVT is another controversy in AIS management.

- *Conscious sedation (CS)* is preferred when feasible due to less hypotension, fewer delays, and better functional outcomes in some observational studies.

- *General anesthesia (GA)* is indicated for:
  - Airway compromise
  - Severe agitation
  - Respiratory failure
  - Complex interventions requiring complete immobility [38]

Canadian stroke guidelines recommend:

- *CS as first choice*, with GA reserved for specific indications.
- *Avoiding hypotension and delays* is critical when GA is used.

Randomized controlled trials are ongoing to further delineate the optimal strategy in different clinical scenarios.

3.12 Neuroprotection Strategies

3.12.1 Effectiveness of Treatments

Neuroprotection remains a largely experimental but promising frontier in acute ischemic stroke (AIS) management. The primary goal is to preserve the penumbra—the area of hypoperfused but salvageable brain tissue—until reperfusion is achieved. Various strategies have been proposed, including pharmacological agents, hypothermia, and metabolic modulation. However, despite strong preclinical evidence, translating these findings into clinical benefit remains elusive [39–42].

3.12.2 Hypothermia

Therapeutic hypothermia has been extensively studied in cardiac arrest and neonatal encephalopathy, showing neuroprotective effects. Its use in stroke, however, remains investigational. Studies have reported feasibility, but complications such as pneumonia, coagulopathy, and shivering limit widespread adoption [40–42].

3.12.3 Pharmacologic Agents [43–48]

Numerous neuroprotective drugs have been evaluated:

- NMDA antagonists (e.g., selfotel, aptiganel): Failed in clinical trials due to poor efficacy and adverse effects [44].
- Free radical scavengers (e.g., NXY-059): Despite promising preclinical data, large trials like SAINT I and II failed to show benefit in human stroke [39].
- Magnesium sulfate, citicoline, and ursodeoxycholic acid have been studied, but none have shown consistent improvement in outcomes [40, 41].

3.12.4 Ongoing Trials

Current research focuses on agents with multimodal mechanisms, including minocycline, remote ischemic preconditioning, and combination therapies. Trials such as ESCAPE-NA1 evaluating nerinetide and RHAPSODY (using activated protein C analogs) represent continued efforts to establish clinically meaningful neuroprotection [43, 45, 48].

3.12.5 Challenges in Translation

- Timing: The therapeutic window for many agents is very narrow [42].
- Heterogeneity: Stroke subtype, collateral status, and comorbidities influence drug response [41, 46].
- Outcome Measures: Many trials use mortality or disability scales, which may not be sensitive to subtle neuroprotective effects [44, 47].

3.12.6 Current Consensus

There is no approved neuroprotective therapy for AIS as of now. Multimodal approaches combining early reperfusion, optimal BP control, and individualized anesthetic and supportive care may serve as the best neuroprotective strategy currently available [42].

3.13 Conclusion

The management of acute ischemic stroke is dynamic and multifaceted, with several controversies that underscore the need for ongoing research and clinical trials. While advances in thrombolytic and endovascular therapies have improved outcomes, questions about patient selection, timing, and the balance between benefits and risks remain. The development of personalized approaches, guided by advanced imaging and biomarkers, holds promise for resolving these controversies and optimizing AIS management.

References

1. Shafaat O, Sotoudeh H. Stroke Imaging. [Updated 2023 May 1]. In: StatPearls [Internet]. Treasure Island (FL): StatPearls Publishing; 2025. Available from: https://www.ncbi.nlm.nih.gov/books/NBK546635/.
2. Simonsen CZ, Yoo AJ, Rasmussen M, et al. Magnetic resonance imaging selection for endovascular stroke therapy: workflow in the GOLIATH trial. Stroke. 2018;49(6):1402–6.
3. Birenbaum D, Bancroft LW, Felsberg GJ. Imaging in acute stroke. West J Emerg Med. 2011;12(1):67–76.

4. Altersberger VL, Sibolt G, Enz LS, et al. Intravenous thrombolysis 4.5–9 hours after stroke onset: a cohort study from the TRISP collaboration. Ann Neurol. 2023.
5. Butcher KS, Saver JL, Goyal M, et al. Intravenous thrombolysis beyond 4.5 hours without thrombectomy. Stroke. 2024;55(1):123–9.
6. Bluhmki E, Danays T, Biegert G, et al. Alteplase for acute ischemic stroke in patients aged >80 years: pooled analyses. Stroke. 2020;51(8):2322–30.
7. Wang Y, Li S, Pan Y, et al. TRACE-2: Tenecteplase vs Alteplase in AIS. Lancet. 2023;401:645–54.
8. Campbell BCV, Mitchell PJ, Churilov L, et al. ATTEST-2: Tenecteplase vs Alteplase within 4.5 h of onset. Lancet Neurol. 2024;23(11):1087–96.
9. Alamowitch S, Turc G, Palaiodimou L, et al. ESO recommendation on Tenecteplase. Eur Stroke J. 2023;8:8–54.
10. Intercollegiate Stroke Working Party. National Clinical Guideline for Stroke for the UK and Ireland. 2023. Available from: www.strokeguideline.org.
11. Campbell BCV, Mitchell PJ, Churilov L, et al. EXTEND-IA TNK part 2 trial. JAMA. 2020;323(13):1257–65.
12. Edwards NJ, Kamel H, Josephson SA. Safety of IV thrombolysis in patients with cerebral aneurysms. Stroke. 2012;43(2):412–6.
13. Virta JJ, Strbian D, Putaala J, Korja M. Risk of aneurysm rupture after thrombolysis. Neurology. 2021;97(18):e1790–8.
14. Beland B, Bala F, Ganesh A. Thrombolysis in patients with premorbid disability: a meta-analysis. Stroke. 2022;53(10):3146–55.
15. Mahmoud NA, Abdalkader M, Kasab SA, et al. Rescue stenting in refractory mechanical Thrombectomy: a review. Adv Neurol. 2024;3(3):3950.
16. Garayzade R, Berlis A, Schiele S, et al. Emergency stenting and Tirofiban use. Cardiovasc Intervent Radiol. 2023;46(3):377–84.
17. Zhu L, Xie F, Li X, et al. Safety of Tirofiban after MT. Am J Transl Res. 2021;13(8):9076–85.
18. Yeo LLL, Andersson T, Waje-Andreassen U, et al. Rescue stenting improves functional outcomes. Stroke. 2024;55(3):812–20.
19. Zhao W, Che R, Shang S, et al. Intracranial rescue stenting feasibility after failed Thrombectomy. Surg Neurol Int. 2022;13:95.
20. Jahan R, Saver JL. Tirofiban and rescue therapy review. Stroke. 2023;54(5):1562–70.
21. Goyal M, Menon BK, van Zwam WH, et al. Endovascular therapy trials: MR CLEAN, ESCAPE, SWIFT PRIME. REVASCAT Summary Stroke. 2016;47(2):548–53.
22. Van der Giessen H, Wilson LC, Coffey S, et al. Detection of PFO: TCD vs Echo. Australas J Ultrasound Med. 2020;23(4):210–9.
23. Rana BS, Thomas MR, Calvert PA. Pathophysiology of PFO and stroke. Am Heart J. 2024;260:123–30.
24. Kim DE, Lee KJ, Bang OY. PFO risk and diagnostic methods: a review. J Neurosonol Neuroimag. 2019;11(1):22–33.
25. Messe SR, Kasner SE. PFO detection and secondary prevention. Stroke. 2023;54(7):2120–9.
26. Kent DM, Ruthazer R. Diagnosis of PFO via imaging modalities. Stroke. 2024;55(4):1456–65.
27. Pareed SA, Vijayaraghavan G, Kartha CC, et al. Antiplatelet drug resistance in Indians. Ann Clin Cardiol. 2020;2(1):36–41.
28. Patel S, Arya V, Saraf A, et al. Aspirin and Clopidogrel resistance in Indian stroke patients. Ann Indian Acad Neurol. 2019;22(2):147–52.
29. Johnston SC, Amarenco P, Denison H, et al. THALES trial. N Engl J Med. 2020;383:207–17.
30. Lun R, Dhaliwal S, Zitikyte G, et al. Network meta-analysis of DAPT strategies. JAMA Neurol. 2022;79(2):141–8.
31. Zhang Y, Fan D, Qiao S, et al. VerifyNow PRU-guided modification of Clopidogrel. Neurol Ther. 2022;11(4):1749–66.
32. Zhang Y, Wang M, Su S. Individualized antiplatelet therapy. J Stroke Cerebrovasc Dis. 2024;33(6):107711.

33. Endo K, Kario K, Koga M, et al. BP variability after thrombolysis: SAMURAI registry. Stroke. 2013;44:816–8.
34. Liu K, Yan S, Zhang S, et al. Systolic BP variability and Hemorrhagic transformation. Transl Stroke Res. 2016;7:186–91.
35. Waltimo T, Haapaniemi E, Surakka IL, et al. BP control post-thrombolysis. Eur J Neurol. 2016;23:1757–62.
36. Anderson CS, Huang Y, Wang JG, et al. ENCHANTED2/MT trial. Stroke. 2024;55(5):1721–32.
37. Yang X, Zhang J, Peng S, et al. SETIN-HYPERTENSION trial: therapeutic induced hypertension. Stroke. 2023;54(9):2643–50.
38. Canadian Stroke Best Practices Advisory Committee. Anesthesia Strategies in EVT. Canadian Stroke Guidelines. 2024. Available from: https://www.strokebestpractices.ca/.
39. Saver JL. Novel neuroprotective strategies in ischemic stroke: unraveling the bench-to-bedside gap. Stroke. 2011;42(1 Suppl):S45–8.
40. Lyden PD. All is not lost: reperfusion and neuroprotection in the penumbra. Stroke. 2021;52(4):e171–8.
41. Hemmen TM, Lyden PD. Multimodal neuroprotective therapy in acute ischemic stroke. Stroke. 2009;40(3 Suppl):S126–8.
42. van der Worp HB, Sena ES, Donnan GA, et al. Hypothermia in animal models of acute ischaemic stroke: a systematic review and meta-analysis. Brain. 2007;130(Pt 12):3063–74.
43. Hill MD, Goyal M, Menon BK, et al. Efficacy and safety of nerinetide for the treatment of acute ischaemic stroke (ESCAPE-NA1): a multicentre, double-blind, randomized controlled trial. Lancet. 2020;395(10227):878–87.
44. Diener HC, Lees KR, Lyden P, et al. NXY-059 for the treatment of acute stroke: pooled analysis of the SAINT I and II trials. Stroke. 2008;39(6):1751–8.
45. Grotta JC, Welch KM, Fagan SC, et al. Clinical trial of uric acid to treat acute stroke (URICO-ICTUS): a randomized double-blind phase 2b/3 trial. Lancet Neurol. 2014;13(5):453–60.
46. Muir KW, Lees KR. Clinical experience with excitatory amino acid antagonist drugs. Stroke. 1995;26(3):503–13.
47. Baron JC. Protecting the ischaemic penumbra as an adjunct to thrombectomy for acute stroke. Nat Rev Neurol. 2018;14(6):325–37.
48. Zonneveld TP, Nederkoorn PJ, Dijkland SA, et al. Safety and outcome of thrombolysis in stroke patients on direct oral anticoagulants: a meta-analysis. Stroke. 2020;51(2):533–41.

Controversies in Management of ICH

4

Saurabh Anand, Prasanna Bidkar,
and Mathangi Krishnakumar

Abstract

Spontaneous intracerebral haemorrhage (ICH) is nontraumatic bleeding in the brain parenchyma, which can extend into the ventricles and the subarachnoid space. There are many dilemmas in the management of ICH, ranging from the management of elevated blood pressure to the surgical management of ICH. This chapter addresses all the controversial issues in light of recent evidence and provides conclusions for the readers on each subtopic.

Blood pressure management forms the cornerstone of ICH treatment, and we have reached the target systolic blood pressure of 140 mm Hg based on current understanding of available evidence.

Similarly, guidelines for the reversal of anticoagulants and antiplatelets are now clear and are outlined in the text, which is derived from the recent stroke guidelines published in 2022.

We have received encouraging news about the surgical management of ICH. We now know that minimally invasive surgery plays a role in the early treatment of ICH. We have chosen not to focus on hyperosmolar therapy for managing ICH as there have been no recent developments in this area. With several new studies underway and the rapidly evolving landscape of ICH, this chapter will soon need to be re-evaluated.

S. Anand (✉)
Neurocritical care and Neuroanaesthesia, Artemis Hospital, Gurugram, Haryana, India

P. Bidkar
JIPMER, Puducherry, Puducherry, India

M. Krishnakumar
Surgical and Neuro Intensive Care Unit, Department of Anaesthesia, St John's Medical College Hospital, Bangalore, Karnataka, India

P. U. Bidkar, M. Krishnakumar (eds.), *Controversies in Neurocritical Care*,
https://doi.org/10.1007/978-981-95-4419-6_4

Keywords

Intracerebral haemorrhage · ICH · Hypertension · Anticoagulation

4.1 Introduction

Spontaneous intracerebral haemorrhage (ICH) denotes bleeding into the brain parenchyma that may, by dissection through tissue planes or via foramina, propagate into the ventricular system and occasionally the subarachnoid space. Globally, ICH contributes approximately one in every seven to ten strokes, with a proportionately heavier burden in low- and middle-income countries [1]. Over recent years, epidemiological observations suggest a relative rise in ICH incidence compared with ischaemic stroke; nevertheless, improvements in systems of care and a more refined understanding of ICH pathobiology have been accompanied by incremental gains in outcome [2].

Clinically, ICH most often presents with abrupt focal neurological deficits coupled with indicators of elevated intracranial pressure (ICP)—nausea and vomiting, headache, reduced level of consciousness—and haemodynamic patterns consistent with the Cushing response (systemic hypertension, reflex bradycardia) alongside disordered respirations when pressure rises rapidly. Symptomatology is shaped by the aetiology and anatomy of bleeding (Fig. 4.1), the pace of haematoma formation, and the secondary mass-effect–related tissue distortion. Although the bedside evaluation can raise a strong suspicion, diagnostic certainty cannot rest on clinical features alone. Emergent neuroimaging is mandatory; non-contrast CT is the frontline

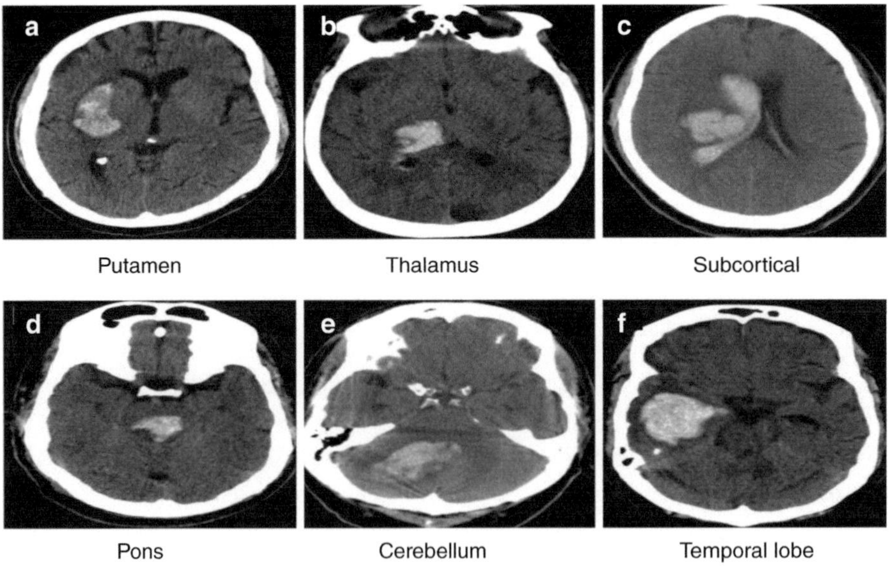

Fig. 4.1 Various locations of bleed

modality for rapid discrimination between haemorrhagic and ischaemic stroke and for quantifying haematoma volume and location, with MRI reserved for diagnostic clarification (e.g. underlying structural lesions) and specific clinical questions.

Management of ICH remains a locus of ongoing debate. Questions begin at the earliest phase—how best to prevent haematoma growth, which patients benefit from rapid blood pressure (BP) reduction, whom to treat with haemostatic therapies, and what to do about pre-injury anticoagulant or antiplatelet exposure. Controversies extend to intraventricular haemorrhage (IVH) care, where external ventricular drainage (EVD) is often necessary, yet functional benefits from adjunctive intraventricular thrombolysis have been difficult to demonstrate definitively. Surgical strategies have undergone extensive testing, particularly for supratentorial haemorrhage, but for many scenarios, the signal for improved functional outcome has been inconsistent despite persuasive mechanistic rationale [3–5]. The following sections synthesise contemporary evidence and offer pragmatic, risk-stratified recommendations, emphasising timing, selection, and execution of key interventions.

4.2 Prevention of Haematoma Expansion

4.2.1 Rationale and Timing

Early haematoma expansion is a central driver of deterioration and poor outcome in ICH. Enlargement is most common in the earliest hours after symptom onset, particularly within the first 6 h [6]. The pathophysiological mechanisms include continued bleeding from the initial ruptured vessel, rebleeding, and "avalanche" effects from mechanical disruption of adjacent fragile vessels. Because the expansion window is narrow, the success of any growth-mitigating strategy depends critically on rapid patient identification, streamlined imaging pathways, fast initiation of interventions, and vigilant avoidance of BP variability or iatrogenic hypoperfusion.

Interventions to prevent further bleeding cluster into three domains: (1) prompt and controlled reduction of BP, (2) targeted haemostatic approaches to stabilise the clot, and (3) reversal of pre-existing anticoagulant effects. Each domain has accumulated randomised evidence; however, interpretation must account for achieved rather than merely assigned physiological targets, treatment-related adverse events, and effect modification by time from onset, baseline volume, and markers of active bleeding.

4.2.1.1 Blood Pressure Control

Evidence from Randomised Trials

INTERACT2 examined whether early intensive BP lowering—targeting systolic BP (SBP) below 140 mm Hg within 6 h—improves outcomes compared with a less aggressive approach (SBP <180 mm Hg). The primary endpoint of death or major disability at 90 days did not differ significantly between groups. Nevertheless, ordinal analyses of functional outcomes suggested a shift in favour of intensive treatment, supporting the concept that—even absent a binary win—controlled lowering may modestly increase the probability of better recovery across the disability spectrum [4].

ATACH-2 pushed the test further by comparing an "ultra-intensive" SBP target (110–139 mm Hg) with a standard intensive target (140–179 mm Hg). Over 3 months, there was no difference in death or disability. Importantly, the more aggressive arm experienced a higher burden of renal adverse events, raising caution about overshooting BP reduction beyond a physiologic sweet spot, particularly in haemodynamically vulnerable patients [5].

Achieved Blood Pressure and What the Trials Really Tested

A key nuance in interpreting these studies lies in the achieved SBP rather than the nominal target. In *ATACH-2*, the mean SBP during the first 24 h settled around ~120 mm Hg in the intensive arm and ~ 140 mm Hg in the standard arm. By contrast, *INTERACT2* achieved ~140–150 mm Hg for the intensive arm and ~ 160 mm Hg for the standard arm. In effect, ATACH-2 compared ultra-intensive versus intensive management, whereas INTERACT2 approximated intensive versus moderate control. This difference in exposure helps explain why ATACH-2 failed to show benefit and flagged safety concerns: pushing SBP into the low-normal range early after ICH may risk insufficient cerebral perfusion, especially in the context of raised ICP or impaired autoregulation [6].

Practical Approach to Targets

The collective evidence supports the safety of lowering SBP to the vicinity of 140 mm Hg soon after ICH. Available data do not support routine acute lowering below ~130 mm Hg, and such reductions could be hazardous when large haematomas or high ICP compromise perfusion. Translating evidence to practice, clinicians can adopt a tiered strategy:

- *Patients with SBP 150–220 mm Hg presenting within 6 h:* It is reasonable and safe to lower SBP towards ~140 mm Hg and maintain values in the 130–150 mm Hg range. Titration should be smooth, avoiding abrupt drops and oscillations, which are associated with worse outcomes.
- *Patients with SBP 150–220 mm Hg presenting after ~ 24 h:* By this time, maximal haematoma volume is often reached. Imaging should guide decisions. In larger haematomas or where ICP concerns are prominent, slightly higher targets around ~160 mm Hg may better protect cerebral perfusion while still discouraging rebleeding. Again, minimising variability is crucial.
- *Patients with SBP > 220 mm Hg or severe ICH within 6 h:* These patients are under-represented in trials and more susceptible to hypoperfusion if aggressive lowering is attempted in the setting of high ICP. A prudent approach is to adopt a more liberal SBP target around ~160 mm Hg in tandem with ICP-lowering strategies and, where feasible, direct ICP monitoring. In operative scenarios, ini-

tiation of BP reduction after haemostatic control (e.g. following clot evacuation) and maintenance around ~140 mm Hg postoperatively may reduce rebleeding risk.

Timing and Execution

Time-to-target matters. Initiating treatment within approximately 2 h of onset and achieving the goal within the subsequent hour are associated with less haematoma growth and better functional outcomes, presumably by truncating the expansion window. Protocolised pathways and pre-approved antihypertensive infusions (e.g. titratable agents with short half-lives) facilitate safer and faster attainment.

4.2.1.2 Haemostatic Agents

The biological rationale for haemostatic therapy is straightforward: enhance clot stability and reduce the likelihood or magnitude of ongoing bleeding. Two agents have been mostly studied in this context—tranexamic acid (TXA), an antifibrinolytic, and recombinant activated factor VII (rFVIIa), a procoagulant that boosts thrombin generation at sites of vascular injury.

Tranexamic Acid (TXA)

TXA, a lysine analogue, binds the lysine site on plasminogen, thereby preventing plasmin from degrading fibrin. This antifibrinolytic action can theoretically stabilise an evolving clot and limit haematoma growth.

- *TICH-2* randomised 2325 patients to receive TXA or a placebo. TXA was associated with a lower rate of haematoma expansion (defined as >6 mL absolute or >33% relative increase)—25% vs 29%—and fewer serious adverse events. Despite those biological signals, TXA did not translate into improved functional outcomes at 90 days, likely because the attenuation of expansion was modest, and the enrolment window (up to 8 h) meant many patients were treated after the period of greatest vulnerability. A prespecified interaction suggested more favourable outcomes among those with baseline SBP <170 mm Hg, hinting that substrate and haemodynamic milieu matter [7].
- *STOP-AUST*, which enriched for patients with the CT "spot sign" (a radiological marker of active bleeding), did not demonstrate a statistically significant reduction in expansion with TXA compared with placebo (44% vs 52%) [8]. The null result underlines the challenge of translating improved haemostatic markers into functional benefit, even in a high-risk subgroup.

Synthesis TXA consistently shows signals of reduced haematoma growth and acceptable safety, but the magnitude of effect has not yet yielded robust functional gains across unselected ICH populations. If TXA is to play a role, it is most plausible in very early presenters—ideally within a 2-h window—where the biology favours impact and before clot stabilisation occurs naturally.

Recombinant Activated Factor VII (rFVIIa)

rFVIIa enhances thrombin generation on activated platelets at sites of tissue factor expression, promoting haemostasis.

- Factor seven for acute haemorrhagic stroke (*FAST*) compared two doses (20 and 80 μg/kg) with placebo when given within 4 h of onset. rFVIIa reduced haematoma growth at 24 h (mean increase 26% with placebo; 18% and 11% with 20 and 80 μg/kg, respectively), with absolute reductions of 2.6 mL and 3.8 mL in volume expansion for the lower and higher doses. However, the 80 μg/kg dose carried an increased risk of arterial thromboembolic events (8% vs 4% with placebo), and neither dose improved the composite of death or severe disability [9].
- A *post hoc* analysis suggested a subgroup that may benefit—patients aged ≤70 years, baseline haematoma volume <60 mL, minimal IVH (<5 mL), and treatment within 2.5 h—where the 80 μg/kg dose was associated with a larger reduction in growth (≈7.3 mL) [10]. The finding is hypothesis-generating but requires prospective confirmation.
- More recent trials, including *SPOTLIGHT* and *STOP-IT*, have not shown a clear benefit [11].

Synthesis Routine administration of rFVIIa is not supported. Its use might be contemplated only in exceptional, tightly selected scenarios with ultra-early presentation and favourable risk profiles, balanced against thrombotic risk.

4.2.1.3 Reversal of Anticoagulant and Antiplatelet Effects

Exposure to anticoagulants and antiplatelets is common amongst patients with ICH and materially influences early haematoma dynamics. Expert guidance from the AHA/ASA (2022) provides a structured approach to reversal [12]; a schematic is often presented in practice (Fig. 4.2).

Vitamin K Antagonists (Warfarin)

- *Prothrombin Complex Concentrates (PCCs):* Four-factor PCC offers rapid and more complete reversal of coagulopathy than fresh frozen plasma (FFP), with lower volume and fewer fluid-related complications. Dosing may be INR- and weight-based (25–50 IU/kg) or follow fixed regimens (e.g. 1500 U for intracranial bleeding), though the optimal strategy awaits larger randomised evaluation [13].
- *Vitamin K:* Intravenous vitamin K (5–10 mg) should be administered to all patients with vitamin K antagonist (VKA)-associated ICH, regardless of whether PCC or plasma is used, ensuring sustained reversal once PCC effects wane [14].

Direct Oral Anticoagulants (DOACs)

- *Factor Xa Inhibitors: Andexanet alfa*, a recombinant modified factor Xa decoy, reverses factor Xa inhibition. In *ANNEXa-I*, andexanet achieved superior haemostatic efficacy compared with usual care (which included PCC in most cases)

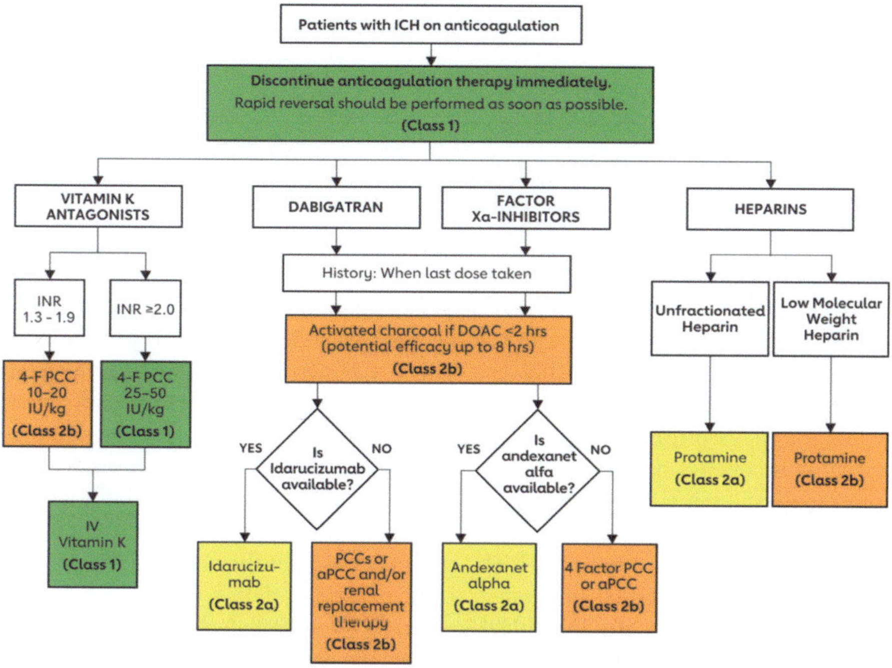

Fig. 4.2 Reversal of anticoagulation

amongst patients with factor Xa inhibitor–associated ICH, aligning with its mechanism as a targeted reversal agent.

- *Dabigatran: Idarucizumab*, a monoclonal antibody fragment, binds dabigatran with high affinity. In a large prospective cohort of patients with serious bleeding or requiring urgent procedures—including a subset with ICH—two 2.5-g boluses (total 5 g) achieved rapid and complete laboratory reversal across demographic and renal function strata. Thrombotic events in the ICH subgroup occurred in roughly 5%, a rate congruent with thrombotic risk when anticoagulation is held [16].

Antiplatelet-Associated ICH

Routine platelet transfusion to reverse antiplatelet effects is not recommended outside neurosurgical contexts. In the *PATCH* trial, platelet transfusion—compared with standard care—led to worse outcomes (higher death or dependence at 3 months) and more serious adverse events, arguing against its use in most patients with antiplatelet-related ICH [17]. Transfusion may be considered peri-operatively when urgent neurosurgery is planned, recognising the balance of bleeding control and transfusion risks.

4.3 Intraventricular Haemorrhage (IVH)

Between one-third and one-half of ICH cases exhibit intraventricular extension. IVH is clinically important because it impairs CSF circulation, predisposes to hydrocephalus, and exacerbates ICP elevation. Three management issues predominate: (1) timely placement of an external ventricular drain (EVD) in the presence of obstructive hydrocephalus or impending herniation, (2) technical aspects of EVD insertion and maintenance, and (3) the role of intraventricular thrombolysis to expedite blood clearance.

EVDs remain the cornerstone for managing elevated ICP in IVH. They provide CSF diversion, permit ICP monitoring, and facilitate sampling. Nonetheless, EVDs do not directly address intraventricular clot burden; hence, adjunctive thrombolysis has been explored to accelerate clot resolution and, in theory, hasten recovery of CSF dynamics.

CLEAR III compared EVD plus intraventricular alteplase with EVD plus saline. While the trial's primary functional endpoint did not favour alteplase, several pre-specified secondary analyses and safety endpoints are noteworthy: mortality was lower in the alteplase group, and rates of serious adverse events (including bacterial ventriculitis) were reduced, supporting the safety of intraventricular thrombolysis under protocolised conditions [18]. The principal caveat is the absence of a parallel improvement in functional outcome, which tempers enthusiasm for routine use. Many centres consequently individualise therapy—employing alteplase where clot burden is high, CSF pathways are occluded, and the neurological trajectory is dominated by hydrocephalus, while recognising that the net functional benefit remains uncertain (Fig. 4.3 offers an algorithmic depiction).

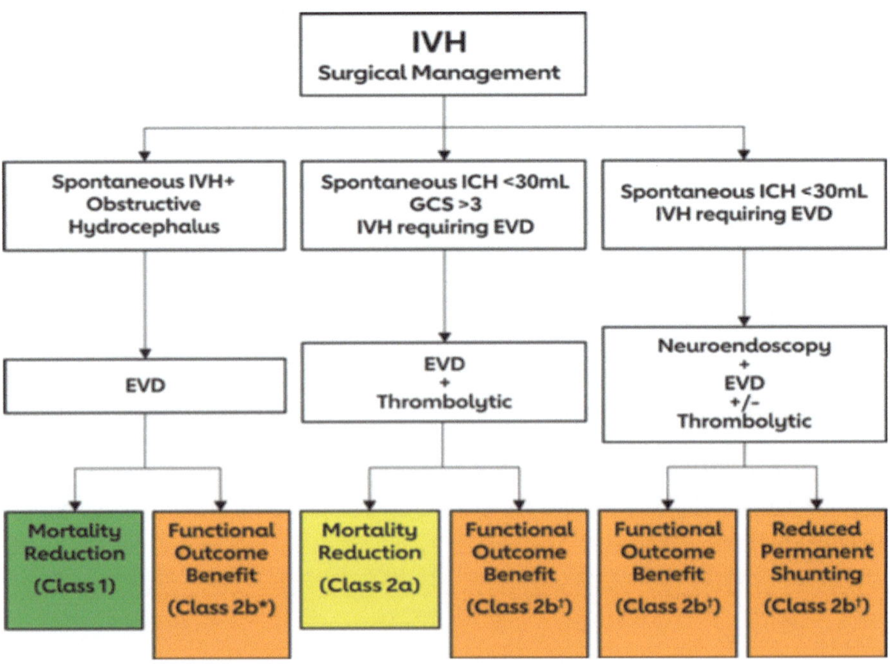

Fig. 4.3 Surgical Management of Intraventricular Haemorrhage

4.4 Haematoma Evacuation

4.4.1 Pathophysiological Rationale

Clot removal in ICH has several theoretical advantages: decompression of adjacent structures, mitigation of midline shift and herniation risk, restoration of local perfusion by reducing ICP and regional tissue pressure, and diminution of neurotoxicity from haemoglobin breakdown products and iron-mediated oxidative injury. Countervailing considerations include surgical trauma, rebleeding risk, and the possibility of disrupting surrounding penumbral tissue. The balance likely varies by haematoma location (lobar vs. deep nuclei), size, presence of IVH, neurological status, and timing relative to onset.

4.4.1.1 Open Craniotomy for Supratentorial ICH

Two landmark trials—*STICH I* and *STICH II*—evaluated early open craniotomy for supratentorial ICH in situations where equipoise existed regarding surgical versus medical treatment. In both, early craniotomy did not improve functional outcomes compared with initial conservative management [19]. These findings do not preclude surgery altogether; rather, they emphasise careful selection. In patients who deteriorate neurologically, develop life-threatening mass effect, or fail to respond to medical measures, craniotomy remains a reasonable life-saving intervention [20, 21]. The expectation, however, should be framed around survival rather than guaranteed functional independence.

4.4.1.2 Minimally Invasive Surgery (MIS)

Technical advances have enabled image-guided aspiration via small corticotomies, often supplemented by intralesional thrombolysis to liquefy and evacuate residual clot.

- *MISTIE III* tested catheter-based aspiration followed by alteplase (typically every 8 h) with the surgical goal of reducing residual volume to ≤15 mL. Compared with standard medical care, MIS did not improve the primary outcome of good functional status at 1 year (modified Rankin Scale 0–3). The procedure did reduce haematoma burden and appeared safe, indicating biological activity even if the clinical signal was muted in the trial's overall population [22].
- *ENRICH* compared early MIS against usual care in a cohort ultimately enriched for lobar haematomas (~70% after an interim decision to stop enrolling deep anterior cases). The trial reported superior functional outcomes with MIS, assessed using a utility-weighted mRS approach, representing one of the clearest positive signals for surgery in lobar ICH to date [23]. The result suggests that anatomy, clot location, and patient selection critically determine the net effect of MIS.

MIS—using endoscopic or stereotactic techniques, with or without adjunctive thrombolytics—is generally safe, reduces clot volume, and may improve outcomes in carefully selected patients, particularly those with lobar haemorrhage and accessible surgical corridors. Evidence for deep haemorrhages remains less persuasive, and trial heterogeneity underscores the need for individualised decision-making.

4.4.1.3 Decompressive Craniectomy

For patients with massive supratentorial ICH, coma, significant midline shift, or refractory intracranial hypertension, decompressive craniectomy (with or without clot evacuation) offers mortality reduction at the cost of a high likelihood of severe disability among survivors. The *SWITCH* trial compared decompressive craniectomy plus best medical management with best medical management alone for severe deep ICH. Although results suggested potential superiority of surgery, confidence intervals were wide and do not exclude no effect. Importantly, harm appears unlikely, but generalizability is limited to the severe deep ICH phenotype studied [24]. Families and clinicians must therefore engage in transparent, values-concordant discussions about expected trajectories.

4.4.1.4 Posterior Fossa (Cerebellar) Haemorrhage

The posterior fossa's tight confines confer a high risk of brainstem compression, hydrocephalus, and herniation with even modest volume increases [25]. For cerebellar haemorrhages meeting criteria (e.g. neurologic decline, brainstem compression, hydrocephalus, or larger volumes), urgent surgical evacuation—often coupled with EVD placement—is recommended over medical management alone to reduce mortality. EVD without evacuation is generally discouraged due to the theoretical risk of upward transtentorial herniation ("reverse herniation") when CSF is diverted in the presence of an unrelieved mass lesion.

4.5 General Care and Additional Controversies

Comprehensive ICH management extends beyond bleeding control and surgery. Protocolised supportive care—antithrombotic decisions, venous thromboembolism prophylaxis, metabolic and temperature targets, and seizure management—has a measurable impact on outcomes and often exhibits less controversy than disease-specific interventions when implemented coherently.

4.5.1 Venous Thromboembolism (VTE) Prophylaxis

Immobility, paresis, systemic inflammatory responses, and central venous catheters converge to elevate VTE risk in ICH. Intermittent pneumatic compression should begin as early as possible. Pharmacologic prophylaxis with low-molecular-weight heparin (LMWH) or low-dose unfractionated heparin is generally introduced once haematoma stability is documented, commonly after 24–48 h, consistent with recommendations from major societies such as the American Heart Association and the Neurocritical Care Society. A randomised controlled trial supports starting pharmacologic prophylaxis as early as 12 h in selected patients, although many centres remain more conservative until repeat imaging confirms stability [26]. The practical recommendation is institutional protocolisation with built-in flexibility for patient-specific haemorrhage dynamics and procedural needs.

4.5.2 Resuming Antithrombotic Therapy

Re-initiation of antithrombotic agents after ICH is nuanced and must incorporate the indication's thrombotic risk, the haemorrhage's characteristics, and the patient's values.

- *Mechanical Heart Valves (MHV):* Evidence is largely observational and indicates that resuming anticoagulation within 2 weeks of ICH is associated with higher haemorrhagic complications. For patients at very high thromboembolic risk (e.g. older generation MHV in the mitral position), some experts consider the earliest restart around day 6, but this is reserved for carefully selected cases after multidisciplinary discussion and usually after imaging confirms stability.
- *Atrial fibrillation (AF):* The *APACHE-AF* study (apixaban versus no anticoagulation) did not yield a definitive conclusion [27]. Guidelines frequently recommend a waiting period of approximately 7–8 weeks before resumption in typical AF-related indications, though decisions should be individualised, considering CHA_2DS_2-VASc and HAS-BLED-like constructs, neuroimaging (microbleeds, cortical superficial siderosis), and patient preference [12].

4.5.3 Glucose and Temperature Control

Hyperglycaemia correlates with poorer outcomes after ICH, and both hypoglycaemia and glucose variability are injurious; thus, most centres adopt moderate glucose targets, avoiding extremes and rapid swings. Fever—particularly central fever—exacerbates metabolic demand and may worsen neuronal injury. A unit-level protocol for early recognition and management of central fever [28] and paroxysmal sympathetic hyperactivity [29] is recommended.

The *INTERACT3* study is notable for testing a bundled care protocol commenced within hours of onset, combining intensive BP lowering with standardised glucose and temperature management and other physiological targets. This multimodal approach improved functional outcomes across a broad ICH population, reinforcing that disciplined delivery of basic physiological care can match or exceed the impact of single-target interventions [30].

4.5.4 Seizure Management

While seizures are not uncommon after ICH—particularly with lobar locations or cortical involvement—routine prophylactic antiepileptic medication is not recommended by contemporary guidelines [12]. Continuous or intermittent electroencephalogram (EEG) monitoring should be used liberally in patients with depressed consciousness, fluctuating examinations, or unexplained deterioration. When clinical or electrographic seizures are detected, they should be treated promptly, with agent selection tailored to organ function, drug interactions, and ease of titration.

4.6 Putting the Evidence Together: A Pragmatic Care Framework

Given the heterogeneity of ICH, a pragmatic framework should:

1. *Confirm diagnosis rapidly and quantify burden.* Immediate non-contrast CT establishes haemorrhage location, volume, intraventricular extension, and mass effect. Where available, CT angiography may identify spot signs or secondary causes requiring targeted management.
2. *Stabilise and prevent early expansion.* Initiate titratable antihypertensives with protocolised pathways aiming for SBP ~140 mm Hg for most patients within 6 h, with individualised targets for late presenters, massive bleeds, or high ICP states. If presentation is ultra-early (≤2 h) and logistics permit, consider TXA after risk–benefit discussion; rFVIIa is not recommended routinely.
3. *Reverse coagulopathy efficiently.* Use four-factor PCC and vitamin K for VKA; deploy specific reversal agents for DOACs (andexanet alfa for factor Xa inhibitors; idarucizumab for dabigatran). Avoid platelet transfusions for antiplatelet-associated ICH except in the neurosurgical setting.
4. *Manage IVH decisively.* Insert EVD for obstructive hydrocephalus and ICP control; consider intraventricular alteplase on a case-by-case basis, acknowledging mortality reduction signals without proven functional gains.
5. *Select surgical candidates thoughtfully.* For lobar haemorrhages with mass effect or clinical decline and accessible corridors, MIS may be favoured given emerging data (e.g. Early minimally-invasive removal of intracerebral hemorrhage (ENRICH trial) (ENRICH)). For deep haemorrhages, evidence remains equivocal; craniotomy typically serves as rescue therapy in deterioration. Decompressive craniectomy is a reasonable option for malignant oedema and refractory ICP when survival with disability aligns with the patient's goals. Cerebellar haemorrhage with mass effect/hydrocephalus warrants urgent evacuation.
6. *Deliver meticulous, supportive care.* Implement care bundles addressing BP variability, glucose, temperature, VTE prophylaxis, airway/ventilation, nutrition, early mobilisation, swallow assessment, and delirium prevention. Standardise protocols while preserving clinician judgement.

7. *Plan for secondary prevention and recovery.* Identify and manage underlying causes (e.g. hypertension, cerebral amyloid angiopathy, cavernous malformations), rehabilitative needs, and psychosocial support. Antithrombotic resumption requires individualised, documented decisions.

4.7 Areas of Active Debate and Future Directions

Despite progress, several domains warrant further investigation:

- *Optimal BP Trajectory:* Beyond a static target, the ideal *trajectory*—rate of decline, avoidance of variability, and interaction with autoregulation—likely influences outcomes. Continuous non-invasive monitoring and adaptive target algorithms may refine care.
- *Hyperacute Haemostatic Windows:* Ultra-early deployment of TXA (or other agents) within the first 60–120 min may produce larger effects than seen in trials with later enrolment. Imaging biomarkers (e.g. spot sign, blend sign) and plasma markers could help identify the subgroup most likely to benefit.
- *Precision Reversal Strategies:* Comparative effectiveness studies for fixed-dose versus weight/INR-based PCC regimens, and cost-effectiveness within resource-constrained settings, remain priorities [13].
- *Surgical Selection and Technique:* The heterogeneity in MIS trials (timing, approach, clot volume thresholds, surgeon experience) complicates generalisation. Future studies should stratify by location (lobar vs deep), incorporate standardised technical competency benchmarks, and measure perioperative physiological control.
- *IVH Thrombolysis and Functional Recovery:* While CLEAR III offers encouraging safety and mortality insights, defining which anatomical patterns and clot burdens translate to functional gains with lytic irrigation remains an unmet need.
- *Care Bundles and Implementation Science:* INTERACT3 underscores that protocolised, scalable interventions can move population outcomes [30]. The challenge is dissemination and fidelity across diverse health systems, particularly in low- and middle-income countries (LMICs), where resource variability is pronounced.

4.8 Conclusion

Intracerebral haemorrhage management has evolved from a series of isolated decisions into an integrated, time-sensitive care pathway. The evidence to date suggests:

- Early, controlled BP reduction to ~140 mm Hg is safe and may modestly enhance functional outcomes when implemented rapidly and smoothly; ultra-intensive reduction below ~130 mm Hg is not supported and may be harmful in selected patients [4–6].

- Antifibrinolytic (TXA) and procoagulant (rFVIIa) therapies reduce haematoma growth but have not demonstrated consistent functional benefit in unselected populations; any role is likely within ultra-early windows and carefully defined subgroups [7, 8–11].
- Reversal of anticoagulation should be prompt, specific, and protocolised—PCC plus vitamin K for warfarin; andexanet alfa for factor Xa inhibitors; idarucizumab for dabigatran; platelet transfusion generally avoided except for urgent neurosurgery [12–17].
- IVH frequently necessitates EVD; intraventricular thrombolysis with alteplase appears safe and may reduce mortality, though functional improvement has not been established [18].
- Surgery remains individualised: open craniotomy offers life-saving decompression without guaranteed functional gains; MIS is safe and likely beneficial in lobar haemorrhage under the right conditions; decompressive craniectomy can reduce mortality in malignant courses at the cost of substantial disability [19–25].
- Protocolised supportive care—BP, glucose, temperature control; early VTE prophylaxis; judicious antithrombotic resumption; seizure detection and treatment—shapes outcomes appreciably, with bundle approaches such as those tested in INTERACT3 delivering broad benefits [26, 27–30].

References

1. GBD 2019 Stroke Collaborators. Global, regional, and national burden of stroke and its risk factors, 1990–2019: a systematic analysis for the global burden of disease study 2019. Lancet Neurol. 2021;20:795–820.
2. Béjot Y, Cordonnier C, Durier J, Aboa-Eboulé C, Rouaud O, Giroud M. Intracerebral haemorrhage profiles are changing: results from the Dijon population-based study. Brain. 2013;136:658–64.
3. Hanley DF, Lane K, McBee N, Ziai W, Tuhrim S, Lees KR, Dawson J, Gandhi D, Ullman N, Mould WA, Mayo SW, Mendelow AD, et al. Thrombolytic removal of intraventricular haemorrhage in treatment of severe stroke: results of the randomised, multicentre, multiregion, placebo-controlled CLEAR III trial. Lancet. 2017;389:603–11. https://doi.org/10.1016/S0140-6736(16)32410-2.
4. Anderson CS, Heeley E, Huang Y, et al. Rapid blood-pressure lowering in patients with acute intracerebral hemorrhage. N Engl J Med. 2013;368:2355–65.
5. Palesch YY, Barsan WG, et al. Intensive blood- pressure lowering in patients with acute cerebral hemorrhage. N Engl J Med. 2016;375:1033–43.
6. Qureshi AI, Palesch YY, Barsan WG, Hanley DF, Hsu CY, Martin RL, et al. Intensive blood-pressure lowering in patients with acute cerebral Hemorrhage. N Engl J Med. 2016;375:1033–43.
7. Sprigg N, Flaherty K, Appleton JP, Al-Shahi Salman R, Bereczki D, Beridze M, Christensen H, Ciccone A, Collins R, Czlonkowska A, et al. TICH- 2 investigators. Tranexamic acid for hyperacute primary IntraCerebral haemorrhage (TICH-2): an international randomised, placebo-controlled, phase 3 superiority trial. Lancet. 2018;391:2107–15. https://doi.org/10.1016/S0140-6736(18)31033-X.
8. Meretoja A, Yassi N, Wu TY, Churilov L, Sibolt G, Jeng JS, Kleinig T, Spratt NJ, Thijs V, Wijeratne T, et al. Tranexamic acid in patients with intracerebral haemorrhage (STOP-AUST): a multicentre, randomised, placebo-controlled, phase 2 trial. Lancet Neurol. 2020;19:980–7. https://doi.org/10.1016/S1474-4422(20)30369-0.

9. Mayer SA, Brun NC, Begtrup K, Broderick J, Davis S, Diringer MN, et al. Efficacy and safety of recombinant activated factor VII for acute intracerebral hemorrhage. N Engl J Med. 2008;358:2127–37. https://doi.org/10.1056/nejmoa0707534.
10. Mayer SA, Davis SM, Skolnick BE, Brun NC, Begtrup K, Broderick JP, et al. Can a subset of intracerebral hemorrhage patients benefit from hemostatic therapy with recombinant activated factor VII? Stroke. 2009;40:833–40. https://doi.org/10.1161/strokeaha.108.524470.
11. Gladstone DJ, Aviv RI, Demchuk AM, Hill MD, Thorpe KE, Khoury JC, Sucharew HJ, Al-Ajlan F, Butcher K, Dowlatshahi D, et al. SPOTLIGHT and STOP-IT investigators and coordinators. Effect of recombinant activated coagulation factor VII on hemorrhage expansion among patients with spot sign-positive acute intracerebral hemorrhage: the SPOTLIGHT and STOP-IT randomized clinical trials. JAMA Neurol. 2019;76:1493–501. https://doi.org/10.1001/jamaneurol.2019.2636.
12. Greenberg SM, Ziai WC, Cordonnier C, Dowlatshahi D, Francis B, Goldstein JN, Hemphill JC 3rd, Johnson R, Keigher KM, Mack WJ, Mocco J, Newton EJ, Ruff IM, Sansing LH, Schulman S, Selim MH, Sheth KN, Sprigg N, Sunnerhagen KS. Guideline for the management of patients with spontaneous intracerebral hemorrhage: a guideline from the American Heart Association/American Stroke Association. Stroke. 2022;53(7):e282–361. https://doi.org/10.1161/STR.0000000000000407.
13. Tomaselli GF, Mahaffey KW, Cuker A, Dobesh PP, Doherty JU, Eikelboom JW, Florido R, Hucker W, Mehran R, Messé SR, et al. 2017 ACC expert consensus decision pathway on management of bleeding in patients on oral anticoagulants: a report of the American College of Cardiology Task Force on expert consensus decision pathways. J Am Coll Cardiol. 2017;70:3042–67. https://doi.org/10.1016/j.jacc.2017.09.1085.
14. Dentali F, Ageno W, Crowther M. Treatment of coumarin-associated coagu- lopathy: a systematic review and proposed treatment algorithms. J Thromb Haemost. 2006;4:1853–63. https://doi.org/10.1111/j.1538-7836.2006.01986.x.
15. Connolly SJ, Sharma MA, Cohen AT, et al. Andexanet for factor Xa inhibitor-associated acute intracerebral hemorrhage. N Engl J Med. 2024;390:1745–55.
16. Pollack CV Jr, Reilly PA, van Ryn J, Eikelboom JW, Glund S, Bernstein RA, et al. Idarucizumab for dabigatran reversal – full cohort analysis. N Engl J Med. 2017;377:431–41.
17. Baharoglu MI, Cordonnier C, Al-Shahi Salman R, de Gans K, Koopman MM, Brand A, Majoie CB, Beenen LF, Marquering HA, Vermeulen M, et al. Platelet transfusion versus standard care after acute stroke due to spontaneous cerebral haemorrhage associated with anti- platelet therapy (PATCH): a randomised, open-label, phase 3 trial. Lancet. 2016;387:2605–13. https://doi.org/10.1016/S0140-6736(16)30392-0.
18. Greenberg SM, Ziai WC, Cordonnier C, et al. Guideline for the management of patients with spontaneous intracerebral hemorrhage: a guideline from the American Heart Association/American Stroke Association. Stroke. 2022;2022(53):e282–361.
19. Mendelow AD, Gregson BA, Rowan EN, Murray GD, Gholkar A, Mitchell PM. Early surgery versus initial conservative treatment in patients with spontaneous supratentorial lobar intracerebral hae- matomas (STICH II): a randomised trial. Lancet. 2013;382:397–408. https://doi.org/10.1016/S0140-6736(13)60986-1.
20. Li M, Mu F, Su D, Han Q, Guo Z, Chen T. Different surgical interventions for patients with spontaneous supratentorial intracranial hemorrhage: a network meta-analysis. Clin Neurol Neurosurg. 2020;188:105617. https://doi.org/10.1016/j.clineuro.2019.105617.
21. Sondag L, Schreuder FHBM, Boogaarts HD, Rovers MM, Vandertop WP, Dammers R, Klijn CJM. Neurosurgical intervention for supratentorial intrace- rebral hemorrhage. Ann Neurol. 2020;88:239–50. https://doi.org/10.1002/ana.25732.
22. Hanley DF, Thompson RE, Rosenblum M, et al. Efficacy and safety of minimally invasive surgery with thrombolysis in intracerebral haemorrhage evacuation (MISTIE III): a randomised, controlled, open-label, blinded endpoint phase 3 trial. Lancet. 2019;393:1021–32.
23. Pradilla G, Ratcliff JJ, Hall AJ, et al. Trial of early minimally invasive removal of intracerebral hemorrhage. N Engl J Med. 2024;390:1277–89.

24. Beck J, Fung C, Strbian D, et al. Decompressive craniectomy plus best medical treatment versus best medical treatment alone for spontaneous severe deep supratentorial intracerebral haemorrhage: a randomised controlled clinical trial. Lancet. 2024; https://doi.org/10.1016/S0140-6736(24)00702-5.
25. Singh SD, Brouwers HB, Senff JR, Pasi M, Goldstein J, Viswanathan A, Klijn CJM, Rinkel GJE. Haematoma evacuation in cerebellar intracerebral haemorrhage: systematic review. J Neurol Neurosurg Psychiatry. 2020;91:82–7. https://doi.org/10.1136/jnnp-2019-321461.
26. Faust AC, Finch CK, Hurdle AC, et al. Early versus delayed initiation of pharmacological venous thromboembolism prophylaxis after an intracranial haemorrhage. Neurologist. 2017;22:166–70.
27. Schreuder FHBM, et al. Apixaban versus no anticoagulation after anticoagulation-associated intracerebral haemorrhage in patients with atrial fibrillation in The Netherlands (APACHE-AF): a randomised, open-label, phase 2 trial. Lancet Neurol. 2021;20(11):907–16. https://doi.org/10.1016/S1474-4422(21)00298-2.
28. Honig A, Michael S, Eliahou R, Leker RR. Central fever in patients with spontaneous intracerebral hemorrhage: predicting factors and impact on outcome. BMC Neurol. 2015;15:6.
29. Xu S, Zhang Q, Li C. Paroxysmal sympathetic hyperactivity after acquired brain injury: an integrative review of diagnostic and management challenges. Neurol Ther. 2024;13:11–20. https://doi.org/10.1007/s40120-023-00561-x.
30. Ma L, Hu X, Song L, et al. The third intensive care bundle with blood pressure reduction in acute cerebral haemorrhage trial (INTERACT3): an international, stepped wedge cluster randomised controlled trial. Lancet. 2023;402:27–40.

Traumatic Spinal Cord Injury

5

Prachi Sharma and Suparna Bharadwaj

Abstract

The treatment of traumatic spinal cord injury (SCI) remains challenging due to its complex pathophysiology and lasting disabilities, including socioeconomic burdens. While current strategies focus on timely surgical interventions and haemodynamic management, recent research in SCI is advancing rapidly, investigating neuroprotective methods and novel biologics. This chapter examines advancements in SCI management, emphasising the "Time is Spine" paradigm for timely surgical decompression. We also address the debated role of steroids, noting their risks and limited benefits. Emerging pharmacological and non-pharmacological neuroprotective strategies, such as therapeutic hypothermia, are discussed. The chapter also sheds light on stem cell therapies and neuromodulation techniques as promising upcoming strategies for promoting neuroregeneration and recovery. Long-term rehabilitation, requiring a multidisciplinary approach, is essential to optimise outcomes, and various strategies proven to be beneficial in SCI have also been highlighted.

Overall, translating proposed innovative management strategies into clinical practice requires further research, robust trials, and collaboration. However, these discoveries are expected to revolutionise SCI management in the next decade if proven beneficial.

P. Sharma
Max Super Speciality Hospital, New Delhi, Delhi, India

S. Bharadwaj (✉)
National Institute of Mental Health and Neurosciences, Bengaluru, Karnataka, India

P. U. Bidkar, M. Krishnakumar (eds.), *Controversies in Neurocritical Care*,
https://doi.org/10.1007/978-981-95-4419-6_5

Keywords

Spinal cord injury · Neuroprotection · Time is spine · Neurorehabilitation Neuromodulation

5.1 Introduction

Significant progress has been made in understanding and treating traumatic spinal cord injury (SCI), yet it continues to cause profound and lasting disabilities. In India, SCI predominantly affects young, healthy adults, leading to substantial financial, psychological, and vocational challenges [1]. The current clinical approaches to treating SCI encompass pharmacological and surgical interventions in the acute phase and rehabilitation focused on restoring function and minimising complications in the subacute and chronic phases. Comprehensive data on long-term functional outcomes, injury severity, and neurological impact are scarce. However, advances in understanding the underlying pathophysiological mechanisms highlight the need for prompt surgical and medical interventions during the critical phase when secondary injury processes occur. The concept of "Time is Spine" has emerged recently as a new paradigm for SCI management [2, 3]. In this chapter, we explore crucial neurological interventions supported by evidence, emerging neuroprotective strategies, neurorehabilitation protocols, neuroregenerative techniques, and controversies in the management of SCI.

5.2 Pathophysiological Mechanisms and the Rationale for Management

The SCI involves interconnected events that often occur simultaneously, complicating treatment [4]. These events lead to motor and sensory dysfunctions due to a cascade of primary and secondary damage [5]. This complexity has hindered the success of many treatment strategies. Therapeutic approaches are broadly categorised into neuroprotective, neuroregenerative, and immune-modulating pathways. Therefore, understanding these pathophysiological mechanisms is critical before understanding the treatment strategies. Figure 5.1 represents the key mechanisms and events in each phase after SCI, providing an overview of the pathophysiology at play.

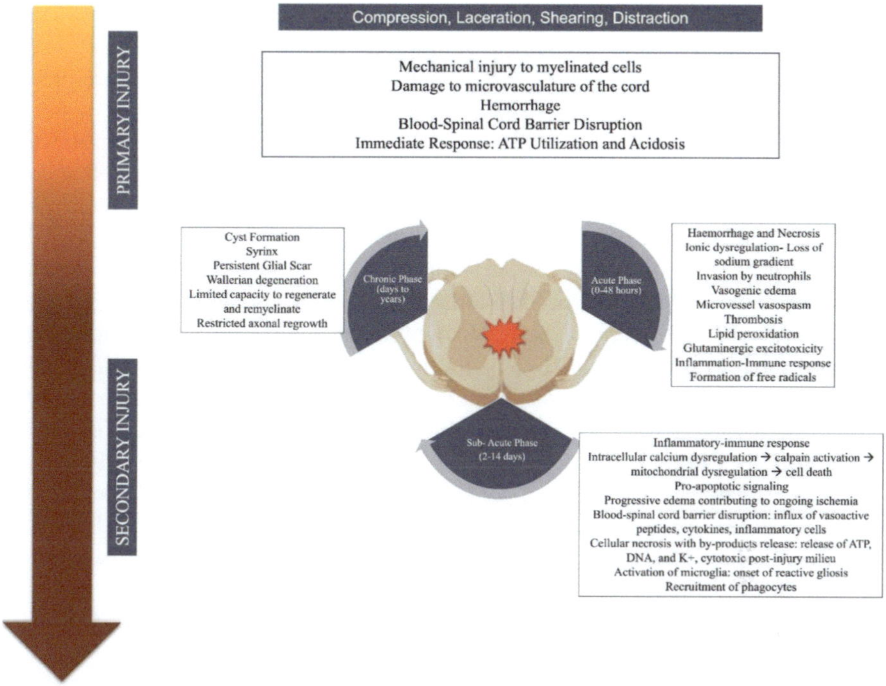

Fig. 5.1 Pathophysiological mechanisms in spinal cord injury, highlighting primary and secondary injuries, and the key mechanisms at play in different phases adenosine tri-phosphate (ATP); potassium (K+); deoxyribonucleic acid (DNA)

5.3 Controversies in Acute Management

Several controversies exist in the management of acute SCI. The following are the most discussed dilemmas.

5.3.1 Early Versus Delayed Surgical Interventions

Traditionally, the acute management of SCI focused on closed reduction and prolonged external immobilisation with minimal emphasis on acute surgical care [6]. However, in recent decades, early surgical intervention has been prioritised, as preclinical evidence indicates that rapid alleviation of spinal cord compression can reduce secondary injury and enhance outcomes [7, 8]. As a result, numerous articles examining the effects of early surgery on patient outcomes have been published in recent years [2, 6, 9] with various time thresholds used to define "early" versus "late" surgical decompression. However, the 24-hour threshold forms the basis for most recent research. A recent phrase in literature is "Time is Spine", which underscores the importance of timely surgical intervention in improving outcomes for patients with SCI.

The Surgical Timing in Acute Spinal Cord Injury Study (STASCIS) trial, was a multicentre, international prospective cohort study, which demonstrated that early decompressive surgery (<24 hours post-injury) for acute cervical SCI significantly improved neurological outcomes, with patients showing a greater likelihood of at least a 2-grade improvement on the American spinal injury association (ASIA) impairment scale (AIS) compared to those who underwent late surgery (≥24 hours post-injury) [10]. More evidence now supports early surgical intervention within 24 hours of injury, as it is linked to better prognosis and functional outcomes without increasing postoperative complications or surgical risks like pressure ulcers, urinary tract infections (UTI), and pneumonia [11, 12]. A recent study has shown results similar to the STASCIS trial, where patients who underwent early surgery had a six-fold higher likelihood of achieving at least a 2-grade improvement in AIS compared to those who had delayed surgery [13]. Early intervention has also shown greater sensorimotor recovery at 1-year follow-up, with significant improvements in not just the motor scores but also pinprick sensation and light touch, while delaying decompression beyond 24–36 hours after injury resulted in a sharp decline in motor recovery [3, 14].

The debate is now shifting from early vs. late to early vs. ultra-early surgery, with some studies indicating that surgery within 8 hours leads to better outcomes than the 8–24-hour window [15]; while others find no significant differences in outcome between interventions at 4 hours vs. 4–24 hours [16]. Overall, meta-analyses have suggested better outcomes with intervention within 8 hours [17].

Additionally, the level and grade of injuries are important when considering effects of timing of surgical decompression on outcomes as ultra-early surgery seems more effective for cervical spine injuries compared to thoracolumbar injuries, and early intervention within the first 12 hours significantly improves outcomes for AIS grade A injuries, while for AIS B to D injuries, delaying decompression up to 24 hours does not seem to affect neurological recovery [18].

In fact, the more recently published SCI-POEM study, which aimed to determine if early (within 12 hours) surgical decompression leads to better recovery a year after injury compared to late (between 12 hours and 14 days) decompression in patients with acute SCI, found no statistically significant or clinically meaningful improvement with early surgery after adjusting for various factors [19]. The non-significant study results may have been influenced by the greater severity as measured by the AIS grades in those treated with early surgery and a greater loss to follow-up in the late surgery group.

Badhiwala et al.'s analysis of data from multiple prospective multicentre studies also indicated that it is the initial 24–36 hours post-injury which is the critical period for performing decompressive surgery to attain optimal neurological outcome in patients with acute SCI [14]. Thus, controversy persists regarding the definition of early decompression and its benefits across different types and levels of SCI. Multiple systematic reviews have demonstrated that, although early surgery is proven to enhance neurological recovery in cervical SCI patients, the evidence for its effectiveness in other SCI populations remains inconsistent [18].

While current guidelines advise spinal decompression in the first 24 hours after SCI, irrespective of level of injury or severity [20], the recommendation may need adjustment when considering specific injury characteristics.

Another important aspect of surgical management to consider besides timing is the adequacy of spinal cord decompression, as the degree of decompression significantly impacts AIS grade conversion [21]. As spinal cord swelling can compromise cerebrospinal fluid (CSF) between the spinal cord and dura, it may lead to increased intrathecal pressure (ITP). Studies have shown that laminectomy combined with duraplasty, compared to laminectomy alone, improves spinal cord perfusion pressure (SCPP) by reducing ITP and secondary ischaemic damage [22].

Summary: Early surgical intervention within 24 hours significantly improves neurological outcomes (STASCIS trial), with recent evidence showing even better results within 8 hours. The SCI-POEM study found no significant difference between early (≤12 hours) and later (12 hours to 14 days) decompression, possibly due to study limitations. Despite some patients arriving at the hospital beyond the initial 24-hour window, we still prioritise early surgery whenever feasible. However, in clinical practice, stabilising patients' haemodynamics due to neurogenic shock sometimes leads to delays. Additionally, complete decompression is crucial for reducing secondary ischaemic damage. Bottom line is: Early action saves spinal function—time is spine!

5.3.2 Steroids in SCI

Steroids, particularly methylprednisolone sodium succinate (MPSS), have been widely researched in traumatic SCI. Animal studies have attributed neuroprotection to mechanisms such as inhibition of calcium influx and lipid peroxidation, with enhanced vascular perfusion [23]. The neuroinflammatory response following SCI has been identified as a significant feature of the secondary injury cascade, capable of both exacerbating damage and facilitating beneficial processes like wound healing and repair. Steroids exert their effects by suppressing this response and inhibiting lipid peroxidation of neuronal cell membranes [24].

However, the administration of steroids in SCI management remains controversial. The landmark National Acute Spinal Cord Injury Studies (NASCIS) played a pivotal role in shaping clinical practice [24–26], exploring the timing and duration of MPSS administration. NASCIS-II revealed improved motor and sensory function when steroids were administered within 8 hours of injury [24], but with increased risk of complications. Moreover, basic errors in subgroup analyses were reported in both NASCIS-II and III trials [27]. Results from NASCIS-III indicated that for patients who received MPSS therapy within 3 hours of injury, a 24-hour treatment duration was sufficient. But if treatment started between 3- and 8-hours post-injury, extending MPSS therapy to 48 hours was linked to better neurological outcomes, albeit with a higher risk of infections, including pneumonia and sepsis [26]. A Cochrane review indicated a slight improvement in AIS motor score with steroids administered within 8 hours [28]. However, a meta-analysis failed to show the effectiveness of high-dose steroids in SCI patients treated within 8 hours of injury [29]. A subsequent meta-analysis published in 2020 reinforced these findings [30]. Currently, there is inadequate scientific evidence to endorse the use of steroids as a neuroprotective therapy after SCI. In fact, several randomised controlled trials (RCT) have indicated not only a lack of benefit but also an increase in overall mortality and complications.

The recommendations on methylprednisolone vary across different guidelines. Evidence-based guidelines typically discourage its use, while consensus-based guidelines often support it [31]. Recent guidelines have shifted away from routine high-dose corticosteroid therapy for SCI patients due to efficacy and safety concerns [32]. AOSpine cautiously recommends a 24-hour MPSS infusion within 8 hours of injury but acknowledges weak evidence [33]. The World Society of Emergency Surgery (WSES) and the European Association of Neurosurgical Societies (EANS) recommend against high-dose corticosteroids in SCI patients with polytrauma [34]. The ASAP Study showed low usage of corticosteroids among respondents [35], and Hejrati et al. found a significant decline in steroid use from 2008 to 2018, correlating with opposing literature and guidelines [36], and a survey has shown that the primary rationale for using steroids in this scenario may stem as much from the belief in the drug's efficacy as from the fear of medical litigation [37].

Summary: There is no solid proof that methylprednisolone is effective for neurological protection in the acute phase of SCI. The NASCIS studies have significant flaws. Steroid use has been linked with a higher risk of sepsis. In clinical practice, while steroids might be considered individually, it is uncommon for the benefits to outweigh the risks. The authors' experience reflects this practice as steroid administration is restricted for patients presenting within 8 hours post-injury, particularly for cervical SCI, in the hope of achieving clinical improvements. Bottom Line: Steroid use is not shown to be beneficial for neurological protection in the acute phase of SCI.

5.3.3 Emerging Neuroprotective Techniques

Given the complex pathophysiology of SCI, a combination of pharmacological interventions and rehabilitation strategies is essential for optimal neuroprotection. Stratifying patients by injury level and personalising treatments are crucial, as different anatomical levels and individual patient characteristics affect treatment efficacy [38].

Multiple pharmacological and non-pharmacological treatments have undergone preclinical and clinical testing, but none have achieved completely satisfactory outcomes, even with combined approaches. Here, we explore some of the more extensively researched treatments.

5.3.3.1 Non-pharmacological Techniques

1. Haemodynamic Management:

   Hemodynamic management has long prioritised maintaining optimal mean arterial pressure (MAP). A 2013 systematic review resulted in a "Level III" recommendation to keep MAP between 85 and 90 mmHg for the first week after injury [39]. However, the neurologic benefits of this specific MAP range are still under debate [40]. Lately, there has been a growing interest in monitoring SCPP, defined as the difference between MAP and either ITP or intraspinal pressure. But currently, there is no agreement on whether SCPP or MAP is more effective for haemodynamic management in acute SCI patients.

   The effect of MAP support on neurological recovery remains uncertain, as two large studies showed mixed results, with Squair et al. finding an association between MAP/SCPP and improved outcomes [41], while Martin et al. found no significant correlation between hypotensive events and motor scores at discharge [42]. MAP augmentation with vasopressors has been shown to produce adverse events such as cardiac arrhythmias and myocardial injury [43]. Similarly, evidence in favour of SCPP-guided management for improved neurological recovery remains inconclusive and of low quality [44], with observational studies suggesting that SCPP targets are more strongly associated with neurological improvement than MAP targets [40]. Amongst the agents used to augment MAP, dopamine has been linked with higher adverse event rates compared to phenylephrine [40]. We did not find studies directly comparing different durations of MAP or SCPP support. Based on the evidence, the latest guidelines recommend maintaining MAP at 75–80 mmHg (not exceeding 90–95 mmHg) for 3–7 days to optimise spinal cord perfusion in acute SCI, with vasopressor or inotrope as per the choice of the attending physician [45].

2. Lumbar Drainage:

   The effect of disrupted autoregulation and increased vascular resistance after SCI results in reduced SCPP due to elevated ITP. Thus, novel interventions like CSF drainage (CSFD) have been tried in attempts to improve cord perfusion. Literature shows mixed results; older studies failed to sufficiently reduce ITP and impact SCPP [46, 47], whereas a recent RCT targeting specific drainage to lower ITP to <10 mmHg demonstrated significant improvement in SCPP and total motor scores over 6 months in the CSFD group without any side effects [48].

3. Therapeutic Hypothermia:

   Hypothermia has been explored for its short-term and prolonged neuroprotective benefits in SCI. It acts through several mechanisms: slowing metabolism, reducing oxygen and glucose consumption, decreasing excitotoxic neurotransmitter release, and minimising free radical formation [49]. Early hypothermia can also inhibit apoptotic and inflammatory pathways, reducing oedema and blood volume at the injury site, thus stabilising the blood-spinal cord barrier.

   Animal studies [50] and some human studies [51] have shown positive outcomes with hypothermia, which can be administered either locally or systemically. Systemic hypothermia is achieved through endovascular heat exchange, administering cold intravenous infusions, or surface cooling. In contrast, local hypothermia involves directly irrigating the extradural or intradural space with cold saline, thereby avoiding systemic side effects. A recent meta-analysis found that 55.8% of patients showed neurological improvement after hypothermia following acute SCI, with no significant difference between local (52.5%) and systemic (70.9%) hypothermia [52]. However, complications such as surgical site infections have been noted, particularly with local hypothermia [53]. Current evidence suggests that modest systemic hypothermia (32–34 °C) may provide neuroprotective benefits without significant morbidity [54], as confirmed by a recent multicentre study showing no increased risk of complications after SCI [55]. The evidence for using hypothermia in severe SCI patients is promising, but there is a need for randomised, multicentre controlled clinical trials to determine if systemic or selective cooling provides clinically significant improvements in acute SCI patients.

4. Hyperbaric Oxygen Therapy (HBOT):

   One of the proposed mechanisms of secondary damage after SCI is ischaemia. HBOT can act by increasing the content of dissolved oxygen and is neuroprotective due to its effects on lowering apoptosis, minimising oxidative stress, reducing inflammation and cord oedema, enhancing angiogenesis, and autophagy [56]. Huang et al. conducted a meta-analysis of all RCTs on HBOT in SCI patients. They found that HBOT significantly improved motor and sensory AIS scores [57]. Most studies used HBOT in a hyperbaric chamber at 1.8–2.0 absolute atmospheres for at least 60 minutes per session [58]. However, there is considerable variability in the timing and duration of HBOT, with no studies directly comparing different treatment protocols. Data indicate that clinical improvements begin within the first 10 days of treatment and can continue to improve for up to 6 months post-surgery [59]. The heterogeneity of these studies currently limits the generalizability of the results.

5.3.3.2 Pharmacological Therapies

Over the years, numerous studies have investigated various treatments for SCI [60–65], and many experimental trials are currently in progress. The primary pharmacological agents that have been the focus of research are included in Table 5.1.

Table 5.2 illustrates the mechanisms, preclinical findings, and clinical trial statuses for various neuroregenerative therapeutic approaches targeting SCI [66–70].

Summary: Maintaining optimal MAP is currently the most crucial neuroprotective strategy for improving the outcome of SCI patients outside of urgent decompression. The latest guidelines recommend keeping MAP at 75–80 mmHg for 3–7 days to optimise spinal cord perfusion, using vasopressors or inotropes as needed, but only augmenting MAP up to 90–95 mmHg. However, in practice, maintaining MAP within the 5 mmHg range of 75–80 and avoiding increases beyond 90–95 is often difficult. The bottom line remains to avoid hypotension. Using evoked potentials in the initial period may help, though it's challenging to implement.

Table 5.1 Pharmacological strategies and the rationale of their use

Drug	Phase of development	Mechanism	Effectiveness
Riluzole	Phase 1 complete [60]; phase 2/3 (RISCIS) terminated [61]	Decreases neuroexcitation, inhibits N-methyl-D-aspartate (NMDA) receptor activation, diminishes microglia activation	Phase 1: Improvements in functional grades in cervical SCI [60]; No reported adverse events in RISCIS. All cervical SCI patient subgroups (AIS grades A, B, and C) treated with riluzole exhibited significant improvement in functional recovery [61]
Minocycline	Phase 2 complete [62]; phase 3 initiated	Increases anti-inflammatory cytokines (IL-10), decreases pro-inflammatory cytokines (NO, TNF-α, IL-1β, IL-6), inhibits microglia activation [63]	Phase 2: 14-point motor score improvement in cervical SCI; no significant effect in thoracic SCI [62]
GM-1 ganglioside	Phase 3 completed [64]	Contributes to neural development, cellular recognition, and neuronal communication	Phase 3: Accelerated motor and bowel/bladder recovery in the first 3 months post-injury; no significant long-term effects [64]
Granulocyte colony-stimulating factor	Phase 3 completed [65]	Stimulates angiogenesis and neurogenesis, reduces inflammation and scar formation	Phase 3: No significant differences in functional improvement at 3 months; trend towards better outcomes at 6 months [65]

RISCIS Riluzole in acute spinal cord injury, *NMDA* N-methyl-D-aspartate, *SCI* spinal cord injury, *AIS* American Spinal Injury Association impairment scale, *IL* interleukins; *NO* nitric oxide, *TNF* tumour necrosis factor

Regarding other neuroprotective strategies, the heterogeneity of SCI and the complexity of its pathophysiology indicate that no single approach is sufficient on its own. Current evidence is of low quality, and while promising, these strategies have a long way to go before transitioning to clinical practice.

5.3.4 Emerging Therapies in SCI

5.3.4.1 Stem-Cell-Based Therapies

After SCI, nerve conduction is disrupted, and neural circuit regeneration is hindered by the inhibitory microenvironment [70]. Thus, progenitor cell transplantation into the injured lesion has been explored for its ability to differentiate into surrogate neurons [31]. Cell transplantation is a novel treatment strategy that leverages the self-renewal and differentiation properties of stem cells in SCI. Cell transplantation

Table 5.2 Clinical Studies of Neuro-regenerative therapies

Therapy	Mechanism	Preclinical findings	Clinical trials
Anti-nogo-A antibody	Neutralises Nogo-A, a major inhibitor of neurite growth in central nervous system (CNS) myelin	Promotes axonal regeneration Improves neurobehavioral recovery [66]	Phase I clinical trial confirmed safety in humans [67]. Ongoing multicentre phase II RCT for acute cervical SCIs
Rho-kinase inhibitor (VX-210)	Inhibits the rho/rho-associated kinase (ROCK) pathway, which affects cytoskeletal dynamics and cell motility	Enhances neuronal regeneration Improves behavioural outcomes in animal models	Phase I/IIa trial showed safety and suggested AIS motor score improvements [68]. Phase IIb/III trial (NCT02669849) ended prematurely due to lack of significant results [69].
Anti-RGMa antibody (Elezanumab)	Neutralises RGMa, which inhibits neurite growth by binding to Neogenin	Promotes neuronal survival Enhances plasticity and corticospinal tract regenerationimproves motor function in rodents and macaques	Double-blind phase II RCT for acute traumatic cervical SCIs and AIS grades A or B ongoing (NCT04295538) [31]

CNS Central nervous system, *RCT* randomised controlled trial, *SCI* spinal cord injury, *AIS* American Spinal Injury Association impairment scale, *RGMa* repulsive guidance molecule A

provides various therapeutic advantages beyond neuroprotection, such as neural relay circuits, tissue replacement, modulating the immune response, and regenerating myelin [71]. The most extensively researched stem cells are mesenchymal (MSCs), neural (NSCs), and haematopoietic (HSCs), detailed in Table 5.3 [72–78].

The numerous therapeutic advantages observed with cell transplantation make it a promising approach for improving outcomes in SCI patients. However, issues such as ethical controversy, cell source availability, immune rejection, timing of intervention, unregulated cell growth, and long-term safety remain barriers to clinical application [79].

5.3.4.2 Neuromodulation

After SCI, the descending motor pathways get disrupted. This loss of supraspinal control makes the spinal neural circuitry below the level of injury inactive, leading to motor deficits. Neuromodulation is a bioengineering technique that uses magnetic or electrical stimulation, pharmacological agents, and optogenetics (modifying light-sensitive transmembrane proteins genetically to control neuron excitability) to target neuronal function [80]. In SCI, neuromodulatory technologies aim to stimulate the spinal motor circuits below the level of injury, with the goal of restoring voluntary motor function. These technologies mainly include stimulation directly at the spinal cord level, the brain, or the use of brain-machine interfaces (which essentially circumvent the damaged areas by capturing signals from the motor cortex and using them to control exoskeletons or prosthetic limbs). They may either directly

Table 5.3 Cell-based therapies in spinal cord injury

Cell type	Benefits	Clinical trials	References
Neural stem cells/neural progenitor cells	Self-renewing differentiation into neurons/ glial cells. Replace damaged tissue. Axon regeneration Functional restoration	Phase I trial of NSI-566 showed safety and potential neurological improvements [72]. Long-term safety and sensory improvements in some patients [73]	Curtis et al. [72], Curt et al. [73]
Mesenchymal stem cells	Ethical acceptability Diverse tissue sources Paracrine activity Trophic support Modulate immune response Promote neuroprotection and fibre regeneration	Stem cell therapy improved bladder sensation, spasticity, and posture control in SCI patients, with 46% showing sustained functional improvement, particularly in thoracic cases with shorter injuries, and varied outcomes based on injury timing and lesion size [74, 75].	El-Kheir et al. [74], Saini et al. [75]
Schwann cells	Reduce tissue injury Enhance neuroprotection Maintain axonal plasticity Acquired from patient's own nerve (reducing rejection risk)	Phase I trials demonstrated safety and some functional improvements in subacute and chronic SCI patients [76].	Anderson et al. [76]
Induced pluripotent stem cells	Avoid ethical issues. Avoid immune rejection. Can be re-programmed to neural stem cells/ neural progenitor cells	Preclinical: Facilitated axon growth and neural circuit reconstruction in rodent models. Potential to promote tumorigenesis is a concern with undifferentiated cells [77, 78].	Lu et al. [77], Ji et al. [78]

stimulate the free endings of the corticospinal tract (cortical stimulation), stimulate the formation of circuits via action on the spared proprio-spinal neurons (spinal cord stimulation), or act by recruiting new afferents. The main technologies utilised in SCI are shown in Table 5.4 [81–92]. Some techniques are also discussed in the rehabilitation section.

Take-Home Points: Stem cell therapies, including mesenchymal, neural, and haematopoietic stem cells, hold exciting potential for SCI treatment by promoting tissue replacement and neuroprotection. However, their clinical application on a large scale faces significant hurdles like ethical concerns, immune rejection, and

Table 5.4 Mechanism of action and a summary of the evidence supporting the use of neuromodulation in the context of spinal cord injury treatment

Therapy	Mechanism	Clinical evidence	References
Brain stimulation techniques			
Transcranial direct current stimulation	Improves the cortical excitability via increasing the discharge rate of active neurons (hyperpolarisation of dendrites and depolarisation of cell body)	Improved grasp function [81], sensory perception [82], and significant improvement in walking [83]	Cortes et al. [81], Murray et al. [82], Simis et al. [83]
Transcranial magnetic stimulation	Repeated application of magnetic pulses over cortical sites to modulate cortical excitability directly affects neurons in the corticospinal tract and activates motor pathways	Improve slower extremity motor scores, reduces spasticity, and enhances gait in patients with motor incomplete SCI [84, 85]	Benito et al. [84], Kumru et al. [85]
Deep brain stimulation	Stimulates brainstem neurons that still have connections to lumbar motor centres	DBS of the ventralis posterior lateralis (VPL) nucleus of the thalamus can reduce phantom sensations and pain after SCI [86], clinical improvement in the gait of patients with incomplete SCI [87].	Katayama et al. [86], Mahlknecht et al. [87].
Spinal cord stimulation techniques			
Transcutaneous spinal cord stimulation	Non-invasive approach of placing electrodes transcutaneously to stimulate the dorsal roots and activate the motor circuits	Clinically significant improvement in upper limb motor scores [88] with mean hand strength improving by >300% [89]	Inanici et al. [88], Freyvert et al. [89]
Epidural electrical stimulation	Electrodes are surgically placed on the dorsal surface of the cord	Requires frequent rehabilitation training for optimal results. Patients have gained independent standing strength [90], trunk stability, improved sensory function in upper limb amputees [91], and facilitated independent walking through task-specific training [92]	Angeli et al. [90], Chandrasekaran et al. [91], Gill et al. [92]

uncontrolled cell proliferation. Despite promising preclinical data and some trials hinting at neurological improvements, the overall quality of evidence remains limited due to methodological flaws, small participant numbers, and short follow-up periods. More extensive trials are necessary to translate preclinical success into clinical reality. As researchers continue to explore and refine these therapies, we can hope for breakthroughs that may transform SCI treatment in the future.

Neuromodulation techniques aim to stimulate spinal circuits and restore voluntary motor function using electrical or magnetic stimulation. Initial studies show promise in improving motor scores and reducing spasticity, but the evidence is still emerging. Further clinical trials are needed to confirm their effectiveness and determine optimal protocols for different types of SCI. Extensive and sustained clinical use of these devices is currently restricted due to factors like limited availability, high cost, and the specialised expertise needed to operate these devices.

Bottom line is that both stem cell therapy and neuromodulation for the management of acute SCI are under investigation.

5.3.5 Other Noteworthy Controversies in SCI Management

5.3.5.1 Airway Management

The goal of airway management in cervical SCI is to prevent further aggravation and secondary damage. Maintaining spinal immobilisation is more important than the specific airway management technique used, although it can complicate securing the airway.

For effective neck immobilisation, using a combination of a hardboard, collar, with sandbags, and tape is the ideal technique [93]. This setup limits neck movement to 5% but makes laryngoscopy difficult. Hard Philadelphia collars work better than soft collars but are less efficacious in limiting neck movement than the hardboard-collar combination [94]. Manual-inline stabilisation (MILS) stabilises the head and torso but can still transmit forces to the mid-cervical spine and worsens the view during intubation [95]. There is limited evidence that MILS reduces the risk of further spinal injury, and it should be removed if intubation is challenging [96]. Similarly, there is limited evidence to support or oppose the use of cricoid force or external laryngeal manipulation. If difficulty in tracheal intubation is encountered when using cricoid force, it should be promptly removed [96]. Recently, the Difficult Airway Society has issued guidelines for managing airways in cervical SCI [96].

Awake tracheal intubation (ATI) was once the preferred method to minimise spine movement, but videolaryngoscopy has become more popular. A study of 252 patients found only 2.3% had ATI with a flexible bronchoscope, while 50% were intubated with videolaryngoscopy, and no neurological deterioration was reported [97]. Current guidelines indicate there is no strong evidence that ATI is better than techniques under general anaesthesia for preventing secondary spinal injury [96]. Likewise, there is no proof that flexible bronchoscope (FOB)-guided intubation is superior to other methods. Videolaryngoscopy is now recommended as the primary technique for patients with suspected or confirmed cervical SCI, with the decision to intubate awake or with FOB being left to the clinician's discretion, being made on a case-by-case basis [96]. The main advantage of FOB is that it permits neurological assessments before and after the procedure to verify that the spinal cord remains undamaged [98].

5.3.5.2 Controversies in Paediatric Spinal Traumatic Spinal Cord Injury

Utilising conservative management approaches is generally favoured for paediatric patients, considering that their expected growth and anatomical development can be hindered by surgical fusion. However, early decompression surgery can be a viable treatment for children with spinal cord hematoma, ongoing compression leading to elevated intraspinal pressure, or progressively worsening symptoms [99].

The NASCIS trials did not include children under 13 years old [100]. Nonetheless, some experts recommend considering steroids within the first 8 hours post-injury due to the potentially higher neurological recovery rates in children compared to adults [99].

For spinal cord injury without radiographic abnormality (SCIWORA), external immobilisation for 12 weeks is recommended, despite some authors reporting no significant difference in outcomes with bracing [101]. No RCTs currently exist to establish the advantage of one management strategy over another for SCIWORA. The universally accepted nonsurgical approach involves immobilising the spine until tenderness resolves, neurological exams are normal, and an MRI shows no instability. All SCIWORA patients should avoid physical activities that could risk re-injury for about 6 months.

Currently, there is a lack of sufficient data to establish specific blood pressure cut-off points for children. It is recommended to maintain blood pressure within age-appropriate ranges [100]. Finally, a systematic review found no evidence to support neuroprotective methods such as hypothermia for paediatric patients [102].

5.4 Long-Term Rehabilitation Protocols in SCI

SCI can result in severe and long-lasting consequences, including loss of sensory function, paralysis, and limited functional mobility. It requires a comprehensive rehabilitation strategy managed by a multidisciplinary team to minimise complications, enhance functionality, and promote maximum independence. Various needs, including physical, metabolic and psychological needs, need to be taken care of. The major goals during the rehabilitation phase are depicted in Fig. 5.2.

5.4.1 Physical Rehabilitation

The techniques and endpoint are decided based on injury severity and the level of injury. These include not only interventions for spasticity and locomotion training but also for respiratory muscle strength training. Rehabilitation should begin in the acute and subacute phase post-injury, typically over a 6–12-week period [103]. The focus during this time should be on preventing complications.

(a) Passive Range of Motion Exercises: Physical therapy is a cornerstone of rehabilitation, employing techniques such as strengthening and passive range of

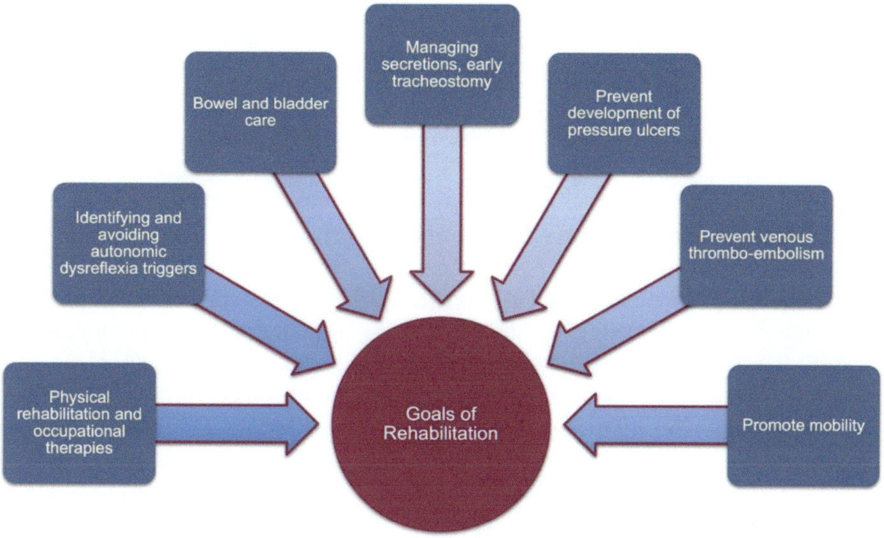

Fig. 5.2 Goals of rehabilitation after spinal cord injury

motion exercises. These have been associated with contracture prevention, promotion of nerve remodelling, and functional improvement via activation of the motor cortex [104]. These exercises are essential for improving muscle strength, joint flexibility, and overall functional capacity. For patients with complete injuries, positioning with sandbags, pillows, or orthotics is essential [105]. Aggressive attempts at mobilisation, initiated early after SCI, are a fundamental principle in the rehabilitation of these patients. Body Weight–Supported Treadmill Training (BWSTT) includes an overhead harness providing partial body weight support, and a moving treadmill belt to assist with leg movements [106]. Systematic reviews provide Level III evidence supporting the effectiveness of BWSTT in improving functional activity in individuals with subacute and chronic SCI.

(b) Functional Electrical Stimulation (FES): FES employs electrical pulses to activate motor neurons or directly stimulate denervated muscle fibres, causing them to contract during specific activities [107]. The objective is to enhance functional recovery by promoting neuroplasticity through the consistent and repeated stimulation of nerves and muscles [108].

FES has been used in addition to other treatment modalities to enhance sensory feedback, reduce atrophy, prevent pressure ulcers, improve trunk stability, and promote cardio-respiratory health. It is not advisable in patients with active thrombosis, seizure disorders and an implanted electrical device.

(c) Epidural spinal cord stimulation aims to activate various central circuits via rhythmic currents. This has been utilised not only in improving mobility but also for improving bladder and bowel control and modulating refractory neuropathic pain after SCI [109]. Krucoff et al. have demonstrated the utility of epidural stimulation at T12-L1 by showing improved motor function in a patient with a complete L1 SCI [110]. A new oscillating field stimulator has demonstrated safety and efficacy in a phase I trial [111].

(d) External motorised orthotic devices or exoskeletons have also been utilised, and a meta-analysis has highlighted improvement in ambulation with their use [112].

5.4.2 Other Components of Rehabilitation

1. Managing spasticity after SCI involves a combination of conservative, pharmacological, and advanced therapeutic approaches. Initially, removing noxious stimuli and using a range of motion exercises, massage, and stretching can help reduce spasticity [113]. Temperature-based therapies like cryotherapy and thermotherapy provide short-term relief, while transcutaneous electrical neuromuscular stimulation (TENS) has shown similar efficacy to oral baclofen [114]. FES and robotic training are also effective in reducing spasticity [115]. Pharmacological treatments include gamma-aminobutyric acid (GABA) agonists such as baclofen and diazepam, alpha-2 adrenergic agonists such as tizanidine, and calcium antagonists like dantrolene [116]. Intrathecal baclofen offers continuous, targeted delivery for severe cases. Local treatments such as botulinum toxin injections and phenol neurolysis provide focal spasticity relief [116]. Emerging non-pharmacological methods like transcranial magnetic stimulation (TMS) and extracorporeal shock wave therapy are also promising in managing spasticity [84, 116].
2. Cardiopulmonary Strength: Aggressive control of secretions is paramount with the use of percussion, assisted coughing, suctioning and vibration techniques to reduce atelectasis and subsequent pneumonia. Respiratory muscle training, early mobilisation, postural changes and breathing exercises are recommended to enhance lung capacity.

   It is estimated that cardiovascular diseases affect 60–70% of individuals with SCI, making them the leading cause of death [117]. Engaging in body-weight–supported training, performing upper limb exercises with moderate to strenuous intensity 3 days a week for at least 6 weeks, and using FES 3 days a week for a minimum of 2 months are suggested strategies to improve cardiovascular health.

   Orthostatic hypotension can be managed with a tilt table, gradually increasing the angle to adapt to sitting and standing [103]. Pharmacological treatment options for autonomic dysreflexia include calcium channel blockers, nitrates, prazosin, and botulinum toxin for refractory cases, in addition to eliminating triggers [118].

   The need for venous thromboembolism (VTE) prophylaxis is also essential. Evidence-based guidelines recommend starting mechanical thromboprophylaxis with intermittent pneumatic compression devices, optionally combined with graduated compression stockings, as soon as possible after acute SCI. Since most VTE events occur within the first 8 weeks following SCI, the Spinal Cord Consortium advises at least 8 weeks of pharmacologic prophylaxis after acute SCI [119].

3. Bladder and Bowel Management: High-cervical injury in SCI patients above T10 leads to impaired oesophageal sphincter control, increased gastro-oesophageal reflux, delayed gastric emptying, and higher gallbladder disease rates [120]. Complete lower cord injuries result in ileus, colonic stasis, and loss of external anal sphincter control. Management includes increasing dietary fluid and fibre to improve stool water content and transit time, using stool softeners, employing bulk-forming laxatives like psyllium or methylcellulose to stimulate peristalsis, and incorporating suppositories, enemas, and rectal stimulation for bowel regularity in complete SCI cases.

   SCI patients often experience functional conus and detrusor-sphincter dyssynergia, leading to involuntary bladder contractions and reduced bladder awareness. Urinary retention is common, increasing the risk of UTIs, kidney stones, hydronephrosis, and kidney failure [121]. Management strategies include early removal of indwelling catheters, scheduled clean intermittent self-catheterisation, and using external or suprapubic catheters. Alternative voiding methods include micturition through straining, sacral root stimulation, and medications like oxybutynin and tamsulosin to reduce bladder spasms and improve emptying [120]. Regular post-void bladder scans and careful monitoring of fluid balance are recommended.

5.5 Conclusion

The management of SCI has advanced significantly, yet it remains a complex field with many challenges. This chapter highlighted the critical need for timely interventions, encapsulated by rapid surgical decompression to prevent secondary damage. The summary of techniques that help in preventing further damage and the general management in the ICU are highlighted in Fig. 5.3. Besides the techniques mentioned in Fig. 5.3, other strategies either remain a controversy or tantalizingly out of reach.

Long-term rehabilitation remains essential, focusing on maximising patient independence and addressing the varied physical and psychological impacts of SCI. A personalised, multidisciplinary approach is crucial for effective rehabilitation. Thus, while significant progress has been made in SCI treatment, continuous research and innovation are necessary.

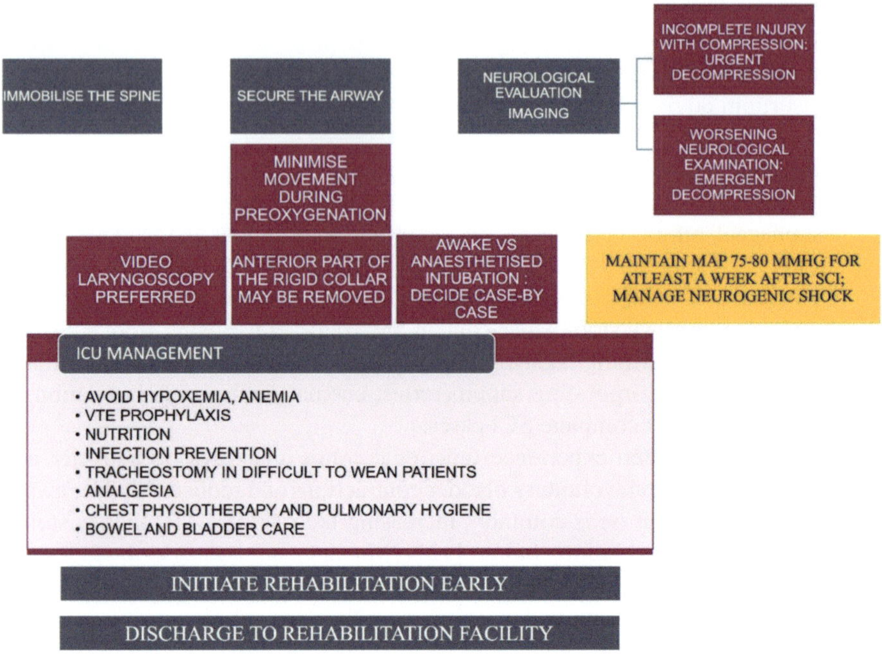

Fig. 5.3 Steps in management of SCI. MAP mean arterial pressure, SCI spinal cord injury, VTE venous thromboembolism

References

1. Mathur N, Jain S, Kumar N, et al. Spinal cord injury: scenario in an Indian state. Spinal Cord. 2015;53(5):349–52.
2. Ahuja CS, Badhiwala JH, Fehlings MG. "Time is spine": the importance of early intervention for traumatic spinal cord injury. Spinal Cord. 2020;58(9):1037–9.
3. Ramakonar H, Fehlings MG. 'Time is Spine': new evidence supports decompression within 24 h for acute spinal cord injury. Spinal Cord. 2021;59(8):933–4.
4. Ahuja CS, Wilson JR, Nori S, et al. Traumatic spinal cord injury. Nat Rev Dis Primers. 2017;3:17018.
5. Anjum A, Yazid MD, Fauzi Daud M, et al. Spinal cord injury: pathophysiology, multimolecular interactions, and underlying recovery mechanisms. Int J Mol Sci. 2020;21(20):7533.
6. Wilson JR, Tetreault LA, Kwon BK, et al. Timing of decompression in patients with acute spinal cord injury: a systematic review. Global Spine J. 2017;7(3 Suppl):95S–115S.
7. Dimar JR 2nd, Glassman SD, Raque GH, et al. The influence of spinal canal narrowing and timing of decompression on neurologic recovery after spinal cord contusion in a rat model. Spine (Phila Pa 1976). 1999;24(16):1623–33.
8. Fehlings MG, Perrin RG. The timing of surgical intervention in the treatment of spinal cord injury: a systematic review of recent clinical evidence. Spine (Phila Pa 1976). 2006;31(11 Suppl):S28–36.

9. Furlan JC, Noonan V, Cadotte DW, et al. Timing of decompressive surgery of spinal cord after traumatic spinal cord injury: an evidence-based examination of preclinical and clinical studies. J Neurotrauma. 2011;28(8):1371–99.
10. Fehlings MG, Vaccaro A, Wilson JR, et al. Early versus delayed decompression for traumatic cervical spinal cord injury: results of the surgical timing in acute spinal cord injury study (STASCIS). PLoS One. 2012;7(2):e32037.
11. Dvorak MF, Noonan VK, Fallah N, et al. The influence of time from injury to surgery on motor recovery and length of hospital stay in acute traumatic spinal cord injury: an observational Canadian cohort study. J Neurotrauma. 2015;32(9):645–54.
12. Xue F, Zhan SZ, Zhang DY, et al. Early versus delayed surgery for acute traumatic cervical/thoracic spinal cord injury in Beijing, China: the results of a prospective, multicenter nonrandomized controlled trial. Orthop Surg. 2021;13(8):2246–54.
13. Quddusi A, Pedro KM, Alvi MA, et al. Early surgical intervention for acute spinal cord injury: time is spine. Acta Neurochir. 2023;165(9):2665–74.
14. Badhiwala JH, Wilson JR, Witiw CD, et al. The influence of timing of surgical decompression for acute spinal cord injury: a pooled analysis of individual patient data. Lancet Neurol. 2021;20(2):117–26.
15. Jug M, Kejžar N, Vesel M, et al. Neurological recovery after traumatic cervical spinal cord injury is superior if surgical decompression and instrumented fusion are performed within 8 hours versus 8 to 24 hours after injury: a single center experience. J Neurotrauma. 2015;32(18):1385–92.
16. Bock T, Heller RA, Haubruck P, et al. Pursuing more aggressive timelines in the surgical treatment of traumatic spinal cord injury (TSCI): a retrospective cohort study with subgroup analysis. J Clin Med. 2021,10(24).5977.
17. Lee DY, Park YJ, Kim HJ, et al. Early surgical decompression within 8 hours for traumatic spinal cord injury: is it beneficial? A meta-analysis. Acta Orthop Traumatol Turc. 2018;52(2):101–8.
18. Yousefifard M, Hashemi B, Forouzanfar MM, et al. Ultra-early spinal decompression surgery can improve neurological outcome of complete cervical spinal cord injury; a systematic review and meta-analysis. Arch Acad Emerg Med. 2022;10(1):e11.
19. Hosman AJF, Barbagallo G. The SCI-POEM Study Group, et al. Neurological recovery after early versus delayed surgical decompression for acute traumatic spinal cord injury. Bone Joint J. 2023;105-B(4):400–11.
20. Fehlings MG, Tetreault LA, Hachem L, et al. An update of a clinical practice guideline for the management of patients with acute spinal cord injury: recommendations on the role and timing of decompressive surgery. Global Spine J. 2024;14(3_suppl):174S–86S.
21. Aarabi B, Sansur CA, Ibrahimi DM, et al. Intramedullary lesion length on postoperative magnetic resonance imaging is a strong predictor of ASIA impairment scale grade conversion following decompressive surgery in cervical spinal cord injury. Neurosurgery. 2017;80(4):610–20.
22. Phang I, Werndle MC, Saadoun S, et al. Expansion duroplasty improves intraspinal pressure, spinal cord perfusion pressure, and vascular pressure reactivity index in patients with traumatic spinal cord injury: injured spinal cord pressure evaluation study. J Neurotrauma. 2015;32(12):865–74.
23. Chen WT, Zhou YP, Zhang GS. The progress and controversies regarding steroid use in acute spinal cord injury. Eur Rev Med Pharmacol Sci. 2023;27(13):6101–10.
24. Bracken MB, Shepard MJ, Collins WF, et al. A randomized, controlled trial of methylprednisolone or naloxone in the treatment of acute spinal cord injury. Results of the second national acute spinal cord injury study. N Engl J Med. 1990;322(20):1405–11.
25. Bracken MB, Shepard MJ, Hellenbrand KG, et al. Methylprednisolone and neurological function 1 year after spinal cord injury. Results of the National Acute Spinal Cord Injury Study. J Neurosurg. 1985;63(5):704–13.

26. Bracken MB, Shepard MJ, Holford TR, et al. Administration of methylprednisolone for 24 or 48 hours or tirilazad mesylate for 48 hours in the treatment of acute spinal cord injury. Results of the third National Acute Spinal Cord Injury Randomized Controlled Trial. National Acute Spinal Cord Injury Study. JAMA. 1997;277(20):1597–604.
27. Hextrum S, Bennett S. A critical examination of subgroup analyses: the National Acute Spinal Cord Injury Studies and beyond. Front Neurol. 2018;9:11.
28. Bracken MB. Steroids for acute spinal cord injury. Cochrane Database Syst Rev. 2012;1(1):CD001046.
29. Liu Z, Yang Y, He L, et al. High-dose methylprednisolone for acute traumatic spinal cord injury: a meta-analysis. Neurology. 2019;93(9):e841–50.
30. Sultan I, Lamba N, Liew A, et al. The safety and efficacy of steroid treatment for acute spinal cord injury: a systematic review and meta-analysis. Heliyon. 2020;6(2):e03414.
31. Fischer G, Bättig L, Stienen MN, et al. Advancements in neuroregenerative and neuroprotective therapies for traumatic spinal cord injury. Front Neurosci. 2024;18:1372920.
32. Miękisiak G, Kloc W, Janusz W, et al. The use of methylprednisolone in the acute phase of spinal cord injury. J Spine Surg. 2013;1:11–24.
33. Fehlings MG, Wilson JR, Tetreault LA, et al. A clinical practice guideline for the management of patients with acute spinal cord injury: recommendations on the use of methylprednisolone sodium succinate. Global Spine J. 2017;7(3 Suppl):203S–11S.
34. Picetti E, Demetriades AK, Catena F, et al. Early management of adult traumatic spinal cord injury in patients with polytrauma: a consensus and clinical recommendations jointly developed by the World Society of Emergency Surgery (WSES) & the European Association of Neurosurgical Societies (EANS). World J Emerg Surg. 2024;19(1):4.
35. Picetti E, Iaccarino C, Coimbra R, et al. The acute phase management of spinal cord injury affecting polytrauma patients: the ASAP study. World J Emerg Surg. 2022;17(1):20.
36. Hejrati N, Aarabi B, Neal CJ, et al. Trends in the use of corticosteroids in the management of acute spinal cord injury in north American clinical trials network sites. J Neurotrauma. 2023;40(17–18):1938–47.
37. Miękisiak G, Łątka D, Jarmużek P, et al. Steroids in acute spinal cord injury: all but gone within 5 years. World Neurosurg. 2019;122:e467–71.
38. Ulndreaj A, Badner A, Fehlings MG. Promising neuroprotective strategies for traumatic spinal cord injury with a focus on the differential effects among anatomical levels of injury. F1000Res. 2017;6:1907.
39. Ryken TC, Hurlbert RJ, Hadley MN, et al. The acute cardiopulmonary management of patients with cervical spinal cord injuries. Neurosurgery. 2013;72(Suppl 2):84–92.
40. Evaniew N, Davies B, Farahbakhsh F, et al. Interventions to optimize spinal cord perfusion in patients with acute traumatic spinal cord injury: an updated systematic review. Global Spine J. 2024;14(3_suppl):58S–79S.
41. Squair JW, Bélanger LM, Tsang A, et al. Spinal cord perfusion pressure predicts neurologic recovery in acute spinal cord injury. Neurology. 2017;89(16):1660–7.
42. Martin ND, Kepler C, Zubair M, et al. Increased mean arterial pressure goals after spinal cord injury and functional outcome. J Emerg Trauma Shock. 2015;8(2):94–8.
43. Readdy WJ, Whetstone WD, Ferguson AR, et al. Complications and outcomes of vasopressor usage in acute traumatic central cord syndrome. J Neurosurg Spine. 2015;23(5):574–80.
44. Chen S, Gallagher MJ, Papadopoulos MC, et al. Non-linear dynamical analysis of Intraspinal pressure signal predicts outcome after spinal cord injury. Front Neurol. 2018;9:493.
45. Kwon BK, Tetreault LA, Martin AR, et al. A clinical practice guideline for the management of patients with acute spinal cord injury: recommendations on hemodynamic management. Global Spine J. 2024;14(3_suppl):187S–211S.
46. Kwon BK, Curt A, Belanger LM, et al. Intrathecal pressure monitoring and cerebrospinal fluid drainage in acute spinal cord injury: a prospective randomized trial. J Neurosurg Spine. 2009;10(3):181–93.

47. Hogg FRA, Gallagher MJ, Kearney S, et al. Acute spinal cord injury: monitoring lumbar cerebrospinal fluid provides limited information about the injury site. J Neurotrauma. 2020;37(9):1156–64.
48. Theodore N, Martirosyan N, Hersh AM, et al. Cerebrospinal fluid drainage in patients with acute spinal cord injury: a Multicenter randomized controlled trial. World Neurosurg. 2023;24:e472.
49. Al-Nashash H, All AH. Neuroprotective role of hypothermia in acute spinal cord injury. Biomedicine. 2022;10(1):104.
50. Batchelor PE, Skeers P, Antonic A, et al. Systematic review and meta-analysis of therapeutic hypothermia in animal models of spinal cord injury. PLoS One. 2013;8(8):e71317.
51. Dididze M, Green BA, Dietrich WD, et al. Systemic hypothermia in acute cervical spinal cord injury: a case-controlled study. Spinal Cord. 2013;51(5):395–400.
52. Shin HK, Park JH, Roh SW, et al. Meta-analysis on the effect of hypothermia in acute spinal cord injury. Neurospine. 2022;19(3):748–56.
53. Gallagher MJ, Hogg FRA, Kearney S, et al. Effects of local hypothermia-rewarming on physiology, metabolism and inflammation of acutely injured human spinal cord. Sci Rep. 2020;10(1):8125.
54. Levi AD, Green BA, Wang MY, et al. Clinical application of modest hypothermia after spinal cord injury. J Neurotrauma. 2009;26(3):407–15.
55. Vedantam A, Jimsheleishvili G, Harrop JS, et al. A prospective multicenter study comparing the complication profile of modest systemic hypothermia versus normothermia for acute cervical spinal cord injury. Spinal Cord. 2022;60(6):510–5.
56. Patel NP, Huang JH. Hyperbaric oxygen therapy of spinal cord injury. Med Gas Res. 2017;7(2):133–43.
57. Huang L, Zhang Q, Fu C, et al. Effects of hyperbaric oxygen therapy on patients with spinal cord injury: a systematic review and meta-analysis of randomized controlled trials. J Back Musculoskelet Rehabil. 2021;34(6):905–13.
58. Siglioccolo A, Gammaldi R, Vicinanza V, et al. Advance in hyperbaric oxygen therapy in spinal cord injury. Chin J Traumatol. 2023;12:348.
59. Sun L, Zhao L, Li P, et al. Effect of hyperbaric oxygen therapy on HMGB1/NF-κB expression and prognosis of acute spinal cord injury: a randomized clinical trial. Neurosci Lett. 2019;692:47–52.
60. Grossman RG, Fehlings MG, Frankowski RF, et al. A prospective, multicenter, phase I matched-comparison group trial of safety, pharmacokinetics, and preliminary efficacy of riluzole in patients with traumatic spinal cord injury. J Neurotrauma. 2014;31(3):239–55.
61. Fehlings MG, Moghaddamjou A, Harrop JS, et al. Safety and efficacy of Riluzole in acute spinal cord injury study (RISCIS): a multicenter, randomized, placebo-controlled, double-blinded trial. J Neurotrauma. 2023;40(17–18):1878–88.
62. Casha S, Zygun D, McGowan MD, et al. Results of a phase II placebo-controlled randomized trial of minocycline in acute spinal cord injury. Brain. 2012;135(Pt 4):1224–36.
63. Shultz RB, Zhong Y. Minocycline targets multiple secondary injury mechanisms in traumatic spinal cord injury. Neural Regen Res. 2017;12(5):702–13.
64. Geisler FH, Coleman WP, Grieco G, et al. The Sygen multicenter acute spinal cord injury study. Spine (Phila Pa 1976). 2001;26(24 Suppl):S87–98.
65. Koda M, Hanaoka H, Fujii Y, et al. Randomized trial of granulocyte colony-stimulating factor for spinal cord injury. Brain. 2021;144(3):789–99.
66. Merkler D, Metz GA, Raineteau O, et al. Locomotor recovery in spinal cord-injured rats treated with an antibody neutralizing the myelin-associated neurite growth inhibitor Nogo-A. J Neurosci. 2001;21(10):3665–73.
67. Donovan J, Kirshblum S. Clinical trials in traumatic spinal cord injury. Neurotherapeutics. 2018;15(3):654–68.

68. Fehlings MG, Theodore N, Harrop J, et al. A phase I/IIa clinical trial of a recombinant rho protein antagonist in acute spinal cord injury. J Neurotrauma. 2011;28(5):787–96.
69. Fehlings MG, Chen Y, Aarabi B, et al. A randomized controlled trial of local delivery of a rho inhibitor (VX-210) in patients with acute traumatic cervical spinal cord injury. J Neurotrauma. 2021;38(15):2065–72.
70. Ahuja CS, Nori S, Tetreault L, et al. Traumatic spinal cord injury-repair and regeneration. Neurosurgery. 2017;80(3S):S9–S22.
71. Assinck P, Duncan GJ, Hilton BJ, Plemel JR, Tetzlaff W. Cell transplantation therapy for spinal cord injury. Nat Neurosci. 2017;20(5):637–47.
72. Curtis E, Martin JR, Gabel B, et al. A first-in-human, phase I study of neural stem cell transplantation for chronic spinal cord injury. Cell Stem Cell. 2018;22(6):941–50.
73. Curt A, Hsieh J, Schubert M, et al. The damaged spinal cord is a suitable target for stem cell transplantation. Neurorehabil Neural Repair. 2020;34(8):758–68.
74. El-Kheir WA, Gabr H, Awad MR, et al. Autologous bone marrow-derived cell therapy combined with physical therapy induces functional improvement in chronic spinal cord injury patients. Cell Transplant. 2014;23(6):729–45.
75. Saini R, Pahwa B, Agrawal D, et al. Efficacy and outcome of bone marrow-derived stem cells transplanted via intramedullary route in acute complete spinal cord injury – a randomized placebo controlled trial. J Clin Neurosci. 2022;100:7–14.
76. Anderson KD, Guest JD, Dietrich WD, et al. Safety of autologous human Schwann cell transplantation in subacute thoracic spinal cord injury. J Neurotrauma. 2017;34(21):2950–63.
77. Lu P, Woodruff G, Wang Y, et al. Long-distance axonal growth from human induced pluripotent stem cells after spinal cord injury. Neuron. 2014;83(4):789–96.
78. Ji P, Manupipatpong S, Xie N, Li Y. Induced pluripotent stem cells: generation strategy and epigenetic mystery behind reprogramming. Stem Cells Int. 2016;2016:8415010.
79. Tian T, Zhang S, Yang M. Recent progress and challenges in the treatment of spinal cord injury. Protein Cell. 2023;14(9):635–52.
80. Hamani C, Moro E. Neuromodulation: a more comprehensive concept beyond deep brain stimulation. Int Rev Neurobiol. 2012;107:1–3.
81. Cortes M, Medeiros AH, Gandhi A, et al. Improved grasp function with transcranial direct current stimulation in chronic spinal cord injury. NeuroRehabilitation. 2017;41(1):51–9.
82. Murray LM, Edwards DJ, Ruffini G, et al. Intensity dependent effects of transcranial direct current stimulation on corticospinal excitability in chronic spinal cord injury. Arch Phys Med Rehabil. 2015;96(4 Suppl):S114–21.
83. Simis M, Fregni F, Battistella LR. Transcranial direct current stimulation combined with robotic training in incomplete spinal cord injury: a randomized, sham-controlled clinical trial. Spinal Cord Ser Cases. 2021;7(1):87.
84. Benito J, Kumru H, Murillo N, et al. Motor and gait improvement in patients with incomplete spinal cord injury induced by high-frequency repetitive transcranial magnetic stimulation. Top Spinal Cord Inj Rehabil. 2012;18(2):106–12.
85. Kumru H, Benito-Penalva J, Valls-Sole J, et al. Placebo-controlled study of rTMS combined with Lokomat® gait training for treatment in subjects with motor incomplete spinal cord injury. Exp Brain Res. 2016;234(12):3447–55.
86. Katayama Y, Yamamoto T, Kobayashi K, et al. Motor cortex stimulation for phantom limb pain: comprehensive therapy with spinal cord and thalamic stimulation. Stereotact Funct Neurosurg. 2001;77(1–4):159–62.
87. Mahlknecht P, Limousin P, Foltynie T. Deep brain stimulation for movement disorders: update on recent discoveries and outlook on future developments. J Neurol. 2015;262(11):2583–95.
88. Inanici F, Samejima S, Gad P, et al. Transcutaneous electrical spinal stimulation promotes long-term recovery of upper extremity function in chronic tetraplegia. IEEE Trans Neural Syst Rehabil Eng. 2018;26(6):1272–8.
89. Freyvert Y, Yong NA, Morikawa E, et al. Engaging cervical spinal circuitry with non-invasive spinal stimulation and buspirone to restore hand function in chronic motor complete patients. Sci Rep. 2018;8(1):15546.

90. Angeli CA, Boakye M, Morton RA, et al. Recovery of over-ground walking after chronic motor complete spinal cord injury. N Engl J Med. 2018;379(13):1244–50.
91. Chandrasekaran S, Nanivadekar AC, McKernan G, et al. Sensory restoration by epidural stimulation of the lateral spinal cord in upper limb amputees. Elife. 2020;9:e54349.
92. Gill ML, Grahn PJ, Calvert JS, et al. Neuromodulation of lumbosacral spinal networks enables independent stepping after complete paraplegia. Nat Med. 2018;24(11):1677–82.
93. Austin N, Krishnamoorthy V, Dagal A. Airway management in cervical spine injury. Int J Crit Illn Inj Sci. 2014;4(1):50–6.
94. Podolsky S, Baraff LJ, Simon RR, et al. Efficacy of cervical spine immobilisation methods. J Trauma. 1983;23(6):461–5.
95. Nolan JP, Wilson ME. Orotracheal intubation in patients with potential cervical spine injuries. An indication for the gum elastic bougie. Anaesthesia. 1993;48(7):630–3.
96. Wiles MD, Iliff HA, Brooks K, et al. Airway management in patients with suspected or confirmed cervical spine injury: guidelines from the difficult airway society (DAS), Association of Anaesthetists (AoA), British Society of Orthopaedic Anaesthetists (BSOA), Intensive Care Society (ICS), Neuro Anaesthesia and Critical Care Society (NACCS), Faculty of Prehospital Care and Royal College of Emergency Medicine (RCEM). Anaesthesia. 2024;79(8):856–68.
97. Holmes MG, Dagal A, Feinstein BA, et al. Airway management practice in adults with an unstable cervical spine: the Harborview Medical Center experience. Anesth Analg. 2018;127(2):450–4.
98. Melesse DY, Tesema TT, Mekonnen ZA, et al. Airway management for individuals with suspected or confirmed traumatic cervical spine injuries: a comprehensive review and analysis. Perioper Care Oper Room Manag. 2024;35(5):100390.
99. Zeng L, Wang YL, Shen XT, et al. Guidelines for management of pediatric acute hyperextension spinal cord injury. Chin J Traumatol. 2023;26(1):2–7.
100. Cunha NSC, Malvea A, Sadat S, et al. Pediatric spinal cord injury: a review. Children (Basel). 2023;10(9):1456.
101. Bosch PP, Vogt MT, Ward WT. Pediatric spinal cord injury without radiographic abnormality (SCIWORA): the absence of occult instability and lack of indication for bracing. Spine (Phila Pa 1976). 2002;27(24):2788–800.
102. Parent S, Mac-Thiong JM, Roy-Beaudry M, et al. Spinal cord injury in the pediatric population: a systematic review of the literature. J Neurotrauma. 2011;28(8):1515–24.
103. Nas K, Yazmalar L, Şah V, et al. Rehabilitation of spinal cord injuries. World J Orthop. 2015;6(1):8–16.
104. Jurkiewicz MT, Mikulis DJ, McIlroy WE, et al. Sensorimotor cortical plasticity during recovery following spinal cord injury: a longitudinal fMRI study. Neurorehabil Neural Repair. 2007;21(6):527–38.
105. Chi JH. Combination therapy improves walking in spinal cord transaction. Neurosurgery. 2009;65(6):N10–1.
106. Lam T, Eng JJ, Wolfe DL, Hsieh JT, Whittaker M. A systematic review of the efficacy of gait rehabilitation strategies for spinal cord injury. Top Spinal Cord Inj Rehabil. 2007;13(1):32–57.
107. Popović DB. Advances in functional electrical stimulation (FES). J Electromyogr Kinesiol. 2014;24(6):795–802.
108. Martin R, Sadowsky C, Obst K, et al. Functional electrical stimulation in spinal cord injury:: from theory to practice. Top Spinal Cord Inj Rehabil. 2012;18(1):28–33.
109. Hachem LD, Ahuja CS, Fehlings MG. Assessment and management of acute spinal cord injury: from point of injury to rehabilitation. J Spinal Cord Med. 2017;40(6):665–75.
110. Krucoff MO, Gramer R, Lott D, et al. Spinal cord stimulation and rehabilitation in an individual with chronic complete L1 paraplegia due to a conus medullaris injury: motor and functional outcomes at 18 months. Spinal Cord Ser Cases. 2020;6(1):96.
111. Shapiro S, Borgens R, Pascuzzi R, et al. Oscillating field stimulation for complete spinal cord injury in humans: a phase 1 trial. J Neurosurg Spine. 2005;2(1):3–10.

112. Miller LE, Zimmermann AK, Herbert WG. Clinical effectiveness and safety of powered exoskeleton-assisted walking in patients with spinal cord injury: systematic review with meta-analysis. Med Devices (Auckl). 2016;9:455–66.
113. Wade D. Upper motor neurone syndrome and spasticity. Clinical management and neurophysiology. J Neurol Neurosurg Psychiatry. 2001;71(6):822.
114. Aydin G, Tomruk S, Keleş I, et al. Transcutaneous electrical nerve stimulation versus baclofen in spasticity: clinical and electrophysiologic comparison. Am J Phys Med Rehabil. 2005;84(8):584–92.
115. Alashram AR, Annino G, Mercuri NB. Changes in spasticity following functional electrical stimulation cycling in patients with spinal cord injury: a systematic review. J Spinal Cord Med. 2022;45(1):10–23.
116. Billington ZJ, Henke AM, Gater DR Jr. Spasticity management after spinal cord injury: the here and now. J Pers Med. 2022;12(5):808.
117. Warburton DE, Eng JJ. Krassioukov A, et al; the SCIRE Research Team. Cardiovascular health and exercise rehabilitation in spinal cord injury. Top Spinal Cord Inj Rehabil. 2007;13(1):98–122.
118. Eldahan KC, Rabchevsky AG. Autonomic dysreflexia after spinal cord injury: systemic pathophysiology and methods of management. Auton Neurosci. 2018;209:59–70.
119. Statements, Potential Conflict-of-Interest. Prevention of venous thromboembolism in individuals with spinal cord injury: clinical practice guidelines for health care providers, 3rd ed.: consortium for spinal cord medicine. Top Spinal Cord Inj Rehabil. 2016;22(3):209–40.
120. Wang TY, Park C, Zhang H, et al. Management of acute traumatic spinal cord injury: a review of the literature. Front Surg. 2021;8:698736.
121. Esclarín De Ruz A, García Leoni E, Herruzo CR. Epidemiology and risk factors for urinary tract infection in patients with spinal cord injury. J Urol. 2000;164(4):1285–9.

Controversies Regarding Different Treatment Modalities for Cortical Sinus Venous Thrombosis

6

Ramamani Mariappan and Mouleeswaran Sundaram

Abstract

Cerebral Sinus Venous Thrombosis (CSVT) constitutes 0.5–3% of all strokes, which primarily affects young women. The clinical presentation is often atypical, with vague symptoms; hence, radiological imaging with computed tomography (CT) and MR venography is considered optimal for diagnosing cerebral venous thrombosis (CVT). Anticoagulation is the mainstay of treatment in these patients, with low-molecular-weight heparin (LMWH) being the preferred agent in the acute stage of the disease, followed by maintenance anticoagulation with warfarin or direct-acting oral anticoagulants (DOACs) for a varying period starting from 3 months to lifelong, based on the associated risk factors (genetic/acquired, provoked/unprovoked). Supportive management includes adequate hydration, reduction of intracranial pressure (ICP) with osmotherapy, cerebrospinal fluid (CSF) drainage, sedation and ventilation, and antiepileptics. In cases of refractory ICP elevation with mass effects and impending herniation, decompressive craniectomy is offered as a therapy to improve outcomes. Endovascular treatment has been shown to have a reasonable safety profile. It should be reserved for patients with poor prognostic scores during admission and for those who deteriorate despite maximal medical care. CSVT in pregnancy is relatively common and requires a multidisciplinary approach because of concerns regarding anticoagulation and contrast-associated teratogenicity, radiation exposure, and prothrombotic state. Management of paediatric and neonatal CSVT is similar to adult management, except that the duration of anticoagulation is shorter for neonates (6–12 weeks) due to the lower rate of propagation and recurrence.

R. Mariappan (✉) · M. Sundaram
Department of Neuroanaesthesia, Christian Medical College, Vellore, Tamil Nadu, India
e-mail: ramamani@cmcvellore.ac.in

P. U. Bidkar, M. Krishnakumar (eds.), *Controversies in Neurocritical Care*,
https://doi.org/10.1007/978-981-95-4419-6_6

Keywords

Anticoagulation · Cerebral sinus venous thrombosis · Decompressive craniectomy · Endovascular therapy · Paediatric and neonatal CSVT · Pregnancy and puerperal CSVT

6.1 Introduction

Cerebral sinus venous thrombosis (CSVT) is characterised by blood clots in the cerebral veins, dural venous sinuses, or both [1]. CSVT represents 0.5–3% of all strokes. It predominantly affects women and patients aged <55 years. A large international study on cerebral venous thrombosis (CVT) (ISCVT), a prospective observational study [2], followed 624 patients with CSVT over 16 months and found that genetic or acquired thrombophilia was the most common cause, followed by oral contraceptives or hormonal replacement therapy (in females). Because of its variable presentation, diagnosis is often delayed; keeping a high index of suspicion and early imaging with CT and MR venography play a vital role in early diagnosis. Anticoagulation is the mainstay of treatment despite its haemorrhagic presentation. This manuscript discusses the controversies regarding the management of CSVT, such as anticoagulation management during the acute, subacute, and chronic stages; duration of anticoagulation; intracranial pressure (ICP) management; the role of decompressive craniectomy (DC); and endovascular thrombectomy for severe CSVT. In addition, the differences in managing paediatric/neonatal CSVT and pregnancy/puerperal CSVT are highlighted. Various new modes of radiological imaging (computed tomography (CT) and magnetic resonance imaging-based) for diagnosing CSVT and its findings are discussed. Important CSVT trials were briefly discussed at the end of this manuscript.

6.2 Controversies Regarding the Anticoagulation Management in CSVT

Anticoagulation is the mainstay of treatment, even in patients presenting with haemorrhagic lesions intracerebral hemorrhage (ICH) or subarachnoid hemorrhage (SAH) due to CSVT. The main goal of anticoagulation is to achieve recanalisation of the occluded vein or sinus, prevent thrombus propagation, and prevent the occurrence of venous thrombosis/embolism elsewhere and their recurrence. Two randomised controlled trials in the 1990s and their meta-analysis compared heparin vs. placebo and showed increased mortality and unfavourable outcomes in patients treated with placebo [3, 4]. Controversies regarding anticoagulation management for CSVT are highlighted in Box 6.1.

Box 6.1: Controversies Regarding Anticoagulation Management

1. *Type of Heparin in the Acute Stage:* Unfractionated heparin (UFH) vs. low molecular weight heparin (LMWH)
2. *Type of Oral Anticoagulation in the Subacute and Chronic Stages*: Vitamin K antagonist (VKAs) vs. Direct oral anticoagulants (DOAC)
3. *Which DOAC?*: Direct Xa inhibitors vs. thrombin inhibitors
4. *Duration of Oral Anticoagulation:* Does this depend on the degree of recanalisation?
5. *Timing of DOAC* initiation: With or without lead-in heparin
6. *The role of antiplatelet agents in secondary prevention after discontinuation of oral anticoagulants*

1. *Unfractionated Heparin (UFH) vs. Low-Molecular-Weight Heparin (LMWH)* [5–8] The American Heart Association/American Stroke Association and European guidelines recommend the initial use of subcutaneous low-molecular-weight heparin (LMWH) over unfractionated heparin (UFH) during the acute stage, followed by oral vitamin K antagonists (VKAs) for varying durations of 3–12 months depending on the presence of transient trigger factors or chronic major risk factors. LMWH is favoured during acute treatment because of the feasibility of its administration, predictability of its anticoagulation effects, and safety because of its lower risk of thrombocytopenia. UFH is prescribed only for specific populations, such as patients who are admitted to the neurointensive care unit (NICU) with the possibility of surgical intervention within a few hours, those who have contraindications to the use of LMWH, such as severe renal insufficiency, and those in whom emergency reversal of anticoagulation is anticipated.
2. *Vitamin K Antagonist (VKA) Versus Direct Oral Anticoagulants (DOAC)?* [9–13] Recent RCTs, systematic reviews, and meta-analyses demonstrated that DOACs are equally effective and safe for the management of CSVT, with a better recanalisation rate than warfarin, a VKA. The functional outcomes, CSVT recurrence, systemic and intracranial haemorrhage, and mortality were comparable between the groups. The better safety profile of DOACs is due to their predictable pharmacokinetics and fewer interactions with other drugs and food. Another advantage of DOACs is that routine coagulation monitoring is not needed, as compared to warfarin, where INR has to be routinely monitored and maintained between 2 and 3. As anticoagulation effects cannot be monitored with DOACs, caution is needed in patients who are at high risk of bleeding, such as the elderly, those who are on antiplatelet therapy, those with low

body weight, and those with renal dysfunction. During pregnancy and breastfeeding, both VKAs and other DOACs should be avoided because they can cause foetal embryopathy and foetal and neonatal bleeding. LMWH is the recommended anticoagulation therapy for pregnancy and breastfeeding. ACTION-CVT study is an international multicentric trial that compared DOACs with warfarin and showed that DOAC treatment was associated with a similar risk of recurrent venous thrombosis (aHR, 0.94 [95% CI, 0.51–1.73]; $P = 0.84$), death (aHR, 0.78 [95% CI, 0.22–2.76]; $P = 0.70$), and rate of partial/complete recanalization (aOR, 0.92 [95% CI, 0.48–1.73]; $P = 0.79$), but a lower risk of significant haemorrhage (aHR, 0.35 [95% CI, 0.15–0.82]; $P = 0.02$) [13]. Fayyaz et al. [14] reviewed and compared VKAs and DOACs, showing that DOACs are non-inferior and safe. A recent randomised trial (CHOICE-CVT trial) compared dabigatran vs. warfarin in 18–80-year-old Chinese patients and showed that dabigatran was safe and efficacious regarding bleeding complications and recurrence [15].

3. *Which DOAC Is Superior for Treating CSVT?* [7, 16] There are no specific recommendations regarding the type of DOAC used to treat CSVT. Studies have shown that the selection of various DOACs depends on the cause of CSVT and associated comorbidities. For patients with a previous history of myocardial infarction (MI), dabigatran should be avoided for treatment because of the increased risk of MI due to the platelet-activating effect of dabigatran. For patients with upper GI bleeding, apixaban or low-dose edoxaban is recommended, as it has been shown to decrease bleeding compared with oral warfarin. Patients who require once-daily dosing are better off starting rivaroxaban or edoxaban. Recently, many randomised controlled trials (RCTs), systematic reviews, and meta-analyses [9–13] demonstrated the efficacy and safety of rivaroxaban in CVT management, compared it with warfarin, and showed that it was non-inferior to warfarin. The RE-SPECT CVT [9] study compared dabigatran with warfarin and showed that both were similar in preventing recurrent venous thromboembolism (VTE) in patients with CVT, and the bleeding complications were comparable between the groups. A study by Wasay et al. [16] compared DOACs (rivaroxaban, dabigatran) with warfarin and showed that DOACs were safe and non-inferior to warfarin. However, DOACs are contraindicated in patients with antiphospholipid syndrome because of the increased recurrence rate of thrombotic events. Therefore, VKA is the drug of choice in this patient population.
4. *Duration of Anticoagulation:* [7, 8] The current guidelines recommend that patients presenting with one CSVT/CVT episode with triggering factors (dehydration, infection, h/o trauma, surgical interventions, or oral contraceptive use) should receive anticoagulation for 3–6 months; patients with one CVT episode without the triggering factor should continue anticoagulation for 6–12 months, and those patients with two or more CVT episodes with severe prothrombotic conditions should continue anticoagulation for lifelong. These recommendations are extrapolated from VTE and pulmonary embolism studies because of the non-availability of RCTs or high-quality observational studies on the duration of

anticoagulation for CSVT/CVT. The effect of anticoagulation duration on the degree of recanalisation over time remains uncertain, and future studies are needed in this regard.

5. *Timing of Starting DOAC*: There is controversy regarding the timing of starting DOAC after the diagnosis of CVT, with or without heparin. Most studies have shown that LMWH and unfractionated heparin are commonly used during the acute stage, followed by oral anticoagulants with either vitamin K antagonists (VKAs) or DOACs. Most RCTs have shown that the average duration of starting oral anticoagulation from the time of diagnosis of CVT is 5–15 days, while observational studies have shown that the time starting oral anticoagulation after heparin is between 3 and 12 days [10, 11, 13, 15]. A preliminary study by Shankar Iyer R [17] started rivaroxaban without heparin during the acute phase and continued for 6 months, which proved safe and efficacious.
6. *Role of Antiplatelets for the Secondary Prevention of CSVT After Stopping oral anticoagulation (OAC):* Studies have shown that aspirin is effective for the secondary prevention of VTE compared to placebo (HR, 0.68 [95% CI, 0.51–0.90]; $P = 0.008$) in patients with a previous history of VTE [18]. However, no studies have used aspirin for the secondary prevention of CSVT. Most patients with CSVT are younger and have to be subjected to prolonged exposure to aspirin and its associated side effects. In addition, the VTE recurrence rate is lower after CSVT. Hence, it is not recommended to start patients with CSVT on antiplatelet therapy routinely for secondary prevention.

6.3 Controversies Regarding the Management of Intracranial Hypertension in CSVT

6.3.1 Do All CSVT Patients Present with Intracranial Hypertension?

Not all CSVT patients present with intracranial hypertension. The incidence of brain swelling in patients with CSVT is around 50%, but the majority of the time, the oedema is minor and does not cause signs of intracranial hypertension [3]. In these patients, systemic anticoagulation is sufficient to re-establish the venous outflow in the thrombosed vein and to reduce the brain oedema and intracranial pressure [19]. Aggressive antiedema therapy is required in only 20% of patients who present with obvious symptoms and signs of intracranial hypertension and brain herniation.

Intracranial hypertension occurs in CSVT as a result of venous obstruction, resulting in cerebral oedema (vasogenic and cytotoxic), haemorrhage, and infarction [20]. Also, it reduces CSF reabsorption, resulting in malabsorptive hydrocephalus [20]. The management of intracranial hypertension is an integral component of the acute management of CSVT, which requires intensive care admission. Following the tiered approach for intracranial pressure-lowering strategies recommended by the Emergency Neurological Life Support (ENLS) is essential. We encourage readers to consult the ENLS protocol for additional information on intracranial pressure-lowering strategies. Controversies regarding the management of intracranial hypertension in CVT are given in Box 6.2.

Box 6.2: Controversies Regarding ICP Management in CSVT

1. Role of osmotherapy and the choice of osmotherapeutic agent for the management of intracranial hypertension.
2. Role of steroids in the treatment of elevated ICP.
3. The role of CSF drainage in patients with intracranial hypertension secondary to CSVT.

1. *Role of Osmotherapy and the Choice of Osmotherapeutic Agent for Treatment of Elevated Intracranial Pressure (ICP)*

   The general principles of osmotherapy should be followed in these groups of patients. Regarding the choice of osmotherapeutic agent, there is no adequate evidence to favour either mannitol or hypertonic saline in this population. Their use is reserved for intracranial hypertension with an impending herniation. Care should be taken to maintain the hydration status of these patients because intravascular dehydration can worsen the viscosity of the blood, potentiating the propagation of cerebral and systemic thrombosis in these patients.
2. *Role of Steroids in the Treatment of Elevated ICP*

   There is no role for glucocorticoid therapy in treating intracranial hypertension in patients with CSVT [8]. No RCTs have evaluated their efficacy in treating patients with CSVT with elevated ICP. ISCVT-cohort analysis showed that glucocorticoids did not offer any benefit, even in the presence of a parenchymal lesion [21]. It is reasonable to continue steroid therapy only in patients with CSVT secondary to inflammatory disorders such as systemic lupus erythematosus and Bechet's disease to treat the underlying disease pathology [22–24].
3. *The Role of CSF Drainage in Patients with Intracranial Hypertension Secondary to CSVT*

   CSF drainage by lumbar puncture can be considered in patients with isolated intracranial hypertension without oedema or mass lesions. CSVT can increase the resistance to CSF absorption, resulting in isolated intracranial hypertension. These patients will not have any obvious radiological abnormalities and will present with elevated ICP and papilledema. An observational study conducted on CSVT patients presenting with isolated intracranial hypertension showed complete recovery in almost 90% of patients, and almost 70% of them received a therapeutic lumbar puncture (LP) [25]. European guidelines recommend therapeutic LP or some form of CSF diversion (shunt procedures) in patients with CSVT presenting with isolated intracranial hypertension, as it prevents vision loss and remarkably improves headache [8].

6.4 Controversies Regarding Reperfusion Strategies for CSVT

The reperfusion strategy aims to establish flow in the thrombosed veins and sinuses at the earliest, thereby preventing fatal consequences of venous thrombosis, such as haemorrhage and infarction. The modalities of endovascular intervention used for reperfusion include transarterial lysis, transvenous thrombectomy (stent retrievers/aspiration), and catheter-directed thrombolysis (alone or in conjunction with thrombectomy). Unlike arterial stroke, reperfusion of the blocked vascular territory is not being done routinely in CSVT due to the lack of widespread evidence in the literature and the fear of haemorrhagic complications in the setting of CSVT. Some of the controversies associated with reperfusion strategies in CSVT are given in Box 6.3.

Box 6.3: Controversies Regarding Reperfusion Strategies in CSVT

1. Is reperfusion of CSVT a therapeutic option?
2. Indications for EVT
3. Is EVT effective as monotherapy?
4. Is there an ideal time for EVT

6.4.1 Role of EVT in CSVT

Transarterial lysis of the CVT is no longer performed, as it is not beneficial and is associated with severe complications. Siddiqui et al. performed a systematic review of all cases of CSVT in which transvenous mechanical thrombectomy was performed with or without intra-sinus thrombolysis. The results of their review showed that endovascular therapy (EVT) resulted in faster and more consistent recanalisation and was associated with good neurological recovery (84% of patients had a modified Rankin scale of 1–2). A new or increased intracerebral haemorrhage was the major complication (approximately 10%). Therefore, they concluded that EVT can be safely performed [26]. A similar review of 235 patients with CVT showed radiographic resolution in 69% of patients with a complication rate of 8.7% (new/worsening intracerebral haemorrhage) [27].

The TO-ACT (Thrombolysis or Anticoagulation for Cerebral Venous Thrombosis) trial was a multicentre RCT conducted in patients with a high risk of poor outcomes. Patients randomly received either EVT along with standard therapy or guideline-based standard therapy. There was no significant improvement in functional outcomes in the EVT group compared with standard therapy [28]. Two more systematic reviews were done, which showed that EVT can be a safe procedure in selective patients and can improve neurological outcomes [29]. The therapy was effective when the endovascular thrombectomy was combined with venous sinus thrombolysis and standard therapy [30].

6.4.2 Recommendations for EVT in Patients with Severe CSVT

Endovascular recanalisation can be considered for patients with CSVT who deteriorate after adequate anticoagulation on a case basis, those with contraindications to standard therapy, or those with risk factors for poor outcomes (CVT prognosis score $\geq$ 3) [31]. Also, it was more effective in the acute phase within the first 24 hours. The procedure should be performed in a specialised neuro-interventional setup after discussion with a multidisciplinary team. Combined therapies (thrombectomy with thrombolysis and anticoagulation) are more effective, and no studies have shown any superiority among the devices used for thrombectomy (aspiration catheter, microcatheter, aspiration systems, and stent retriever) [7].

6.5 Controversies Regarding Decompressive Craniectomy (DC) for Severe CSVT

Four per cent of patients with supratentorial haemorrhagic venous infarctions due to CSVT develop high intracranial pressure and present with the clinical and radiological features of brain herniation. Brain herniation is a common cause of mortality in CSVT patients. Various retrospective studies have shown that the mortality rate in CSVT ranges from 11–30%. Low venous collateral score, malignancy, and small juxtacortical haemorrhage (concave haemorrhage measuring <20 mm on the cortical surface) are the primary independent risk factors contributing to the development of intracranial herniation in patients with CVST.

As collateral venous drainage decreases, hydrostatic pressure in the cortical vein increases, leading to brain oedema and haemorrhage; hence, a low venous collateral score is an independent predictor of brain herniation. Juxtacortical haemorrhage is seen at the junction of the superficial and deep venous drainage systems, and it is specific for patients with cortical vein thrombosis and superior sagittal sinus thrombosis. The cortical vein drains into the superior sagittal vein; hence, thrombosis involving the cortical or superior sagittal vein increases the hydrostatic pressure in the cortical vein, leading to the rupture of those veins and causing juxtacortical haemorrhage.

Decompressive craniectomy (DC) is performed in CVST patients to prevent the progression of brain herniation leading to brain death. It helps to improve the cortical collateral venous drainage, thereby helping to reduce the ICP and improve the cerebral perfusion pressure (CPP). Patients undergoing DC for CSVT have a better prognosis than those undergoing DC for stroke. This could be due to its pathology; DC for CSVT is performed due to venous congestion-induced venous infarct, while it is performed for ischaemic stroke due to cytotoxic oedema-induced arterial infarct. The role of DC for traumatic brain injury (TBI) and stroke is well established based on RCTs, but for CSVT, the recommendation is based on various small retrospective and small prospective cohort studies and case series [32–36]. RCT is unavailable because of its rarity and ethical reasons; hence, DC is considered Class

IIb; Level of Evidence C; to improve outcomes and reduce mortality in patients with malignant CSVT [37]. Controversies regarding DC for severe CSVT are shown in Box 6.4.

Box 6.4: Controversies Regarding DC for Severe CSVT

1. Indications for Decompressive Craniectomy: Clinical vs. radiological signs
2. Type of DC Technique: External or internal decompression technique for CSVT
3. Timing of DC: Prophylactic Vs therapeutic to reduce the ICP for malignant CSVT
4. Timing of re-initiation of anticoagulation after DC

1. *Indications for Decompressive Craniectomy: Clinical vs. Radiological Signs of Elevated ICP*

   Rapid deterioration of consciousness with signs of raised ICP (hypertension, bradycardia, pupillary abnormality, and abnormal respiration) despite all medical measures is a *clinical indication* for DC. The presence of venous infarction with significant oedema causes a mass effect on the underlying brain with midline shift >5 mm, uncal herniation, effacement of basal cisterns, and hypodensity in the PCA territory due to herniation, causing PCA territory ischaemia, is a *radiological indication* for decompressive craniectomy (DC). The decision to proceed with DC should be based on clinical and radiological factors [33]. In a recent prospective international cohort study, *Decompressive Surgery for Patients with Cerebral Venous Thrombosis, Part 2 (DECOMPRESS-2)*, 118 consecutive CVT patients with severe symptoms, including coma (31%), dilated pupil(s) (18%), large haemorrhagic/ischaemic lesions with a median maximal diameter 6.5 cm, and imaging evidence of impending herniation (37%) were subjected to DC and were evaluated at discharge and at 6 and 12 months after surgery. Two-thirds (66%) of the patients with severe CVT were alive, and more than one-third (37%) were independent at 12 months after DC. Based on the results of this study, DC is indicated in patients with CSVT who present with signs of an impending herniation [38].
2. *Type of Decompressive Craniectomy*

   DC involves a large frontotemporoparietal bone flap removal (12 × 15 × 15 cm in length) extending into the temporal floor or a bifrontal bone flap removal with a dural opening with or without duroplasty. This surgical technique is referred to as external decompression. Bone flap removal combined with resection of infarcted cerebral tissue or selective decompression of a haematoma is termed internal decompression. External decompression is commonly performed for CSVT-induced brain herniation. However, both techniques have been shown to improve the outcome [32–34].

3. *Timing of Decompressive Craniectomy*

   From the year 2000 to the present, various studies (retrospective and prospective cohort studies) have shown a definitive improvement in functional outcomes after DC in selective patients with CSVT, with signs and symptoms of raised ICP or those who fail to improve despite medical measures. Mahale et al. [39] showed that DC is a lifesaving intervention in patients with malignant CVST. More than two-thirds of the patients showed favourable outcomes. In that study, they showed that patients with CSVT with age > 50 years, midline shift >10 mm, and total effacement of basal cisterns are some of the predictors of poor outcomes following DC for CSVT [39]. Few case reports and meta-analyses [36, 40] have shown that even in patients with a significant increase in ICP causing bilateral dilatation of the pupil, performing DC improved the outcome. Jose M Ferro demonstrated that patients with low GCS at presentation and bilateral lesions showed poor functional outcomes (mRS 3–5) following DC [40]. A retrospective study comparing medical treatment versus medical treatment and DC showed 100% mortality with medical treatment compared to 23% with medical treatment and DC [41]. Prophylactic DC is not indicated in patients who show improvement in medical measures.
4. *Timing of Reinitiation of Anticoagulation Therapy After DC*

   Despite the lack of high-quality studies, a systematic review involving a large case series has shown that patients with CVST undergoing DC, anticoagulation therapy, can safely resume after 48 hours. Smaller case series have shown that starting anticoagulation with half the therapeutic dose or at a prophylactic dose, even at 12 hours after DC, did not increase morbidity [42]. The authors recommended that anticoagulation be safely initiated or resumed 24–48 hours postoperatively after DC for CSVT (Box 6.5).

6.6 Controversies Regarding CVT Management During Pregnancy and Puerperium

Box 6.5 Controversies Regarding CVT Management During Pregnancy and Puerperium

1. Imaging modalities for the diagnosis of CVT during pregnancy
2. Differences in managing CVT during pregnancy and puerperium compared to non-pregnant women
3. Safety of future pregnancies in patients with a previous h/o CVT

Pregnancy is a prothrombotic state associated with an increased risk of CVT. Pregnancy- and puerperium-associated CVT accounts for 5–20% of all CVT cases. Venous strokes cause 6–64% of all maternal strokes during pregnancy and puerperium. The incidence of pregnancy and puerperium-associated CVT ranges from 1 in 2500 deliveries to 1 in 10,000 deliveries in Western countries (OR 1.3–13.0). In Asian countries, the reported incidence is high, ranging from 400 to 500/100,000 deliveries. The third trimester and first 4–6 weeks of the puerperium period are the most significant periods of risk for CVT. Apart from the physiological changes that promote a prothrombotic state during pregnancy, dehydration, excessive vomiting, prolonged bed rest, pregnancy-induced hypertension, lower segment caesarean section, anaemia, infection, younger age (14–25 years), and genetic factors of thrombophilia are some of the independent risk factors for the development of obstetric CVT [43, 44].

Gazioglu S et al. [45] compared the clinical and radiological presentation and risk factors and the prognosis of CVT occurring during pregnancy and puerperium with non-pregnant women. Eighty per cent of CVT occurred during the puerperal period, especially during the first 4 weeks after delivery. The remaining 20% of cases occurred during the third trimester. Patients in the pregnant and puerperium groups were younger compared to non-pregnant women; apart from this, all other clinical, radiological, and other risk factors, including genetic thrombophilia, were comparable between the groups. Hence, they recommended screening for additional risk factors, such as genetic thrombophilia, in patients presenting with CVT during pregnancy and puerperium. This study also compared the functional outcome using mRS; more patients in the pregnancy and puerperium groups had better functional outcomes (mRS score 0–2) than the non-pregnant group. However, the difference was not statistically significant because of a smaller sample size.

1. *Radiological Imaging to Confirm CVT During Pregnancy*

   Regarding imaging techniques for diagnosing CSVT/CVT during pregnancy, it is important to choose a method that yields the maximum potential for diagnosis while minimising ionising radiation and avoiding the use of intravenous contrast agents, including gadolinium. Magnetic resonance imaging (MRI) and magnetic resonance venography (MRV) using non-contrast techniques such as 2-dimensional (2D) time-of-flight or 3D phase-contrast venography are reliable tools for detecting thrombosis involving the sinuses and large cerebral veins. SWI and diffusion-weighted imaging (DWI) sequences of MRI help diagnose CVT without contrast in the acute and subacute stages. Computed tomography (CT) venography is a reliable alternative to MRV in patients with contraindications to MRV or in centres lacking MRI facilities.
2. *Differences in the Management of CVT During Pregnancy and Puerperium Between Pregnant and Non-pregnant Women*

   Managing CVT during pregnancy and puerperium requires a multidisciplinary team approach involving an obstetrician, neurologist, and neurosurgeon. The care includes general supportive care with analgesics, adequate hydration, and management of elevated intracranial pressure with anti-oedema measures, seizures with anti-seizure medication, and prevention of progression of thrombosis with anticoagulation management using LMWH with enoxaparin, as it has a long plasma half-life and high bioavailability. It does not cross the placenta nor is it secreted into breast milk [8]. Oral anticoagulants such as VKA (warfarin) and direct-acting oral anticoagulants (apixaban, edoxaban, rivaroxaban, and dabigatran) and unfractionated heparin are contraindicated as they can cause foetal embryopathy and bleeding in the foetus and neonates during pregnancy and puerperium [7, 46, 47]. endovascular therapy (EVT) and DC should be offered for life-threatening and debilitating cases of obstetric CSVT that fail to improve with anticoagulation measures, to save the lives of mothers. A case report in which the authors performed a literature review reported 12 cases of malignant CSVT for which endovascular thrombectomy was performed. Almost 75% of the patients (9/12) had good functional outcomes (mRS -0–2). No RCT is available comparing the outcomes following endovascular thrombectomy and conventional anticoagulation management because of ethical issues and the rarity of the disease. Radiation exposure to the foetus during an endovascular procedure is minimal because of the distance between the mother's head and the uterus. The absorbed foetal radiation dose during EVT is approximately 2.8 mGy, which has little effect on the foetus. Kashkoush K et al. [48] in their pooled systematic review on CVT during pregnancy and puerperium concluded that clinical status at the time of treatment is the most important predictive factor for excellent outcomes. Hence, early diagnosis and treatment with anticoagulation before clinical deterioration are needed to achieve a good outcome. They also suggested that intra-arterial thrombolysis with mechanical thrombectomy is a safe and effective adjunct to anticoagulation for patients who are moribund or have clot propagation.

Although the prognosis for obstetric CVT is better than that for other causes of stroke, the reported mortality rate varies from 4% to 33%. Patients presenting with an acute fulminant course, bilateral haemorrhagic venous infarction, and diffuse cerebral oedema with a low Glasgow coma scale score (GCS <9), involvement of the deep cerebral venous system, and underlying systemic diseases such as malignancy and systemic infection have a poor prognosis.

3. *Safety of Future Pregnancies in Women with Previous h/o CVT*

The ISCVT-2 Pregnancy Study is the most extensive study to evaluate the safety of pregnancy after CVT [49]. They found that the incidence of recurrent CVT during subsequent pregnancies was 12 per 1000 with a 95% CI of 2–66%. In that study, the authors found that among the 82 pregnancies, one patient developed CVT during the first trimester (10 weeks), with the identified risk factors of oral contraceptive use and protein S deficiency. The patient received a prophylactic dose of LMWH at the time of CVT diagnosis. Pregnancy is further complicated by intrauterine growth restriction and preterm labour. The mother received a therapeutic dose of LMWH after the diagnosis of CVT and recovered fully without any neurological sequelae during further follow-up [49]. The incidence of noncerebral VTE is approximately 24 per 1000 pregnancies (95% CI, 7–85). The incidence of spontaneous abortion was 17%, which was significantly lower in patients who received heparin during the first trimester. The study concluded that prior CVT was not a contraindication for future pregnancies. A systematic review (17 studies and 393 pregnancies) found that the recurrence rate for CVT was 8 per 1000 pregnancies (95% CI, 3–22) and for the noncerebral VTEs was 22 per 1000 pregnancies (95% CI, 11–43) (Fig. 6.1).

There was a trend toward a lower rate of recurrent thrombotic events and spontaneous abortions in women who received antithrombotic prophylaxis during pregnancy and puerperium with LMWH. Considering the results of various studies and the meta-analysis, pregnancy is not contraindicated in women with a history of CVT (Box 6.6).

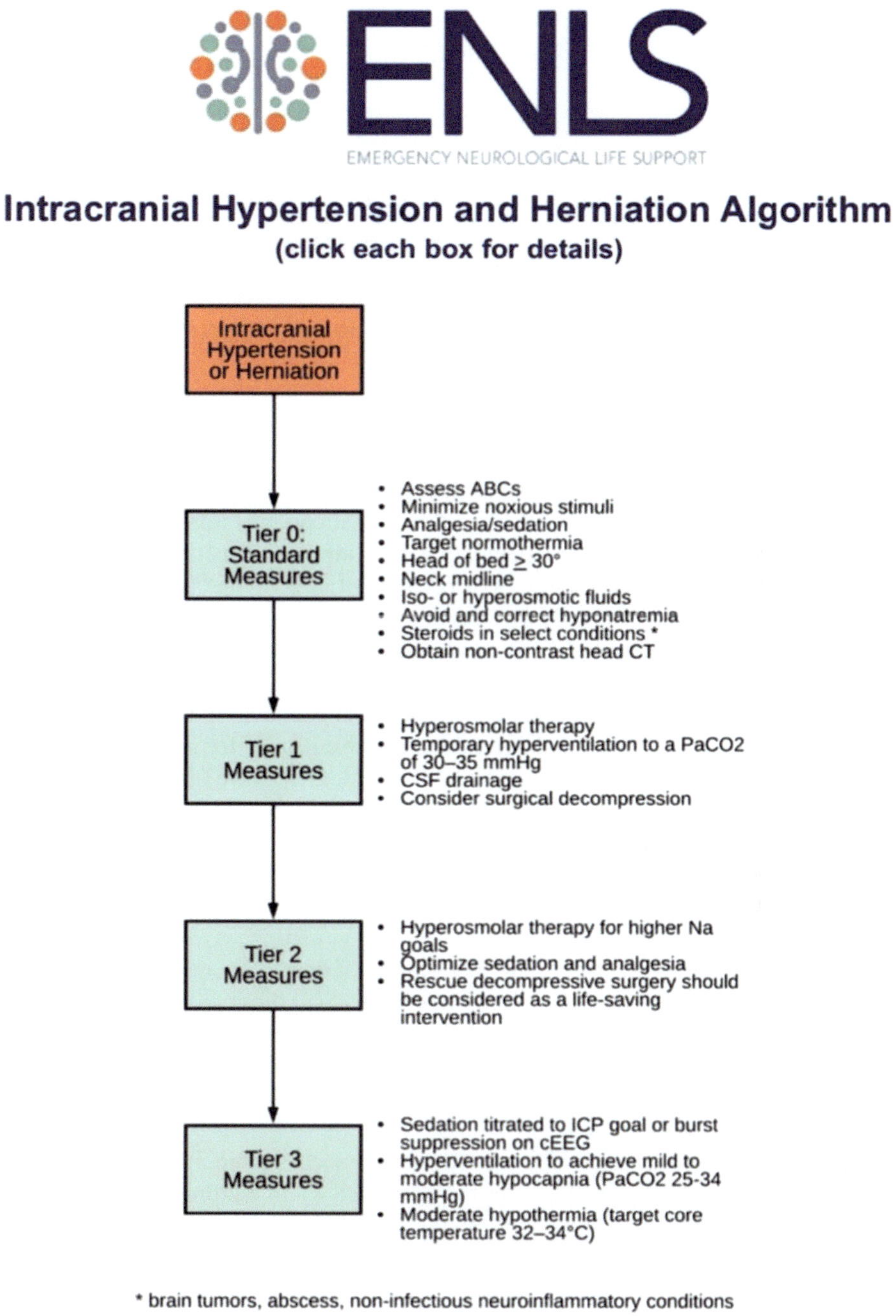

Fig. 6.1 Emergency neurological life support—intracranial hypertension and herniation algorithm

6.7 Controversies Involved in Paediatric and Neonatal CSVT Diagnosis and Management

Box 6.6: Controversies Involved in Paediatric and Neonatal CSVT Diagnosis and Management

1. Safety of anticoagulation in the acute phase of CSVT in children
2. Efficacy of anticoagulation during the acute phase of CSVT
3. Anticoagulation regimen
4. The duration of anticoagulation

1. *Safety of Anticoagulation*

   Studies have shown that children and neonates with or without ICH treated with anticoagulation have lower mortality rates. (Class IIa evidence in children and Class IIb evidence in neonates). The International Paediatric Stroke Study (IPSS)—CSVT cohort analysis showed that children (aged >28 days to 19 years) with CSVT treated with anticoagulation had improved functional outcomes at discharge and long-term follow-up. Children with CSVT due to trauma or intracranial surgery are less likely to receive anticoagulation therapy. Children who present with an infarct are likely to have an unfavourable outcome [50].

   There is variable practice worldwide regarding anticoagulation treatment for neonates. Conservative management without anticoagulation is practised in the USA, whereas LMWH or unfractionated heparin is used for anticoagulation in Canada and Europe. Neonates with CSVT without ICH have been shown to have decreased mortality. Pre-treatment ICH, elevated systemic blood pressure, thrombocytopenia, and supratherapeutic anticoagulant regimen cerebral atrophy are the risk factors for increased bleeding in children who are on anticoagulation for CSVT [51] (Class I, level of evidence B).
2. *Efficacy of Anticoagulation*

   Children treated with anticoagulants have a reduced risk of thrombus propagation and enhanced recanalisation. The incidence of thrombus propagation was 37% in untreated children treated with anticoagulants and decreased to 7% in children treated with anticoagulants. Anticoagulation treatment reduces the incidence of clot propagation in neonates from 25–30% to 3%.
3. *Duration of Anticoagulation*

   Studies have shown that 50% of recurrences occur within 3 months, and two-thirds occur within 6 months after the initial CSVT in children. Hence, a 3–6-month period has been proposed as the standard duration of anticoagulation therapy in most studies in children. CSVT in neonates is often due to acute obstetric causes without any systemic illness; the recanalisation rate is faster, and the recurrence rate is lower. Hence, neonates require a shorter anticoagulation duration of approximately 6–12 weeks. Children aged >2 years with a chronic thrombogenic pathology and failure to recanalise after 6 months, especially those carrying the F2 mutation, are at high risk for recurrence. These children often need prolonged anticoagulation or prophylactic anticoagulation when there is another risk factor found, such as dehydration and prolonged immobilisation [52, 53].

4. *Types of Anticoagulation:* There are no data comparing the safety and efficacy of a particular anticoagulant agent for treating paediatric CSVT. Children with CSVT are often treated with unfractionated heparin (UFH) (target APTT 60-85), low-molecular-weight heparin (LMWH) (Xa level 0.4–1 U/ml) during the acute stage, followed by oral anticoagulation with warfarin to maintain the INR between 2 and 3 or by continuing the LMWH. Recently, DOAC has been non-inferior to VKA regarding safety and efficacy in children with CSVT/CVT. EINSTEIN-Jr CVT study studied the safety and effectiveness of rivaroxaban in paediatric CVT and showed that rivaroxaban is safe, with the risk of VTE recurrence and clinically relevant bleeding being low in the rivaroxaban group [54].

6.8 Controversies Involved in the Accurate Diagnosis of CSVT/CVT Using Various Radiological Imaging

Box 6.7: Controversies Involved in the Accurate Diagnosis of CSVT/CVT Using Various Radiological Imaging

1. Which diagnostic modality is superior for the accurate diagnosis?: Computed tomography (CT) based Vs. magnetic resonance imaging (MRI) based Vs. digital subtraction angiography (DSA) based imaging modalities for accurate diagnosis.
2. What are the newer modalities of radiological imaging for the diagnosis of CSVT?

Diagnosing CSVT/CVT based on clinical presentation is often challenging because of varied atypical presentations. This requires a high degree of suspicion in high-risk patients. Radiological imaging modalities are crucial for establishing a definitive diagnosis, treatment progression, and the diagnosis of CSVT-related complications. Recently, various CT and MRI-based techniques have been used to establish diagnosis [7, 55–57]. Subacute to chronic haemorrhage appears hypodense on CT and shows a rim-like contrast enhancement. It is often misdiagnosed as an abscess, which delays the treatment of CSVT. Hence, multiple imaging modalities must be utilised and clinically correlated for correct diagnosis. Thorough knowledge of the various imaging modalities, their principles, imaging findings, and the advantages and disadvantages of each imaging modality will help neurointensive care physicians choose an appropriate test with high sensitivity and specificity. Studies have shown that a delay in diagnosis or misdiagnosis can lead to deleterious consequences. Table 6.1 discusses the various imaging modalities, their findings

Table 6.1 Showing various CT and MRI-based diagnostic modalities and their findings

Various CT technologies for diagnosing CSVT and CVT		
Non-contrast CT brain	*Direct signs:* Direct visualisation of thrombus on thin-slice CT. *Dense vessel sign or dense clot sign*: increase in protein factor of haemoglobin within the red blood cells; this sign is *specific to venous sinus thrombosis.* *Dense triangle sign:* Hyperattenuation in sagittal sinus or deep cerebral veins in a triangle shape. *Cord or string sign*—serpiginous or linear hyperdensity within a vein: *specific to cortical venous thrombosis.* *Attenuated vein sign*: hyperattenuated appearance of the affected veins, *specific to deep venous sinus thrombosis*	*Advantages:* Easily available even in small hospitals. Fast; hence, diagnosis is not delayed. Reduced motion artefact. *Disadvantages:* Radiation hazards; Use of contrast medium and its complications, Poor detection of small parenchymal abnormalities. Low sensitivity in small cortical and deep thrombosis. High haematocrit values can cause hyperattenuation of a vein which results in a false positive diagnosis of CVT. Anaemia may result in false negative diagnosis. Subacute thrombosis (7–14 days) also result in a false negative diagnoses since the density of thrombi gets attenuated over time and becomes isodense or even hypodense. Based on the recent meta-analysis overall, CT has a sensitivity of 0.79 (95% CI, 0.76–0.82) and specificity of 0.90 (95% CI, 0.89–0.91) for diagnosing cortical venous thrombosis. For the diagnosis of sinus venous thrombosis, the pooled sensitivity and specificity of CT were 81% (95%CI 78–84%) and 89% (95%CI 88–91%), respectively. Widespread availability and cost effectiveness is an advantage of the CTV. CTV was found to be reliable for diagnosing sinus venous thrombosis with a sensitivity and specificity of both 100% CTV has a lower sensitivity (6–75%) for diagnosing cortical vein thrombosis
Contrast-enhanced—CT brain	*Direct Signs:* after administration of contrast, the *presence of filling defects* indicates venous sinus thrombosis. *Empty delta sign or dense triangle sign:* Thrombosed sinus seen as triangular area of enhancement with relatively low-attenuation centre– *specific to superior sagittal sinus thrombosis.* *Indirect Signs: Unilateral hypodensity*- not conforming to the arterial territories or sparing the overlying cortex. *Bilateral hypodensities:* Bilateral parasagittal hemispheric hypodense lesions—*specific to superior sagittal sinus thrombosis;* Bilateral thalamic hypodensity - *specific to deep cerebral vein thrombosis* Temporo-occipital hypodensity - *specific for transverse sinus thrombosis* *Haemorrhagic transformation*- within regions of hypodensity. *Intracerebral haemorrhage*- (40%) associated with subarachnoid or subdural haemorrhages. *Cashew nut sign, a juxtacortical C-shaped hyperdensity- (12%)* at the junction of superficial and deep venous system—*specific for cortical venous thrombosis with sagittal sinus thrombosis*	
CT- venography (CTV)-	*Mass effects*: CTV is a *contrast-enhanced* *helical CT examination performed with a time-optimised contrast bolus*, allows direct visualization of a thrombosed cerebral vein. *Filling defects* in the superficial and deep venous system indicates thrombosis. *"Empty delta sign"* in CTV is specific to superior sagittal sinus thrombosis. The *'missing cortical vein'* due to contrast filling defect is often difficult to distinguish from physiological variations in venous anatomy	
Newer CT techniques Multidetector row CT (MDCT) State of the art techniques include mask-subtraction and dual energy Photon-counting CT	MDCT—Thin slices are obtained with the use of less contrast and shorter scanning time allowing better image quality without significantly increasing overall radiation dose. With mask-subtraction, a low-dose non-enhanced CT is subtracted from the contrast-enhanced vascular (CTV) acquisition. With dual-energy techniques, bone removal is obtained by postprocessing a dual-energy CT data set that is simultaneously acquired with a low and high kilovoltage, where difference in x-ray absorption of different materials depends on x-ray energy Improved visualization of CVT using this technique	

Subacute and chronic CVT	Isodense and hypodense on CT with rim-like contrast enhancement. It is often misdiagnosed as abscess	
Various magnetic resonance based imaging technique for diagnosing venous sinus thrombosis (VST) and CVT		
Non-contrast-enhanced flow related MRI (a) Time-of-flight MRV (TOF MRV) (2D or 3D) (b) Phase-contrast MRV (PC MRV)	Absence of normal flow patterns indicates thrombosis Flow related enhancement, sensitive to low flow, time-of-flight (TOF) MRV technique is highly reliable for diagnosing VST and CVT involving larger cerebral veins. It is not sensitive for diagnosing CVT involving smaller veins. Works on the principle of velocity induced phase shift of spins	*Advantages:* No ionizing radiation exposure, contrast medium not needed for TOF and phase-contrast sequence MRI. Good visualization of brain parenchyma Good for detection of cortical and deep cerebral vein thrombosis. Non-contrast-enhanced MRI is the imaging modality of choice in pregnant patients and patients with breast feeding. *Disadvantages of MRI techniques:* Time consuming Motion artefact can degrade images. Reduced availability Contraindicated in some patients (Cardiac devices, medically unstable) A meta-analysis showed conventional MRI sequences have sensitivity of 0.82 (95% CI, 0.78–0.85) and specificity of 0.92 (95% CI, 0.91–0.94) in diagnosing CVT
Native contrast thrombus MRI	The presence of paramagnetic deoxyhaemoglobin, methaemoglobin, or hemosiderin indicates thrombosis. On MRI of the brain—visualization of the thrombus in the T1-weighted images. *In the acute phase* (first 5 days after CVT) the thrombus is isointense on T1W images and hypointense on T2W images. *In the subacute phase* (from 5 to 15 days), the thrombus becomes hyperintense on T1W and T2W images. *In the chronic phase* (after 15 days, it becomes homogeneous and isointense on T1W imaging, and iso to hyperintense on T2W image	
MR—Black blood thrombus Imaging	It is a native contrast thrombus imaging, which helps to differentiate the acute and chronic CVT	
Contrast-enhanced MRV	Presence of filling defect indicates thrombosis. The diagnostic performance of contrast-enhanced MRV was better than that of non-contrast-enhanced TOF and PC MRV	
Gradient recalled Echo susceptibility weighted (GRE-SWI) images	Blood breakdown products such as (methaemoglobin, deoxyhaemoglobin) can cause exaggerated signal drop-out by which the thrombus is detected	
Brush sign in paramagnetic sensitive MRI brain sequences	Brush sign is abnormal hypointensity of the subependymal and deep medullary veins seen in thrombosis involving the deep venous system. The deep medullary veins are located adjacent to the atrium and posterior body of the lateral ventricle, draining the white matter of the cerebral hemispheres to the subependymal veins of the lateral ventricles. Brush sign indicates higher thrombus load and ipsilateral parenchymal lesions. This sign may be a marker of CVT severity. These patients need close monitoring during the acute phase of CVT	
Digital subtraction angiography (DSA)	DSA is not routinely indicated for the diagnosis of sinus venous thrombosis (SVT) or CVT. DSA is indicated only when the therapeutic intervention is planned	*Advantages:* Considered gold standard test for diagnosing CVT. *Disadvantages:* The incidence of neurologic complications following DSA is about 1.3%. The incidence of permanent neurological damage is about 0.5%. Radiation exposure, allergic reaction, and iodinated contrast agents induced nephrotoxicity

and the advantages and disadvantages of each modality. Among all modalities, CT Venography and contrast-enhanced MR venography are optimal tests for confirming the diagnosis of CVT with high sensitivity and specificity. Although digital subtraction angiography (DSA) is the gold standard, it is used only when invasive treatment is considered because of the associated complications (Box 6.7).

6.9 Conclusion

Anticoagulation is the mainstay of treatment for patients with CSVT, even in the presence of haemorrhage. Based on recent evidence, LMWH is the drug of choice in the acute stage, except in patients with a definite contraindication for use or in whom urgent reversal is needed. Oral anticoagulants (VKAs or DOACs) are started after the initial bridging with heparin. There is a recent trend towards selecting DOACs over warfarin because of their better safety profiles. There are no current recommendations regarding the start of DOACs without lead in heparin in the acute stage and no specific DOAC over others. Its selection depends on risk factors for CSVT and the associated comorbidities. Current guidelines recommend 3 months to lifelong administration of anticoagulation, depending on the cause of CSVT (provoked/unprovoked), except for neonatal CSVT, in which short-term anticoagulation for 6–12 weeks is warranted.

Regarding the management of intracranial hypertension, a three-tiered approach is followed; no specific osmotherapeutic agents are recommended, and there is no role for steroids. DC is recommended for severe CSVT with clinical and radiological signs of impending herniation. EVT is indicated for patients who deteriorate rapidly and fail to recanalise despite adequate anticoagulation therapy. The availability of various new modes of radiological imaging aids in diagnosing and assessing treatment progression, reducing morbidity and mortality.

References

1. Saposnik G, Barinagarrementeria F, Brown RD, Bushnell CD, Cucchiara B, Cushman M, et al. Diagnosis and management of cerebral venous thrombosis: a statement for healthcare professionals from the American Heart Association/American Stroke Association. Stroke. 2011;42(4):1158–92.
2. Ferro JM, Canhão P, Stam J, Bousser MG, Barinagarrementeria F. ISCVT Investigators. Prognosis of cerebral vein and dural sinus thrombosis: results of an international study on cerebral vein and dural sinus thrombosis (ISCVT). Stroke. 2004;35(3):664–70.
3. Einhäupl KM, Masuhr F. Cerebral venous and sinus thrombosis – an update. Eur J Neurol. 1994;1(2):109–26.
4. de Bruijn SF, Stam J. Randomised placebo-controlled trial ofanticoagulantt treatment with low-molecular-weight heparin for cerebral sinus thrombosis. Stroke. 1999;30(3):484–8.
5. Misra UK, Kalita J, Chandra S, Kumar B, Bansal V. Low molecular weight heparin versus unfractionated heparin in cerebral venous sinus thrombosis: a randomized controlled trial. Eur J Neurol. 2012;19(7):1030–6.

6. Coutinho JM, Ferro JM, Canhão P, Barinagarrementeria F, Bousser MG, Stam J, et al. Unfractionated or low-molecular weight heparin for the treatment of cerebral venous thrombosis. Stroke. 2010;41(11):2575–80.
7. Saposnik G, Bushnell C, Coutinho JM, Field TS, Furie KL, Galadanci N, et al. Diagnosis and Management of Cerebral Venous Thrombosis: a scientific statement from the American Heart Association. Stroke. 2024;55(3):e77–90.
8. Ferro JM, Bousser MG, Canhão P, Coutinho JM, Crassard I, Dentali F, et al. European stroke organization guideline for the diagnosis and treatment of cerebral venous thrombosis – endorsed by the European academy of neurology. Eur J Neurol. 2017;24(10):1203–13.
9. Ferro JM, Coutinho JM, Dentali F, Kobayashi A, Alasheev A, Canhão P, et al. Safety and efficacy of dabigatran Etexilate vs dose-adjusted warfarin in patients with cerebral venous thrombosis: a randomized clinical trial. JAMA Neurol. 2019;76(12):1457–65.
10. Bharath SP, Arshad H, Song YB, Kirmani JF. Long-term anticoagulation with Apixaban in patients with cerebral venous thrombosis. Clin Appl Thromb. 2023;29:10760296221129591.
11. Field TS, Dizonno V, Almekhlafi MA, Bala F, Alhabli I, Wong H, et al. Study of rivaroxaban for cerebral venous thrombosis: a randomized controlled feasibility trial comparing anticoagulation with rivaroxaban to standard-of-Care in Symptomatic Cerebral Venous Thrombosis. Stroke. 2023;54(11):2724–36.
12. Nepal G, Kharel S, Bhagat R, Ka Shing Y, Ariel Coghlan M, Poudyal P, et al. Safety and efficacy of direct OralAnticoagulantss in cerebral venous thrombosis: a meta-analysis. Acta Neurol Scand. 2022;145(1):10–23.
13. Yaghi S, Shu L, Bakradze E, Salehi Omran S, Giles JA, Amar JY, et al. Direct OralAnticoagulantss versus warfarin in the treatment of cerebral venous thrombosis (ACTION-CVT): a Multicenter international study. Stroke. 2022;53(3):728–38.
14. Fayyaz M, Abbas F, Kashif T. The role of warfarin and rivaroxaban in the treatment of cerebral venous thrombosis. Cureus. 2019;11(5):e4589.
15. Ma H, Gu Y, Bian T, Song H, Liu Z, Ji X, et al. Dabigatran etexilate versus warfarin in cerebral venous thrombosis in Chinese patients (CHOICE-CVT): an open-label, randomized controlled trial. Int J Stroke Off J Int Stroke Soc. 2024:17474930241234749.
16. Wasay M, Khan M, Rajput HM, Farooq S, Memon MI, AlRukn SA, et al. New OralAnticoagulantss versus warfarin for cerebral venous thrombosis: a multi-Center. Observational Study J Stroke. 2019;21(2):220–3.
17. Shankar Iyer R, Tcr R, Akhtar S, Muthukalathi K, Kumar P, Muthukumar K. Is it safe to treat cerebral venous thrombosis with oral rivaroxaban without heparin? A preliminary study from 20 patients. Clin Neurol Neurosurg. 2018;175:108–11.
18. Simes J, Becattini C, Agnelli G, Eikelboom JW, Kirby AC, Mister R, et al. Aspirin for the prevention of recurrent venous thromboembolism: the INSPIRE collaboration. Circulation. 2014;130(13):1062–71.
19. Ameri A, Bousser MG. Cerebral venous thrombosis. Neurol Clin. 1992;10(1):87–111.
20. Khan M, Kamal AK, Wasay M. Controversies of treatment modalities for cerebral venous thrombosis. Stroke Res Treat. 2010;2010:956302.
21. Canhão P, Cortesão A, Cabral M, Ferro JM, Stam J, Bousser MG, et al. Are steroids useful to treat cerebral venous thrombosis? Stroke. 2008;39(1):105–10.
22. Hatemi G, Silman A, Bang D, Bodaghi B, Chamberlain AM, Gul A, et al. Management of Behçet disease: a systematic literature review for the European league against rheumatism evidence-based recommendations for the management of Behçet disease. Ann Rheum Dis. 2009;68(10):1528–34.
23. Vidailhet M, Piette JC, Wechsler B, Bousser MG, Brunet P. Cerebral venous thrombosis in systemic lupus erythematosus. Stroke. 1990;21(8):1226–31.
24. Aguiar de Sousa D, Mestre T, Ferro JM. Cerebral venous thrombosis in Behçet's disease: a systematic review. J Neurol. 2011;258(5):719–27.
25. Biousse V, Ameri A, Bousser MG. Isolated intracranial hypertension as the only sign of cerebral venous thrombosis. Neurology. 1999;53(7):1537–42.

26. Siddiqui FM, Dandapat S, Banerjee C, Zuurbier SM, Johnson M, Stam J, et al. Mechanical thrombectomy in cerebral venous thrombosis: systematic review of 185 cases. Stroke. 2015;46(5):1263–8.
27. Ilyas A, Chen CJ, Raper DM, Ding D, Buell T, Mastorakos P, et al. Endovascular mechanical thrombectomy for cerebral venous sinus thrombosis: a systematic review. J Neurointerventional Surg. 2017;9(11):1086–92.
28. Coutinho JM, Zuurbier SM, Bousser MG, Ji X, Canhão P, Roos YB, et al. Effect of endovascular treatment with medical management vs standard care on severe cerebral venous thrombosis: the TO-ACT randomized clinical trial. JAMA Neurol. 2020;77(8):966–73.
29. Bücke P, Hellstern V, Cimpoca A, Cohen JE, Horvath T, Ganslandt O, et al. Endovascular treatment of intracranial vein and venous sinus thrombosis—a systematic review. J Clin Med. 2022;11(14):4215.
30. Lewis W, Saber H, Sadeghi M, Rajah G, Narayanan S. Transvenous endovascular recanalization for cerebral venous thrombosis: a systematic review and meta-analysis. World Neurosurg. 2019;130:341–50.
31. Weimar C, Beyer-Westendorf J, Bohmann F, Hahn G, Halimeh S, Holzhauer S, et al. New recommendations on cerebral venous and dural sinus thrombosis from the German consensus-based (S2k) guideline. Neurol Res Pract. 2024;6(1):23.
32. Zuurbier SM, Coutinho JM, Majoie CBLM, Coert BA, van den Munckhof P, Stam J. Decompressive hemicraniectomy in severe cerebral venous thrombosis: a prospective case series. J Neurol. 2012;259(6):1099–105.
33. Keller E, Pangalu A, Fandino J, Könü D, Yonekawa Y. Decompressive craniectomy in severe cerebral venous and dural sinus thrombosis. Acta Neurochir Suppl. 2005;94:177–83.
34. Mohamed MWF, Aung SS, Mereddy N, Ramanan SP, Hamid P. Role, effectiveness, and outcome of Decompressive Craniectomy for cerebral venous and Dural sinus thrombosis (CVST): is surgery really an option? Cureus. 2020;12(12):e12135.
35. Qi M, Qu X, Wang N, Jiang LD, Cheng WT, Chen WJ, et al. Role of Decompressive Craniectomy in the treatment of malignant cerebral venous sinus thrombosis: a single Center consecutive case series study in China. World Neurosurg. 2024;181:e867–74.
36. Théaudin M, Crassard I, Bresson D, Saliou G, Favrole P, Vahedi K, et al. Should decompressive surgery be performed in malignant cerebral venous thrombosis?: a series of 12 patients. Stroke. 2010;41(4):727–31.
37. Lechanoine F, Janot K, Herbreteau D, Maldonado IL, Velut S. Surgical Thrombectomy combined with bilateral Decompressive Craniectomy in a life-threatening case of coma from cerebral venous sinus thrombosis: case report and literature review. World Neurosurg. 2018;120:485–9.
38. Aaron S, Ferreira JM, Coutinho JM, Canhão P, Conforto AB, Arauz A, et al. Outcomes of Decompressive surgery for patients with severe cerebral venous thrombosis: a DECOMPRESS2 observational study. Stroke. 2024;55(5):1218–26.
39. Mahale R, Mehta A, Varma RG, Hegde AS, Acharya PT, Srinivasa R. Decompressive surgery in malignant cerebral venous sinus thrombosis: what predicts its outcome? J Thromb Thrombolysis. 2017;43(4):530–9.
40. Ferro JM, Crassard I, Coutinho JM, Canhão P, Barinagarrementeria F, Cucchiara B, et al. Decompressive surgery in cerebrovenous thrombosis: a multicenter registry and a systematic review of individual patient data. Stroke. 2011;42(10):2825–31.
41. Baharvahdat H, Ahmadi S, Ganjeifar B, Etemadrezaie H, Zabyhian S, Sasannejad P, et al. Malignant cerebral venous infarction: Decompressive Craniectomy versus medical treatment. World Neurosurg. 2019;128:e918–22.
42. Salottolo K, Bartt R, Frei DF, Bellon RJ, Atchie B, McCarthy K, et al. Timing of anticoagulation in patients with cerebral venous thrombosis requiring Decompressive surgery: systematic review of the literature and case series. World Neurosurg. 2020;137:408–14.
43. Sharma N, Sharma SR, Hussain M. An audit of cerebral venous thrombosis associated with pregnancy and puerperium in teaching hospital in north eastern India. J Fam Med Prim Care. 2019;8(3):1054–7.

44. Algahtani H, Bazaid A, Shirah B, Bouges RN. Cerebral venous sinus thrombosis in pregnancy and puerperium: a comprehensive review. Brain Circ. 2022;8(4):180–7.
45. Gazioglu S, Dinc G. Cerebral venous sinus thrombosis in pregnancy and puerperium. Acta Neurol Belg. 2021;121(4):967–72.
46. Kamel H, Navi BB, Sriram N, Hovsepian DA, Devereux RB, Elkind MSV. Risk of a thrombotic event after the 6-week postpartum period. N Engl J Med. 2014;370(14):1307–15.
47. Fang T, Shu L, Elnazeir M, Zubair AS, Kasab SA, Antonenko K, et al. Characteristics and outcomes of postpartum cerebral venous sinus thrombosis: a subgroup analysis of the ACTION-CVT study. J Stroke Cerebrovasc Dis Off J Natl Stroke Assoc. 2022;31(12):106865.
48. Kashkoush AI, Ma H, Agarwal N, Panczykowski D, Tonetti D, Weiner GM, et al. Cerebral venous sinus thrombosis in pregnancy and puerperium: a pooled, systematic review. J Clin Neurosci Off J Neurosurg Soc Australas. 2017;39:9–15.
49. Aguiar de Sousa D, Canhão P, Crassard I, Coutinho J, Arauz A, Conforto A, et al. Safety of pregnancy after cerebral venous thrombosis: results of the ISCVT (international study on cerebral vein and Dural sinus thrombosis)-2 PREGNANCY study. Stroke. 2017;48(11):3130–3.
50. Felling RJ, Hassanein SMA, Armstrong J, Aversa L, Billinghurst L, Goldenberg NA, et al. Treatment and outcome of childhood cerebral sinovenous thrombosis. Neurol Clin Pract. 2020;10(3):232–44.
51. Moharir MD, Shroff M, Stephens D, Pontigon AM, Chan A, MacGregor D, et al. Anticoagulantss in pediatric cerebral sinovenous thrombosis: a safety and outcome study. Ann Neurol. 2010;67(5):590–9.
52. Kenet G, Kirkham F, Niederstadt T, Heinecke A, Saunders D, Stoll M, et al. Risk factors for recurrent venous thromboembolism in the European collaborative paediatric database on cerebral venous thrombosis: a multicentre cohort study. Lancet Neurol. 2007;6(7):595–603.
53. Lebas A, Chabrier S, Fluss J, Gordon K, Kossorotoff M, Nowak-Göttl U, et al. EPNS/SFNP guideline on theanticoagulantt treatment of cerebral sinovenous thrombosis in children and neonates. Eur J Paediatr Neurol. 2012;16(3):219–28.
54. Connor P, Sánchez van Kammen M, Lensing AWA, Chalmers E, Kállay K, Hege K, et al. Safety and efficacy of rivaroxaban in pediatric cerebral venous thrombosis (EINSTEIN-Jr CVT): for the EINSTEIN-Jr cerebral venous thrombosis trial investigators. Blood Adv. 2020;4(24):6250–8.
55. van Dam LF, van Walderveen MAA, Kroft LJM, Kruyt ND, Wermer MJH, van Osch MJP, et al. Current imaging modalities for diagnosing cerebral vein thrombosis – a critical review. Thromb Res. 2020;189:132–9.
56. Liberman AL. Diagnosis and treatment of cerebral venous thrombosis. Contin Minneap Minn. 2023;29(2):519–39.
57. Kashyap PV, Kashyap M, Dhiran A, Yadav A. Missed cerebral venous thrombosis: a diagnostic challenge. Ann Neurosci. 2023;30(3):197–204.

Controversies in the Management of Nontraumatic Weakness in the ICU

7

Prasanna Udupi Bidkar and Rajasekar Ramadurai

Abstract

Acute nontraumatic weakness has a varied etiology and presentation. Myasthenia gravis and Guillain–Barré Syndrome are the two most widely discussed diseases of this subgroup. However, their management is still riddled with a few obscurities that need validation. The choice between plasmapheresis and intravenous immunoglobin in the management of acute nontraumatic weakness, the decision to continue or withhold acetylcholinesterase inhibitors during myasthenic crisis, the Implications of the second dose of IVIg in neurocritical care, the role of non-invasive ventilation (NIV) in neuromuscular weakness, and the search for ideal weaning strategy in patients requiring ventilatory support are a few gray areas which are bound to be addressed. A comprehensive review of recent literature and recommendations from professional bodies on the above subjects has been made and presented in the following chapter.

Keywords

Acute nontraumatic weakness · Myasthenia gravis · Guillain–Barré Syndrome IVIg vs. Plasma exchange (PLEX) · Anticholinesterase · NIV in neuromuscular weakness

Acute nontraumatic weakness (ANTW) is the sudden onset of weakness in any degree in any part of the body, occurring due to a disruption in some areas of the motor pathway, from pyramidal cells to peripheral muscles. ANTW is of heterogeneous etiology, and the presentation may range from trivial weakness to

P. U. Bidkar (✉) · R. Ramadurai
JIPMER, Puducherry, Puducherry, India

P. U. Bidkar, M. Krishnakumar (eds.), *Controversies in Neurocritical Care*, https://doi.org/10.1007/978-981-95-4419-6_7

life-threatening respiratory failure and autonomic dysfunction. Likewise, the disease course is variable, and patients may deteriorate rapidly despite prompt treatment. Hence, a comprehensive clinical evaluation to localize the disease, complemented by laboratory tests and neuroimaging, is warranted [1]. Synchronous resuscitative measures, investigative workup, and evidence-based treatment strategies individualized to every condition form the cornerstones of management [2]. A list of common causes of acute nontraumatic weakness with appropriate localization is enumerated in Table 7.1. It is outside the purview of the chapter to review all the diseases in their entirety, and hence it would primarily revolve around the two most important among them: Myasthenia gravis (MG) and Guillain–Barré syndrome (GBS).

Table 7.1 List of common causes of acute nontraumatic weakness with anatomical localization

Anatomical region involved	Causes of ANTW
Brain	Intracranial mass
	Acute ischemic stroke
	Todd's paresis
	Hypertensive encephalopathy
	Hemiplegic migraine
Spinal cord	Spinal cord infarction
	Aortic dissection
	Brown Sequard syndrome
	Transverse myelitis
	Amyotrophic lateral sclerosis (ALS)
Peripheral nerves	Guillain–Barré syndrome (GBS)
	Vasculitic neuropathy
	Toxin induced neuropathy
	Heavy metal toxicity
	Nerve compression syndromes
Neuromuscular junction	Botulism
	Tick paralysis
	Organophosphate toxicity
	Myasthenia gravis
	Lambert-Eaton syndrome
Muscle	Dermatomyositis
	Muscular dystrophy
Systemic causes	Hypo/hyperglycemia
	Hypo/hypernatremia
	Hypermagnesemia
	Hypophosphatemia
	Periodic paralysis
Miscellaneous	Envenomation
	Locked-in syndrome
	Acute porphyria
	Psychiatric illness
	Intensive care unit (ICU)-acquired weakness

ICU care plays a crucial role in the management of nontraumatic weakness. However, the various management strategies in neurocritical care are not without controversies. The salient controversies that are to be discussed in the chapter are as follows.

1. Plasmapheresis vs. intravenous immunoglobulin in the management of acute nontraumatic weakness in the ICU
2. To continue or withhold acetylcholinesterase inhibitors during myasthenic crisis
3. Implications of the second dose of IVIg in neurocritical care
4. Role of noninvasive ventilation (NIV) in neuromuscular weakness
5. Weaning strategies in patients requiring ventilatory support

7.1 IVIg Versus PLEX: A Never-Ending Saga

Myasthenic respiratory crisis is one of the dreaded complications of MG, which usually warrants admission to the intensive care unit (ICU). Intravenous immunoglobulin (IVIg) and plasma exchange (PLEX) are the two rescue therapies employed currently to prevent rapid myasthenic worsening when a fast response to treatment is deemed necessary or when the other treatment modalities are ineffective. PLEX removes the destructive antibodies and replaces them with a replacement fluid, such as plasma, which is disease-free. The mode of action of IVIg in MG is yet to be fully understood. The postulated mechanism is that IVIg binds to the pathological antibodies directly and offsets them. The efficacy and superiority of one technique over the other have been debated for ages.

The latest International Consensus Guidelines on the management of MG consider both treatment options as equally effective in severe generalized MG and advise choosing between PLEX and IVIg based on patient-specific factors and on the availability of therapeutics [3]. Patient comorbidity is an important determinant of the therapy choice; PLEX cannot be utilized in sepsis due to the hemodynamic derangements associated with it, and conditions such as hypercoagulable states, renal failure, or hypersensitivity contraindicate the use of IVIg. The procedural complications of PLEX cannot be overlooked. Most of its complications are attributed to the venous access route and could be averted using peripheral access, as an alternative to central.

Both techniques are equally efficacious in most settings, and there is no clear evidence of superiority [4, 5]. However, for ocular MG, the efficacy of IVIg is less certain, and in terms of MuSK MG, PLEX has the edge over IVIg. The usefulness of IVIg in maintenance therapy is also noteworthy; it has a definitive role in patients with refractory MG and in whom immunosuppressants are contraindicated. A comparative description of the pros and cons of both modalities is given in Table 7.2.

The recent evidence comparing the safety and efficacy of PLEX versus IVIg in Myasthenia management must be reviewed before drawing conclusions. In a systematic review by Pavlekovics et al., in patients with moderate-to-severe MG, the results failed to show any significant difference. However, a faster efficacy of PLEX

Table 7.2 Pros and cons of the two major treatment options for GBS and MG

	Advantages	Disadvantages
Plasma exchange	1. Immediate intervention possible 2. Rapid removal of autoimmune antibodies	1. Requires invasive venous access for establishing therapy 2. Requires expert personnel and special equipment for therapy
Intravenous immunoglobulin	1. Immediate intervention possible 2. Minimally invasive intervention 3. Suitable for daycare settings	1. Expensive therapy 2. Availability issues

in the initial 2 weeks of treatment was evident [6]. This inclination can have therapeutic significance in critical clinical situations like the MG crisis. Also, the side effect profile did not significantly differ between the two modalities. Concerning the invasiveness associated with PLEX, it did not result in significantly higher adverse events. In yet another review by Tina et al. [7], patients with acute myasthenic crisis and patients undergoing thymectomy manifested a higher response rate with PLEX than IVIg. Though no mortality differences between the two treatment options were noted, fewer adverse events were reported with IVIg use. They also added that there might be a tip in the favorability of PLEX when a rapid response is warranted, since rapid responses and briefer ventilatory hours are more likely with PLEX. Conversely, IVIg should be the ideal choice for patients with infections, renal failure, and cardiovascular disease.

On the other end of the spectrum, treatment options for severely affected Guillain–Barré syndrome (GBS) patients are again perplexed between PLEX and IVIg. The recent literature pertaining to GBS outcomes after treatment with PLEX and/or IVIg consists primarily of case reports or case series from developing countries where the choice between PLEX and IVIg is biased by economic considerations. A recent systematic review and meta-analysis by Zaki et al. [8] suggests that IVIg and PE have comparable curative rates, reductions in ICU and hospitalization length, and complication rates. They recommended that IVIg be preferred over PE for treating patients with severe GBS due to the ease of administration. However, this recommendation was offered with the caution that the simplicity of the IVIg should not tempt physicians to treat GBS without sufficient and appropriate intensive care facilities. Small-volume plasma exchange (SVPE) is a viable alternative treatment for GBS, particularly in low- and middle-income countries where pricing is the limiting and decisive factor for the treatment choice. SVPE is comparable in terms of efficacy and safety in GBS [9]. In the pediatric population, PLEX had an advantage over IVIg by showing a reduction in the duration of ICU stay and hospitalization [10].

In recent years, novel techniques for plasmapheresis, such as immunoadsorption and double-filtration plasmapheresis (DFPP), have provided the advantage of more selective removal of toxic substances, rendering the need for plasma supplementation futile. A recent meta-analysis proposes that DFPP can be recommended for the short-term alleviation of MG [11]. It is crucial to highlight the rapid therapeutic agents, such as complement inhibitor therapies and anti-FcRn antibody therapy, as potential future management strategies for the MG crisis [12]. It is beyond the scope of the current chapter to provide a detailed note of these novel treatment possibilities.

In summary, recent literature and recommendations from professional bodies strongly imply that PLEX has superior utility in the management of acute MG. The side effect profile should also be considered, but no discernible pattern of major adverse events or increased mortality rates has been seen across studies. To add on, the outcomes of PLEX can grow further bounds with early intervention and initiation via peripheral venous access. From the economic standpoint, a cost-minimization analysis of plasma exchange versus IVIg done in 2022 states that PLEX was half as costly when compared to IVIg therapy and warranted the need for the development of more plasma exchange units in neurology centers [13]. It is mandated that the choice of treatment should be patient-tailored and decided based on the available clinical resources. Overall, most literature asserts the need for better-designed studies to provide higher-quality evidence. Future studies in this premise should ideally be prospective, with well-defined and standardized protocols. The inclusion of quality-of-life assessments as a study objective for different treatments would shed more light on the evaluation of the long-term benefits.

7.2 Second Dose IVIg: Is It Worth It?

IVIg has been used for decades in the field of autoimmune disorders; however, the mechanism by which it produces its clinical effect remains unascertained [14]. The mechanism of action appears to be different for individual disorders. Direct immunomodulating effects like reduction in T-cell proliferation, suppression of pro-inflammatory cytokines, and B-cell differentiation; inhibition of complement-mediated antibody production are a few mechanisms postulated [15]. IVIg is one of the keystones of treatment in GBS, along with PLEX. It has been proven beneficial and should be commenced as early as possible before irreversible neuronal injury commences. IVIg is the preferred treatment for GBS in many centers due to its availability, ease of administration, and avoidance of the adverse effects associated with PLEX, as narrated in detail in the previous section of this chapter.

In patients severely affected by GBS, recovery from the disease may take months, coinciding with the onset of axonal regeneration. However, a few continue to deteriorate in spite of all supportive and immunomodulatory therapy. This could be attributed to a severe, prolonged immune-mediated attack resulting in severe axonal damage. It remains cryptic how to manage such patients who persistently worsen or worsen after early signs of improvement [16]. IVIg is usually administered as a single-dose regimen of 400 mg/kg/day for 5 days. Repeated cycles of IVIg are an option to be considered for the treatment of such severe forms of GBS refractory to the first course. It is credible to treat patients again who exhibit signs of relapse after an initial positive response; however, there are no existing guidelines for patients who continue to deteriorate [17]. On the downside, IVIg is costly, and there is a possibility that the uncommon severe side effects will become more frequent due to repeated administration. Despite this, 25% of patients with GBS are re-treated with IVIg when no clinical improvement is seen after initial therapy [18].

The efficacy of repeated IVIg in severe GBS, especially in subtypes with severe axonal damage, has been reported in the literature as early as 1997 by Farcas et al. [17]. They highlighted that the standard doses of IVIg are universally not sufficient. Following the standard dosing, it is reported that 20% of patients remain non-ambulatory after 6 months, 20–30% of patients are ventilator dependent, and 3–7% die [19]. The regimen of IVIg administration in GBS—2gm/day in divided doses over 5 days was ascertained primarily by deriving from studies on autoimmune disorders of the blood [20, 21]. Raphael et al. reported that a high-dose therapy of IVIg (2.4 g/kg) was more efficacious than a lower dose (1.2 g/kg), with a rapid recovery rate in GBS [22]. In addition, reports showing a lower increase in the immunoglobulin level after 2 weeks of IVIg infusions, leading to poor outcomes, emphasize the fact that the pharmacokinetic profile of IVIg is highly variable and hence warrants repeat doses [21].

A few small studies by Godoy et al. and Alboudi et al. recommended a second cycle of IVIg for the treatment of severe GBS [23, 24]. A second IVIg dose administered in the initial days of the disease, before irreversible neuronal injury has occurred, might benefit, although the evidence in this regard is scant [18, 25]. The 2008 European Federation of Neurological Sciences guidelines with respect to IVIg in the treatment of neurological diseases state that patients who initially improve after IVIg and then later relapse should preferentially be provided with a second course. However, in patients who are unresponsive to the primary course of IVIg, a trial of a second course may be given, but supportive evidence for such a strategy is deficient [26]. This lack of proper evidence called for further multicenter trials using a repeat course of IVIg to strengthen the current guidelines and recommendations, and the landmark SID-GBS trial came as an answer to it [27].

The SID-GBS study was carried out at 59 hospitals in the Netherlands, in which 327 patients aged 12 years and older with GBS were included. After a standard initial treatment dosing with IVIg 2 g/kg total for 5 consecutive days, patients who had a poor prognosis (mEGOS score > 6) were further randomized 7 to 9 days after the first day of initial treatment to receive either a placebo or a second course of IVIg over 5 days. The outcome measures included the GBS disability scale score at 4 weeks after the start of the initial course, the duration of ventilator dependency, and mortality. The study concluded that no significant clinical benefit was found in patients with poor prognosis following a second IVIg course administered shortly after the first standard IVIG dose. Additionally, the IVIg group had more serious adverse events, including thromboembolic events and four mortalities.

The results of the SID-GBS study were in accordance with earlier studies, which showed no benefits in GBS after additional immunotherapy [28, 29]. Contrary to the belief that a sizable rise in serum IgG concentration after IVIg treatment was attributed to a more substantial recovery [21], it seems probable that IVIg in GBS is primarily effective early in the disease course, and no benefit could be reaped by prolonging a high serum IgG concentration. Thromboembolic events are a rare, albeit familiar side effect of IVIg, which is believed to be due to the increase in plasma viscosity, which is dose-dependent [30]. Additional factors, which include sepsis, immobility, dehydration, and leukocytosis, can also contribute to an increase in plasma viscosity, thereby leading to serious adverse events. Also, the events must be solely attributed to the second IVIg course rather than the serum IgG concentrations, since patients with thromboembolic events failed to exhibit a higher IgG concentration after one standard course of IVIg or after a second dose.

To conclude, repeated cycles of IVIG should be contemplated as a therapeutic option only in highly selected patients who are refractory to the first course of treatment and with close monitoring for serious thromboembolic and cardiovascular complications. The cost of management with such repeat therapy is also a considerable factor. In addition, it can be recommended to consider novel agents acting through a different mechanism than IVIg, such as IgG-degrading enzymes (NCT03943589) and complement inhibitors (NCT04035135).

7.3 Acetylcholinesterase Inhibitors in Myasthenic Crisis: To Persist or Desist?

Myasthenia gravis (MG) is a rare but the most common disease of autoimmune etiology affecting the neuromuscular junction, characterized by fluctuating muscle weakness [31]. Extraocular and bulbar muscle groups are usually at risk, and the symptoms are generally triggered by various stressors such as infections, steroids, surgeries, etc. [32]. Unlike in the past, the mortality rates of MG have drastically reduced from 40% to 5% in the last decade [33]. This has been made possible with the advent of multimodal therapeutic options, which include immunosuppressive agents, steroids, plasma exchange, IVIg, and thymectomy. However, Acetylcholinesterase Inhibitors (AChEI) are considered the magic bullet and have been consistently used for almost a century now in the management of MG.

Acetylcholinesterase inhibitors were discovered and introduced in the treatment of MG as early as 1934. Pyridostigmine, a synthetic acetylcholinesterase inhibitor, is currently the most commonly used AChEI in clinical practice. It inhibits acetylcholine hydrolysis in the synaptic cleft and thereby expands the number of interactions between the acetylcholine and its receptor in the neuromuscular junction. Also, pyridostigmine lacks central nervous system toxicity, since it does not traverse the blood–brain barrier. The standard starting dose of pyridostigmine is 60 mg every 6 hours and is usually escalated up to 60–120 mg every 3 hours depending on the clinical response. Caution is advised at higher doses as side effects are anticipated [34].

Myasthenic crisis (MC) is a life-threatening complication of MG presenting with worsening muscle weakness, which may result in respiratory failure, warranting mechanical ventilation. Severe affection of the bulbar muscles is the hallmark of MC. The treatment strategy for myasthenic crisis consists of the following:

- Stabilization and initiation of supportive care
- Removal of trigger and stressor factors
- Differentiation from other conditions that may mimic myasthenic crisis
- Continuous treatment of underlying MG

With prompt treatment and the wide range of therapeutic agents available currently for MC, the prognosis is great, and patients can attain near total recovery with proper therapy [35].

After stabilization of the airway, hemodynamics, and respiratory parameters, IVIg or PLEX is usually considered as the first-line of definitive management [35]. In the past, AChEIs continued to augment the other therapeutic measures [36, 37]. However, recent guidelines suggest discontinuation of AChEI during the initial phase of MC due to the possibility of worsening from increased bronchial secretions and to rule out the mimic of cholinergic crisis (CC) [38]. But it also must be noted that these recommendations were derived from small observational studies only. Hence, the question of whether to continue or withhold AChEI during MC remains debatable. This part of the chapter is intended to answer the following questions:

1. Should AChEI be continued in MC?
2. If yes, what type, route, and dosage of AChEI should be administered, and whether it can serve as the sole treatment option during MC?
3. What is the ideal time to administer AChEI during MC?
4. What are the advantages and disadvantages of adding AChEI to the other therapeutic options in MG?

Cholinergic Crisis occurs due to an overdose of anticholinesterase medications, resulting in muscle weakness mimicking a myasthenic crisis. The possibility that muscle weakness and respiratory failure are caused by CC is usually excluded by temporarily stopping AChEI while the treatment of MC is continued. Acute treatment is supportive in both entities, though theoretically, the management differs. Though CC is an important differential, it is uncommon and has been rarely diagnosed [39]. Although retrospective studies have found no patients with cholinergic crisis mimicking MC [40], AChEI may be recommended to be significantly lowered or withheld to avoid superabundant secretions in the purview of respiratory distress [41].

Apart from the disadvantage of bronchorrhea mentioned previously, AChEI, if continued during the crisis phase, may interfere with the assessment of other treatment modalities and, if used in excess, can exacerbate muscle weakness [31]. Hence, a period of withdrawal is recommended to augment the response to other medications [33]. These medications are reported to provide only symptomatic relief and do not have any disease-altering benefits [41]. Nevertheless, AChEI can be restarted during the recovery phase when substantial muscle strength has recovered after a course of IVIg or PLEX and can be titrated for symptomatic relief [31, 41]. A stop-start strategy or AChEI holiday is considered to improve the sensitivity of the postsynaptic membranes and might be beneficial during the resumption of the drug prior to weaning [42]. However, recent reviews in the same context reveal that a benefit was perceived whether the drug was administered during or before weaning or extubation of patients with MC [43].

Case reports documenting the positive effects of higher oral doses of pyridostigmine in MC without any IVIg or PLEX are available in the literature [44]. Though IVIg and PLEX are considered the first-line of management in MC, it is a fact that, aside from their side effects, the cost and need for technical expertise for their administration and dependence on equipment limit their use in underdeveloped countries [31]. AChEI is a low-cost, easy-to-get, and easy-to-administer drug and can serve as a plausible alternative; however, no RCTs that determine the efficacy and safety of AChEI in MC are available, mainly due to ethical constraints. A recent systematic review stated that the addition of AChEI may shorten the crisis duration among patients with MG [43]. Nevertheless, most of the studies included in the review utilized PLEX, IVIg, or immunomodulators as cointerventions. In a study by Berrouschot, the clinical outcome and complication of giving AChEI alone were found to be not statistically different from giving PLEX [37].

The onset of oral pyridostigmine is 15–30 minutes and may last up to 3–4 hours; however, responses vary for individual patients. Intravenous formulations are equally efficacious with 1 mg of intravenous pyridostigmine equaling 30 mg of oral pyridostigmine, and hence have been considered alternatively as infusions at 1–2 mg per hour during crisis. Despite having similar efficacy to that of PLEX, continuous infusions of pyridostigmine are not considered ideal due to the increased risk of life-threatening cardiac arrhythmia associated with it [37, 45]. To circumvent the adverse effects, intramuscular pyridostigmine doses that are equally effective have also been used. The other alternative form of long-acting pyridostigmine tablets is reserved only for nocturnal use in MG and is not recommended in MC because of variable absorption [33].

To conclude, it is ideal to withhold AChEI during the initial phase of MC due to its deleterious effects of bronchorrhea and worsening weakness. However, it may be beneficial in the weaning phases in conjunction with other measures. Both oral and intravenous formulations are equally efficacious, but caution is warranted for the latter due to its arrhythmogenic properties. The addition of AChEI in MC to other measures can be beneficial, but its role as a solitary agent is yet to be evaluated, and further studies are necessary to reach a verdict.

7.4 NIV in Patients with Neuromuscular Disorders: Lifesaver or Prolonging the Inevitable?

Various neuromuscular diseases eventually lead to respiratory failure and require mechanical ventilation at some point during the course of the disease. The etiopathogenesis of the disease plays a major role in deciding the ventilatory strategy of these patients and thereby plays a role in altering the prognosis itself [46]. Noninvasive ventilation (NIV) is a plausible prospect in patients with neuromuscular respiratory failure. The advantage of NIV lies in its potential to achieve physiological effects similar to those of invasive mechanical ventilation without the risks associated with the use of an artificial airway. Though its role is better validated in chronic neuromuscular pathologies like amyotrophic lateral sclerosis [47], NIV can also benefit patients with acute exacerbation of chronic conditions like MG [48, 49].

The critical factors deciding the utility and beneficence of NIV in neuromuscular respiratory failure are the diagnosis per se and the timing of initiation of therapy. Certain conditions are well-suited for the application of NIV, whereas it can turn dangerous in a few other conditions. Also, the timing of NIV initiation plays a major role. Application of NIV in patients with respiratory fatigue and severe hypercapnia may lead to ventilatory failure and fatal complications. Hence, it is pivotal to identify the clinical features early and understand the pathophysiology involved in neuromuscular respiratory failure to aid in the prompt initiation of ventilatory care [50, 51]. Frequent reassessment of the clinical parameters is also of paramount importance to ensure the appropriateness of NIV. This chapter aims to highlight the pros and cons of NIV in major neuromuscular disorders encountered in neurocritical care settings.

The eye for clinical acumen in neuromuscular respiratory failure is the foremost tool for diagnosis. Patients with neuromuscular respiratory failure present with tachypnea and labored breathing. Inability to clear oropharyngeal secretions and a weak cough accompanies them—the use of accessory muscles and paradoxical breathing points toward impending respiratory failure. A detailed neurological examination gives more diagnostic clues. Recognition of bulbar weakness is a priority, as it may lead to aspiration. Signs like ophthalmoplegia and ptosis may point toward MG, and the absence of reflexes may occur in GBS. Bulbar weakness is typical of both GBS and Myasthenia and may warrant immediate airway intervention. Pulmonary examination might reveal signs of atelectasis and aspiration if any. Bedside spirometry, blood gases, and chest radiographs aid in the diagnosis.

Neuromuscular diseases produce a restrictive form of respiratory failure. Respiratory muscle weakness leads to atelectasis of the alveoli, causing increased work of breathing. As respiratory fatigue sets in, alveolar hypoventilation ensues. An initial compensation with increased respiratory rates keeps the pCO2 in check; however, it spirals into hypercapnic acidosis and hypoxemia in due course due to respiratory pump impairment. The level of compensation is especially high in patients with chronic disorders. Prompt usage of NIV could avert the increased workload of respiratory muscles and help evade the need for invasive tracheal intubation. NIV in combination with a cricothyroid mini-tracheostomy has been proven to be an effective and safer alternative to endotracheal intubation in patients with neuromuscular disorders who develop respiratory failure [52].

NIV in continuous positive airway pressure (CPAP) mode reduces the upper airway resistance and prevents alveolar collapse, thereby improving oxygenation. However, it does not address the needs of respiratory muscle fatigue. Hence, bilevel positive airway pressure (BiPAP) is deemed ideal. The ventilatory parameters are to be tailored to the individual for better outcomes [53]. The success of NIV delivery lies in the mask fitting, which should balance patient comfort and air leak [54].

Optimal fit also prevents pressure sores, which might be a limiting factor in NIV acceptance in the long run. Oronasal interfaces are more ideal than nasal-only, as most of the patients with respiratory fatigue are oral breathers, rendering nasal interfaces ineffective [55].

NIV is most useful in acute myasthenic crisis, which usually warrants ventilatory assistance. MG with anti-muscle-specific tyrosine kinase antibodies usually exhibits bulbar palsy and ends up in respiratory failure [56]. The typical recovery of muscle power following rest in MG applies to the respiratory muscle group as well, and NIV can help in recovering from weakness [49]. Timely intervention with BiPAP therapy has been proven to reduce the need for tracheal intubation [48], thereby reducing the incidence of pulmonary complications and the length of hospital stay [49]. As discussed earlier, the timing of intervention is key since the rate of NIV failure increases proportionally with the onset of hypercapnia [48, 49]. Hence, it is recommended that the treating physician has a lower threshold for NIV initiation based primarily on clinical parameters since the bedside pulmonary function tests are inconsistent due to the waxing and waning nature of the disease. The role of NIV extends to the recovery phase of the disease as well [57]. NIV plays a significant part in reducing the extubation failure rates, which are otherwise high in MG [58]. Overnight trials of NIV in patients with weak muscle power post-extubation are beneficial in terms of preventing alveolar collapse occurring due to impaired muscle tone during sleep [59]. NIV coupled with cough assist devices can also aid in the extubation of patients with ICU-acquired weakness [60].

Unlike MG, GBS has a rapidly progressive course, which may lead to acute respiratory failure due to diaphragmatic and bulbar weakness. There are reports of successful management of GBS using NIV in the absence of bulbar weakness [61]. Nevertheless, once the stage of respiratory paralysis is reached, the further course is expected to spiral down, and measures like NIV are only going to delay the inevitable [62]. Moreover, the autonomic disturbances associated with GBS can be complicated in the event of emergency intubation [63]. Hence, it is recommended to intubate electively in patients with impending failure in GBS as assessed by clinical parameters and bedside spirometry tools, which is more reliable in these settings than MG [64]. Also, NIV may not be appropriate since a long duration of mechanical ventilation is anticipated. However, NIV can be beneficial during the recovery phase of GBS where autonomic instability is not expected. It has been successfully used in weaning patients from mechanical ventilation [65, 66].

The presence of bulbar weakness is an important confounder in the introduction of NIV in neuromuscular weakness. In the event of preserved bulbar function, the use of NIV in conjunction with manual cough assistance devices can be successfully used to clear the airway of secretions and avoid endotracheal intubation [67, 68]. Though the risk of aspiration and airway obstruction prevails, it should not always necessitate intubation in patients with bulbar palsy. Such patients do tolerate NIV in early reversible stages of respiratory failure [69]. Favorably, bulbar weakness makes NIV easier by reducing the resistance to inspiratory pressures. Agitated patients who require sedation are usually not ideal candidates for NIV. However, in the setting of neuromuscular weakness, agitation is a result of hypercapnia and hypoxia, and NIV can actually be the cure. Nonetheless, the pooling of secretions is always a dangerous sign, but does not contraindicate NIV [70]. NIV, together with secretion clearance techniques in patients with myasthenia gravis or GBS, is still a feasible option [71].

Thus, NIV can be a valuable tool in the armamentarium of neurointensivists in patients admitted to the ICU with neuromuscular weakness. However, it is imperative to be cognizant of which patients and at what point of the disease course would benefit from it. It is of immense benefit in early myasthenia crisis; however, it must be used with caution in GBS. If NIV is deemed necessary, patient selection and close monitoring are the keys to successful management. Literature in this regard is sparse, with only a few studies comparing the effectiveness of NIV in these patient subgroups, despite a compelling reason to use it, and more studies are mandated.

7.5 Weaning Strategies in Patients with Neuromuscular Weakness

7.5.1 Is There One Optimal Technique?

Weaning patients with neuromuscular respiratory failure from mechanical ventilation is a complex and multifaceted process requiring a thorough understanding of both the underlying neuromuscular condition and the principles of respiratory care. The goal of weaning is to transition the patient from mechanical support to spontaneous breathing while ensuring safety and minimizing discomfort or complications. This process involves several stages, including assessment, optimization of respiratory function, gradual reduction of ventilatory support, and close monitoring.

Successful weaning is traditionally defined as the ability to maintain spontaneous ventilation without warranting for any reintubation and invasive mechanical ventilation for 48 hours post-extubation, and this definition can be slightly altered in patients with neuromuscular weakness, as the absence of requiring a tracheostomy and mechanical ventilation for 5 days following extubation [72]. Conventional weaning from mechanical ventilation is generally challenging in patients with neuromuscular weakness and hence can lead to a higher incidence of extubation failures, prolonged mechanical ventilation, and tracheostomies. Vigilant monitoring is expected in the post-extubation period to catch the signs of extubation failure and the need for reintubation, as listed in Table 7.3.

Traditionally, the weaning process is conducted in one of the three following protocols:

- T-piece-based weaning with a progressive increase in spontaneous ventilation time
- Continuous positive airway pressure (CPAP) technique with titrated reduction of applied pressure
- Pressure-support technique with gradual reduction of the support pressure

Table 7.3 Possible signs of weaning failure in patients with neuromuscular weakness

Respiratory rate > 35 rpm
Respiratory acidosis (pH < 7.35 with PaCO2 > 45 mm Hg)
SpO2 < 90% or PaO2 < 60 mm Hg despite FiO2 > 50%
Use of accessory muscles of respiration
Paradoxical movement of the abdominal wall
Decreased level of consciousness
Restlessness
Excessive sweating

Table 7.4 Attributes of different weaning protocols in patients with neuromuscular weakness

Technique	Description	Advantages	Challenges
T- piece trials	The patient breathes through a T-piece connected to the ventilator circuit, receiving humidified oxygen without ventilatory support	Allows complete assessment of the patient's ability to breathe without assistance	Patients with neuromuscular weakness may fatigue quickly, necessitating close monitoring
PSV	The patient breathes spontaneously with a preset level of pressure support to assist in inspiratory efforts	Reduces the work of breathing by providing support during inspiration	Determining the optimal level of pressure support can be complex, and patients may require gradual reduction
CPAP	Maintains a constant positive airway pressure throughout the respiratory cycle	Keeps airways open and reduces the work of breathing	May not be sufficient for patients with significant muscle weakness who require inspiratory support

Usually, at the end of the protocols, a spontaneous breathing trial (SBT) is assessed for readiness for extubation [73].

This section of the chapter will deal with the attributes of different weaning protocols in patients with neuromuscular weakness (Table 7.4), how the various protocols can affect weaning success, length of ICU stay, hospital stay, morbidity, and mortality, and whether any technique can be deemed the ideal one based on these characteristics.

Weaning predictor indices are an integral part of weaning readiness assessments. The commonly used indices that have high accuracy in predicting weaning outcomes include:

1. Frequency/tidal volume (f/VT)
2. Maximum inspiratory pressure with unidirectional valve (P_{Imax} (UV))
3. Tension-time index of inspiratory muscles (TT_{mus})
4. Integrative weaning index (IWI)
5. Timed inspiratory effort (TIE).

In patients with neuromuscular disease, the TIE index is considered to have a better performance than the other weaning indices mentioned above [74].

The ideal time to wean these patients and discontinue mechanical ventilation (MV) is critical. Premature liberation is associated with high rates of reintubation, whereas delayed weaning has its own cons. Diaphragm function assessment during the process of weaning in critically ill neuromuscular disease patients hastens weaning. The modalities available to study diaphragmatic dysfunction include fluoroscopy, trans-diaphragmatic pressure, phrenic nerve conduction study, and ultrasound-based evaluation, such as diaphragm thickening fraction (DTF) [75]. The electrical activity of the diaphragm (Edi) and diaphragm excursion changes have been recently proven to be efficacious and can guide the weaning trials in neuromuscular disease [76].

Concerning the available literature, no quality evidence exists in support or against any of the weaning protocols as per a recent review by Bernardes et al. [72]. Sun et al. [77] investigated weaning success using SBT with a gradual reduction of support pressure in patients with myasthenia gravis crisis. Rapid and shallow breathing index (RSBI) and diaphragm thickening fraction (DTF) were also measured to assess the outcomes. Their findings suggested that weaning protocol using pressure support aided by DTF and RSBI during SBT could provide a good predictive value for weaning failure. Vianello et al. [78] assessed the utility of NIV post-extubation in comparison to standard therapy in patients who underwent weaning through SBT in PSV mode. Though the patients were judged to be ready for extubation by the PSV protocol in both groups, the need for reintubation and tracheostomy was greater in the standard group. Their findings highlight the usefulness of NIV in weaning and, on the other hand, question the efficacy of PSV protocols in deciding extubation readiness. The pursuit of the ideal weaning strategy in this subset of patients ultimately led researchers to change their concern toward the use of NIV to supplement weaning from mechanical ventilation [65]. The combination of invasive MV with NIV has led to a reduction in weaning failures, as discussed in the previous section of this chapter.

Mechanical insufflation-exsufflation (MIE), or cough assist, is particularly beneficial for patients with neuromuscular weakness who have ineffective coughs. MIE alternates between positive and negative pressures to simulate a cough and clear secretions. It enhances secretion clearance, preventing atelectasis and respiratory infections. However, the usage requires patient cooperation and proper technique to be effective. In conjunction with NIV, its role in weaning is superlative [68]. Inspiratory muscle training (IMT) is another auxiliary technique that promotes weaning. It involves specific exercises designed to strengthen the respiratory muscles, particularly the diaphragm, by creating resistance during inspiration. With consistent practice and patient motivation, the success rates are high [79].

Apart from the ventilatory challenges, the other factors to be considered regarding the weaning of patients with neuromuscular weakness are

1. Residual Muscle Weakness:
   - Persistent muscle weakness can prolong the weaning process. Inspiratory muscle training and gradual reduction of support are crucial.
2. Bulbar Dysfunction:

- Patients with bulbar involvement may struggle with secretion management and airway protection. Mechanical insufflation-exsufflation (MIE) and suctioning can be beneficial.

3. Dysphagia:
   - Swallowing difficulties increase the risk of aspiration. Modified diets, swallowing therapy, and enteral feeding may be necessary.
4. Autonomic Dysfunction:
   - Conditions like GBS can involve autonomic instability, affecting heart rate and blood pressure control. Hence, close monitoring is essential.
5. Psychological Support:
   - Anxiety and depression are common and can impact the weaning process. Psychological support and pharmacological interventions are often required.

In conclusion, the absence of structured studies does not allow us to provide any verdict on the advantage of any specific weaning protocol for neuromuscular weakness. Nevertheless, the lack of proof of effectiveness is not proof that the interventions are ineffective. Proper assessment of readiness for extubation guided by the various indices, utilization of ancillary techniques like NIV and cough assist device, assessment of diaphragmatic function, and vigilant monitoring during weaning can improve the success irrespective of the weaning protocol employed.

References

1. Jangra K, Bhagat H, Takkar A. Acute nontraumatic muscle weakness. J Neuroanaesth Crit Care. 2019/09/11 ed. 2019;6(3):236–56.
2. Caulfield AF, Flower O, Pineda JA, Uddin S. Emergency neurological life support: acute nontraumatic weakness. Neurocrit Care. 2017;27(S1):29–50.
3. Sanders DB, Wolfe GI, Benatar M, Evoli A, Gilhus NE, Illa I, et al. International consensus guidance for management of myasthenia gravis: executive summary. Neurology. 2016;87(4):419–25.
4. Achiron A, Barak Y, Miron S, Sarova-Pinhas I. Immunoglobulin treatment in refractory myasthenia gravis. Muscle Nerve. 2000;23(4):551–5.
5. Qureshi AI, Choudhry MA, Akbar MS, Mohammad Y, Chua HC, Yahia AM, et al. Plasma exchange versus intravenous immunoglobulin treatment in myasthenic crisis. Neurology. 1999;52(3):629.
6. Pavlekovics M, Engh MA, Lugosi K, Szabo L, Hegyi P, Terebessy T, et al. Plasma exchange versus intravenous immunoglobulin in worsening myasthenia gravis: a systematic review and meta-analysis with special attention to faster relapse control. Biomedicine. 2023;11(12):3180.
7. Ipe TS, Davis AR, Raval JS. Therapeutic plasma exchange in myasthenia gravis: a systematic literature review and meta-analysis of comparative evidence. Front Neurol. 2021;12:662856.
8. Zaki HA, Iftikhar H, Najam M, Masood M, Al-Marri NDR, Elgassim MAM, et al. Plasma exchange (PE) versus intravenous immunoglobulin (IVIG) for the treatment of Guillain-Barré syndrome (GBS) in patients with severe symptoms: a systematic review and meta-analysis. eNeurologicalSci. 2023;31:100468.
9. Balili K, Louhab N, Adarmouch L, Chraa M, Hachimi A, Belbachir A, et al. Guillain–Barre syndrome: small-volume plasmapheresis versus intravenous immunoglobulin—3rd level hospital experience. Egypt J Neurol Psychiatry Neurosurg. 2024;60(1):45.

10. Savithri Nandeesha S, Kasagga A, Hawrami C, Ricci E, Hailu KT, Salib K, et al. Treatment efficacy of plasmapheresis versus intravenous immunoglobulin in Guillain-Barré syndrome management: a systematic review. Cureus [Internet]. 2024.
11. Liu C, Liu P, Ma M, Yang H, Qi G. Efficacy and safety of double-filtration plasmapheresis treatment of myasthenia gravis: a systematic review and meta-analysis. Medicine (Baltimore). 2021;100(17):e25622.
12. Zhu LN, Hou HM, Wang S, Zhang S, Wang GG, Guo ZY, et al. FcRn inhibitors: a novel option for the treatment of myasthenia gravis. Neural Regen Res. 2023;18(8):1637–44.
13. Klemencic Kozul T, Yudina A, Donovan C, Pinto A, Osman C. Cost-minimisation analysis of plasma exchange versus IVIg in the treatment of autoimmune neurological conditions. BMC Health Serv Res. 2022;22(1):904.
14. Dalakas MC. The use of intravenous immunoglobulin in the treatment of autoimmune neuromuscular diseases: evidence-based indications and safety profile. Pharmacol Ther. 2004;102(3):177–93.
15. Buchwald B, Ahangari R, Weishaupt A, Toyka KV. Intravenous immunoglobulins neutralize blocking antibodies in Guillain-Barré syndrome. Ann Neurol. 2002;51(6):673–80.
16. Arcila-Londono X, Lewis R. Guillain-Barré Syndrome. Semin Neurol. 2012;32(03):179–86.
17. Farcas P, Avnun L, Frisher S, Herishanu YO, Wirguin I. Efficacy of repeated intravenous immunoglobulin in severe unresponsive Guillain-Barré syndrome. Lancet Lond Engl. 1997;350(9093):1747.
18. Verboon C, Doets AY, Galassi G, Davidson A, Waheed W, Péréon Y, et al. Current treatment practice of Guillain-Barré syndrome. Neurology. 2019;93(1):e59–76.
19. van den Berg B, Walgaard C, Drenthen J, Fokke C, Jacobs BC, van Doorn PA. Guillain-Barré syndrome: pathogenesis, diagnosis, treatment and prognosis. Nat Rev Neurol. 2014;10(8):469–82.
20. Dalakas MC. Mechanisms of action of IVIg and therapeutic considerations in the treatment of acute and chronic demyelinating neuropathies. Neurology. 2002;59(12 Suppl 6):S13–21.
21. Kuitwaard K, De Gelder J, Tio-Gillen AP, Hop WCJ, Van Gelder T, Van Toorenenbergen AW, et al. Pharmacokinetics of intravenous immunoglobulin and outcome in Guillain-Barré syndrome. Ann Neurol. 2009;66(5):597–603.
22. Raphael JC, Chevret S, Harboun M, Jars-Guincestre MC, French Guillain-Barré Syndrome Cooperative Group. Intravenous immune globulins in patients with Guillain-Barré syndrome and contraindications to plasma exchange: 3 days versus 6 days. J Neurol Neurosurg Psychiatry. 2001;71(2):235–8.
23. Godoy DA, Rabinstein A. Is a second cycle of immunoglobulin justified in axonal forms of Guillain-Barré syndrome? Arq Neuropsiquiatr. 2015;73(10):848–51.
24. Alboudi AM, Sarathchandran P, Geblawi SS, Kayed DM, Inshasi J, Purayil SP, et al. Rescue treatment in patients with poorly responsive Guillain–Barre syndrome. SAGE Open Med. 2019;7:205031211984019.
25. Walgaard C, Lingsma HF, Ruts L, van Doorn PA, Steyerberg EW, Jacobs BC. Early recognition of poor prognosis in Guillain-Barre syndrome. Neurology. 2011;76(11):968–75.
26. Elovaara I, Apostolski S, van Doorn P, Gilhus NE, Hietaharju A, Honkaniemi J, et al. EFNS guidelines for the use of intravenous immunoglobulin in the treatment of neurological diseases: EFNS task force on the use of intravenous immunoglobulin in the treatment of neurological diseases. Eur J Neurol. 2008;15(9):893–908.
27. Walgaard C, Jacobs BC, Lingsma HF, Steyerberg EW, van den Berg B, Doets AY, et al. Second intravenous immunoglobulin dose in patients with Guillain-Barré syndrome with poor prognosis (SID-GBS): a double-blind, randomised, placebo-controlled trial. Lancet Neurol. 2021;20(4):275–83.
28. Verboon C, van den Berg B, Cornblath DR, Venema E, Gorson KC, Lunn MP, et al. Original research: second IVIg course in Guillain-Barré syndrome with poor prognosis: the non-randomised ISID study. J Neurol Neurosurg Psychiatry. 2020;91(2):113–21.

29. van Koningsveld R, Schmitz PIM, Meché FGA, Visser LH, Meulstee J, van Doorn PA, et al. Effect of methylprednisolone when added to standard treatment with intravenous immunoglobulin for Guillain-Barré syndrome: randomised trial. Lancet Lond Engl. 2004;363(9404):192–6.
30. Kapoor M, Spillane J, Englezou C, Sarri-Gonzalez S, Bell R, Rossor A, et al. Thromboembolic risk with IVIg: incidence and risk factors in patients with inflammatory neuropathy. Neurology. 2020;94(6):e635–8.
31. Ahmed S, Kirmani JF, Janjua N, AlKawi A, Khatri I, Yahia AM, et al. An update on myasthenic crisis. Curr Treat Options Neurol. 2005;7(2):129–41.
32. Bershad EM, Feen ES, Suarez JI. Myasthenia gravis crisis. South Med J. 2008;101(1):63–9.
33. Kirmani JF, Yahia AM, Qureshi AI. Myasthenic crisis. Curr Treat Options Neurol. 2004;6(1):3–15.
34. Farmakidis C, Pasnoor M, Dimachkie MM, Barohn RJ. Treatment of myasthenia gravis. Neurol Clin. 2018;36(2):311–37.
35. Bedlack RS, Sanders DB. How to handle myasthenic crisis: essential steps in patient care. Postgrad Med. 2000;107(4):211–22.
36. Godoy DA, Mello LJVD, Masotti L, Napoli MD. The myasthenic patient in crisis: an update of the management in neurointensive care unit. Arq Neuropsiquiatr. 2013;71(9A):627–39.
37. Berrouschot J, Baumann I, Kalischewski P, Sterker M, Schneider D. Therapy of myasthenic crisis. Crit Care Med [Internet]. 1997;25(7).
38. Goti P, Spinelli A, Marconi G, Duranti R, Gigliotti F, Pizzi A, et al. Comparative effects of plasma exchange and pyridostigmine on respiratory muscle strength and breathing pattern in patients with myasthenia gravis. Thorax. 1995;50(10):1080.
39. Lacomis D. Myasthenic crisis. Neurocrit Care. 2005;3(3):189–94.
40. Thomas CE, Mayer SA, Gungor Y, Swarup R, Webster EA, Chang I, et al. Myasthenic crisis: clinical features, mortality, complications, and risk factors for prolonged intubation. Neurology. 1997;48(5):1253–60.
41. Juel VC. Myasthenia gravis: management of myasthenic crisis and perioperative care. Semin Neurol. 2004;24(1):75–81.
42. Sonkar KK, Bhoi SK, Dubey D, Kalita J, Misra UK. Direct and indirect cost of myasthenia gravis: a prospective study from a tertiary care teaching hospital in India. J Clin Neurosci. 2017;38:114–7.
43. Prado MB, Adiao KJ. Acetylcholinesterase inhibitors in Myasthenic crisis: a systematic review of observational studies. Neurocrit Care. 2021;35(2):528–44.
44. Mishra SK, Krishnappa S, Bhat RR, Badhe A. Role of intermittent noninvasive ventilation in anticholinesterase dose adjustment for Myasthenic crisis. Acta Anaesthesiol Taiwanica. 2010;48(1):53–4.
45. Mayer SA, Thomas CE. Therapy of myasthenic crisis. Crit Care Med. 1998;26(6):1136–7.
46. Cabrera Serrano M, Rabinstein AA. Causes and outcomes of acute neuromuscular respiratory failure. Arch Neurol. 2010;67(9):1089–94.
47. Radunovic A, Annane D, Rafiq MK, Mustfa N. Mechanical ventilation for amyotrophic lateral sclerosis/motor neuron disease. Cochrane Database Syst Rev. 2013;3:CD004427.
48. Rabinstein A, Wijdicks EFM. BiPAP in acute respiratory failure due to myasthenic crisis may prevent intubation. Neurology. 2002;59(10):1647–9.
49. Seneviratne J, Mandrekar J, Wijdicks EFM, Rabinstein AA. Noninvasive ventilation in myasthenic crisis. Arch Neurol [Internet]. 2008.
50. Rabinstein AA, Wijdicks EFM. Warning signs of imminent respiratory failure in neurological patients. Semin Neurol. 2003;23(1):97–104.
51. Rabinstein AA. Update on respiratory management of critically ill neurologic patients. Curr Neurol Neurosci Rep. 2005;5(6):476–82.
52. Vianello A, Bevilacqua M, Arcaro G, Gallan F, Serra E. Non-invasive ventilatory approach to treatment of acute respiratory failure in neuromuscular disorders. A comparison with endotracheal intubation. Intensive Care Med. 2000;26(4):384–90.

53. Nava S, Hill N. Non-invasive ventilation in acute respiratory failure. Lancet Lond Engl. 2009;374(9685):250–9.
54. Gregoretti C, Pisani L, Cortegiani A, Ranieri VM. Noninvasive ventilation in critically ill patients. Crit Care Clin. 2015;31(3):435–57.
55. Rabinstein AA. Noninvasive ventilation for neuromuscular respiratory failure: when to use and when to avoid. Curr Opin Crit Care. 2016;22(2):94–9.
56. Deymeer F, Gungor-Tuncer O, Yilmaz V, Parman Y, Serdaroglu P, Ozdemir C, et al. Clinical comparison of anti-MuSK- vs anti-AChR-positive and seronegative myasthenia gravis. Neurology. 2007;68(8):609–11.
57. Rabinstein AA, Wijdicks EFM. Weaning from the ventilator using BiPAP in myasthenia gravis. Muscle Nerve. 2003;27(2):252–3.
58. Seneviratne J, Mandrekar J, Wijdicks EFM, Rabinstein AA. Predictors of extubation failure in myasthenic crisis. Arch Neurol [Internet]. 2008.
59. Irfan M, Selim B, Rabinstein AA, St Louis EK. Neuromuscular disorders and sleep in critically ill patients. Crit Care Clin. 2015;31(3):533–50.
60. Bach JR, Gonçalves MR, Hamdani I, Winck JC. Extubation of patients with neuromuscular weakness: a new management paradigm. Chest. 2010;137(5):1033–9.
61. Pearse RM, Draper A, Grounds RM. Non-invasive ventilation to avoid tracheal intubation in a patient with Guillain-Barré syndrome. Br J Anaesth. 2003;91(6):913–6.
62. Wijdicks EFM, Roy TK. BiPAP in early guillain-barré syndrome may fail. Can J Neurol Sci J Can Sci Neurol. 2006;33(1):105–6.
63. Henderson RD, Lawn ND, Fletcher DD, McClelland RL, Wijdicks EFM. The morbidity of Guillain-Barré syndrome admitted to the intensive care unit. Neurology. 2003;60(1):17–21.
64. Lawn ND, Fletcher DD, Henderson RD, Wolter TD, Wijdicks EF. Anticipating mechanical ventilation in Guillain-Barré syndrome. Arch Neurol. 2001;58(6):893–8.
65. Craig VJ, Ford V, Chakrabarti B, Parker R, Duffy N, Ward K, et al. Non invasive ventilation in the weaning of patients with acute Guillain Barre syndrome requiring invasive ventilation. In: B50 Critical care: beyond the ventilator-non-invasive ventilation, high flow oxygen, and non-conventional ventilation [Internet]. American Thoracic Society; 2017. p. A3691. [cited 2024 Jul 5] (American Thoracic Society International Conference Abstracts).
66. Choi WA, Kang SW, Kim D, Won YH, Cho HE, Lee JW, et al. Weaning protocol using non-invasive ventilator in ventilator dependent Guillain Barre syndrome patients. In: C40 ARDS and acute respiratory failure: mechanism, risk, and outcomes [Internet]. American Thoracic Society; 2024. p. A5501. [cited 2024 Jul 10]. (American Thoracic Society International Conference Abstracts).
67. Rafiq MK, Bradburn M, Proctor AR, Billings CG, Bianchi S, McDermott CJ, et al. A preliminary randomized trial of the mechanical insufflator-exsufflator versus breath-stacking technique in patients with amyotrophic lateral sclerosis. Amyotroph Lateral Scler Front Degener. 2015;16(7–8):448–55.
68. Vianello A, Corrado A, Arcaro G, Gallan F, Ori C, Minuzzo M, et al. Mechanical insufflation-exsufflation improves outcomes for neuromuscular disease patients with respiratory tract infections. Am J Phys Med Rehabil. 2005;84(2):83–8. discussion 89–91
69. Bourke SC, Tomlinson M, Williams TL, Bullock RE, Shaw PJ, Gibson GJ. Effects of non-invasive ventilation on survival and quality of life in patients with amyotrophic lateral sclerosis: a randomised controlled trial. Lancet Neurol. 2006;5(2):140–7.
70. Mehta S. Neuromuscular disease causing acute respiratory failure. Respir Care. 2006;51(9):1016–21. discussion 1021–1023
71. Scala R, Pisani L. Noninvasive ventilation in acute respiratory failure: which recipe for success? Eur Respir Rev. 2018;27(149):180029.
72. Bernardes Neto SCG, Torres-Castro R, Lima Í, Resqueti VR, Fregonezi GAF. Weaning from mechanical ventilation in people with neuromuscular disease: a systematic review. BMJ Open. 2021;11(9):e047449.
73. Zein H, Baratloo A, Negida A, Safari S. Ventilator weaning and spontaneous breathing trials; an educational review. Emerg Tehran Iran. 2016;4(2):65–71.

74. De Souza LC, Guimarães FS, Lugon JR. The timed inspiratory effort: a promising index of mechanical ventilation weaning for patients with neurologic or neuromuscular diseases. Respir Care. 2015;60(2):231–8.
75. American Thoracic Society/European Respiratory Society. ATS/ERS statement on respiratory muscle testing. Am J Respir Crit Care Med. 2002;166(4):518–624.
76. Krishnakumar M, Muthuchellappan R, Chakrabarti D. Diaphragm function assessment during spontaneous breathing trial in patients with neuromuscular diseases. Neurocrit Care. 2021;34(2):382–9.
77. Sun Q, Shan F, Dong H, Jiang Y, Sun Y, Sun Y. Predictive value of ultrasonic diaphragm thickening fraction on successful weaning for patients with myasthenia gravis crisis. Zhonghua Wei Zhong Bing Ji Jiu Yi Xue. 2017;29(7):619–23.
78. Vianello A, Arcaro G, Braccioni F, Gallan F, Marchi MR, Chizio S, et al. Prevention of extubation failure in high-risk patients with neuromuscular disease. J Crit Care. 2011;26(5):517–24.
79. Elkins M, Dentice R. Inspiratory muscle training facilitates weaning from mechanical ventilation among patients in the intensive care unit: a systematic review. J Physiother. 2015;61(3):125–34.

Seizures in ICU

8

Jayanth R. Seshan, Prasanna Udupi Bidkar, and Adethen Gunasekaran

Abstract

Seizures in the intensive care unit may occur in 3–34% of patients based on the etiology. This chapter intends to provide an overview of controversies regarding management, highlighting recent evidence from the literature and the latest guidelines. Continuous monitoring of the electroencephalograph (EEG) is helpful for early detection and guiding the management of nonconvulsive status epilepticus in high-risk etiologies. Despite the introduction of newer antiepileptic medications, phenytoin and levetiracetam continue to be used in routine clinical practice, although the use of phenytoin may be declining. Evidence continues to emerge regarding the optimal drugs, time duration of treatment, and weaning of anesthetic medications for refractory status epilepticus. The treatment protocol of nonconvulsive status epilepticus remains largely extrapolated from the same for convulsive status epilepticus, although newer agents like topiramate, perampanel, and lacosamide continue to be explored. Long-term seizure prophylaxis in acute brain injury can be guided by clinical and electrographic risk scores.

Keywords

EEG · Status epilepticus · Nonconvulsive seizures · Antiepileptic drugs · Seizures

J. R. Seshan · P. U. Bidkar (✉) · A. Gunasekaran
JIPMER, Puducherry, Puducherry, India

P. U. Bidkar, M. Krishnakumar (eds.), *Controversies in Neurocritical Care*,
https://doi.org/10.1007/978-981-95-4419-6_8

8.1 Introduction

A seizure is usually a transient occurrence of signs/ symptoms due to abnormal, excessive, or synchronous neuronal activity in the brain [1]. The incidence of seizures in the intensive care unit (ICU) varies from 3% to 34%, based on underlying etiology [2]. Seizures may remain a controlled, isolated event or progress to severe forms like status epilepticus due to multiple causes. This chapter provides an overview of certain important aspects of the management of seizures in the ICU, while readers are encouraged to refer to the resources provided at the end for a comprehensive understanding.

8.2 Continuous Versus Intermittent (Routine) EEG Monitoring

8.2.1 Need for EEG Monitoring

Nonconvulsive seizures (electrographic seizures without clinically evident seizures) occur in up to 10–48% of patients in the ICU. According to a recent meta-analysis, the estimated prevalence of nonconvulsive seizure, nonconvulsive status epilepticus (NCSE), or either of them in the ICU by routine and continuous EEG monitoring is 3.1%, 6.2%, 6.3%, and 17.9%, 9.1% and 15.6%, respectively [3, 4]. The role of EEG monitoring in the ICU includes:

1. Seizure detection and management, including titration of antiseizure medications
2. Monitoring for cerebral ischemia
3. Neuroprognostication
4. Diagnosis of seizure mimics
5. Titration of anesthetics (sedation monitoring and during withdrawal of anesthetics in the management of status epilepticus)

8.2.2 Definition of Routine and Continuous EEG Monitoring

Routine EEG (also known as spot EEG) conventionally refers to a minimum of 20 minutes of technically satisfactory (artifact-free) recordings of the electrical activity of the brain, which also includes the use of activation procedures like hyperventilation (barring specific contraindications) and photic stimulation [5, 6]. Continuous EEG monitoring usually lasts for several hours to days and is commonly used in epilepsy units and in critically ill patients at risk of seizures. cEEG may include simultaneous video recordings to improve electroclinical correlation and rule out seizure mimics [7].

8.2.3 Indications for Continuous EEG Monitoring

The incidence of seizures in patients admitted to the ICU with encephalopathy, coma, or other disorders of consciousness following traumatic brain injury (TBI), subarachnoid (SAH) or intracerebral hemorrhage (ICH), meningoencephalitis, brain tumors, post-neurosurgical procedures, sepsis, or even cardiac arrest is about 15% [8]. Hence, monitoring for detection assumes significance. The American Clinical Neurophysiology Society (ACNS) has recommended continuous monitoring of the EEG for the following indications [9].

1. Persistently altered mental status following clinically evident seizures or generalized convulsive status epilepticus, or acute supratentorial brain injury
2. Fluctuations or unexplained alteration of mental status without known acute brain injury
3. EEG patterns of periodic discharges and lateralized rhythmic delta activity, which are suggestive of an ictal-interictal continuum
4. Situations like extracorporeal membrane oxygenation (ECMO) or targeted temperature management for cardiac arrest, which require pharmacological paralysis, potentially mask the risk of clinical seizures
5. Paroxysmal clinical events with a suspicion of possible seizures

8.2.4 Continuous Versus Routine: How to Choose?

Since Neurocritical Care Society (NCS) detection in the ICU is the major role of EEG monitoring, stratification of patients for risk of seizures may help in identifying those who require continuous/prolonged EEG monitoring. The *2HELPS2B* score has been validated to predict the probability of subsequent seizure risk based on the findings of the initial EEG recordings and the patient's history. The constituents include frequency exceeding *2 Hz*, independent sporadic *e*pileptiform discharges, *l*ateralized rhythmic or periodic patterns, *p*lus features like superimposed rhythmic fast or sharp activity, prior *s*eizure history, epilepsy, or suspicion of acute clinical seizure, and *b*rief ictal rhythmic discharges. Of the above, one point is accorded for all except brief rhythmic discharges, which are given two points. Accordingly, the predicted seizure risk for points 0–5 is <5%, 12%, 27%, 50%, 73%, and 88% respectively. Based on the score, patients with >2 points on the initial hour of EEG monitoring are considered high-risk and benefit from continuous EEG monitoring [10, 11].

8.2.5 cEEG in aSAH

The incidence of seizures in aneurysmal subarachnoid hemorrhage (aSAH) was previously reported to be around 26%. This has been refined in recent times due to the advent of EEG monitoring, and recent studies project the incidence to be

7.8–15.2% with a 2.3% incidence of early postoperative seizure [12, 13]. Depressed mental status, ruptured middle cerebral artery (MCA), high-grade SAH, ICH, hydrocephalus, and cortical infarcts are reasonable indications to institute cEEG monitoring for the detection of seizures [14]. Continuous EEG monitoring can detect delayed cerebral ischemia (DCI) with findings such as a change in total power of the quantitative EEG [15], decreased relative alpha variability [16], and post-stimulation reduction in the ADR (alpha power/delta power) by >50% [17].

8.2.6 cEEG in TBI

Incidence of electrographic seizures (NCS) detected by cEEG in TBI patients ranges between 3.8% and 33%. The most recent literature demonstrated ictal-interictal (IIC) patterns in 74 out of 152 patients (49%), [18–20] Faster frequency lateralized rhythmic delta activity (LRDA) or generalized periodic discharges (GPD), lateralized periodic discharges, or electrographic seizures were the features suggestive of severe IIC and were present in 22 (14%) patients. Such severe features occurred either earlier than 4 hours or later than 48 hours of injury in seven patients each and between 4 and 48 hours in the rest (36%), suggesting the need for continuous and prolonged EEG monitoring. Absence of PDR or N2 sleep transients and presence of background delta activity are the risk factors associated with poor functional outcome [19].

8.2.7 Post-cardiac Arrest

The role of EEG monitoring in comatose patients following resuscitation after cardiac arrest is probably the least disputed. Monitoring brain activity during targeted temperature management, determining the extent of brain injury after cardiac arrest, and identifying epileptiform activity are the major indications. Generalized EEG suppression (<10 μV) and synchronous patterns with >50% suppression are features of poor neurological recovery with low sensitivity (50%) but high specificity (100%) up to 24 hours after cardiac arrest [21–23]. Conversion from rEEG to cEEG should be considered on identification of factors predicting a favorable prognosis—brainstem reflexes, evoked potentials, brain imaging, or rEEG showing continuous background EEG activity [24].

Table 8.1 summarizes the recent evidence regarding continuous vs intermittent monitoring of EEG in neurocritical care settings.

8.2.8 Practical Considerations

Key aspects to consider are the rapid availability of EEG, technical expertise to analyze an enormous amount of data generated by continuous monitoring, and, as such, the availability of such equipment adequately in resource-limited settings.

Table 8.1 Continuous vs intermittent EEG monitoring- summary of recent evidence

Type of study	Author (year)	Objectives	Sample size	Definitions	Results	Conclusions.
Systematic review and meta-analysis	Limotai et al. [3] (2019)	Pooled prevalence of NCS, NCSE and epileptiform activity detected by different EEG types in critically ill and compare detection rates	78 cross-sectional studies (16,707 patients) and 8 comparative studies (4894 patients)	rEEG (routine)- 20 minutes; cEEG (continuous)- 12 hours or longer	rEEg vs cEEG prevalence of NCS, NCSE, EA- 3.1%, 6.2%, 6.3% and 17.9%, 9.1% and 15.6% respectively. Odds Ratio of detection by cEEG vs rEEG for paired data (patients initially monitored with rEEG and then by cEEG) was 2.57 (1.11–5.96)	Higher prevalence of seizures detected by cEEG; especially in post-convulsive status epilepticus, CNS infections and post-cardiac arrest
Systematic review	Kondziella et al. [25] (2014)	Diagnostic accuracy of cEEG for detecting nonconvulsive seizure, including NCSE, and DCI in patients with aneurysmal SAH	18 studies (481 patients) with aneurysmal SAH	Duration of cEEG not defined	cEEG incidence of NCS, and NCSE was 7–18% and 3–13% respectively. Duration of cEEG monitoring- 5 days (range 1–60 days). Diagnosis of DCI established in 20–46% of patients.	Increased detection of subclinical seizures with cEEG monitoring following SAH. cEEG may predict DCI in advance
Systematic review	Guo et al. [26] (2020)	Diagnostic accuracy and predictive factors of cEEG for detecting seizure and DCI following aSAH	23 studies with 3675 patients. 1224 underwent cEEG monitoring		cEEG incidence of NCS and NCSE was 6.4% each; 119 and 104 patients respectively. cEEG monitoring duration ranged from 0 to 60 days. 214 patients (27%) diagnosed with DCI with qEEG; detection was 7 hours- 1.9 days prior to standard diagnosis by imaging or TCD.	cEEG is an effective monitoring tool for early detection of DCI and seizures

(continued)

Table 8.1 (continued)

Type of study	Author (year)	Objectives	Sample size	Definitions	Results	Conclusions.
Prospective cohort (post-hoc analysis of INTREPID RCT)	Lee et al. [19] (2019)	Prevalence of electrographic seizures after moderate–severe TBI and correlate cEEG with functional outcome	152 underwent cEEG monitoring	Median of 70 hours (42–101) starting 10 (8–14) hours after injury	Ictal-interictal continuum and electrographic seizures in 22 (14%) and 4 (2.6%) patients respectively.	Incidence of IIC features did not affect functional outcome
RCT	Rossetti et al. (2020) [27]—CERTA trial	Assess whether cEEG is associated with reduced mortality when compared with rEEG in a mixed ICU population	364 patients randomized to cEEG and rEEG	cEEG- 30-48 hours vs rEEG 20–30 minutes 48-hours apart	IIC detection cEEG vs rEEG- 128 (69.2%) vs 102 (55.7%). Seizures/SE- 29 (15.7%) vs 8 (4.4%) respectively. 6-month mortality- 89 (48.9%) vs 88 (48.4%) (*P* 0.92)	cEEG led to higher detection of epileptiform activity but no effect on mortality
RCT (post-hoc analysis of CERTA trial)	Urbano et al. [22] (2022)	Relationship of cEEG and rEEG on outcome in post-cardiac arrest patients	112 patients- cEEG- 60 (53.6%) and rEEG- 52 (46.4%)	cEEG- 30-48 hours vs rEEG 20–30 minutes 48-hours apart	Mortality in the groups cEEG vs rEEG- 39 (65%) vs 29 (55.8%) respectively. (*P* 0.318) Detection of seizures/SE and IIC were comparable in the groups. [12(20%) vs 5 (9.6%) (*P* 0.127] and [11 (18.3%) vs 7 (13.5%) (*P* 0.484)] respectively.	cEEG and repeat rEEG lead to comparable outcomes in comatose patients following cardiac arrest

Based on evidence available so far, it may be reasonable to consider cEEG for a duration of up to 12–24 hours in patients with recent seizures or status epilepticus (SE). The addition of video-EEG adds to the detection of NCS and treatment surveillance in such patients. For those with unproven ictal events, rEEG may be considered initially, and risk stratification scores may be employed to determine the need for further monitoring. If no abnormal activity is noted in the rEEG, a repeat EEG may be considered after 24–48 hours based on the evolving clinical condition [28].

Despite conclusively contributing to increased detection of NCS/NCSE, epileptiform activity, and features of ictal-interictal continuum, current evidence does not give a clear indication favoring the use of cEEG monitoring in the ICU to improve the outcome in neurocritical care. Use of EEG monitoring should be encouraged for titration of antiseizure medications, including anesthetics. Resource-limited settings should consider the use of routine EEGs whenever applicable until such time as more reliable evidence supports the superiority of continuous EEG monitoring and recommends the same.

8.3 First-Line Antiepileptic Drugs (AED) in Neurocritical Care

The initiation of AED depends on the type and nature of seizure as well as the etiology. The most common indications of AED initiation in neurocritical care include termination of acute seizure/convulsive status epilepticus, nonconvulsive seizures, or as prophylaxis for certain etiologies like TBI, Stroke–ICH, ischemic stroke, and SAH, and in neuroinfections. Table 8.2 provides a summary of the pharmacological properties of the commonly used AEDs.

8.3.1 Status Epilepticus (SE) and Refractory Status Epilepticus (RSE)

Emergency management of status epilepticus involves the use of intravenous benzodiazepines, antiseizure medications, and progressive escalation to anesthetic agents based on the stage of SE being dealt with.

8.3.1.1 Stage I: Early Status Epilepticus

Intravenous Lorazepam, diazepam, intramuscular or buccal midazolam, or rectal diazepam form the established first-line AEDs to terminate seizures [2]. If seizures continue for 5 minutes after the first dose, a second dose should be considered. Though IV is the preferred route, other routes of administration are acceptable and equally effective, provided appropriate doses are given. The use of diazepam is discouraged in the presence of other alternatives. Despite its fast onset of action, the similarly fast redistribution increases the risk of seizure recurrence [29].

Table 8.2 Properties of conventional AEDs and anesthetic drugs used in RSE

Drugs	Mechanism of action	Route of administration	Metabolism & Elimination	Loading dose	Maximum tolerated Maintenance dose	Adverse effects
AEDs- Second and third generation						
Levetiracetam	SV2A receptor	IV, PO	Renal (unchanged)	60 mg/kg	1500 mg TDS	Behavioral and psychiatric issues
Fosphenytoin	Na channel	IV, PO	Hepatic	20 mg/kg	100 mg TDS	Purple glove syndrome, cardiac arrhythmias, sedation
Lacosamide	Na channel	IV, PO	Renal (unchanged)	8 mg/kg	200 mg TDS	Dizziness, diplopia, sedation
Brivaracetam	SV2A	IV, PO	Hepatic metabolism	4 mg/kg	100 mg TDS	Sedation (only in severe overdose)
Perampanel	AMPAR	PO	Hepatic metabolism	8–24 mg	12 mg OD	Sedation
Anesthetic medications						
Midazolam	GABA-A	IV/ IM	Oxidation and glucuronidation	0.2 mg/kg	2 mg/kg/hour	Respiratory depression, hypotension, tachyphylaxis
Propofol	GABA-A	IV		1–2 mg/kg	5 mg/kg/hour	Respiratory depression, hypotension myocardial suppression, propofol infusion syndrome
Ketamine	NMDA	IV		1–2 mg/kg	10–15 mg/kg/hour	Cardiovascular and respiratory stimulation
Thiopentone	GABA-A	IV		2–5 mg/kg	5 mg/kg/hour	Respiratory depression, hypotension, myocardial suppression, paralytic ileus, higher risk of infections due to immunosuppression

8.3.1.2 Stage II: Established Status Epilepticus

This stage involves the use of a non-sedating AED administered usually along with a benzodiazepine. The AEDs available for use at this stage include phenytoin, fosphenytoin, valproate, and levetiracetam. Newer agents like Lacosamide and Brivaracetam are less well studied [30].

8.3.1.3 Stage III: Refractory Status Epilepticus

Progression to refractory seizures—non-responsiveness to Stage I and II treatment occurs in about 30% of those with seizures [31, 32]. Management of RSE depends on the type of seizures. Generalized convulsive RSE requires ICU admission and administration of anesthetics. A similar management strategy is extrapolated for NCSE as these patients tend to be intubated due to the altered mental status, permitting ease of administration of anesthetic medications. For focal RSE, non-sedative AEDs may be safely used to manage such patients even outside the ICU setting. Newer medications like topiramate and perampanel have found use in this regard [33].

Management of RSE is described in the latter part of this chapter.

8.3.2 AEDs for Seizure Prophylaxis/Management in Acute Brain Injury

8.3.2.1 Traumatic Brain Injury

The risk factors for seizures following TBI have been defined in the Brain Trauma Foundation guidelines. The most recent guideline, published in 2016, emphasized the use of phenytoin as prophylaxis to reduce the incidence of early post-traumatic seizures (PTS) (less than 7 days of injury). It also outlined the insufficient evidence to recommend the use of levetiracetam over phenytoin regarding the efficacy in the prevention of early PTS and the toxicity profile [34].

More recently, the Neurocritical Care Society (NCS) has provided guidelines for seizure prophylaxis in adults with moderate–severe TBI [35].

1. It is suggested that either prophylactic AED or no AED may be used in moderate–severe TBI *(weak recommendation, low quality of evidence).*
2. If the use of a prophylactic AED is warranted, levetiracetam may be suggested over phenytoin or fosphenytoin *(weak recommendation, low quality of evidence).*
3. When AEDs are used, it is suggested to prefer a short duration (<7 days) of treatment over a longer duration *(weak recommendation, low quality of evidence).*

It may be noted that the definition of early PTS is inclusive of a 14-day duration since the trauma, considering the average duration of hospitalization of 2 weeks in such cases.

8.3.3 Stroke

Post-stroke seizures and epilepsy have an incidence of about 3–6% with a higher risk in hemorrhagic stroke. The European Stroke Organization (ESO) recommendations guide the current practice of seizure prophylaxis in stroke. The recent recommendations summarized below are plagued by low-quality evidence and weak strength of recommendation [36].

1. Primary AED prophylaxis is not recommended to prevent acute symptomatic seizures.
2. Immediate secondary AED prophylaxis is not recommended to treat acute symptomatic seizures or prevent recurrence of unprovoked seizures.
3. Use of an AED in order to improve functional outcome or reduce mortality after stroke is not recommended.
4. Secondary AED prophylaxis may be considered after one post-stroke unprovoked seizure.

8.3.3.1 Acute Ischemic Stroke

The American Heart Association (AHA), in its recommendations for the early management of patients with acute ischemic stroke, opined the following regarding the management of seizures [37].

1. Recurrent seizures after stroke should be treated similarly to seizures occurring in other neurological conditions and require selection of AEDs based on specific patient characteristics *(Level I evidence; Class C: limited data*)
2. Prophylactic use of AED is not recommended (*Level III; Class B*)

Evidence from guidelines was supported by a recent Cochrane review, which found insufficient evidence to support the routine use of AEDs for the primary prevention and treatment of post-stroke seizures [38]. Contrary to the guidelines, a recent decision analysis suggested benefits from the use of a short-term secondary AED prophylaxis (1 week) and restarted later and continued for life, only in the case of the patient developing a late seizure [39].

8.3.3.2 Subarachnoid Hemorrhage

The AHA/ ASA guidelines (2023) regarding the management of patients with aSAH elaborate on the primary and secondary seizure prophylaxis [40].

1. Use of AEDs for primary prophylaxis is considered reasonable in aSAH with high-risk features for seizures (MCA aneurysm, high-grade SAH, ICH, hydro-

cephalus, cortical infarcts) (*Level 2b*), while no benefit is offered in patients without high-risk features (*Level 3*).
2. Phenytoin for primary and prophylaxis in seizures is associated with increased risk of mortality and morbidity (*Level 3*).

8.3.3.3 Spontaneous Intracerebral Hemorrhage

The AHA/ ASA guidelines (2022) regarding the management of spontaneous ICH elaborate on the primary and secondary seizure prophylaxis [41].

1. AEDs *should be* administered to reduce morbidity in patients with spontaneous ICH, impaired consciousness, and confirmed electrographic seizures (*Level I recommendation*)
2. AEDs are recommended to improve functional outcomes and prevent recurrent seizure-induced brain injury in patients with spontaneous ICH and clinical seizures (*Level I recommendation*)
3. Prophylactic AEDs are not beneficial to improve functional outcomes, long-term seizure control, or mortality in patients with spontaneous ICH without evidence of seizures (*Level 3 recommendation*)

8.3.3.4 Clinical Practice Variations

Prescription of AEDs in aSAH also tends to depend on the severity of radiological grading and the treatment modality for securing the aneurysm, clipping> coiling [42]. In line with the recommendation against phenytoin, most patients in this study were prescribed levetiracetam, and no association was found between the use of AED and morbidity or mortality at 6-month duration. Levetiracetam is now commonly used as the first-choice AED for prophylaxis in acute brain injury in vulnerable groups [43–45].

8.4 Management of Refractory Status Epilepticus

The International League Against Epilepsy (ILAE), established to classify and assign appropriate terminologies, has provided definitions and stages of epileptic events based on the duration of these events. "*Status Epilepticus is a condition resulting from either failure of the mechanisms responsible for seizure termination or from the initiation of such mechanisms, which lead to abnormally prolonged seizures (T1). It can lead to long-term consequences (T2) including neuronal death, neuronal injury and alteration of neuronal networks, depending on the type and duration of seizures,*" [46]

8.4.1 Refractory Status Epilepticus

Refractory status epilepticus (RSE) refers to the persistence of status epilepticus despite the administration of at least two appropriately selected and dosed parenteral medications, including a benzodiazepine, and not specified by a time duration. The incidence of RSE was found to be 3.0–7.2 per 100,000 adults per year [47, 48]. Older age and female gender are associated with a higher incidence of status epilepticus—79.9 and 89.6 per 1,00,000 adults, respectively, with mortality rates of up to 22.5% in females [49]. Needless to say, the risk of mortality increases with status epilepticus refractory to initial management. Status epilepticus may stem from cerebrovascular disorders, trauma, infections, alcohol and drug-induced conditions, or may be a result of low antiseizure medication levels in patients with preexisting epilepsy disorder.

8.4.2 Controversies in the Management of RSE

1. Selection of anesthetic medications—risk vs. benefit
2. Anesthetic drugs and the time duration of seizure freedom
3. Weaning of anesthetic medications
4. Role of ketamine

8.4.3 Selection of Anesthetics

Midazolam, propofol, and barbiturates are commonly used medications as continuous infusions for the management of RSE (Table 8.2). Lately, ketamine, used in the management of SRSE, is also being used for RSE. Except for ketamine, all the other medications are prone to cause significant respiratory depression and require endotracheal intubation for mechanical ventilation. The choice of individual agents also depends on the other side-effect profile, especially with a longer duration of administration required for effective seizure control. Increased risk of complications and mortality has been found in observational studies, and there is a clear lack of high-grade evidence owing to the nonavailability of RCTs. Current evidence suggests that midazolam may be the most commonly used, while barbiturates exhibit better efficacy in seizure control, albeit with a higher risk of complications and longer duration of mechanical ventilation [50].

8.4.4 Duration of Administration for Seizure Freedom

The goal of seizure freedom is achieved with boluses of anesthetic agents followed by maintenance infusions. Current guidelines suggest a duration of 24–48 hours of maintenance of anesthetic infusions with burst suppression for the management of RSE [51, 52]. This guideline is not based on high-quality evidence from the literature but on expert opinions. The duration may be guided by continuous EEG monitoring to demonstrate a lack of seizure activity or burst suppression. Recent literature has challenged this current concept by providing evidence that shorter duration and deeper anesthetic levels may be more beneficial and that every 12 additional hours of therapeutic coma increases the risk of seizure recurrence by 20% [53].

8.4.5 Protocol for Weaning

The major consideration regarding weaning from induced coma is the risk of withdrawal seizure. Also, breakthrough seizures (occurrence of nonconvulsive seizures during the course of treatment) necessitate the use of cEEG monitoring. Currently, there is no available evidence to define the weaning protocols accurately. It may be reasonable to allow progressive weaning over a period of several hours to minimize the risk of complications. Rapid weaning protocols are also described, which mandate dose escalation and longer duration of treatment in case of relapse [54]. An acceptable protocol for midazolam would be to wean at a rate of 1–2 mg/hour from the maximal dose of 2 mg/kg/hour, which would allow a total duration of 24–48 hours for the cessation of drug administration.

8.4.6 Role of Ketamine

Ketamine is an NMDA receptor antagonist, differing from the action of other anesthetic medications, and thereby offers a different strategy for treatment. Until recently, ketamine has been considered in the management of SRSE, while recent evidence, though based on small reports, may provide the clinician with the option of earlier initiation. This may be due to the lack of respiratory and cardiovascular depressant properties. A combination of ketamine with midazolam or propofol may negate the latter's negative circulatory effects and provide superior efficacy.

Table 8.3 provides consolidated evidence of recent trials regarding anesthetic drugs in the management of RSE.

Table 8.3 Summary of recent evidence on anesthetic drugs for management of RSE

Type of study	Author (year)	Objectives	Sample size	Results	Conclusions
Systematic review	Au et al. [50] (2024)	Comparison of various anesthetic drugs for RSE with clinical outcomes	66 studies with 1637 patients. Midazolam (838), Propofol (619), Pentobarbital (66), Ketamine (10)	1. Duration of SE in midazolam, propofol and barbiturate group were 2.2, and 0.4 days respectively 2. Mortality rates with midazolam, propofol and barbiturates were 37%, 20% and 40.3% respectively 3. Complications like short-term failure and hypotension in the three groups were 23.4%, 42.3%, 10.4% and 44.1%, 39.9%, 81.9% respectively	Choice of initial AED is associated with treatment failure and adverse events but not mortality
RCT	Rossetti et al. [55] (2011)	Propofol vs barbiturates for the control of RSE	24 (14 received propofol and 9 received barbiturates); target sample size- 150	1. Primary endpoint: propofol vs barbiturate- 43% vs 22% (*P* 0.40) 2. Similar rates of infection and arterial hypotension between the groups 3. No difference in mortality- 43% vs 34% 4. Longer duration of mechanical ventilation in barbiturate group	Significant morbidity and mortality in patients undergoing treatment for RSE. Underpowered trial emphasizing the need for multi-centric data
RCT	Masapu et al. [56] (2018)	Compare the efficacy of midazolam and propofol (TCI) in patients with RSE	23 (Propofol-11, midazolam-12)	1. Overall seizure control: 34.8%; propofol vs midazolam- 45% vs 25% 2. Mortality: propofol vs midazolam: 72.7% vs 58.3% (*P* 0.667)	Choice of anesthetic agent does not affect overall outcome in RSE

Systematic review	Yan et al. [57] (2024)	Efficacy of Ketamine for the treatment of super-refractory status epilepticus	11 studies with 307 patients including RSE and SRSE	1. Response to ketamine was observed in 36.36–91% of patients across studies 2. Mortality ranged between 0% and 54%	Early administration of ketamine is advised after detailed analysis of individual patient characteristics
Systematic review	Adhikari et al. [58] (2024)	Role of ketamine in children and adults with SRSE	19 studies with 336 participants	1. Seizure resolution rates between 40% and 100% 2. Latency to ketamine use ranged from 6 hours to 122 days and duration of use was 6 hours to 30 days 3. Mortality across the larger studies included were 38.8–59.5%	Ketamine is safe and effective in SRSE, provides neuroprotection and reduces vasopressor requirements
Retrospective cohort	Muhlhofer et al. [53] (2019)	Define an optimal window for therapeutic coma to provide sustained seizure control and minimal complications	182 patients with various types of SE treated with propofol and midazolam infusions	1. Seizure recurrence observed in 44 (24.2%) patients 2. Seizure recurrence group had a longer duration of treatment than nonrecurrence group (27.2 vs 15.6 hours, P 0.02) 3. Longer duration of treatment was associated with increased rate of complications (P 0.002) with no effect on mortality (P 0.32)	Shorter duration of deeper therapeutic coma may be more effective and safer than the conventional duration of 24–48 hours

8.5 Nonconvulsive Seizures: Detection and Implications

Nonconvulsive seizures (NCS) refer to a heterogeneous clinical condition defined by a paroxysmal change in behavior from baseline without convulsive activity and EEG evidence of continuous paroxysmal activity or electrographic discharges [59]. Nonconvulsive status epilepticus (NCSE) is defined as a continuous NCS lasting for 10 minutes or more (shortened from the prior interval of 30 minutes) without recovery of sensory, motor, or cognitive functions in between [60]. The terms NCS and NCSE are commonly interchangeable with electrographic seizures and electrographic status epilepticus, respectively. NCS may be present in 8–30% of patients with altered mental status, while NCSE accounts for 21–47% of status epilepticus in the ICU. The most common causes include underlying epilepsy, acute brain injury, acute systemic insults, and drugs.

8.5.1 Salzburg Consensus Criteria

The following EEG patterns are recognized as diagnostic of NCS/ NCSE [61].

1. Epileptiform discharges (spikes, polyspikes, sharp waves, and, sharp and slow wave complexes) > 2.5 Hz; or
2. Epileptiform discharges <2.5 Hz or rhythmic delta/ theta activity (>0.5 Hz) along with
   (a) EEG as well as clinical improvement after treatment with intravenous AED
   (b) Subtle clinical ictal phenomena observed during the EEG patterns described
   (c) Typical spatiotemporal evolution

8.5.2 Implications of NCS/ NCSE in the ICU

Among the known causes, epilepsy is the most commonly associated with NCS, and a significant proportion of critically ill convulsive status epilepticus patients (30–50%) transform into NCSE and may be the result of inadequate early treatment [62]. The incidence of AIS, ICH, TBI, and aSAH, and the role of EEG monitoring in detection have been described in Table 8.1.

8.5.3 Management of NCS/ NCSE

The pharmacological management of NCS/ NCSE largely follows the protocol for the treatment of convulsive status because of inadequate evidence. Initial management consists of benzodiazepine administration followed by second-line treatment with adequately dosed AEDs. Since NCS includes focal seizures and those with absence of coma, a few drugs like topiramate, perampanel, and lacosamide are beneficial, apart from the use of older-generation AEDs (Table 8.4). If uncontrolled, the third step in the management would proceed with anesthetic drugs with similar objectives to those in convulsive SE.

Table 8.4 Summary of evidence for the use of newer AEDs for NCS/ NCSE

Type of study	Author (year)	Objectives	Sample size	Results	Conclusions
RCT: Treatment of Recurrent Electrographic Nonconvulsive Seizures (TRENdS)	Husain et al. [63] (2018)	Compare Lacosamide and Fosphenytoin for electrographic cessation of NCS using cEEG	74 (37 subjects in each group)	1. Primary end point achieved in 19 (63%) vs 16 (50%) (*P* 0.02) in lacosamide vs fosphenytoin group 2. Similar adverse effect profile: 25.7% vs 24.3% in both groups	Lacosamide is non-inferior to Fosphenytoin in the treatment of NCS detected by cEEG
Retrospective Study	Rohracher et al. [64] (2018)	Efficacy and safety of perampanel as add-on treatment in RSE and SRSE	30	1. High-dose approach 24 mg (16–32) in 14 patients (vs standard dose of 4 mg in 16 patients) 2. Termination of SE in 5 (17%) patients 3. Unfavorable neurological outcome in 13 (43%) patients-56% in high-dose group	Oral perampanel was tolerated in high doses but no significant efficacy
Retrospective Study	Fechner et al. [65] (2019)	Resolution of SE after initiation of topiramate	106 patients	1. Response to treatment in 29 (27.6%) patients. [21 (31.8%) in RSE] 2. Hyperammonemia observed in 38 (35.8%) patients	Topiramate can be an alternative option in treating RSE and SRSE

8.5.4 Prognosis in NCSE

NCSE without coma generally results in a better prognosis. For those with a coma, it is recommended to treat aggressively with first- and second-line medications and proceed to make a rapid assessment of response prior to initiation of anesthetic drugs. Prognostic clinical scores may be employed to assess the seizure burden and proceed with management accordingly. The status epilepticus severity score (STESS) is a six-point scoring system that relies on four parameters: age (0–1 points), prior seizure history (0–1 points), extent of consciousness impairment (0–1 points), and type of seizure (0–2 points) with low scores (0–2) indicating a favorable prognosis. The outcomes are largely dependent on the primary etiology and early detection of NCS; therefore, it becomes vital in patients with severe acute brain injury [66, 67].

8.6 Long-Term Management of Epilepsy After Brain Injury

Epilepsy is a recognized complication of various acute neurological injuries, including traumatic brain injury, stroke, and CNS infections.

8.6.1 TBI

Epilepsy following TBI usually correlates with the severity of the initial injury, but it is known to occur even after mild TBI. The incidence of seizures after TBI increases from 1% in 1 year to up to 4% in 9 years following the initial trauma [68]. A recent systematic review estimated that individuals who suffered a TBI were 4.25 times at a higher risk of epilepsy than those without TBI and that such risk is highest till 5 years after the trauma [69].

8.6.2 Management

Despite evidence from the literature regarding the incidence and risk, current guidelines do not support the long-term use of AED prophylaxis. Prophylaxis may be employed for the prevention of early PTS, but has no significant effect on late PTS. This may be partly due to the significant adverse effects of such drugs, resulting in neuropsychiatric effects and influence on functional outcomes.

8.6.3 Stroke

Stroke constitutes a major cause of new-onset epilepsy in older adults. Both ischemic and hemorrhagic strokes can lead to post-stroke epilepsy (PSE) with an incidence ranging between 2–14% and 10–20%, respectively [70, 71]. Post-stroke inflammation, blood–brain-barrier disruptions, and maladaptive neuronal plasticity are the major mechanisms attributed to post-stroke epilepsy [72].

8.6.4 Risk Factors

Volume of tissue involved, cortical affection, hemorrhagic transformation, stroke severity, and early seizures after stroke are the major risk factors for long-term epilepsy. Reperfusion therapy is not a proven risk factor [73, 74]. Major risk factors have been evaluated in the development of scoring systems for prognostic significance. The CAVE scoring system for hemorrhagic stroke incorporates cortical hemorrhage, age, volume of intracranial hemorrhage, and early seizures, and has been shown to have PSE in up to 34.8% and 46.2% in those with scores 3 and 4, respectively, during long-term follow-up [75]. As regards ischemic stroke, the SeLECT score, which includes stroke severity, presence of large artery atherosclerosis, occurrence of early seizure, involvement of cortical regions, and the middle cerebral artery territory, estimates the risk of delayed seizures at 45%, 65%, and 83% for scores of 7,8, and 9, respectively [76].

8.6.5 Pathophysiology

Early and late PSE generally have different mechanisms and so do hemorrhagic and ischemic strokes. Neuronal excitation secondary to tissue damage is the reason for early PSE in ischemic stroke, whereas late PSE is secondary to gliotic scarring and disruption of neuronal networks. On the other hand, the pathogenesis of epileptogenesis after hemorrhagic stroke includes albumin extravasation into the brain parenchyma and iron deposition (from the extravasated blood). The resultant cytotoxicity has come to be known as ferroptosis and is mediated by reactive oxygen species [77, 78].

8.6.6 Management

Despite an abundance of data regarding risk factors and the evolution of multiple scoring systems for risk stratification, current guidelines do not recommend AED prophylaxis for long-term management of post-stroke epilepsy. This may be due to the possible formation of epileptic foci in the initial hours after stroke onset, where treatment with AEDs tends to result in adverse effects and drug reactions. Currently, the only class of drugs with reliable evidence regarding lowered risk of epilepsy in stroke is statins. Their neuroprotective effects and possible anticonvulsant properties are attributed to the suppression of proinflammatory cytokines and modulation of endothelial nitric oxide synthase activity [79, 80].

8.6.7 aSAH

The incidence of late postoperative seizures in aSAH is 5.5% [81]. Risk factors include MCA aneurysms, microsurgical clipping over endovascular coiling, and high-grade aneurysms. Despite the risk, routine AED use does not seem to prevent seizures in SAH. Accordingly, current guidelines do not recommend long-term AED prophylaxis in patients with aneurysmal subarachnoid hemorrhage.

1. Patients with aSAH and seizures have a reasonable benefit from treatment with AED for <7 days to reduce the risk of complications in the postoperative period (*level 2a*)
2. Treatment with AEDs for aSAH patients with seizures and no prior epilepsy beyond 7 days is not effective for reducing the future risk of seizures (*Level 3*).

8.6.8 Clinical Practice Variation in the Long-Term Management of Epilepsy After Acute Brain Injury

Use of multiple AEDs for prophylaxis was noted in a clinical practice survey regarding the management of TBI. Phenytoin continued to be the first-choice AED, followed by levetiracetam. Duration of treatment varies between 1 week and 3 months, and decision-making on withdrawal also varies between radiological resolution, clinical status, and EEG evidence. Dual AEDs were also used in cases of prior history of seizure, severe TBI, temporal lobe injury, alcoholism, or post-craniotomy status [82]. In stroke, real-world cohort data suggested use of newer Generation AEDs for the treatment of PSE (predominantly levetiracetam) without significant risk of seizure recurrence or requirement of change of initial AED [83].

8.7 Withdrawal of AEDs: Timing and Process

Withdrawal of AEDs generally utilizes an individualized approach to risk-benefit assessment for decision-making. Common indications for drug withdrawal include prevention or management of side effects, potential teratogenicity of certain AEDs, effect on concurrent drug metabolism, and partially to lessen financial burdens. Generally, patients with epilepsy are considered for drug withdrawal not before a 2-year seizure-free period.

Tapering or withdrawal of conventional AEDs is highly unlikely to be considered during the course of ICU management, as a 2-year seizure-free period is advised for the same. Furthermore, a gradual course of tapering over a period of 6 months is advised [84–86].

8.7.1 Non-anesthetic AEDs

Limited evidence exists regarding tapering/ withdrawal of non-anesthetic AEDs. One retrospective study found that the incidence of seizure relapse was 17% in patients with successful termination of NCS/NCSE followed by weaning of non-anesthetic AEDs during the same hospitalization, compared to 13% (*P* 0.77) in patients who did not undergo such weaning [87]. No protocol has been described for such weaning, while it was observed that the median number of AEDs in the two groups at the time of seizure control was 4 (3, 4) and 3 (2, 3) ($P < 0.001$), respectively. The duration of hospital stays and the median number of AEDs at discharge were 14 (11–24) [vs 11 (6–19)- *P* 0.02] and 2 (2, 3) [vs 3(2–3)- *P* 0.40] in the group with AED wean, signifying a longer duration of hospital stay.

Similar retrospective data suggested weaning initiation as early as 1 week after hospital discharge, with successful control of new-onset status epilepticus. Weaning was done in 44 (34.4%) patients from at least one AED in the study, with a reported seizure recurrence rate of 13.6%. Younger patients and those with refractory NCS, as compared with convulsive status, tended to be considered for weaning [88].

Weaning protocol for anesthetic medications as AEDs in the ICU has been described in the section on refractory status epilepticus.

8.8 Conclusion

- This chapter has strived to describe systematically the important aspects of management of seizures in neurocritical care and the controversies surrounding them.
- Despite the evident role of continuous EEG monitoring in severe acute brain injury, newer techniques like the rapid EEG are upcoming, which, when combined with the risk-scoring systems, may likely alter the management methods in ABI.
- Levetiracetam is steadily emerging as the first-line AED in neurocritical care over phenytoin due to its relative safety. Newer anticonvulsants with neuroprotective properties, like perampanel, when available in IV formulations, have the potential to be the mainstays in the management of status epilepticus.
- A combination of ketamine and midazolam for RSE/SRSE needs further research.
- Early identification of nonconvulsive status and an adequately dosed antiepileptic regimen is essential in severe anoxic brain injury.
- Current guidelines do not provide recommendations for the prophylaxis of seizures in acute brain injury except in spontaneous intracerebral hemorrhage; this is not bereft of clinical practice variations.
- Weaning of AEDs in the ICU is currently applicable only to anesthetic medications, and in the absence of high-quality evidence, current protocols for 24–48-hour administration followed by gradual weaning may continue to be employed.

References

1. Fisher RS, van Emde BW, Blume W, Elger C, Genton P, Lee P, et al. Epileptic seizures and epilepsy: definitions proposed by the International League Against Epilepsy (ILAE) and the International Bureau for Epilepsy (IBE). Epilepsia. 2005;46(4):470–2.
2. Boggs JG. Seizure Management in the Intensive Care Unit. Curr Treat Options Neurol. 2021;23(11):36.
3. Limotai C, Ingsathit A, Thadanipon K, McEvoy M, Attia J, Thakkinstian A. How and whom to monitor for seizures in an ICU: a systematic review and meta-analysis. Crit Care Med. 2019;47(4):e366–73.
4. Claassen J, Taccone FS, Horn P, Holtkamp M, Stocchetti N, Oddo M, et al. Recommendations on the use of EEG monitoring in critically ill patients: consensus statement from the neurointensive care section of the ESICM. Intensive Care Med. 2013;39(8):1337–51.
5. Sinha SR, Sullivan L, Sabau D, San-Juan D, Dombrowski KE, Halford JJ, et al. American clinical neurophysiology society guideline 1: minimum technical requirements for performing clinical electroencephalography. J Clin Neurophysiol. 2016;33(4):303.
6. Sharma S, Nunes M, Alkhachroum A. Adult critical care electroencephalography monitoring for seizures: a narrative review. Front Neurol [Internet]. 2022 Jul 15; [cited 2024 Jun 14];13. Available from: https://www.frontiersin.org/journals/neurology/articles/10.3389/fneur.2022.951286/full
7. Beniczky S, Schomer DL. Electroencephalography: basic biophysical and technological aspects important for clinical applications. Epileptic Disord. 2020;22(6):697–715.
8. Rosenthal ES. Seizures, status epilepticus, and continuous EEG in the intensive care unit. Contin Minneap Minn. 2021;27(5):1321–43.
9. Herman ST, Abend NS, Bleck TP, Chapman KE, Drislane FW, Emerson RG, et al. Consensus statement on continuous EEG in critically ill adults and children, part I: indications. J Clin Neurophysiol Off Publ Am Electroencephalogr Soc. 2015;32(2):87–95.
10. Struck AF, Ustun B, Ruiz AR, Lee JW, LaRoche SM, Hirsch LJ, et al. Association of an Electroencephalography-Based Risk Score with Seizure Probability in hospitalized patients. JAMA Neurol. 2017;74(12):1419–24.
11. Struck AF, Tabaeizadeh M, Schmitt SE, Ruiz AR, Swisher CB, Subramaniam T, et al. Assessment of the validity of the 2HELPS2B score for inpatient seizure risk prediction. JAMA Neurol. 2020;77(4):500–7.
12. Claassen J, Vespa P, Participants in the International Multi-disciplinary Consensus Conference on Multimodality Monitoring. Electrophysiologic monitoring in acute brain injury. Neurocrit Care. 2014;21(Suppl 2):S129–47.
13. Chen DF, Kumari P, Haider HA, Ruiz AR, Lega J, Dhakar MB. Association of epileptiform abnormality on electroencephalography with development of epilepsy after acute brain injury. Neurocrit Care. 2021;35(2):428–33.
14. Connolly ES, Rabinstein AA, Carhuapoma JR, Derdeyn CP, Dion J, Higashida RT, et al. Guidelines for the management of aneurysmal subarachnoid hemorrhage. Stroke. 2012;43(6):1711–37.
15. Labar DR, Fisch BJ, Pedley TA, Fink ME, Solomon RA. Quantitative EEG monitoring for patients with subarachnoid hemorrhage. Electroencephalogr Clin Neurophysiol. 1991;78(5):325–32.
16. Vespa PM, Nuwer MR, Juhász C, Alexander M, Nenov V, Martin N, et al. Early detection of vasospasm after acute subarachnoid hemorrhage using continuous EEG ICU monitoring. Electroencephalogr Clin Neurophysiol. 1997;103(6):607–15.
17. Claassen J, Hirsch LJ, Kreiter KT, Du EY, Connolly ES, Emerson RG, et al. Quantitative continuous EEG for detecting delayed cerebral ischemia in patients with poor-grade subarachnoid hemorrhage. Clin Neurophysiol Off J Int Fed Clin Neurophysiol. 2004;115(12):2699–710.
18. Aquino L, Kang CY, Harada MY, Ko A, Do-Nguyen A, Ley EJ, et al. Is routine continuous EEG for traumatic brain injury beneficial? Am Surg. 2017;83(12):1433–7.

19. Lee H, Mizrahi MA, Hartings JA, Sharma S, Pahren L, Ngwenya LB, et al. Continuous electroencephalography after moderate to severe traumatic brain injury. Crit Care Med. 2019;47(4):574–82.
20. Ronne-Engstrom E, Winkler T. Continuous EEG monitoring in patients with traumatic brain injury reveals a high incidence of epileptiform activity. Acta Neurol Scand. 2006;114(1):47–53.
21. Ruijter BJ, Tjepkema-Cloostermans MC, Tromp SC, van den Bergh WM, Foudraine NA, Kornips FHM, et al. Early electroencephalography for outcome prediction of postanoxic coma: a prospective cohort study. Ann Neurol. 2019;86(2):203–14.
22. Urbano V, Alvarez V, Schindler K, Rüegg S, Ben-Hamouda N, Novy J, et al. Continuous versus routine EEG in patients after cardiac arrest: analysis of a randomized controlled trial (CERTA). Resuscitation. 2022;176:68–73.
23. Rossetti AO, Carrera E, Oddo M. Early EEG correlates of neuronal injury after brain anoxia. Neurology. 2012;78(11):796–802.
24. Fenter H, Rossetti AO, Beuchat I. Continuous versus routine electroencephalography in the intensive care unit: a review of current evidence. Eur Neurol. 2024;87(1):17–25.
25. Kondziella D, Friberg CK, Wellwood I, Reiffurth C, Fabricius M, Dreier JP. Continuous EEG monitoring in aneurysmal subarachnoid hemorrhage: a systematic review. Neurocrit Care. 2015 Jun;22(3):450–61.
26. Guo Y, Fang S, Wang J, Wang C, Zhao J, Gai Y. Continuous EEG detection of DCI and seizures following aSAH: a systematic review. Br J Neurosurg. 2020;34(5):543–8.
27. Rossetti AO, Schindler K, Sutter R, Rüegg S, Zubler F, Novy J, et al. Continuous vs routine electroencephalogram in critically ill adults with altered consciousness and no recent seizure: a Multicenter randomized clinical trial. JAMA Neurol. 2020;77(10):1225–32.
28. Rossetti AO, Lee JW. What's new on EEG monitoring in the ICU. Minerva Anestesiol. 2021;87(10):1139–45.
29. Kienitz R, Kay L, Beuchat I, Gelhard S, von Brauchitsch S, Mann C, et al. Benzodiazepines in the management of seizures and status epilepticus: a review of routes of delivery, pharmacokinetics, efficacy, and tolerability. CNS Drugs. 2022;36(9):951–75.
30. Rossetti AO, Claassen J, Gaspard N. Status epilepticus in the ICU. Intensive Care Med. 2024;50(1):1–16.
31. Outin H, Lefort H, Peigne V. Guidelines the FG for SE. Guidelines for the management of status epilepticus. Eur J Emerg Med. 2021;28(6):420.
32. Glauser T, Shinnar S, Gloss D, Alldredge B, Arya R, Bainbridge J, et al. Evidence-based guideline: treatment of convulsive status epilepticus in children and adults: report of the guideline Committee of the American Epilepsy Society. Epilepsy Curr. 2016;16(1):48–61.
33. Beuchat I, Novy J, Rosenow F, Kellinghaus C, Rüegg S, Tilz C, et al. Staged treatment response in status epilepticus: lessons from the SENSE registry. Epilepsia. 2024;65(2):338–49.
34. Carney N, Totten AM, O'Reilly C, Ullman JS, Hawryluk GWJ, Bell MJ, et al. Guidelines for the management of severe traumatic brain injury, Fourth edition. Neurosurgery. 2017;80(1):6–15.
35. Frontera JA, Gilmore EJ, Johnson EL, Olson D, Rayi A, Tesoro E, et al. Guidelines for seizure prophylaxis in adults hospitalized with moderate-severe traumatic brain injury: a clinical practice guideline for health care professionals from the Neurocritical care society. Neurocrit Care. 2024;40(3):819–44.
36. Holtkamp M, Beghi E, Benninger F, Kälviäinen R, Rocamora R, Christensen H, et al. European stroke organisation guidelines for the management of post-stroke seizures and epilepsy. Eur Stroke J. 2017;2(2):103–15.
37. Powers WJ, Rabinstein AA, Ackerson T, Adeoye OM, Bambakidis NC, Becker K, et al. Guidelines for the early Management of Patients with acute ischemic stroke: 2019 update to the 2018 guidelines for the early management of acute ischemic stroke: a guideline for healthcare professionals from the American Heart Association/American Stroke Association. Stroke. 2019;50(12):e344–418.
38. Chang RS, Leung WC, Vassallo M, Sykes L, Battersby Wood E, Kwan J. Antiepileptic drugs for the primary and secondary prevention of seizures after stroke. Cochrane Database Syst Rev. 2022;2(2):CD005398.

39. Jones FJS, Sanches PR, Smith JR, Zafar SF, Hernandez-Diaz S, Blacker D, et al. Anticonvulsant primary and secondary prophylaxis for acute ischemic stroke patients: a decision analysis. Stroke. 2021;52(9):2782–91.
40. Hoh BL, Ko NU, Amin-Hanjani S, Chou SHY, Cruz-Flores S, Dangayach NS, et al. 2023 guideline for the management of patients with aneurysmal subarachnoid hemorrhage: a guideline from the American Heart Association/American Stroke Association. Stroke. 2023;54(7):e314–70.
41. Greenberg SM, Ziai WC, Cordonnier C, Dowlatshahi D, Francis B, Goldstein JN, et al. 2022 guideline for the management of patients with spontaneous intracerebral hemorrhage: a guideline from the American Heart Association/American Stroke Association. Stroke. 2022;53(7):e282–361.
42. Carnegie V, Schweikert S, Anstey M, Wibrow B, Delaney A, Flower O, et al. A multicentre observational study of the use of antiseizure medication in patients with aneurysmal subarachnoid haemorrhage in the PROMOTE-SAH study. J Clin Neurosci. 2022;103:20–5.
43. Naidech AM, Beaumont J, Jahromi B, Prabhakaran S, Kho A, Holl JL. Evolving use of seizure medications after intracerebral hemorrhage: a multicenter study. Neurology. 2017;88(1):52–6.
44. Menon RG. Use of prophylactic antiepileptics following aneurysmal subarachnoid hemorrhage: time to relook. Neurol India. 2020;68(3):593.
45. Savalia K, Sekar P, Moomaw CJ, Koch S, Sheth KN, Woo D, et al. Effect of primary prophylactic antiseizure medication for seizure prevention following intracerebral hemorrhage in the ERICH study. J Stroke Cerebrovasc Dis. 2022;31(1):106143.
46. Trinka E, Cock H, Hesdorffer D, Rossetti AO, Scheffer IE, Shinnar S, et al. A definition and classification of status epilepticus–report of the ILAE task force on classification of status epilepticus. Epilepsia. 2015;56(10):1515–23.
47. Kantanen AM, Sairanen J, Kälviäinen R. Incidence of the different stages of status epilepticus in eastern Finland: a population-based study. Epilepsy Behav EB. 2019;101(Pt B):106413.
48. Schubert-Bast S, Zöllner JP, Ansorge S, Hapfelmeier J, Bonthapally V, Eldar-Lissai A, et al. Burden and epidemiology of status epilepticus in infants, children, and adolescents: a population-based study on German health insurance data. Epilepsia. 2019;60(5):911–20.
49. Leitinger M, Trinka E, Giovannini G, Zimmermann G, Florea C, Rohracher A, et al. Epidemiology of status epilepticus in adults: a population-based study on incidence, causes, and outcomes. Epilepsia. 2019;60(1):53–62.
50. Au YK, Kananeh MF, Rahangdale R, Moore TE, Panza GA, Gaspard N, et al. Treatment of refractory status epilepticus with continuous intravenous Anesthetic drugs: a systematic review. JAMA Neurol. 2024;81(5):534–48.
51. Brophy GM, Bell R, Claassen J, Alldredge B, Bleck TP, Glauser T, et al. Guidelines for the evaluation and management of status epilepticus. Neurocrit Care. 2012;17(1):3–23.
52. Meierkord H, Boon P, Engelsen B, Göcke K, Shorvon S, Tinuper P, et al. EFNS guideline on the management of status epilepticus in adults. Eur J Neurol. 2010;17(3):348–55.
53. Muhlhofer WG, Layfield S, Lowenstein D, Lin CP, Johnson RD, Saini S, et al. Duration of therapeutic coma and outcome of refractory status epilepticus. Epilepsia. 2019;60(5):921–34.
54. Rubin DB, Angelini B, Shoukat M, Chu CJ, Zafar SF, Westover MB, et al. Electrographic predictors of successful weaning from anaesthetics in refractory status epilepticus. Brain. 2020;143(4):1143–57.
55. Rossetti AO, Milligan TA, Vulliémoz S, Michaelides C, Bertschi M, Lee JW. A randomized trial for the treatment of refractory status epilepticus. Neurocrit Care. 2011;14(1):4–10.
56. Masapu D, Gopala Krishna KN, Sanjib S, Chakrabarti D, Mundlamuri RC, Manohar N, et al. A comparative study of midazolam and target-controlled propofol infusion in the treatment of refractory status epilepticus. Indian J Crit Care Med. 2018;22(6):441–8.
57. Yan M, Sun T, Liu J, Chang Q. The efficacy and safety of ketamine in the treatment of super-refractory status epilepticus: a systematic review. J Neurol. 2024;271(7):3942–52.
58. Adhikari A, Yadav SK, Nepal G, Aryal R, Baral P, Neupane P, et al. Use of ketamine in super refractory status epilepticus: a systematic review. Neurol Res Pract. 2024;6:33.

59. Meierkord H, Holtkamp M. Non-convulsive status epilepticus in adults: clinical forms and treatment. Lancet Neurol. 2007;6(4):329–39.
60. Sutter R, Semmlack S, Kaplan PW. Nonconvulsive status epilepticus in adults – insights into the invisible. Nat Rev Neurol. 2016;12(5):281–93.
61. Beniczky S, Hirsch LJ, Kaplan PW, Pressler R, Bauer G, Aurlien H, et al. Unified EEG terminology and criteria for nonconvulsive status epilepticus. Epilepsia. 2013;54(Suppl 6):28–9.
62. Laccheo I, Sonmezturk H, Bhatt AB, Tomycz L, Shi Y, Ringel M, et al. Non-convulsive status epilepticus and non-convulsive seizures in neurological ICU patients. Neurocrit Care. 2015;22(2):202–11.
63. Husain AM, Lee JW, Kolls BJ, Hirsch LJ, Halford JJ, Gupta PK, et al. Randomized trial of lacosamide versus fosphenytoin for nonconvulsive seizures. Ann Neurol. 2018;83(6):1174–85.
64. Rohracher A, Kalss G, Neuray C, Höfler J, Dobesberger J, Kuchukhidze G, et al. Perampanel in patients with refractory and super-refractory status epilepticus in a neurological intensive care unit: a single-center audit of 30 patients. Epilepsia. 2018;59(Suppl 2):234–42.
65. Fechner A, Hubert K, Jahnke K, Knake S, Konczalla J, Menzler K, et al. Treatment of refractory and superrefractory status epilepticus with topiramate: a cohort study of 106 patients and a review of the literature. Epilepsia. 2019;60(12):2448–58.
66. Wang X, Yang F, Chen B, Jiang W. Non-convulsive seizures and non-convulsive status epilepticus in neuro-intensive care unit. Acta Neurol Scand. 2022;146(6):752–60.
67. Rossetti AO, Logroscino G, Milligan TA, Michaelides C, Ruffieux C, Bromfield EB. Status epilepticus severity score (STESS): a tool to orient early treatment strategy. J Neurol. 2008;255(10):1561–6.
68. DeGrauw X, Thurman D, Xu L, Kancherla V, DeGrauw T. Epidemiology of traumatic brain injury-associated epilepsy and early use of anti-epilepsy drugs: an analysis of insurance claims data, 2004–2014. Epilepsy Res. 2018;146:41–9.
69. Sui S, Sun J, Chen X, Fan F. Risk of epilepsy following traumatic brain injury: a systematic review and meta-analysis. J Head Trauma Rehabil. 2023;38(4):E289–98.
70. Sen A, Jette N, Husain M, Sander JW. Epilepsy in older people. Lancet Lond Engl. 2020;395(10225):735–48.
71. Pitkänen A, Roivainen R, Lukasiuk K. Development of epilepsy after ischaemic stroke. Lancet Neurol. 2016;15(2):185–97.
72. Tanaka T, Ihara M, Fukuma K, Mishra NK, Koepp MJ, Guekht A, et al. Pathophysiology, diagnosis, prognosis, and prevention of Poststroke epilepsy: clinical and research implications. Neurology. 2024;102(11):e209450.
73. Ferreira-Atuesta C, Döhler N, Erdélyi-Canavese B, Felbecker A, Siebel P, Scherrer N, et al. Seizures after ischemic stroke: a matched Multicenter study. Ann Neurol. 2021;90(5):808–20.
74. Zelano J, Holtkamp M, Agarwal N, Lattanzi S, Trinka E, Brigo F. How to diagnose and treat post-stroke seizures and epilepsy. Epileptic Disord Int Epilepsy J Videotape. 2020;22(3):252–63.
75. Haapaniemi E, Strbian D, Rossi C, Putaala J, Sipi T, Mustanoja S, et al. The CAVE score for predicting late seizures after intracerebral hemorrhage. Stroke. 2014;45(7):1971–6.
76. Galovic M, Döhler N, Erdélyi-Canavese B, Felbecker A, Siebel P, Conrad J, et al. Prediction of late seizures after ischaemic stroke with a novel prognostic model (the SeLECT score): a multivariable prediction model development and validation study. Lancet Neurol. 2018;17(2):143–52.
77. Cacheaux LP, Ivens S, David Y, Lakhter AJ, Bar-Klein G, Shapira M, et al. Transcriptome profiling reveals TGF-beta signaling involvement in epileptogenesis. J Neurosci. 2009;29(28):8927–35.
78. Yan HF, Zou T, Tuo QZ, Xu S, Li H, Belaidi AA, et al. Ferroptosis: mechanisms and links with diseases. Signal Transduct Target Ther. 2021;6(1):1–16.
79. Freiman S, Hauser WA, Rider F, Gulyaeva N, Guekht A. Post-stroke epilepsy: from clinical predictors to possible mechanisms. Epilepsy Res. 2024;199:107282.
80. Zhao L, Li J, Kälviäinen R, Jolkkonen J, Zhao C. Impact of drug treatment and drug interactions in post-stroke epilepsy. Pharmacol Ther. 2022;233:108030.

81. Raper DMS, Starke RM, Komotar RJ, Allan R, Connolly ES. Seizures after aneurysmal subarachnoid hemorrhage: a systematic review of outcomes. World Neurosurg. 2013;79(5–6):682–90.
82. Gopalan H, Krishnakumar P, Arun S. Use of anti-epileptic drugs for post traumatic seizure: a global survey. Ann Neurosci. 2023;30(1):26–32.
83. Tanaka T, Fukuma K, Abe S, Matsubara S, Motoyama R, Mizobuchi M, et al. Antiseizure medications for post-stroke epilepsy: a real-world prospective cohort study. Brain Behav. 2021;11(9):e2330.
84. Beghi E, Giussani G, Grosso S, Iudice A, La Neve A, Pisani F, et al. Withdrawal of antiepileptic drugs: guidelines of the Italian league against epilepsy. Epilepsia. 2013;54(Suppl 7):2–12.
85. Gloss D, Pargeon K, Pack A, Varma J, French JA, Tolchin B, et al. Antiseizure medication withdrawal in seizure-free patients: practice advisory update summary: report of the AAN guideline subcommittee. Neurology. 2021;97(23):1072–81.
86. Laue-Gizzi H. Discontinuation of antiepileptic drugs in adults with epilepsy. Aust Prescr. 2021;44(2):53–6.
87. Creed JA, Son J, Farjat AE, Swisher CB. Early withdrawal of non-anesthetic antiepileptic drugs after successful termination of nonconvulsive seizures and nonconvulsive status epilepticus. Seizure. 2018;54:45–50.
88. Chakraborty T, Hocker S. Weaning from antiseizure drugs after new onset status epilepticus. Epilepsia. 2019;60(5):979–85.

Neuroinfections

9

Soumya Madhusudhan, Mathangi Krishnakumar, and Moses Charles D. Souza

Abstract

Central nervous system (CNS) infections are complex entities caused by pathogens like bacteria, fungi, and viruses. They necessitate early recognition, diagnosis, and prompt treatment strategies, which are crucial in reducing the morbidity and mortality associated with CNS infections. Clinicians face countless challenges in acute care settings because of several dilemmas inherent to the presentation, diagnosis, and management of CNS infections. This chapter addresses these controversies and reviews evidence-based solutions to overcome these clinical obstacles.

Keywords

Meningitisexternal ventricular drain (EVD) · Intrathecal antibiotics · Blood–brain barrier · Steriods in meningitis

9.1 Introduction

Central nervous system infection is divided into three broad categories: meningitis, encephalitis, and brain abscess. The extent of the neurovascular space involved determines the type of infection. The worldwide incidence of bacterial meningitis in low-income countries is 80 per 100,000 individuals, and the mortality rate is up to 54%. Out of this, 24% develop several neurological sequelae in the form of hearing loss and focal neurological deficits[1]. Meningitis is the inflammation of the membranous envelope composed of pia, arachnoid, dura mater, and CSF within the

S. Madhusudhan (✉) · M. Krishnakumar · M. C. D. Souza
Surgical and Neuro Intensive Care Unit, Department of Anaesthesia, St Johns Medical College, Bengaluru, Karnataka, India

P. U. Bidkar, M. Krishnakumar (eds.), *Controversies in Neurocritical Care*,
https://doi.org/10.1007/978-981-95-4419-6_9

subarachnoid space. It is always secondary to bacterial, viral, and fungal infections. Bacterial meningitis has an acute presentation. The most common organisms causing adult bacterial infection are *Neisseria meningitides*, *Streptococcus pneumoniae*, *Listeria monocytogenes*, and *Haemophilus influenzae* type B [2].

Herpes simplex virus (HSV) and varicella-zoster virus (VZV) are common neurotropic viruses that cause viral meningitis. Viral meningitis presents with less clinical severity than bacterial meningitis.

They progress to involve the brain parenchyma and result in meningoencephalitis. Tuberculous meningitis is more common in low-income groups and must be suspected in all high-risk patients presenting with focal neurological deficits, hydrocephalus and hyponatraemia [3].

Each of the above infections has a different clinical presentation, complications, ability of diagnostic tests to isolate the pathogen and response to treatment. Therefore, proper diagnosis, imaging, testing, treatment, follow-up, and surveillance are not just essential but also the responsibility of clinicians to improve outcomes in CNS infections.

Case Scenario 1

A 32-year-old engineer complained of a fever associated with a headache for 4 days. He visited his general practitioner, who prescribed him antipyretics and antibiotics. However, he failed to respond even after antibiotics. His fever spiked to 104° F, and he noticed a stiff neck and could not open his eyes in bright light. On examination, he was conscious oriented no.

Neurological deficits were documented. A working diagnosis of CNS infection was made.

What must be the next appropriate step?

Diagnosis of meningitis requires a combined approach involving detailed clinical examination, imaging and appropriate laboratory investigations. Lumbar puncture and analysis of the CSF are the gold standard tests to confirm the diagnosis of meningitis. Inflammation of the meninges leads to increased blood–brain barrier permeability and vasogenic oedema. Cerebral oedema leads to reduced perfusion and an increase in intracranial pressure. Lumbar puncture in patients with raised ICP can precipitate herniation and poor outcomes. CT imaging can guide the clinician about the safety of performing a lumbar puncture, and it must be considered. However, the flip side is a delay in obtaining the imaging; not all centres have facilities for CT scans, and there is further delay in starting treatment.

9.2 Controversy 1: Is Imaging Warranted Before Lumbar Puncture in All Patients?

A lumbar puncture can be safely performed without prior CT imaging when we do not suspect increased intracranial pressure or other CNS diseases. Imaging before lumbar puncture leads to unnecessary delay in initiating antibiotic treatment [4].

Table 9.1 Indications to perform imaging before lumbar puncture

GCS less than 12
Papilledema
Seizures prior to lumbar puncture
Focal neurological deficits

Delays in obtaining CSF samples also reduce rates of isolating pathogens, prolonged hospital stays, and increased mortality [5]. There has been controversy regarding herniation following lumbar puncture in cases of meningitis. The risk of brain herniation is about 5%, with a mortality rate of 30% in these cases [6]. Brain imaging can pick up CNS pathologies and features of raised ICP, but a routine CT scan before a lumbar puncture does not make it a safe procedure.

The increased rate of imaging is probably due to irrational fear of herniation, even in patients with no features of increased intracranial pressure. A lumbar puncture can hasten herniation only when features of the brain shift, like tense dura mater, effaced cisterns, flattened gyri, and sulci, are present. During a lumbar puncture, CSF escapes; this removes counterpressure from below, and the brain shift increases, causing herniation. It is never instantaneous but gradually sets in within 48 hours with clinically overlapping features of increased headache, neck stiffness, pupillary abnormalities, bradycardia and apnoea [7]. The need for imaging before lumbar puncture must be assessed on a case-by-case basis, considering the clinical presentation. The indications for imaging (CT scan brain) before lumbar puncture are listed in Table 9.1 [8].

There should be no delay in the initiation of treatment; however, every attempt should be made to perform a lumbar puncture within 1 hour of arrival at the hospital.

9.3 Controversy 2: Lumbar Puncture Is Mandatory Before Starting Antibiotics

Lumbar puncture and CSF analysis are desirable before starting antibiotics. When doing LP is delayed at presentation, empirical antibiotics must be started. The choice of antibiotics is based on common bacterial species that cause meningitis, the patient's age group, and a local antibiogram. Apart from logistical reasons, the delay in performing LP is due to specific clinical conditions that warrant the delay in the procedure (Refer to Table 9.2).

Once the patient is clinically stable, LP can still be performed up to 4 hours after initiating treatment. However, the probability of isolating the organisms rapidly declines after that. A delay in starting intravenous antibiotics exponentially increases mortality [9].

LP in a patient on anticoagulation increases the risk of subdural hematoma. Low molecular weight heparin must be stopped 12 hours before performing LP and can be restarted after 4 hours. Unfractionated heparin is relatively safe to start within an hour of LP. The risk of reversing warfarin must be weighed against the benefit of doing LP, and other clinical tests can diagnose meningitis. An INR > 1.5 and a platelet count of less than 40,000 must be considered contraindications for LP [10].

Table 9.2 Contraindications to perform lumbar puncture

Clinically unstable patient (cardiac or respiratory compromise)
Papilledema
Abnormal dolls eye phenomenon
Shock
Infection at the site of infection
Anticoagulation
Thrombocytopenia; INR >1.5
Severe sepsis

Clopidogrel inhibits platelets for the entire lifespan of platelets, 9–10 days. When LP is needed for clinical management in these patients, it is prudent to perform LP after a transfusion of platelets [11]. The reason for not performing LP must be reassessed every 12 hours and performed as soon as possible to increase the diagnostic yield of the procedure. The common contraindications to perform LP are enumerated in Table 9.2.

9.4 Controversy 3: Does a Negative Gram Stain and CSF Culture Rule Out Bacterial Meningitis?

The CSF sample must constantly be subjected to culture in patients undergoing LP regardless of cell count and chemistry. The sensitivity of Gram stain for detecting *Listeria Monocytogenes* is 25%, while it is about 90% for *Streptococcus pneumoniae*. Sensitivity declines by 50% if patients have already received antibiotics [12]. A positive culture is always 100% specific to bacterial meningitis. However, sensitivity varies with the pathogen and time elapsed between antibiotics and culture. The common organisms identified in the Meningo-Encephalitis Panel are listed in Table 9.3.

CSF culture has variable sensitivity ranging from 80–90%, but to our surprise, in practice, it can be as low as 40% [13]. Within 2 hours of starting treatment, *Neisseria meningitidis* becomes undetectable in CSF, whereas *Streptococcal pneumonia* can be detected up to 8 hours after antibiotic treatment. Although culture can yield the growth of the bacteria, the turnaround time for culture results is long, which may not add to the management time frame. CSF PCR (polymerase chain reaction) helps identify the fastidious organisms in patients who have received prior antibiotics. A multiplex PCR test called BioFire Film Array meningitis/encephalitis panel (FA-MEP) is an FDA-approved PCR test for rapid bacterial diagnosis. It identifies bacteria, viruses and fungi. This assay runs for about 5 minutes, and results can be obtained in 60 minutes. The tests perform nucleic acid extraction and 2-stage amplification to increase specificity [14].

Although PCR testing helps obtain results rapidly, it cannot replace traditional CSF testing.

The drawback of this testing is that it can identify only common organisms causing meningitis but cannot detect many pathogens affecting post-neurosurgical and

Table 9.3 Organisms identified in the ME panel

Bacteria	Virus	Fungi
E.coli Ki capsular subtype	HSV-1 and -2	*C.neoformans/gattii*
Haemophilus influenzae	VZV	
L.monocytogenes	CMV	
N.meningitidis	HHV-6	
S.Agalactiae	Enterovirus	
S.Pneumoniae		

immunocompromised patients. Regional organisms like Borrelia and West Nile virus cannot be picked up by PCR testing.

PCR testing cannot differentiate between chronic and acute infections associated with the herpes virus. Detection of the organism does not always translate to causative action. These tests are advocated for confirmation in clinical settings of unexpected negative or positive results of traditional testing.

9.5 Controversy 4: The Time to Antibiotics (TTA): Is this the Game Changer?

Bacterial meningitis is a life-threatening emergency. Appropriate antibiotics and adjuvants like steroids are lifesaving. Practice guidelines for meningitis indicate that there is insufficient data to establish the optimal timing for antibiotics and their association with death and neurological sequelae [15]. In a meta-analysis study including data from four different centres, the UK, Australia and Denmark, the risk of death was associated with TTA [16]. The risk of death increased when TTA was more than 2 hours (OR 2.29, 95%CI 1.28–4.09) and increased exponentially as the time lag increased. Greater than 3 hours was associated with increased neurological sequelae. Therefore, starting antibiotics in suspected neuroinfections as early as possible and within 2 hours of hospital presentation is imperative to reduce mortality and neurological sequelae [17].

9.6 Controversy 5: Treatment of CNS Infection with Adjuvant Corticosteroids: The Pendulum That Swings Back and Forth: USE Versus Do Not USE

Adjuvant corticosteroid therapy is proven beneficial in specific bacterial meningitis but can be detrimental in several other CNS infections. Here, we describe the role of corticosteroids in each subgroup of infections caused by bacteria, viruses and in immunocompromised hosts.

Acute Bacterial Meningitis: Bacterial invasion into the meninges disrupts the blood–brain barrier. Bacteria actively replicate in this space, and leaky blood vessels lead to the infiltration of fluids, leucocytes, and other large particles. This provokes an intense inflammatory response, leading to sensory neural hearing, venous infarct, seizures and raised ICP. Steroid administration helps to reduce this response. However, these benefits are demonstrated in animal studies and extrapolated to use in humans. A large study involving 300 patients diagnosed with meningitis were enrolled in a large study. The effect of dexamethasone was compared with the placebo group. At 8 weeks of follow-up, the mortality rate was lower in the steroid group (7% vs. 15%) than in the other group, and the rate of unfavourable outcomes was 15% vs. 25% in the placebo group [18].

A 2013 Cochrane review concluded that the use of dexamethasone in pneumococcal meningitis has mortality benefits and has reduced rates of hearing loss. This benefit was not demonstrated in other etiologies of meningitis [19]. In the 2015 update on the Cochrane review, dexamethasone reduced neurological sequelae and hearing loss but not overall mortality. This result was seen in high-income countries but not in low-income countries. This could be due to a delay in starting steroids or a delayed presentation at the hospital. Dexamethasone was associated with recurrent fever [20]. Present practice guidelines recommend starting 10 mg of dexamethasone every 6 hours before or simultaneously with antibiotics. When culture results identify *Streptococcus pneumoniae,* dexamethasone must be continued for another 4 days. If other causes are identified, steroids must be promptly discontinued [8]. *Listeria Monocytogenes* meningitis is seen more commonly after the age of 50 years and in immunocompromised individuals. When *Listeria Monocytogenes* is isolated, steroids must promptly be discontinued, as it is associated with worse outcomes and increased mortality [21]. Steroids have no role in *N. meningitidis* infection [22].

Encephalitis: Herpes simplex (HSV) virus is the most common causative pathogen in sporadic cases of encephalitis. HSV-1 is associated with encephalitis, whereas HSV-2 leads to meningitis [23]. Starting a high dose of acyclovir is the standard of care and is continued for 21 days in both immunocompetent and immunocompromised hosts. Data from mouse models and preclinical studies have shown that starting dexamethasone along with acyclovir has a beneficial effect in reducing virus multiplication [24]. No human studies have shown the same beneficial role of steroids along with acyclovir. However, in clinical practice, dexamethasone is still used as a magic bullet to reduce intracranial pressure and cerebral oedema in severe cases of encephalitis.

West Nile encephalitis (WNE) is an arthropod-borne disease spread via mosquito bites. The virus multiplies locally and spreads via lymphatic tissue into the CNS. Less than 1% of the cases have neuroinvasiveness, which can range from meningitis to myelitis [25]. WNE has a mortality rate of 15–18%. Presently, there are no FDA-approved drug regimens or recommendations for managing WNE. High-dose corticosteroids have been successfully used in patients with WNE and have shown dramatic improvement. This is reported in only one case report [26]. A study from Colorado included 228 patients and compared mortality among patients who received dexamethasone. The patient group receiving dexamethasone had fewer deaths compared to the placebo group [27]. Due to the lack of consistent data at present, no formal recommendations are made regarding adjuvant steroid therapy in WNE.

Autoimmune Encephalitis: Primary autoimmune encephalitis is caused by an innate immune response against the cell surface proteins. Paraneoplastic autoimmune encephalitis is associated with underlying malignancy; encephalitis is collateral damage due to the immune reaction to the cancerous growth. Corticosteroids, mainly methylprednisolone, are the drug of choice and are included among the first-line agents of initial immunotherapy [28]. Steroids, although they reduce the immune response, cause exaggeration of depression, insomnia, and

psychosis due to their potential neurodegenerative effects on chronic use [29]. The most common parasitic infection in the CNS is Neurocysticercosis, caused by the *Taenia solium* tapeworm [30]. IDSA (Infectious Disease Society of America) strongly recommends the use of steroids to mitigate the effects of antiparasitic drugs [31]. Steroids help to reduce the frequency of seizures in these cases. Steroids reduce the inflammatory reaction secondary to antiparasitic drugs. Single-enhancing lesions due to NCC are always associated with perilesional oedema secondary to antiparasitic treatment. Steroids are recommended in the management of cerebral oedema. However, in calcified NCC, where there is not much cerebral oedema, steroids are not routinely recommended. However, in cysticercal encephalitis with cerebral oedema, IDSA recommends corticosteroid-only administration without the use of antiparasitic drugs, as they result in excessive cerebral oedema and worsening of the symptoms [30].

Toxoplasmosis: *Toxoplasma gondii* is a single-cell parasite that causes encephalitis. The first-line of management in this parasitic infection is sulfadiazine with pyrimethamine. Steroids have no role where cerebral oedema is not associated with the ring-enhancing lesions. It is indicated only when the abscess is well-formed and has significant mass effects [32].

Cryptococcal meningitis is a CNS infection most prevalent in HIV patients. It is caused by *cryptococcal neoformans* and, less commonly, by *Cryptococcus gattii*. Cryptococcal infections are always associated with low CD4 counts [33]. In a randomised controlled trial consisting of 451 patients in the acute phase of cryptococcal meningitis, the effect of adjuvant dexamethasone with amphotericin B was compared against only amphotericin B. Patients received steroids with amphotericin B for 6 weeks. The trial was prematurely stopped due to safety concerns. The trial results were not in favour of dexamethasone. The rate of mortality in the dexamethasone group was higher (47% as compared to 41%) in the placebo group. This mortality rate increased in the next 6 months to 57% against 47% in the no-steroids group. Based on these trials, steroids are not recommended during the acute phase of cryptococcal meningitis [34]. *Cryptococcus gattii* is a new globally identified neurotropic pathogen. Unlike C. neoformans, which affects immunocompromised hosts, *C. gattii* is seen in immunocompetent patients [35]. The hallmark of *C. gattii* infection is the presence of raised ICP. However, these warning signs are always absent on CT scans, adding to the clinical dilemma of correct diagnosis. The cryptococcosis in the brain can mimic malignancy and always cause delays in diagnosis and treatment [36]. The clinical presentation must be meticulously analysed, and signs of raised ICP must be picked up at the bedside and managed appropriately with aggressive antiedema measures, including CSF diversion procedures and steroids. Intraparenchymal deposition of polysaccharide capsule leads to low brain compliance, leading to raised ICP. This state is described as a "frozen brain state" [37]. This frozen brain state causes the imaging and clinical presentation disparity. Immune reconstitution syndrome secondary to antifungal therapy usually responds to steroid therapy.

Brain Abscess: There is a higher incidence of brain abscess in HIV/AIDS patients. The first-line of management is aspirations and the start of appropriate antibiotics. Mortality is higher in brain abscesses due to repeated aspirations and the ineffectiveness of antibiotics [38]. Dexamethasone is added to the regimen to reduce perilesional oedema around the abscess and decrease the severity of post-neurological sequelae [39]. On the contrary, the administration of steroids was associated with immunosuppression in an already compromised host and reduced penetration of antibiotics [40]. In a meta-analysis demonstrating the influence of dexamethasone in patients with brain abscesses, results inferred that steroids do not affect overall mortality [41]. No strong recommendations are made for the use of steroids in the brain abscess. Instead, the use of steroids in the management of abscesses must be based on the physician's discretion.

9.7 Antibiotic Regimen for CNS Infections: A Multifaceted Challenge

The blood–brain barrier is selective for antibiotic penetration, which presents a challenge to antibiotic selection. The commonly used antimicrobials and their CNS penetration features are described in Table 9.4. The capillary spaces in the brain comprise tight junctions that prevent the passage of large molecules into the CSF.

These tight junctions are absent in a few areas around the hypothalamus and floor of the fourth ventricle. They prevent the diffusion of hydrophilic molecules, limiting the number of antibiotics available to treat CNS infection. The unfortunate complication of highly effective antibiotics that enter CSF readily and establish drug levels is that they are severely toxic to the brain, causing encephalopathy and seizures.

Community-acquired bacterial meningitis (CABM) is a CNS infection without recent hospitalisation, head trauma or indwelling devices. The incidence of CABM is rapidly reducing due to increased vaccination rates. *Streptococcus Pneumoniae* (Pneumococcus), *Neisseria meningitidis* (Meningococcus), and *Listeria Monocytogenes* are the most common organisms implicated as causative agents. Meningitis due to *H. Influenzae*

occurs most commonly in patients predisposed to ear or sinus infections [42]. Penicillin resistance was first detected in pneumococcus and has recently emerged in meningococcus. Penicillin has poor penetrability in CNS tissues and requires large doses and continuous infusions. Third-generation cephalosporin is the preferred first-line antibiotic for empirical cover untill definitive sensitive patterns are available. Due to the development of resistance to third-generation cephalosporins, adding vancomycin can provide adequate cover for these resistant isolates.

Table 9.4 Antimicrobial class and its CNS penetration

Antimicrobial agent	CSF penetration	Antivirals	CSF penetration	Antifungals	CSF penetration
Aminoglycosides	Poor	Acyclovir	Good	Fluconazole	Good
First Generationcephalosporin Second generation Third generation Fourth generation	Poor Poor Fair Fair	Cidofovir	Poor	Itraconazole	Poor
Aztreonam	Fair	Foscarnet	Fair	Voriconazole	Good
Betalacatams	Fair	Famciclovir	Unknown	Posaconazole	Poor
Tetracyclines	Poor	Ganciclovir	Unknown		
Tigecycline	Insufficient data	Valacyclovir	Fair		
Vancomycin					
Carbepenam	Fair				

Fluoroquinolones are an effective alternative to third-generation cephalosporins. Levofloxacin and moxifloxacin have good CNS penetration [43]. *H. Influenzae* and *L.monocytogenes* account for less than 10% of CABM cases. Ampicillin is the drug of choice for Listeria Monocytogenes. Third- or fourth-generation cephalosporin has been the mainstay of treatment for these agents [44]. Healthcare-associated meningitis and ventriculitis always occur following neurosurgical procedures, trauma, and indwelling infected devices. Common pathogens causing infections are *Coagulase-negative Staphylococcus, Staphylococcus aureus, Enterobacter, Pseudomonas and Acinetobacter* [45]. The treatment strategy for managing healthcare-associated meningitis includes empirical antibiotics (Tables 9.5 and 9.6), removal of infected devices, and direct administration of antibiotics via intraventricular route (IVT) or intrathecally into the thecal sac. Bacteria form a biofilm on these devices, and the colonies multiply in the polysaccharide matrix, protecting the microorganisms from exposure to the host immune system [46]. *Acinetobacter baumanii* is commonly associated with biofilm formation. The biofilm is immature and

Table 9.5 Empirical antimicrobial regimen in community-acquired bacterial meningitis in adults

	Pathogen	Empirical	Alternative therapy
Community-acquired bacterial meningitis	Streptococcus pneumoniae Nesseria meningitidis Haemophilus influenzae Listeria monocytogenes Staphylococcal aureus	Third generation cephalosporin + Vancomycin + Ampicillin	Levofloxacin Moxifloxacin Fosfomycin TMP/SMX

Table 9.6 Antimicrobial agents for the management of healthcare-associated meningitis/ventriculitis

Pathogen	Standard therapy	Alternative therapies
Staphylococci Methicillin resistant Methicillin sensitive	Vancomycin naficillin	Vancomycin Daptomycinor linezolid
Propionibacterium acnes	Penicillin G	Third-generation cephalosporin, vancomycin, daptomycin, or linezolid
Extended spectrum β-lactamase-producing gram-negative bacilli	Meropenam	Cefepime or a fluoroquinolone
Pseudomonas	Cefepime, ceftazidime, or meropenem	Aztreonam or ciprofloxacin
Acinetobacter baumannii	Meropenem	Colistin /polymyxin B
Other enterobacteriaceae	Third-generation cephalosporin	Meropenem, aztreonam, trimethoprim-sulfamethoxazole or ciprofloxacin

amenable to antibiotics within 6 weeks of infection. Device removal may not be required in this phase, but as the biofilm matures, the removal of the device is needed, as antibiotics are ineffective at this stage.

9.8 External Ventricular Drain (EVD): A Catheter of Constant Worry. Do Antibiotics Have a Preemptive Role in Preventing Ventriculostomy-Related Infections (VRI)?

VRI is a common complication after EVD placement. The incidence of VRI is high, as much as 20–30% and is associated with high mortality [47]. This makes it a logical approach to start preemptive antibiotics before insertion. Several randomised and retrospective studies have compared the results of prior versus durational antibiotics (continued throughout EVD placement) [48]. The results of these studies are inconclusive because there is a positive correlation between the duration of the catheter in place and the risk of infection. In a randomised trial study of 228 patients, prior doses of antibiotics were compared to the duration group (received antibiotics for the entire duration of EVD) and observed that the incidence of disease was less in the duration group [49]. The results are confounding because the durational antibiotic group received a broader spectrum of antibiotics, whereas the prior group received a single dose of essential antibiotics like ampicillin /sulbactam. A Cochrane database showed a reduction in VRI by 50% by administration of periprocedural antibiotics [50]. They also observed an increase in the isolation of resistant organisms from the durational group. There is burning evidence against the emergence of antibiotic resistance and the increased incidence of Clostridium difficile infections due to prolonged and injudicious use of antibiotics. There is a conditional recommendation for using a single dose of antibiotics before insertion, whereas a strong recommendation exists against using antibiotics for the duration of EVD [51]. A local antibiogram must guide the choice of antibiotics.

9.9 Does Antimicrobial-Impregnated EVD/VP Shunt Reduce the Rate of VRI

Antibiotic-coated catheters contain rifampicin along with clindamycin or minocycline [52]. These catheters with pharmacological agents prevent bacterial colonisation and reduce the rate of VRI compared to the routine catheter [53]. These agents have a spectrum of activity only against gram-positive organisms. There is nil gram-negative cover; hence, they are ineffective in reducing gram-negative VRI. Antimicrobial-impregnated catheters can be recommended to reduce the rates of VRI. However, their use depends on practitioners, the availability of the device and financial resources.

9.10 Change of the External Ventricular Drain: Calendar-Based or Need-Based

EVD, when handled with meticulous sterile technique, colonisation of bacteria usually begins from the seventh to the tenth day. After that, it plateaus, and further colonisation is unlikely to occur. In a randomised control trial, the rate of infection in patients in whom the EVD was regularly changed once in 5 days was observed against the control group in whom EVD was changed on clinical demand. The results showed that the infection rate was alarmingly high, about 7.6% in the repetitive changing group compared to 3.8% in the control group [54]. In another retrospective study involving 269 EVD cases, when a multiple logistic regression model was applied, they observed that multiple EVD placements were statistically significant risk factors for VRI. Each additional EVD placement increased the risk of infection by fourfold (odds ratio = 4.6, 95% CI 2.3–9.1, $p = 0.0001$) [55]. To summarise, the scheduled catheter change offers no clinical benefit. It can be kept as long as clinically indicated. Adhering to sterile protocol, following care bundles, sampling CSF when indicated, and promptly removing the EVD as soon as possible are crucial elements in preventing VRI.

9.11 Controversy: XDR, MDR, DTR: Tough Cookies to Crack

Nosocomial bacterial meningitis/ventriculitis is a hospital-acquired infection of the central nervous system that occurs after head or spinal trauma and neurosurgery. *Staphylococcus* was the most commonly implicated organism then, but the etiological agent has changed to gram-negative pathogens [56]. *Acinetobacter baumani* is the most common organism, accounting for about 30% of infections, with a high mortality of about 56%. This is followed by Coagulase-negative staphylococci, 21% and *S.Aureus*, 15% [57]. The development of multidrug resistance patterns among these pathogens narrows the treatment options and increases mortality risk. The terms multidrug-resistant (MDR), Extensively drug-resistant (XDR) and pandrug-resistant (PDR) were devised by an international expert committee CDC to describe the antibiotic resistance pattern in *Staphylococcus aureus*, Enterococcus spp., Enterobacteriaceae (other than *Salmonella* and *Shigella*), *Pseudomonas aeruginosa* and *Acinetobacter*. These pathogens are critical threats as they are prone to antibiotic resistance.

MDR is defined as acquired non-susceptibility to at least one agent in three or more antimicrobial categories.

XDR is defined as non-susceptibility to at least one agent in all but two or fewer antimicrobial categories (i.e. bacterial isolates remain susceptible to only one or two categories), and PDR is defined as non-susceptibility to all agents in all antimicrobial categories [58]. Current guidelines recommend starting empirical antibiotics until the pathogen is isolated. Vancomycin and carbapenems or antipseudomonal cephalosporins are recommended. Aztreonam and fluoroquinolones can be effective alternatives to beta-lactams [45]. Antimicrobial agents differ in their ability to cross the blood–brain barrier to reach the CSF space and achieve sufficient drug concentration. This is a limitation in managing gram-negative infections due to extensive resistance patterns. Therefore, direct instillation of antibiotics into the CSF space has been tried in difficult-to-treat cases. Intraventricular instillation ensures uniform distribution of the drug in the CSF spaces, but this is not true during intrathecal administration. The dose of the drug to be instilled depends on the size of the ventricles and the estimated clearance rate of CSF [59].

9.12 Is Intraventricular/Intrathecal Administration of Antibiotics the Last Resort? The Holy Grail of Treating Infections

The FDA has approved only intravenous administration of antibiotics [60]. However, the need for intrathecal administration has emerged due to increased resistance patterns among pathogens. Guidelines recommend administering intrathecal antibiotics (Table 9.7) in patients with ventriculitis only when there is a poor response to systemic antibiotics alone. A meta-analysis on patients with ventriculitis secondary to gram-negative pathogens included 11 studies, totalling 348 cases. It concluded that combined intrathecal and intravenous therapy was superior to intravenous treatment alone in managing carbapenem-resistant organisms. The eradication of pathogens was satisfactory via the intraventricular route (odds ratio 10.06; 95% confidence interval [CI], 2.62–38.65), and overall mortality (OR, 0.22; 95% CI, 0.08 to 0.60). However, similar results were not seen when there were other pathogens [61]. The duration of intrathecal antibiotics is individualised, and no formal recommendations exist. In uncomplicated cases, intrathecal therapy can be stopped after 48–72 hours of culture being negative. In cases where the CSF repeatedly isolates pathogens, IDSA recommends continuing intrathecal treatment for 10–14 days from the last positive culture [45]. Treatment of multidrug-resistant (MDR) and nosocomial CNS infections by the intraventricular route is a challenging intervention with almost no large clinical trials and no current recommended or approved therapy. The use of bilateral OMAYA reservoirs for the instillation of antibiotics, endoscopic lavage of ventricles, and saline irrigation has recently been tried to manage MDR infections.

Management of CNS Infection in the Immunocompromised Host CNS infection in immunocompromised hosts usually presents as a new onset of confusion and requires admission into the ICU. The success of transplantation and newer modalities of treatment in HIV-infected patients, as well as in haematological malignancies, has increased the proportion of survivors and, hence, the incidence of opportunistic infection in them. The three most critical opportunistic infections in immunocompromised hosts are toxoplasmosis, Mycobacterium tuberculosis and cryptococcal meningitis [62] (Table 9.8). Increased incidence of infection is seen when CD4 counts fall below 200. In the HIV group of patients with low CD4, coma is a strong predictor of poor outcomes.

Table 9.7 List of Antibiotic agents administered via intraventricular/intrathecal route

	Antibacterial spectrum	Dose	Duration	Adverse effects
Colistin/ polymyxin	*Acinetobacter baumannii, A. Calcoaceticus, Pseudomonas aeruginosa, Klebsiella pneumoniae, Neisseria catarrhalis,*	50,000–250,000 IU (first day) 10,000 IU OD	5–6 days	Meningeal irritation Seizures, anorexia, irritability
Amikacin	*Acinetobacter baumannii, Mycobacterium Tuberculosis, Escherichia coli, Pseudomonas aeruginosa*	5 mg–20 mg/day	6 weeks–9 M	Minor hearing loss
Gentamycin	*Mycobacterium tuberculosis, Pseudomonas aeruginosa,* Klebsiella spp Propionibacterium spp Enterococcus	1–5 mg/day	30 days	Aseptic meningitis, hearing loss, seizures, Eosinophilic granulocytosis of CSF
Vancomycin	*Staphylococcus epidermidis, S. aureus,* Enterococcus spp *Listeria monocytogenes, Streptococcus sanguis, Corynebacterium*	5–20 mg/day	18 days–3 weeks	Sensory neural hearing loss

Solid organ transplantation with chronic immunosuppression increases the risk of CNS infection in the first year. CNS aspergillosis is common in post-solid organ transplant patients [63]. Haematological malignancies also predispose to opportunistic infections during the phase of stem cell transplantation and post-chemotherapy-associated leucopenia [64]. Severe bacterial meningitis occurs in these subsets of patients. The most common pathogens causing meningitis are gram-negative organisms and *Streptococcus pneumoniae* [65]. The management of CNS infections in immunocompromised hosts has several challenges due to their atypical presentation and associated primary illness. The classical features like fever and leucocytosis are always absent. There are several confounders, like drug interactions, organ dysfunction, and metabolic disturbances, adding to the diagnostic dilemma. Although the

Table 9.8 CNS infections in immunocompromised hosts

CNS infections	Pathogen	Clinical features	Imaging	Laboratory diagnosis	Treatment
Toxoplasmosis	*Toxoplasma gondii* (Protozoan)	Headache, altered sensorium, status epilepticus, focal deficit,	Multiple ring-enhancing lesions in basal ganglia, grey matter	PCR detection of *Toxoplasma Gondii* Sensitivity: 50%. Specificity: 90–100%	Pyrimethamine Sulfadiazine Folinic acid
Aspergillosis	*Aspergillus fumigatus*	Brain abscess	Multiple ring-enhancing lesions, infarction with vascular insult	CSF galactomannan positive	Voriconazole Adjuvant corticosteroids may be harmful
Cryptococcus	*Cryptococcus neoformans* *Cryptococcus gattii*	Subacute meningitis Raised ICP	Ring like lesions	CSF cryptococcal antigen positive Sensitivity: 96%. Specificity: 100%	Amphotericin B Flucytosine
Tuberculosis	*Mycobacterium complex*	Headache, CN palsy	Meningeal enhancements Hydrocephalus Basal exudates	Direct examination PCR detection of Mycobacterium tuberculosis complex	4D-regimen for 2 months HRZE 10 months dual therapy isoniazid, rifampicin

incidence of CNS infections is lower, they are associated with increased morbidity and mortality. Aggressive management of raised intracranial pressure and cerebral oedema is of paramount importance. Increasing the CD4 count through continuous antiretroviral therapy and improving immunity reduces the burden of the disease. Reducing immunosuppression to reduce the sequelae of infection in post-transplant patients must be weighed against the risk of graft failure.

Conclusion: The current approach for treating central nervous system infections is complex, incorporating evidence-based and practice-based recommendations. Further research is required to fill these knowledge gaps.

Based on clinical history, preliminary gram stain, PCR testing, and imaging, the immediate decision to start appropriate antibiotics and steroids must be prioritised. The CNS space presents a unique challenge in selecting antibiotics due to their differential permeability, which must be accounted for before starting antibiotics.

The management approach must target early diagnosis, treatment, and strategies to prevent hearing loss and improve outcomes.

References

1. Hasbun R. Progress and challenges in bacterial meningitis: a review. JAMA [Internet]. 2022;328(21):2147. [cited 2024 Jul 24]. Available from: https://jamanetwork.com/journals/jama/fullarticle/2799148
2. Bowers KM, Mudrakola VV. Neuroinfections: presentation, diagnosis, and treatment of meningitis and encephalitis. EMJ Neurol [Internet]. 2020:93–102. [cited 2024 Jul 24]. Available from: https://www.emjreviews.com/neurology/article/neuroinfections-presentation-diagnosis-and-treatment-of-meningitis-and-encephalitis/
3. Davis A, Meintjes G, Wilkinson RJ. Treatment of tuberculous meningitis and its complications in adults. Curr Treat Options Neurol. 2018;20(3):5.
4. Carter E, McGill F. The management of acute meningitis: an update. Clin Med [Internet]. 2022;22(5):396–400. [cited 2024 Jul 25]. Available from: https://linkinghub.elsevier.com/retrieve/pii/S1470211824026526
5. McGill F, Griffiths MJ, Bonnett LJ, Geretti AM, Michael BD, Beeching NJ, et al. Incidence, aetiology, and sequelae of viral meningitis in UK adults: a multicentre prospective observational cohort study. Lancet Infect Dis. 2018;18(9):992–1003.
6. Joffe AR. Lumbar puncture and brain herniation in acute bacterial meningitis: a review. J Intensive Care Med. 2007;22(4):194–207.
7. van Crevel H, Hijdra A, de Gans J. Lumbar puncture and the risk of herniation: when should we first perform CT? J Neurol. 2002;249(2):129–37.
8. McGill F, Heyderman RS, Michael BD, Defres S, Beeching NJ, Borrow R, et al. The UK joint specialist societies guideline on the diagnosis and management of acute meningitis and meningococcal sepsis in immunocompetent adults. J Infect. 2016;72(4):405–38.
9. Michael B, Menezes BF, Cunniffe J, Miller A, Kneen R, Francis G, et al. Effect of delayed lumbar punctures on the diagnosis of acute bacterial meningitis in adults. Emerg Med J EMJ. 2010;27(6):433–8.
10. Working Party:, Association of Anaesthetists of Great Britain & Ireland, Obstetric Anaesthetists' Association, Regional Anaesthesia UK. Regional anaesthesia and patients with abnormalities of coagulation: the association of anaesthetists of Great Britain & Ireland the obstetric anaesthetists' association regional anaesthesia UK. Anaesthesia. 2013;68(9):966–72.

11. Patel IJ, Davidson JC, Nikolic B, Salazar GM, Schwartzberg MS, Walker TG, et al. Consensus guidelines for periprocedural management of coagulation status and hemostasis risk in percutaneous image-guided interventions. J Vasc Interv Radiol JVIR. 2012;23(6):727–36.
12. Gray LD, Fedorko DP. Laboratory diagnosis of bacterial meningitis. Clin Microbiol Rev. 1992;5(2):130–45.
13. Piquet AL, Cho TA. The clinical approach to encephalitis. Curr Neurol Neurosci Rep. 2016;16(5):45.
14. Kanjilal S, Cho TA, Piantadosi A. Diagnostic testing in central nervous system infection. Semin Neurol. 2019;39(3):297–311.
15. Tunkel AR, Hartman BJ, Kaplan SL, Kaufman BA, Roos KL, Scheld WM, et al. Practice guidelines for the management of bacterial meningitis. Clin Infect Dis Off Publ Infect Dis Soc Am. 2004;39(9):1267–84.
16. Stockdale AJ, Weekes MP, Aliyu SH. An audit of acute bacterial meningitis in a large teaching hospital 2005–10. QJM Mon J Assoc Physicians. 2011;104(12):1055–63.
17. Eisen DP, Hamilton E, Bodilsen J, Køster-Rasmussen R, Stockdale AJ, Miner J, et al. Longer than 2 hours to antibiotics is associated with doubling of mortality in a multinational community-acquired bacterial meningitis cohort. Sci Rep [Internet]. 2022;12(1):672. [cited 2024 Jul 26]. Available from: https://www.nature.com/articles/s41598-021-04349-7.
18. de Gans J, van de Beek D. European dexamethasone in adulthood bacterial meningitis study investigators. Dexamethasone in adults with bacterial meningitis. N Engl J Med. 2002;347(20):1549–56.
19. Brouwer MC, McIntyre P, Prasad K, van de Beek D. Corticosteroids for acute bacterial meningitis. Cochrane Database Syst Rev. 2013;(6):CD004405.
20. Brouwer MC, McIntyre P, Prasad K, van de Beek D. Corticosteroids for acute bacterial meningitis. Cochrane Database Syst Rev. 2015;2015(9):CD004405.
21. Hasbun R. Update and advances in community acquired bacterial meningitis. Curr Opin Infect Dis. 2019;32(3):233–8.
22. Heckenberg SGB, Brouwer MC, van der Ende A, van de Beek D. Adjunctive dexamethasone in adults with meningococcal meningitis. Neurology. 2012;79(15):1563–9.
23. Bradshaw MJ, Venkatesan A. Herpes simplex Virus-1 encephalitis in adults: pathophysiology, diagnosis, and management. Neurother J Am Soc Exp Neurother. 2016;13(3):493–508.
24. Meyding-Lamadé UK, Oberlinner C, Rau PR, Seyfer S, Heiland S, Sellner J, et al. Experimental herpes simplex virus encephalitis: a combination therapy of acyclovir and glucocorticoids reduces long-term magnetic resonance imaging abnormalities. J Neurovirol. 2003;9(1):118–25.
25. Colpitts TM, Conway MJ, Montgomery RR, Fikrig E. West Nile virus: biology, transmission, and human infection. Clin Microbiol Rev. 2012;25(4):635–48.
26. Leis AA, Sinclair DJ. Lazarus effect of high dose corticosteroids in a patient with West Nile virus encephalitis: a coincidence or a clue? Front Med. 2019;6:81.
27. Bode AV, Sejvar JJ, Pape WJ, Campbell GL, Marfin AA. West Nile virus disease: a descriptive study of 228 patients hospitalized in a 4-county region of Colorado in 2003. Clin Infect Dis Off Publ Infect Dis Soc Am. 2006;42(9):1234–40.
28. Shin YW, Lee ST, Shin JW, Moon J, Lim JA, Byun JI, et al. VGKC-complex/LGI1-antibody encephalitis: clinical manifestations and response to immunotherapy. J Neuroimmunol. 2013;265(1–2):75–81.
29. Shin YW, Lee ST, Park KI, Jung KH, Jung KY, Lee SK, et al. Treatment strategies for autoimmune encephalitis. Ther Adv Neurol Disord. 2018;11:1756285617722347.
30. García HH, Gonzalez AE, Rodriguez S, Tsang VCW, Pretell EJ, Gonzales I, et al. Neurocysticercosis: unraveling the nature of the single cysticercal granuloma. Neurology. 2010;75(7):654–8.
31. White AC, Coyle CM, Rajshekhar V, Singh G, Hauser WA, Mohanty A, et al. Diagnosis and treatment of Neurocysticercosis: 2017 clinical practice guidelines by the Infectious Diseases Society of America (IDSA) and the American Society of Tropical Medicine and Hygiene (ASTMH). Clin Infect Dis Off Publ Infect Dis Soc Am. 2018;66(8):e49–75.

32. Pereira-Chioccola VL, Vidal JE, Su C. Toxoplasma gondii infection and cerebral toxoplasmosis in HIV-infected patients. Future Microbiol. 2009;4(10):1363–79.
33. Rajasingham R, Rhein J, Klammer K, Musubire A, Nabeta H, Akampurira A, et al. Epidemiology of meningitis in an HIV-infected Ugandan cohort. Am J Trop Med Hyg. 2015;92(2):274–9.
34. Beardsley J, Wolbers M, Kibengo FM, Ggayi ABM, Kamali A, Cuc NTK, et al. Adjunctive dexamethasone in HIV-associated Cryptococcal meningitis. N Engl J Med. 2016;374(6):542–54.
35. Chen SCA, Slavin MA, Heath CH, Playford EG, Byth K, Marriott D, et al. Clinical manifestations of Cryptococcus gattii infection: determinants of neurological sequelae and death. Clin Infect Dis Off Publ Infect Dis Soc Am. 2012;55(6):789–98.
36. Tan CT, Kuan BB. Cryptococcus meningitis, clinical–CT scan considerations. Neuroradiology. 1987;29(1):43–6.
37. Bach MC, Tally PW, Godofsky EW. Use of cerebrospinal fluid shunts in patients having acquired immunodeficiency syndrome with cryptococcal meningitis and uncontrollable intracranial hypertension. Neurosurgery. 1997;41(6):1280–2. discussion 1282–1283
38. Brouwer MC, Tunkel AR, McKhann GM, van de Beek D. Brain abscess. N Engl J Med. 2014;371(5):447–56.
39. Schroeder KA, McKeever PE, Schaberg DR, Hoff JT. Effect of dexamethasone on experimental brain abscess. J Neurosurg. 1987;66(2):264–9.
40. Hasdemir MG, Ebeling U. CT-guided stereotactic aspiration and treatment of brain abscesses. An experience with 24 cases. Acta Neurochir. 1993;125(1–4):58–63.
41. Simjian T, Muskens IS, Lamba N, Yunusa I, Wong K, Veronneau R, et al. Dexamethasone administration and mortality in patients with brain abscess: a systematic review and meta-analysis. World Neurosurg. 2018;115:257–63.
42. Figueiredo AHA, Brouwer MC, van de Beek D. Acute community-acquired bacterial meningitis. Neurol Clin. 2018;36(4):809–20.
43. Nau R, Sörgel F, Eiffert H. Penetration of drugs through the blood-cerebrospinal fluid/blood-brain barrier for treatment of central nervous system infections. Clin Microbiol Rev. 2010;23(4):858–83.
44. Nau R, Seele J, Djukic M, Eiffert H. Pharmacokinetics and pharmacodynamics of antibiotics in central nervous system infections. Curr Opin Infect Dis. 2018;31(1):57–68.
45. Tunkel AR, Hasbun R, Bhimraj A, Byers K, Kaplan SL, Scheld WM, et al. 2017 infectious diseases society of America's clinical practice guidelines for healthcare-associated Ventriculitis and meningitis. Clin Infect Dis Off Publ Infect Dis Soc Am. 2017;64(6):e34–65.
46. Conen A, Raabe A, Schaller K, Fux CA, Vajkoczy P, Trampuz A. Management of neurosurgical implant-associated infections. Swiss Med Wkly [Internet]. 2020 Apr 24; [cited 2024 Aug 6]; Available from: https://smw.ch/index.php/smw/article/view/2772.
47. Lozier AP, Sciacca RR, Romagnoli MF, Connolly ES. Ventriculostomy-related infections: a critical review of the literature. Neurosurgery. 2002;51(1):170–81. discussion 181–182
48. Saini N, Dewan Y, Grewal S. Efficacy of periprocedural vs extended use of antibiotics in patients with external ventricular drains—a randomized trial. Indian J Neurotrauma. 2012;9:30–2.
49. Poon WS, Ng S, Wai S. CSF antibiotic prophylaxis for neurosurgical patients with ventriculostomy: a randomised study. Acta Neurochir Suppl. 1998;71:146–8.
50. Ratilal B, Costa J, Sampaio C. Antibiotic prophylaxis for surgical introduction of intracranial ventricular shunts. Cochrane Database Syst Rev. 2006;2006(3):CD005365.
51. Fried HI, Nathan BR, Rowe AS, Zabramski JM, Andaluz N, Bhimraj A, et al. The insertion and Management of External Ventricular Drains: an evidence-based consensus statement: a statement for healthcare professionals from the Neurocritical care society. Neurocrit Care. 2016;24(1):61–81.
52. Zabramski JM, Whiting D, Darouiche RO, Horner TG, Olson J, Robertson C, et al. Efficacy of antimicrobial-impregnated external ventricular drain catheters: a prospective, randomized, controlled trial. J Neurosurg. 2003;98(4):725–30.
53. Parker SL, McGirt MJ, Murphy JA, Megerian JT, Stout M, Engelhart L. Comparative effectiveness of antibiotic-impregnated shunt catheters in the treatment of adult and pediatric hydro-

cephalus: analysis of 12,589 consecutive cases from 287 US hospital systems. J Neurosurg. 2015;122(2):443–8.
54. Wong GKC, Poon WS, Wai S, Yu LM, Lyon D, Lam JMK. Failure of regular external ventricular drain exchange to reduce cerebrospinal fluid infection: result of a randomised controlled trial. J Neurol Neurosurg Psychiatry. 2002;73(6):759–61.
55. Lo CH, Spelman D, Bailey M, Cooper DJ, Rosenfeld JV, Brecknell JE. External ventricular drain infections are independent of drain duration: an argument against elective revision. J Neurosurg. 2007;106(3):378–83.
56. Beer R, Lackner P, Pfausler B, Schmutzhard E. Nosocomial ventriculitis and meningitis in neurocritical care patients. J Neurol [Internet]. 2008;255(11):1617–24. [cited 2024 Aug 7]. Available from: http://link.springer.com/10.1007/s00415-008-0059-8
57. Sipahi OR, Nazli Zeka A, Taşbakan M, Pullukçu H, Arda B, Yamazhan T, et al. Pooled analysis of 899 nosocomial meningitis episodes from Turkey. Turk J Med Sci. 2017;47(1):29–33.
58. Falagas ME, Koletsi PK, Bliziotis IA. The diversity of definitions of multidrug-resistant (MDR) and pandrug-resistant (PDR) Acinetobacter baumannii and Pseudomonas aeruginosa. J Med Microbiol. 2006;55(Pt 12):1619–29.
59. Ziai WC, Lewin JJ. Improving the role of intraventricular antimicrobial agents in the management of meningitis. Curr Opin Neurol [Internet]. 2009;22(3):277–82. [cited 2024 Aug 7]. Available from: https://journals.lww.com/00019052-200906000-00014
60. Van De Beek D, Drake JM, Tunkel AR. Nosocomial bacterial meningitis. N Engl J Med [Internet]. 2010;362(2):146–54. [cited 2024 Aug 7]. Available from: http://www.nejm.org/doi/abs/10.1056/NEJMra0804573
61. Karvouniaris M, Brotis AG, Tsiamalou P, Fountas KN. The role of intraventricular antibiotics in the treatment of nosocomial ventriculitis/meningitis from gram-negative pathogens: a systematic review and meta-analysis. World Neurosurg. 2018;120:e637–50.
62. Lanoy E, Guiguet M, Bentata M, Rouveix E, Dhiver C, Poizot-Martin I, et al. Survival after neuroAIDS: association with antiretroviral CNS penetration-effectiveness score. Neurology. 2011;76(7):644–51.
63. van Veen KEB, Brouwer MC, van der Ende A, van de Beek D. Bacterial meningitis in solid organ transplant recipients: a population-based prospective study. Transpl Infect Dis Off J Transplant Soc. 2016;18(5):674–80.
64. Wright AJ, Fishman JA. Central nervous system syndromes in solid organ transplant recipients. Clin Infect Dis Off Publ Infect Dis Soc Am. 2014;59(7):1001–11.
65. van Veen KEB, Brouwer MC, van der Ende A, van de Beek D. Bacterial meningitis in hematopoietic stem cell transplant recipients: a population-based prospective study. Bone Marrow Transplant. 2016;51(11):1490–5.

Care of the Postsurgical Patient

10

Manikandan Sethuraman, Ranganatha Praveen, and Revikrishnan Sreekumar

Abstract

Effective postoperative management for neurosurgical patients is crucial for optimizing outcomes and minimizing complications. This chapter discusses the multidisciplinary strategies involved in caring for patients after neurosurgical procedures. It emphasizes the significance of individualized patient assessment, early recognition, and intervention for complications such as intracranial hematoma, pneumocephalus, cerebral edema, seizures, cerebrospinal fluid (CSF) leak, and venous thromboembolism. The chapter also explores the systemic complications alongside anesthesia-related challenges, including delayed awakening, pain, airway issues, and postoperative delirium. It highlights the role of advanced multimodal monitoring, targeted physiological goals, and early mobilization strategies while incorporating evidence-based prophylactic and therapeutic interventions in a patient-centered, protocol-driven approach for successful neurosurgical outcomes.

Keywords

Postoperative neurosurgical careperioperative complications · Intracranial pressure management · Multimodal monitoring · Neurosurgical outcomes

10.1 Introduction

The outcome of patients after neurosurgery is contingent upon their comprehensive perioperative care. Various factors, such as the patient's comorbid medical conditions, effective management of intraoperative complications (surgical, blood loss,

---

M. Sethuraman · R. Praveen (✉) · R. Sreekumar
Neuroanesthesia and Critical care, Sree Chitra Tirunal Institute for Medical Sciences and Technology, Trivandrum, Kerala, India

P. U. Bidkar, M. Krishnakumar (eds.), *Controversies in Neurocritical Care*,
https://doi.org/10.1007/978-981-95-4419-6_10

venous air embolism), and postoperative complications, determine the overall outcome [1]. It is imperative to optimize the comorbidities of the patient preoperatively and to understand and minimize the surgical complications for safe perioperative management. A comprehensive understanding of the various postoperative complications following neurosurgery is essential for optimizing patient care and improving overall treatment outcomes.

10.2 Overview of Immediate Postoperative Management

The meticulous postoperative management necessitates a multidisciplinary team's approach from the preoperative phase, considering patient comorbidities and adherence to intraoperative targeted physiological goals. The traditional practice of early recovery of neurosurgical patients in intensive care units (ICUs) is limited only to patients who are anticipated to require elective mechanical ventilation for at least 24 h [2]. Other patients can be nursed in the dedicated areas that allow for early recognition of neurological complications [3].

Smooth emergence from anesthesia and extubation would minimize coughing and prevent acute surges in blood pressure (BP), thereby avoiding a sudden rise in intracranial pressure (ICP).

Nursing the patients at a 30-degree angle (head up) would prevent obstruction to cerebral venous outflow. Morbidly obese patients with underlying obstructive sleep apnea (OSA) who are at higher risk of postoperative airway collapse can be appropriately supported by high-flow nasal cannula (HFNO) or noninvasive ventilation (NIV) unless contraindicated.

Factors to consider for postoperative ventilation include depressed level of consciousness, brainstem or cranial nerve dysfunction, and worsening neurological deficit, while aiming for the ventilation strategies that would prevent secondary cerebral insults, hypoxemia, and hypercarbia.

Neurological assessments would cover the consciousness level, cranial nerve functions, pupillary responses, limb power, and new-onset focal neurological deficit, with an urgent cranial computed tomography (CT) scan in case of its variations. Glasgow Coma Scale (GCS) and the Full Outline of Unresponsiveness score (FOUR score) aid in repetitive quantitative reporting of neurological status [4].

Advanced multimodal neuromonitoring encompassing variables such as ICP, cerebral blood flow, and cerebral oxygenation can be utilized to anticipate cerebral ischemia and can guide prophylactic measures. Progress in neuromonitoring has enabled the adoption of a patient-specific approach [5].

Intracranial hemorrhage and worsening of cerebral edema can occur in the immediate postoperative period with acute surges in BP, thereby requiring stringent monitoring. Other hidden causes for its surge, like acute pain, urinary retention, shivering, and hypercarbia, need to be appropriately addressed. Hemodynamically unstable patients require invasive BP monitoring and transthoracic echocardiographic examination to assess cardiac function.

Apart from continuous monitoring of oxygen saturation, monitoring end-tidal carbon dioxide (EtCO2) for intubated patients is essential. Monitoring the partial pressures of CO2 (PaCO2) levels upon admission to the ICU and at regular intervals, as well as during any instances of neurological deterioration, avoids hypo and hypercapnia, both of which can have detrimental effects.

Acute post-craniotomy pain is a prevalent issue in more than 60% of patients, which is moderate-to-severe in the initial 48 h following surgery. Analgesic management needs to prioritize facilitating swift recovery without impacting neurological function [6].

About 3.5% of malignant brain tumor patients and 7% of them with a preoperative functional dependence are reported to develop venous thromboembolism. Use of mechano-prophylaxis and pharmaco-prophylaxis has been shown to reduce its risk, while pharmaco-prophylaxis can only be initiated after 48 h of uncomplicated intracranial surgery, whose initiation and duration are tailored to each patient [7].

While hypothermia after prolonged surgery can delay recovery, hyperthermia and rapid rewarming can cause detrimental effects on the neurological outcomes [8]. Early initiation of enteral feeding is preferred, with more caution in patients susceptible to cranial nerve deficiency, particularly following infratentorial procedures. Assessing swallowing function is imperative for at-risk patients before oral feeding is resumed.

10.3 Complications Following Neurosurgery

Postoperative complications are seen in 45% of the patients within 24 h following neurosurgery, of which 13–27% of patients suffer major complications [9]. They can be broadly classified into surgically related, medically related, and other complications, including anesthesia-related (Fig. 10.1).

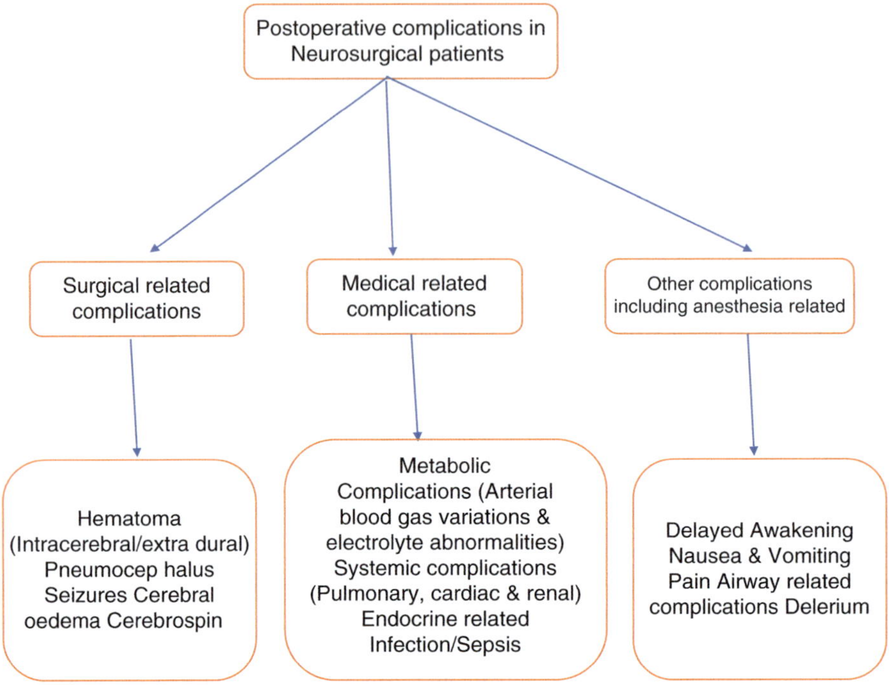

Fig. 10.1 Postoperative complications in neurosurgical patients

10.4 Demography and Management of Various Complications

10.4.1 Surgical-Related Complications

10.4.1.1 Hematoma

It is the intracranial collection of blood following neurosurgery and can be seen in 0.8–50% of patients, with 3–7% of them requiring surgical intervention upon clinical deterioration [10]. After a craniotomy, the critical time frame for the clinical manifestation of post-surgical hematoma is typically within 6 h. Subsequent management should be predicated upon serial clinical examination [10].

This complication primarily occurs at the surgical site (Fig. 10.2) due to inadequate hemostasis, complex tumor resection, hypertensive episodes during recovery, prolonged retraction, regional blood flow alterations following arteriovenous malformation (AVM) surgery, and from the residual tumor [1].

Hematomas can occur in areas remote from the surgical site, such as subdural and epidural hematomas. Hematoma can develop at the pin site or secondary to negative intracranial pressure following significant CSF loss after tumor resection or ventriculoperitoneal shunt [11]. Bleeding disorders, vascular disease,

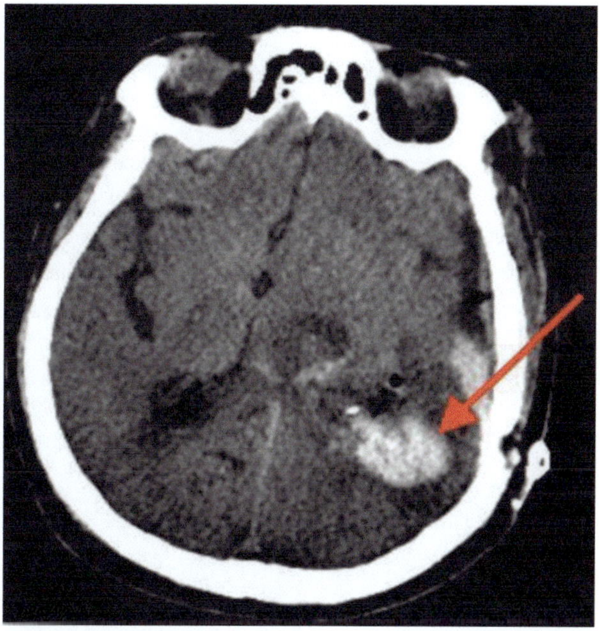

Fig. 10.2 CT scan of the brain showing the operative site hematoma (arrow)

uncontrolled hypertension, antiplatelet and anticoagulant use, and hypothermia are predisposing factors for postoperative hematoma [10, 12].

Clinical deterioration after full recovery from anesthesia, such as altered mental state, consciousness, pupillary response, new neurological deficits, and a decrease in GCS, along with brain stem reflex changes, may indicate an intracranial bleed. An immediate CT scan would confirm the diagnosis [12]. Immediate surgical evacuation is recommended for postoperative hematoma leading to elevated intracranial pressure and clinical deterioration [10].

Meticulous hemostasis with Valsalva and mild elevation of BP above baseline following tumor resection, minimizing sudden loss of CSF and filling of saline in the deficient area caused by extensive tumor resection, dural tenting sutures are primary preventive measures for postoperative hematoma.

Balanced transfusion of red blood cell (RBC), plasma, and platelets during massive blood loss, avoiding intraoperative hypothermia, maintaining postoperative BP well within that during hemostasis, minimizing coughing during emergence, maintaining BP toward low normal following AVM resection, optimizing preoperative BP, and appropriate stoppage of antiplatelets and anticoagulants with bridging therapy as guided before surgery would also prevent postoperative hematoma [10, 12].

10.4.1.2 Pneumocephalus

Pneumocephalus denotes the presence of air within the cranial cavity, commonly observed in post-neurosurgical procedures, which typically manifests without overt symptoms and tends to resolve spontaneously. It can occur following traumatic brain injury (TBI) involving dural laceration, skull base fractures, mastoiditis,

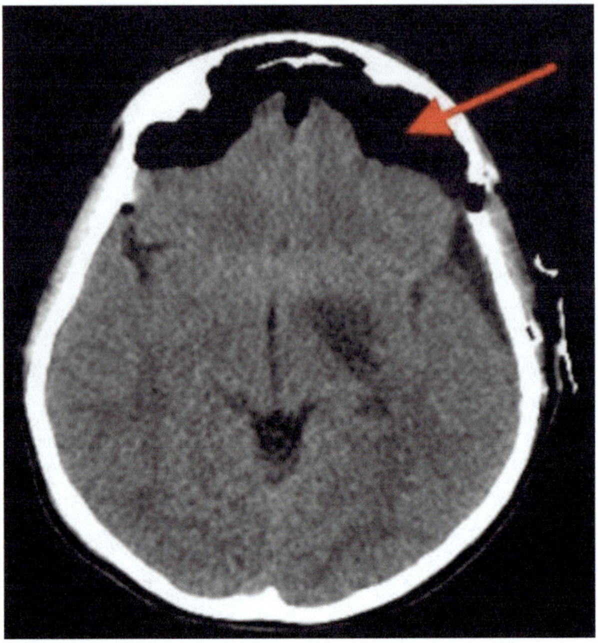

Fig. 10.3 CT scan brain showing bifrontal pneumocephalus—Mount Fuji sign (arrow)

spinal surgeries, and lumbar punctures [12]. In prone-position neurosurgeries, the occurrence rate is 57%, while it is 100% in sitting-position neurosurgeries [13].

It can occur within 72 h (acute) or after 72 h (chronic) of surgery, with the most common site being the frontal and most frequently in the subdural space (Fig. 10.3). It can also occur in intracerebral, epidural, intraventricular, and subarachnoid spaces [13]. Predisposing factors include significant hydrocephalus, osmotherapy, sitting-position surgery, nitrous oxide use, prolonged surgery (> 4.5 h), male, elderly age, working ventriculoperitoneal shunt, and hyperventilation [14].

Trapped air in the cranial cavity rarely causes symptoms. Tension pneumocephalus (0.11% to 3% of cases) occurs if increased pressure develops from trapped air. Symptoms are seen with >60 ml of air, while <20 ml is usually asymptomatic [14]. Multiple potential mechanisms have been proposed, including the one-way ball valve effect, through which extracranial air ingress occurs via cerebrospinal fluid (CSF) leakage. Additionally, a relatively negative ICP, stemming from CSF leak, external drainage, or continuous intraoperative loss, facilitates the ingress of air (manifesting as bubbles) into the intracranial cavity through a dural defect, thereby replacing CSF and reaching equilibrium with the extracranial atmosphere [13].

Delayed emergence, decreased consciousness, restlessness, and seizures are the clinical features associated with the detection of air in the CT scan (which can detect as little as 0.5 ml of air) [12].

Postoperative pneumocephalus is often asymptomatic and can be treated with oxygen through a mask for extubated patients and by maintaining a high fractional inspired oxygen pressure (FiO2) for intubated patients. According to a mathematical model, 30% and 72% of intracranial air can be absorbed in 48 h with oxygen levels of 0.4 and 1.0 FiO2, respectively. CSF leak, when present, needs to be surgically addressed. Tension pneumocephalus should be addressed on an emergency basis with the twist drill burr hole and evacuation of air [14].

Minimizing CSF loss during surgery, subdural injection of saline prior to dural closure can reduce the formation of pneumocephalus.

10.4.1.3 Seizures

Seizures in the postoperative period have a quicker onset and can present in various clinical forms, with a lesser likelihood of progressing to status epilepticus. Non-convulsive seizures (identifiable in EEG alone) have also been observed as a cause of altered consciousness [15, 16].

It occurs in 5–10% of patients after supratentorial or posterior fossa surgery (requiring external ventricular drainage for intraoperative release of CSF) [15]. Surgical complications such as pneumocephalus, hematoma, prolonged retractor use, brain tissue traction, and edema are common causes [1]. Preoperative history of epilepsy, lesions involving temporal, frontal, and insula, supratentorial tumor (meningioma having the highest propensity, near motor area), perioperative electrolyte abnormalities, hypoxia, hyperglycemia, and traumatic brain injury are a few of thc prcdisposing factors [1, 12, 15].

Diagnosed clinically, and a CT scan would identify the primary cause, which is managed by supplementing with oxygen, benzodiazepines such as lorazepam, a loading dose of antiepileptics, securing the airway, and elective mechanical ventilation while addressing the primary cause when identified from the CT scan.

Intraoperative continuation of antiepileptics for patients who are already on these medications is desirable [15].

10.4.1.4 Cerebral Edema

One of the causes of delayed emergence following neurosurgery is cerebral edema. It can be due to pre- and intraoperative cerebral edema or postoperative factors leading to its development within 5 h following craniotomy, and may peak by 48–72 h [1, 12]. Preoperative cerebral edema from TBI, poor-grade subarachnoid hemorrhage (SAH), and large tumors with mass effect contribute to intraoperative brain bulge. Excessive neck flexion, factors associated with increased intrathoracic pressures, and the use of nitrous oxide also play a role [12].

Improper placement of support during prone and lateral positioning, prolonged brain retraction during surgery, the extent of coagulation used, the choice of anesthetics, and damage to cerebral veins or dural venous sinuses can all contribute to the development of cerebral edema. Furthermore, postoperative seizures, hematoma, and venous infarction can exacerbate cerebral edema [1].

Patients may be asymptomatic or present with altered consciousness, seizures, and worsening focal deficits. CT scan features include loss of gray-white matter differentiation, mass effect, and hypodensities. Patients with minimal reduction in consciousness levels may be observed with osmotherapy and continued dexamethasone treatment for several days. However, edema secondary to hematoma or venous infarct (with significant mass effect on the brain or signs of impending uncal herniation) would require urgent surgical intervention.

10.4.1.5 CSF Leak

Leakage of CSF from the craniotomy site and nose is a distressing issue that can occur postoperatively. Since the dura mater is opened in most neurosurgeries, this complication is inevitable unless a tight closure is ensured at the end of the procedure. CSF leak can give way to various other secondary complications such as meningitis, infection of the surgical wound, its delayed healing, and intracranial hypotension [17].

It can occur in up to 13% of routine neurosurgeries, being more common in posterior fossa tumor surgeries as compared to supratentorial (5.8% vs. 2.9%). Among supratentorial tumor procedures, it is more common in open skull base tumor procedures as compared to endoscopic procedures (6.2% vs. 2.8%). High hydrostatic pressure associated with posterior fossa lesions causes more stress on the suture line, and difficulty in accessing the skull base area technically leads to increased chances of CSF leak. It is more common in craniectomy procedures than in craniotomies and relatively less common in the pediatric population [17, 18].

Risk factors include intraventricular tumor location, hydrocephalus, intraoperative blood loss, and non-watertight technique of dural closure [19]. These patients have a prolonged hospital stay with high chances of wound and brain infections. Most of the postoperative CSF leaks are treated with conservative measures such as bed rest, pressure dressing, and lumbar drain placement with appropriate use of antibiotics. However, surgical correction is required in 3% of these patients [17].

Achieving watertight dural closure and performing ventriculoperitoneal shunt preoperatively for hydrocephalus would significantly reduce the onset of postoperative CSF leak [19].

10.5 Medical-Related Complications

10.5.1 Metabolic Complications

Post-neurosurgical metabolic complications mostly include hyperlactatemia, metabolic acidosis, hyponatremia, or hypernatremia. Lactic acid level of >2 mmol/liter in the postoperative period was observed in >50% of brain tumor patients, which resolved by itself in the first 24 h and mostly did not result in metabolic acidosis [20].

Predisposing factors include the type of tumor (glioblastoma), prolonged surgery, age, dexamethasone, and hyperglycemia [20]. Hyperlactatemia was not associated with new-onset neurological deficits or increased 6-month mortality but was linked to prolonged hospital stay. Aggressive management is not recommended [20, 21].

Intraoperative fluid shifts secondary to blood loss and resuscitation with normal saline (hyperchloremia) and blood products can cause postoperative metabolic acidosis, with intraoperative use of mannitol and hypertonic saline contributing to it [21]. Correcting metabolic acidosis and its causes and electrolyte abnormalities is important. Intraoperative use of balanced salt solution is preferred.

Hypo- or hypernatremia is also common in the postoperative period following neurosurgery, which needs to be appropriately taken care of (Table 10.1) [22].

Table 10.1 Details of sodium disturbances in the postoperative period following neurosurgery [16–19]

	SIADH	CSW	DI
Causes	Of the 50% of SAH patients who had developed hyponatremia, 71% had SIADH, 15% of moderate-to-severe TBI patients, 3–25% of patients after transsphenoidal pituitary tumor surgery, and brain tumors/intracranial hematoma	Few patients following TBI,SAH,ICH, AVM, and brain tumor surgery	Postpituitary surgery (18–38%) for craniopharyngioma/pituitary adenoma/Rathkes cyst, and TBI
Etiology	Increased release of ADH	Release of brain natriuretic peptide (BNP)	Decreased secretion of ADH
Intravascular volume	Increased/normal	Decreased	Decreased
Serum Osmolality	Decreased	Decreased	Increased
Serum sodium	Decreased	Decreased	Increased
Urine output	Decreased	Normal	Increased
Urine osmolality	High	High	Low
Urine sodium	>40 mEq/L	>40 mEq/L	<15 mEq/L
Treatment	Fluid restriction; hypertonic saline (3%); slow infusion (when $Na^+$is acutely <125 mm/L); correction not to exceed 12 mmol/L over a day, to be stopped once the level reaches 130 mm/L Vaptans	0.9% sodium chloride fluid to maintain positive balance, sometimes requires 3% saline infusion very slowly Fludrocortisone	Awake patients are encouraged to drink water, avoiding negative fluid balance and intravenous fluids in intubated patients. For urine output exceeding 1litre in 4 h with low urine specific gravity, vasopressin (intramuscular or subcutaneous) is used. Many centers now use small doses of desmopressin (intranasal or intravenous)

Neurosurgical hyponatremia can be euvolemic—syndrome of inappropriate antidiuretic hormone secretion (SIADH), adrenocorticotropic hormone (ACTH) deficiency, hypovolemic—cerebral salt-wasting syndrome (CSWS), negative intravenous fluid balance, or hypervolemic hyponatremia (excessive intravenous fluid administration) [22–24].

Diabetes insipidus (DI) with hypernatremia is very common after pituitary tumor surgery. However, a very recent study reported the occurrence of postoperative hypernatremia in 14.9% of patients after elective craniotomy and its association with increased complications and death. This report has warranted the timely management of hypernatremia in the postoperative period after craniotomy procedures in order to minimize adverse outcomes [25]. Sometimes, postoperative DI can have a triple-phase response. In the first 48 h, it can manifest as acute DI, after which the release of preformed vasopressin (from damaged neurons) leads to hyponatremia for days. Neuronal gliosis follows thereafter, resulting in long-standing DI [23, 26].

10.6 Endocrine-Related Complications

Patients with skull base tumors, pituitary tumors, and craniopharyngioma often experience neuroendocrine disturbances due to hypothalamo-pituitary axis disruptions, which can also be caused by TBI and SAH, leading to acute or chronic manifestations [27]. Intracranial surgery and medications (steroids, diuretics) also contribute to the above complications. These neuroendocrine disturbances can manifest at any time during the perioperative period.

Hypocortisolism is common in pituitary tumors, necessitating preoperative steroid supplementation. Pituitary apoplexy requires intravenous steroids and sometimes vasopressors. Preoperative hormonal assessment and postoperative steroid supplementation are crucial for effective management. Hypothyroidism may require thyroxine supplementation, and monitoring free T4 levels would be beneficial, as delayed awakening may be expected [22].

Maintaining blood glucose levels between 140 and 180 mg/dL in the postoperative period is crucial for optimal wound healing and a shorter hospital stay. Transient use of insulin infusion would sometimes be desired to achieve the same.

10.7 Systemic Complications

10.7.1 Pulmonary

Neurosurgical patients with comorbidities such as chronic obstructive pulmonary disease (COPD) and obesity with obstructive sleep apnea (OSA) are at high risk for postoperative pulmonary complications, including reintubation, prolonged mechanical ventilation, atelectasis, pneumonia, respiratory depression, and pulmonary embolism. They are more sensitive to opioids and residual anesthetic effects, thereby increasing the risk of CO2 retention, airway infections, and reintubation. This risk applies mainly to pituitary surgery, cervical spine surgery, procedures in various positions, and surgeries involving the lower cranial nerve and the brain stem in posterior fossa tumors. The coexisting coronary artery disease in them predisposes them to pulmonary edema and embolism.

Perioperative use of bronchodilators/steroid nebulization, and incentive spirometry with the use of reverse Trendelenburg position, along with immediate use of high-flow nasal cannula (HFNC) or NIV after extubation when permitted, can minimize these complications in them. Use of opioid-free multimodal analgesia and endoscopically guided insertion of a nasopharyngeal cannula can help reduce these complications. Use of high positive end-expiratory pressure (PEEP) in morbidly obese intubated patients helps prevent lung atelectasis. Early tracheostomy for patients with lower cranial nerve dysfunction can also minimize complications [28].

10.7.2 Cardiovascular

Postoperative hypertension can be a part of Cushing's reflex, a preexisting hypertensive patient, or following brain-stem–related surgeries, hypercarbia, and pain, which can predispose to intracranial hemorrhage and cerebral edema can be detrimental following AVM surgeries. Postoperative hypotension can be a sequel of intraoperative massive blood loss and also secondary to new-onset intracranial hemorrhage. Hypotension can compromise cerebral blood flow and further elevate ICP, which eventually contributes to poor outcomes [22].

SAH patients can manifest with a reversible cardiac dysfunction known as neurogenic stunned myocardium (brain–heart crosstalk) with electrocardiogram (ECG) manifestation (ST-T wave changes, QTc prolongation), left ventricular dysfunction (regional wall motion abnormalities, global hypokinesia), and cardiac troponin level elevation in 20–40% of cases. Following a reduction in ICP, it is found that these cardiac changes resolve completely or partially, thereby requiring transient vasopressor or inotropic support in the postoperative period. Higher level of cardiac troponin is associated with poor-grade SAH, which in turn is associated with poor functional outcome [22, 29].

A recent study reported cardiac arrest in 36.5% of non-trauma emergency craniotomy patients with American Society of Anesthesiologists (ASA) >3. And 18% of these cardiac arrests were witnessed from the intraoperative period up to within 24 h of postoperative stay, with a high mortality rate [30]. In patients with three or more revised cardiac risk index factors, use of beta-blockers with utmost careful titration in the postoperative period is being suggested in order to minimize the risk of perioperative adverse cardiac events [28].

Use of advanced minimally invasive hemodynamic monitors for precise volume management in patients with high cardiac risks is also suggested to minimize postoperative adverse cardiac events. Maintaining a liberal hemoglobin threshold during blood transfusion is found to benefit these cardiac comorbid patients [28].

10.8 Cardiopulmonary

10.8.1 Venous Air Embolism

Venous air embolism is more common during surgeries in the sitting position (39–76%), craniosynostosis, deep brain stimulator placement, and complex spine fusion. Increased pulmonary artery pressures cause ventilation-perfusion mismatch, leading to increased PaCO2 and reduced end-tidal carbon dioxide (ETCO2). Clinical severity depends on volume and speed of entry of air, manifesting from $ETCO_2$ drop, oxygen desaturations, right heart strain, myocardial ischemia, arrhythmias, pulmonary hypertension, bronchoconstriction, and hypotension.

A large air volume can result in its locking and obstructing the right ventricular outflow tract completely, resulting in cardiopulmonary arrest requiring cardiopulmonary resuscitation to break the airlock. These patients require close monitoring, including invasive monitors, in the postoperative period with the requirement of vasopressor or inotropic support and transthoracic echocardiographic assessment. Use of transesophageal echocardiography, precordial doppler, and $ETCO_2$ monitor would help in early detection and efficient management of this complication [29].

10.8.2 Acute Kidney Injury (AKI)

AKI was reported in 1.16% of patients following craniotomy, which developed within 24 h or within 48 h following surgery [31, 32]. American Society of Anesthesiologists (ASA) status >III, intraoperative hypotension, preoperative mannitol use, hyperglycemia, hypertension, COPD, chronic kidney disease, body mass index (BMI) >30 were all implicated as risk factors for postoperative AKI and should be optimized.

10.9 Infection/Sepsis

10.9.1 Surgical Site Infections (SSIs)

Central nervous system infections, such as wound and bone-flap infection, subdural empyema, meningitis, and brain abscess following neurosurgery, were previously reported between 1% and 18%, until a recent study which reported 1.1% in elective neurosurgical patients.

Risk factors included postoperative CSF leakage, prolonged surgery, male sex, redo-operations, ASA grade (>2), and hyperglycemia, with craniotomy for brain metastasis, meningioma, and subdural hematoma being at increased risk. Surprisingly, age and steroid use were not directly linked to SSI.

The common organisms implicated were Staphylococcus aureus, Pseudomonas aeruginosa, Enterococcus, and Klebsiella. Prophylactic use of cefazolin and vancomycin antibiotics, along with modification of the possible risk factors, has been found to minimize the SSI [33, 34].

10.9.2 Sepsis

Sepsis occurs in 0.87–1.35% of elective neurosurgical patients, with a mortality rate between 7.69% and 11.16% and septic shock in 0.65%. ASA grade III, BMI >35/underweight, functional dependence, male sex, increasing age, prolonged operative time, COPD, bleeding disorder, prolonged steroid use, and disseminated malignancy are all predisposing factors for postoperative sepsis.

Modification of the possible risk factors prior to elective surgery is desirable in order to minimize this complication [35, 36].

10.10 Other Complications, Including Anesthesia-Related

10.10.1 Delayed Awakening

It is the delay in the recovery of consciousness beyond 60 min of complete discontinuation of anesthetic agents. Residual effects of anesthetic agents like inhalational, opioids, and muscle relaxants are implicated in prolonged surgeries. Hypothermia and hypocalcemia worsen the problem, especially in hypothyroid patients. Other potential causes include acidosis from fluid shifts during surgery, blood loss, vasopressor use, hypercarbia, and abnormalities of sodium hypo or hyperglycemia.

Surgical complications such as pneumocephalus, cerebral edema, hematoma/venous infarct, seizures, and surgeries affecting the reticular activating system pathways may lead to delayed awakening. Neonates/elderly, epilepsy, reduced cognition, stroke, obstructive sleep apnea, hypothyroidism, obesity, and larger brain lesions are predisposing factors for delayed awakening.

Opioid overdose can be reversed with naloxone and patient warming. Additional levothyroxine may be administered via a nasogastric tube, and neuromuscular weakness can be monitored and appropriately managed. Both metabolic and surgical causes need to be individually addressed [12].

10.11 Postoperative Nausea and Vomiting (PONV)

Postoperative nausea and vomiting occur in 40–50% of neurosurgical patients, potentially leading to increased intracranial pressure and complications. Risk factors include female sex, surgeries beyond an hour, young age, posterior fossa/

retro-mastoid surgery, CSF leak, inhalational anesthetics, and opioids. Post-craniotomy PONV management involves addressing preoperative risk factors, dexamethasone and ondansetron prophylaxis, maintaining normo-volemia, dexmedetomidine, and scalp block (minimizes opioid use) [37].

10.12 Postoperative Delirium (POD)

POD refers to changes in consciousness, attention, and cognitive functions in patients immediately following surgery, which can persist for up to 7 days. Its incidence varies from 12% to 26% in the neurosurgical population, with 19% being reported from a very recent study and a meta-analysis.

Several factors, such as age, prolonged surgery, type and site of intracranial lesion, preoperative cognitive issues, reduced hemoglobin, education, functional status, emergence delirium, reduced oxygen saturation upon admission, prolonged immobilization, postoperative pain, fever, postoperative hematoma, and electrolyte imbalances, can predispose individuals to complications after surgery.

Neuroinflammation and oxidative stress are the implicated mechanisms, and among neurosurgeries, it is most common in neurovascular surgeries (42%). No specific anesthetics (inhalational vs propofol) are implicated; however, use of remifentanil showed less incidence of POD as compared to other opioid use. Preoperative cognitive decline and the emergence of delirium are risk factors for POD in neurosurgical patients. POD can lead to significant morbidity and longer ICU and hospital stays.

Identifying the risk factors and appropriately addressing them, including modification of surgical technique, would help in minimizing POD. The use of regional anesthesia techniques and EEG-guided anesthetic titration has shown potential in reducing postoperative delirium in non-neurosurgical patients, but further research is needed in neurosurgical populations [38, 39].

10.13 Airway-Related Complications

Cushing's and acromegalic patients (with morbid obesity, OSA history, and contraindication to postoperative CPAP), airway edema after prolonged prone-position for upper cervical spine surgery, posterior fossa surgery involving brain stem and lower cranial nerves, and anterior cervical spine surgery (possible recurrent laryngeal nerve injury) pose a definitive challenge during extubation.

Use of endoscopically guided nasopharyngeal airway in transnasal surgery, cuff leak test to assess airway edema, and tracheostomy, where lower cranial nerve palsy is expected, would minimize reintubation-related complications in them [22, 40].

10.14 Pain

Postoperative pain can cause increased heart rate and blood pressure, which can have deleterious effects on patients with multiple comorbidities, predisposing them to hematoma. Hence, pain management becomes an important aspect of postoperative care. Also, patients with posterior fossa surgery are known to suffer more pain as compared to their supratentorial counterparts.

In the absence of gold standard analgesic therapy, a multimodal approach is recommended. Opioids, the commonly used analgesics, are most effective but not without side effects. Patient-controlled analgesia (PCA) is found to offer superior pain control and overall patient satisfaction, but the evidence is limited [6]. Tramadol, while less likely to cause respiratory depression, is not as effective as morphine and has a higher risk of nausea and vomiting. The scalp nerve blocks may afford longer and higher-quality analgesia akin to morphine. The use of nonsteroidal anti-inflammatory drugs here is debatable. Acetaminophen, gabapentin, or dexmedetomidine have been found to reduce postoperative opioid consumption [6, 22, 29].

10.15 Clinical Pitfalls

A very recent report was an eye-opener in the management of tension pneumocephalus. Following an uneventful posterior fossa meningioma (abutting the right transverse sinus) surgery and anesthesia in a 59-year-old woman, there was no recovery of consciousness, with pupils becoming fixed and dilated in the early postoperative period. A CT scan revealed pneumocephalus distorting and flattening the ventral surface of the pons. Amidst the dilemma between surgical decompression vs. conservative approach, she was administered 100% oxygen in the sitting position to facilitate the movement of air through the prepontine cisternal space to the supratentorial subarachnoid compartment. Subsequently, pupillary dilation was reversed as the ventral pons was relieved of compression and the patient was eventually extubated. Surgical decompression would not have benefited but rather worsened this scenario, as air would have recollected again after the procedure [41].

Though routine intraoperative antiepileptic prophylaxis is not being recommended for neurosurgical patients, small randomized controlled data are indicating the benefits of prophylactic antiepileptics, especially in patients who are at a high risk of postoperative seizures [15, 16].

Surprising cases of postoperative intracranial hematoma unimaginably remote from surgical sites are described. The first patient showed clinical deterioration in the postoperative period with a surgical drain containing CSF along with blood. A similar picture was noticed following excision of a large temporal meningioma. A third scenario involved deterioration in consciousness 1.5 h following thoracic Pancoast tumor excision. CT scan showed hemorrhage in the cerebellar sulci (zebra sign). CSF loss would have resulted in mechanical shifting of the cerebellum with posterior fossa venous occlusion, transiently, thereby forming a hemorrhagic venous infarct. Subarachnoid pleural fistula was the cause of CSF loss after Pancoast tumor excision [1, 42].

Hyperlactemia, which is common after neurosurgery (>50%), does not need aggressive management (until metabolic acidosis prevails), as it was neither associated with new-onset neurological deficits nor increased 6-month mortality. However, overzealous fluid administration to correct lactic acid levels resulted in pulmonary complications [21].

Hypernatremia following elective neurosurgery was independently associated with an increase in 30-day mortality, and the rate increased with the severity of hypernatremia. However, even mild hypernatremia is also at risk as per a recent study and needs to be corrected [25]. As per a study, 15% of the TBI patients developed hyponatremia, and >80% of them had low plasma cortisol levels, thereby suggesting ACTH deficiency [23].

Amidst various risk factors mentioned for the development of postoperative delirium, a very recent study and meta-analysis have identified preoperative cognitive decline and emergence of delirium as the only major causes and indicated optimizing them [38, 39].

Age and steroid use were not considered as risk factors for the development of surgical site infections following craniotomy [33, 34].

Nursing postoperative neurosurgical patients with the head of bed (HOB) elevated beyond 30° was a concern due to the fear of a reduction in cerebral blood flow, which can be detrimental in neuro patients. However, few obese neurosurgical patients need to be nursed in the HOB position beyond 30° to minimize postoperative pulmonary complications. To address this problem, a recent study supports safe nursing with HOB up to 60° when guided by cerebral blood flow and cerebral oxygenation monitoring, and in patients who do not require cerebral perfusion pressure–guided management [43].

10.16 Conclusion

With the paradigm shifts in the understanding of various risk factors that contribute to postoperative complications following neurosurgery, a thorough knowledge would improve the quality of their management. A comprehensive multidisciplinary approach beginning from the preoperative period, adherence to intraoperative surgical and anesthetic protocols, along with the incorporation of advanced multimodal neuro-monitoring, would help in their safe management.

References

1. Fugate JE. Complications of neurosurgery. Continuum (Minneap Minn). 2015;21:1425–44.
2. Wong DJN, Popham S, Wilson AM, Barneto LM, Lindsay HA, Farmer L, et al. Postoperative critical care and high-acuity care provision in the United Kingdom, Australia, and New Zealand. Br J Anaesth. 2019;122:460–9.

3. Errico M, Luoma AMV. Postoperative care of neurosurgical patients: general principles. Anaesth Intensive Care Med. 2023;24:282–90.
4. Wijdicks EFM, Bamlet WR, Maramattom BV, Manno EM, McClelland RL. Validation of a new coma scale: the FOUR score. Ann Neurol. 2005;58:585–93.
5. Smith ME, Smith M. Neuromonitoring. Anaesth. Intensive Care Med. 2017;18:224–9.
6. Vadivelu N, Kai AM, Tran D, Kodumudi G, Legler A, Ayrian E. Options for perioperative pain management in neurosurgery. J Pain Res. 2016;9:37–47.
7. Wan AWZ, Luoma AMV. Postoperative care of neurosurgical patients: general principles. Anaesth Intensive Care Med. 2020;21:349–55.
8. Burkhart CS, Strebel SP, Steiner LA. Post-operative care of neurosurgical patients. In: Matta BF, Menon DK, Smith M, editors. Core topics in neuroanaesthesia and neurointensive care [Internet]. 1st ed. Cambridge University Press; 2011. p. 301–14.
9. Lonjaret L, Guyonnet M, Berard E, Vironneau M, Peres F, Sacrista S, et al. Postoperative complications after craniotomy for brain tumor surgery. Anaesth Crit Care Pain Med. 2017;36:213–8. https://doi.org/10.1016/j.accpm.2016.06.012.
10. Seifman MA, Lewis PM, Rosenfeld JV, Hwang PY. Postoperative intracranial haemorrhage: a review. Neurosurg Rev. 2011;34:393–407. https://doi.org/10.1007/s10143-010-0304-3.
11. George J, Praveen R, Vimala S, Sethuraman M. Anesthetic uncertainties in a child with multiple epidural hematoma immediately following brain tumour resection. Med J Armed Forces India. 2024;80:121–2. https://doi.org/10.1016/j.mjafi.2022.02.009.
12. Prabhakar H, editor. Complications in Neuroanesthesia. Academic Press; 2016.
13. Dabdoub CB, Salas G, Silveira Edo N, Dabdoub CF. Review of the management of pneumocephalus. Surg Neurol Int. 2015;6:155. https://doi.org/10.4103/2152-7806.166195.
14. Machetanz K, Leuze F, Mounts K, Trakolis L, Gugel I, Grimm F, Tatagiba M, Naros G. Occurrence and management of postoperative pneumocephalus using the semi-sitting position in vestibular schwannoma surgery. Acta Neurochir. 2020;162:2629–36. https://doi.org/10.1007/s00701-020-04504-5.
15. Ersoy TF, Ridwan S, Grote A, Coras R, Simon M. Early postoperative seizures (EPS) in patients undergoing brain tumour surgery. Sci Rep. 2020;10:13674. https://doi.org/10.1038/s41598-020-70754-z.
16. Sakakura K, Ishikawa E, Matsuda M, Akutsu H, Masuda Y, Zaboronok A, et al. Postoperative epileptic seizures after brain tumor surgery. Interdiscip Neurosurg Adv Tech Case Manag. 2020;19:100549.
17. Coucke B, Van Gerven L, De Vleeschouwer S, Van Calenbergh F, van Loon J, Theys T. The incidence of postoperative cerebrospinal fluid leakage after elective cranial surgery: a systematic review. Neurosurg Rev. 2022;45:1827–45. https://doi.org/10.1007/s10143-021-01641-y.
18. Slot EMH, van Baarsen KM, Hoving EW, Zuithoff NPA, van Doormaal TPC. Cerebrospinal fluid leakage after cranial surgery in the pediatric population-a systematic review and meta-analysis. Childs Nerv Syst. 2021;37:1439–47. https://doi.org/10.1007/s00381-021-05036-8.
19. Hirbo Guyolla Y, Biluts Mersha H, Tesfaye AF. Predictors of cerebrospinal fluid leakage after elective cranial surgery. Interdiscip Neurosurg. 2023;31:101704.
20. de Smalen PP, van Ark TJ, Stolker RJ, Vincent AJPE, Klimek M. Hyperlactatemia after intracranial tumor surgery does not affect 6-month survival: a retrospective case series. J Neurosurg Anesthesiol. 2020;32:48–56.
21. Klimek M, de Smalen P, Janssen J. Hyperlactatemia and other perioperative metabolic disturbances in neuroanesthesia. Curr Opin Anaesthesiol. 2022;35:537–42.
22. Panda N, Mahajan S, Chouhan R. Management of postoperative neurosurgical patients. J Neuroanaesthesiol Crit Care. 2019;6:80–6.
23. Hannon MJ, Thompson CJ. Neurosurgical Hyponatremia. J. Clin Med. 2014;3:1084–104.
24. Cuesta M, Hannon MJ, Thompson CJ. Diagnosis and treatment of hyponatraemia in neurosurgical patients. Endocrinol Nutr. 2016;63:230–8. English, Spanish. https://doi.org/10.1016/j.endonu.2015.12.007.
25. Li T, Zhang Y, Chen X, Jia L, Tian Y, He J, He M, Chen L, Hao P, Xiao Y, Peng L, Chong W, Hai Y, You C, Fang F. Association of postoperative hypernatremia with outcomes after elective craniotomy. J Clin Anesth. 2024;92:111294. https://doi.org/10.1016/j.jclinane.2023.111294.

26. Bhat R, Baldeweg SE, Wilson SR. Sodium disorders in neuroanaesthesia and neurocritical care. BJA Educ. 2022;22:466–73. https://doi.org/10.1016/j.bjae.2022.08.001.
27. Bajwa SJ, Haldar R. Endocrinological disorders affecting neurosurgical patients: an intensivists perspective. Indian J Endocrinol Metab. 2014;18:778–83.
28. Algahtani R, Merenda A. Multimorbidity and critical care neurosurgery: minimizing major perioperative cardiopulmonary complications. Neurocrit Care. 2021;34:1047–61. https://doi.org/10.1007/s12028-020-01072-5.
29. Prabhakar H, Ali Z, editors. Textbook of neuroanesthesia and neurocritical care. Singapore: Springer; 2019.
30. Quinn TD, Brovman EY, Aglio LS, Urman RD. Factors associated with an increased risk of perioperative cardiac arrest in emergent and elective craniotomy and spine surgery. Clin Neurol Neurosurg. 2017;161:6–13.
31. Li J, Zhao Y, Yan X, Li R, Zhang X, Zeng M, Dong J, Li S, Peng Y, Han R. Perioperative risk factors associated with acute kidney injury in patients after brain tumor resection. J Neurosurg Anesthesiol. 2022;34:51–6.
32. Chung S, Brovman EY, Aglio LS, Beutler SS, Urman RD. Risk factors and associated complications of acute kidney injury in adult patients undergoing a craniotomy. Clin Neurol Neurosurg. 2020;190:105642. https://doi.org/10.1016/j.clineuro.2019.105642.
33. McClelland S 3rd, Hall WA. Postoperative central nervous system infection: incidence and associated factors in 2111 neurosurgical procedures. Clin Infect Dis. 2007;45:55–9.
34. Corsini Campioli C, Challener D, Comba IY, Shah A, Wilson WR, Sohail MR, Van Gompel JJ, O'Horo JC. Overview and risk factors for postcraniotomy surgical site infection: a four-year experience. Antimicrob Steward Healthc Epidemiol. 2022;2:e14. https://doi.org/10.1017/ash.2021.258.
35. Pertsch NJ, Tang OY, Seicean A, Toms SA, Weil RJ. Sepsis after elective neurosurgery: incidence, outcomes, and predictive factors. J Clin Neurosci. 2020;78:53–9.
36. Zhang J, Li YI, Pieters TA, Towner J, Li KZ, Al-Dhahir MA, Childers F, Li YM. Sepsis and septic shock after craniotomy: predicting a significant patient safety and quality outcome measure. PLoS One. 2020;15:e0235273. https://doi.org/10.1371/journal.pone.0235273.
37. Uribe AA, Stoicea N, Echeverria-Villalobos M, Todeschini AB, Esparza Gutierrez A, Folea AR, Bergese SD. Postoperative nausea and vomiting after craniotomy: an evidence-based review of general considerations, risk factors, and management. J Neurosurg Anesthesiol. 2021;33:212–20.
38. Kappen PR, Kakar E, Dirven CMF, van der Jagt M, Klimek M, Osse RJ, Vincent APJE. Delirium in neurosurgery: a systematic review and meta-analysis. Neurosurg Rev. 2022;45:329–41.
39. Chakrabarti D, Bharadwaj S, Akash VS, Wadhwa A, Konar S, Kamath S, Gopalakrishna KN. Postoperative delirium after intracranial neurosurgery: a prospective cohort study from a developing nation. Acta Neurochir. 2023;165:1473–82.
40. Murselović T, Makovšek A. Airway management in neuroanesthesia. Acta Clin Croat. 2023;62:119–24.
41. Ghare A, Dhaliwal J, Al-Mohammad A, Waraich M, Samandouras G. Acute, life-threatening postoperative pneumocephalus: emergency diagnostic and therapeutic steps with underlying pathophysiology. Br J Anaesth. 2023;131:e39–41. https://doi.org/10.1016/j.bja.2023.04.027.
42. Brockmann MA, Nowak G, Reusche E, Russlies M, Petersen D. Zebra sign: cerebellar bleeding pattern characteristic of cerebrospinal fluid loss. Case report. J Neurosurg. 2005;102:1159–62.
43. Baskar N, Sethuraman M, Praveen R, Hrishi AP, Vimala S, Prathapadas U, Abraham M. Evaluation of cerebral perfusion pressure, cerebral blood flow, and cerebral oxygenation at different head of bed positions using transcranial Doppler and near-infrared spectroscopy in postoperative neurosurgical patients. Cureus. 2024;16:e51923. https://doi.org/10.7759/cureus.51923.

Hemodynamic Management in Neuro ICU: Controversies

11

Mathangi Krishnakumar, Sharmishtha Pathak, and Jaya Lal

Abstract

Optimal hemodynamic management in the neuro-intensive care unit is vital to prevent secondary brain injury in patients with acute brain insults such as ischemic stroke, intracerebral hemorrhage, subarachnoid hemorrhage, traumatic brain injury, and spinal cord injury. This chapter highlights key controversies in fluid therapy, blood pressure targets, cerebral perfusion pressure optimization, and the use of vasopressors and advanced hemodynamic monitoring. Individualized strategies, guided by multimodal monitoring—including intracranial pressure, cerebral autoregulation (PRx), cerebral oxygenation, and spinal cord perfusion pressure—are emphasized over generalized protocols. The utility of goal-directed therapy (GDT), transfusion thresholds, and coagulopathy management in neurocritical care is also discussed. While technological advances support personalized care, many recommendations remain based on moderate-quality evidence, underscoring the need for further high-quality research.

Keywords

Advanced hemodynamic monitoring · Multimodal neuromonitoring · Goal-directed therapy · Pressure reactivity index · Cerebral perfusion pressure

M. Krishnakumar (✉)
Surgical and Neuro Intensive Care Unit, Department of Anaesthesia, St John's Medical College Hospital, Bengaluru, Karnataka, India

S. Pathak
Anaesthesiology, Pain Medicine and Critical Care, JPNATC, AIIMS, New Delhi, India

J. Lal
Pediatric Trauma and Orthopaedics, Royal Machester Children's Hospital, Manchester, UK

P. U. Bidkar, M. Krishnakumar (eds.), *Controversies in Neurocritical Care*,
https://doi.org/10.1007/978-981-95-4419-6_11

11.1 Introduction

Prevention of secondary brain injury in patients admitted to the neuro-intensive care unit (NICU) requires rigorous management of the hemodynamics. The cerebral autoregulation may be impaired in patients suffering from acute injuries to the brain, such as acute ischemic stroke (AIS), intracranial hemorrhage (ICH), subarachnoid hemorrhage (SAH), and traumatic brain injury (TBI). Along with impaired cerebral autoregulation, brain perfusion and oxygenation may also be adversely affected. The occurrence of these pathologies renders the brain highly dependent on variations in systemic blood pressure to meet its metabolic requirements. Consequently, suboptimal hemodynamic management—including fluids, vasoactive drugs, and hemodynamic monitoring—can exacerbate ischemic areas, promote hemorrhagic evolution, and lead to secondary brain injury [1, 2].

Hemodynamic management in the NICU involves maintaining cerebral perfusion pressure (CPP) and managing intracranial pressure (ICP) to optimize brain oxygenation and prevent further injury. CPP is influenced by systemic blood pressure (BP) and ICP, making the control of these parameters essential in neurocritical care. Disturbances in cerebral autoregulation, a common feature in acute brain injury (ABI) patients, complicate the management of these variables. Autoregulation refers to the brain's ability to maintain consistent blood flow despite changes in systemic BP. In conditions such as AIS, ICH, SAH, and TBI, this regulatory mechanism is often disrupted, making the brain more susceptible to fluctuations in systemic BP [3, 4].

Managing ICP and CPP is essential for preventing secondary brain injury. Elevated ICP can reduce CPP and compromise cerebral perfusion, leading to further neuronal damage. Maintaining adequate CPP is critical, especially in conditions like TBI, where impaired autoregulation is common. The recommended CPP targets vary, with some guidelines suggesting 60–70 mmHg, while others advocate for higher targets in certain populations. Monitoring cerebrovascular autoregulation using techniques like the pressure reactivity index (PRx) can help tailor CPP targets to individual patients, yet the widespread adoption of such personalized approaches is still evolving [5, 6].

Ensuring adequate cardiac output and oxygen delivery is fundamental to supporting brain metabolism in neurocritical care patients. Noninvasive methods, such as transthoracic echocardiography, and advanced hemodynamic monitoring technologies, like transpulmonary thermodilution and pulse contour analysis, provide valuable insights into cardiac function and guide interventions [7]. However, the utility and impact of these monitoring methods on patient outcomes remain subjects of ongoing research and debate. Advanced monitoring tools offer detailed hemodynamic assessments but are complex and costly. Their integration into clinical practice is challenged by questions about cost-effectiveness and the potential for over-reliance on technical data. Despite these concerns, some clinicians argue that the comprehensive data provided by these technologies justify their use, especially in critically ill patients [8, 9].

The strategies for hemodynamic management rely on moderate to low-quality evidence obtained from relatively small studies [10]. As a result, strong recommendations are often absent in the most recent consensus guidelines. Hemodynamic monitoring and target-setting, as well as fluid management strategies, must account for the unique physiological characteristics of patients with acute brain injury (ABI) [11]. These patients often exhibit disturbed cerebral autoregulation, a propensity for increased ICP, and decreased CPP. Furthermore, patients with acute cardiac dysfunction associated with sympathetic stimulation and catecholamine release present additional challenges that must be carefully managed to optimize outcomes [12, 13].

11.2 Hemodynamic Targets in Different Conditions

Hemodynamic management in the Neuro ICU involves complex decision-making to maintain optimal cerebral perfusion and systemic stability while preventing secondary brain injury (Table 11.1). The management strategies are often influenced by the type of acute brain injury, with distinct considerations for conditions such as acute ischemic stroke (AIS), intracerebral hemorrhage (ICH), subarachnoid

Table 11.1 Hemodynamic targets in different neurocritical conditions

Condition	Primary hemodynamic target	Suggested target values	Notes
Traumatic brain injury (TBI)	Cerebral perfusion pressure (CPP)	60–70 mmHg	Individualize based on PRx
Acute ischemic stroke (AIS)	Blood pressure (BP)	<180 mmHg (without thrombolysis), <140 mmHg (with thrombolysis)	Balance risk of hemorrhagic transformation and perfusion
Intracerebral hemorrhage (ICH)	Blood pressure (BP)	<140 mmHg	Prevent hematoma expansion while maintaining perfusion
Subarachnoid hemorrhage (SAH)—aneurysm secured	Blood pressure (BP)	120–160 mmHg	Prevent rebleeding and manage vasospasm
Subarachnoid hemorrhage (SAH)—aneurysm unsecured	Blood pressure (BP)	<140 mmHg	Minimize risk of aneurysm rupture
Subarachnoid hemorrhage (SAH)—vasospasm	Cerebral blood flow (CBF)	Optimize CBF using advanced monitoring	Prevent delayed cerebral ischemia
Acute spinal cord injury (SCI)	Mean arterial pressure (MAP)	MAP-85–90 mmHg	Maintain spinal cord perfusion
Brain death	Systemic blood pressure (BP), organ perfusion	Maintain MAP >65 mmHg	Ensure organ viability for transplantation

hemorrhage (SAH), traumatic brain injury (TBI), and acute spinal cord injury (SCI). Despite advancements in monitoring and therapeutic interventions, controversies persist regarding the optimal hemodynamic targets for these conditions. This section will address these controversies through recent evidence and trials.

11.2.1 Acute Ischemic Stroke (AIS)

1. *Controversy: What is the optimal blood pressure target in AIS to balance the risk of hemorrhagic transformation against maintaining adequate cerebral perfusion?*

Elevated blood pressure (BP) is frequently observed in patients suffering from acute ischemic stroke (AIS) and is believed to be a compensatory mechanism to maintain cerebral perfusion in the ischemic penumbra. However, the optimal management of BP in AIS remains controversial due to the risk of hemorrhagic transformation associated with elevated BP and the need to maintain perfusion.

Current guidelines often recommend a strategy of permissive hypertension, where BP is allowed to remain elevated for a certain period to support cerebral perfusion. The AHA/ASA guidelines suggest maintaining systolic BP below 220 mmHg in the acute phase of AIS, based on limited evidence [14]. This recommendation aims to avoid the risk of hemorrhagic transformation while supporting penumbral perfusion.

On the other hand, some clinicians advocate for more aggressive BP control. The ENCHANTED trial (Enhanced Control of Hypertension and Thrombolysis Stroke Study) compared intensive BP lowering (target systolic BP 130–140 mmHg) with standard BP management (target systolic BP <180 mmHg) in patients receiving thrombolysis. The trial did not reveal any significant difference in death or disability at 90 days between the two groups; however, fewer hemorrhagic transformations were observed in the intensive BP control group [15].

Given the conflicting evidence, individualized BP management strategies are being explored. Factors such as baseline BP, comorbidities, and the extent of ischemic damage may influence the optimal BP target for individual patients. Continuous monitoring and dynamic adjustment of BP targets based on real-time data are essential to optimize outcomes [16].

11.2.2 Intracerebral Hemorrhage (ICH)

2. *Controversy: Should intensive BP lowering be universally applied in ICH, or should targets be individualized?*

In patients with intracerebral hemorrhage (ICH), BP management is crucial to minimize hematoma expansion and prevent secondary brain injury. The optimal BP target, however, remains a subject of debate.

The INTERACT2 trial (Intensive Blood Pressure Reduction in Acute Cerebral Hemorrhage Trial) suggested that intensive BP lowering (target systolic BP <140 mmHg) could improve functional outcomes in patients with ICH compared to standard BP management (target systolic BP <180 mmHg). The trial found a non-significant reduction in death or major disability at 90 days, but significant improvements in functional status and quality of life [17, 18].

Conversely, the ATACH-II trial (Antihypertensive Treatment of Acute Cerebral Hemorrhage II) did not demonstrate significant benefits from aggressive BP reduction. The trial compared intensive BP lowering (target systolic BP 110–140 mmHg) with standard BP management (target systolic BP 140–180 mmHg) and observed no significant difference in the primary outcome of death or severe disability at 90 days. Moreover, the intensive treatment group experienced more adverse renal events [19].

Given the mixed results from these trials, an individualized approach to BP management in ICH is recommended. Factors such as the size and location of the hematoma, the patient's baseline BP, and comorbid conditions should be considered when determining the BP target. Continuous monitoring and frequent reassessment are critical to ensure that BP management strategies are tailored to the needs of each patient [20].

11.2.3 Subarachnoid Hemorrhage (SAH)

3. *Controversy: Is Triple H therapy (hypervolemia, hypertension, hemodilution) still the best approach for managing cerebral vasospasm in SAH, or are more conservative strategies preferable?*

Subarachnoid hemorrhage (SAH) is often complicated by cerebral vasospasm, which can lead to delayed cerebral ischemia. Traditionally, Triple H therapy has been used to prevent and treat vasospasm by maintaining high blood volume, BP, and hemodilution. However, the safety and efficacy of this approach have been questioned.

Triple H therapy has been the cornerstone of SAH management for decades. The rationale is to increase cerebral perfusion pressure and prevent ischemia. However, it is connected with significant risks, including pulmonary edema, myocardial ischemia, and electrolyte imbalances [21]. Recent studies and expert opinions suggest that a more conservative approach may be equally effective and safer. There is no role for prophylactic hemodynamic management in SAH [22].

The current trend is toward individualized therapy based on dynamic assessments of cerebral hemodynamics. Advanced monitoring techniques, such as transcranial Doppler ultrasonography and cerebral blood flow monitoring, can help tailor BP management to the needs of each patient. Maintaining euvolemia and avoiding aggressive hypervolemia and hypertension are increasingly recommended [22].

11.2.4 Traumatic Brain Injury (TBI)

4. *Controversy: How should cerebral perfusion pressure (CPP) targets be determined in TBI, and should these targets be adjusted based on individual cerebrovascular autoregulation?*

Cerebral perfusion pressure (CPP) is an indispensable parameter in the management of traumatic brain injury (TBI). The optimal CPP target, however, is still debated, particularly in the context of impaired cerebral autoregulation [23].

Traditional guidelines have recommended maintaining CPP between 60–70 mmHg to ensure adequate cerebral perfusion while minimizing the risk of increased intracranial pressure (ICP). However, this approach of one-size-fits-all may be inappropriate for TBI patients [6].

Recent evidence suggests that CPP targets should be individualized based on assessments of cerebrovascular autoregulation. The pressure reactivity index (PRx), which measures the relationship between ICP and mean arterial pressure (MAP), can help determine the optimal CPP for individual patients. Studies have shown that maintaining CPP within the optimal range defined by PRx monitoring is associated with better outcomes [11, 23].

Continuous monitoring of autoregulation and dynamic adjustment of CPP targets are increasingly advocated. This approach involves using advanced monitoring techniques to tailor CPP management to the individual patient's needs, thereby optimizing cerebral perfusion and minimizing secondary injury. In addition, the use of cerebral oxygenation and ICP for optimizing CPP is also advocated [9].

11.2.5 Acute Spinal Cord Injury (SCI)

5. *Controversy: What are the optimal hemodynamic targets in acute spinal cord injury (SCI) to improve neurological outcomes and minimize complications?*

Hemodynamic management in acute spinal cord injury (SCI) aims to maintain spinal cord perfusion and prevent further ischemic damage. The optimal targets for blood pressure and perfusion pressure in SCI are subjects of ongoing debate [24].

Current guidelines recommend maintaining mean arterial pressure (MAP) in the range of 85–90 mmHg for the initial 7 days following acute SCI to ensure adequate spinal cord perfusion [12]. This recommendation is based on limited evidence, primarily from retrospective studies and expert consensus. The rationale is to enhance spinal cord perfusion and potentially improve neurological recovery. Use of norepinephrine for upper thoracic and cervical injuries and phenylephrine or norepinephrine for mid- to lower thoracic injuries should be considered [25, 26].

The concept of spinal cord perfusion pressure (SCPP), similar to cerebral perfusion pressure (CPP), is gaining attention. SCPP is calculated as MAP minus intrathecal pressure (ITP), with higher SCPP believed to improve spinal cord oxygenation.

However, the lack of robust clinical evidence to define optimal SCPP targets warrants further research for validation [27].

Given the variability in patient responses and injury characteristics, individualized hemodynamic management strategies are recommended. Continuous monitoring of MAP and ITP, along with assessments of spinal cord perfusion using advanced imaging and monitoring techniques, can help tailor interventions to optimize outcomes [27].

11.3 Multimodal Monitoring: General to Personalized Hemodynamic Targets

The application of multimodal monitoring is essential for precise hemodynamic management in neurocritical care (Fig. 11.1). Integrating various monitoring techniques allows for a comprehensive understanding of a patient's hemodynamic status and facilitates personalized treatment strategies. This section addresses the controversies surrounding general versus personalized hemodynamic targets, supported by recent evidence and clinical trials.

6. *Controversy: Is multimodal monitoring superior to traditional monitoring in improving outcomes for neurocritical care patients?*

Traditional hemodynamic monitoring primarily involves basic parameters such as blood pressure (BP), heart rate, central venous pressure (CVP), and urine output. These parameters, while crucial, provide limited information about the complexities of cerebral and systemic hemodynamics.

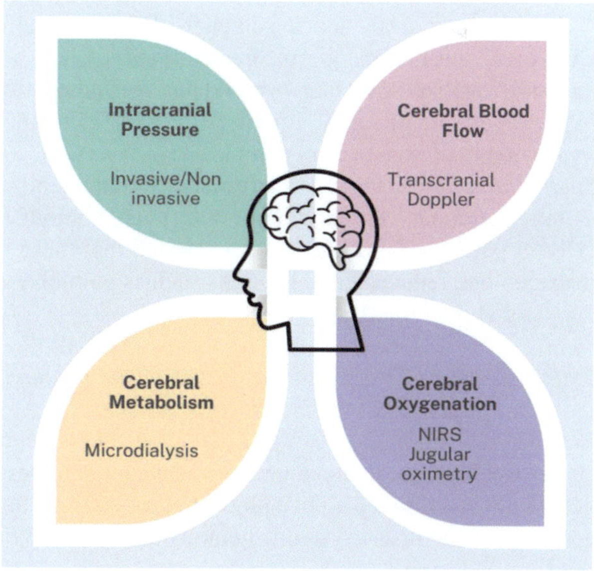

Fig. 11.1 Multimodal neuromonitoring

Continuous arterial BP monitoring via an indwelling arterial catheter is standard practice in the Neuro ICU. Monitoring CVP helps assess fluid status and guide fluid therapy. However, CVP alone may not adequately reflect the true hemodynamic status, as it does not provide information on cardiac output or tissue perfusion [28]. These general monitoring techniques often fail to capture the full complexity of hemodynamic disturbances in neurocritical care, leading to the need for advanced multimodal monitoring strategies [7].

11.3.1 Advanced Hemodynamic Monitoring Techniques

Transpulmonary Thermodilution This technique measures cardiac output, global end-diastolic volume, and extravascular lung water. It provides a comprehensive assessment of cardiac preload and fluid responsiveness, crucial for optimizing fluid therapy and avoiding complications such as pulmonary edema [29]. Studies have shown that transpulmonary thermodilution can improve the management of critically ill patients by providing accurate and dynamic measurements of hemodynamic parameters [30].

Pulse Contour Analysis Pulse contour analysis calculates cardiac output and stroke volume variation by analyzing the arterial pressure waveform. It is less invasive than transpulmonary thermodilution and offers continuous, real-time data. This technique is particularly useful in guiding fluid resuscitation and vasopressor therapy [31].

Echocardiography Both transthoracic (TTE) and transesophageal echocardiography (TEE) are valuable tools in the Neuro ICU. Echocardiography provides detailed information about cardiac function, including ventricular function, valvular abnormalities, and fluid status. Its noninvasive nature and ready availability at bedside make it a versatile and accessible monitoring tool [32].

Studies have evaluated the impact of multimodal monitoring, including ICP, CPP, PRx, and PbtO2, on outcomes in patients with severe TBI. The study found that individualized CPP targets based on PRx and continuous monitoring of cerebral oxygenation significantly improved patient outcomes, reducing mortality and improving neurological function [11, 33].

Studies have shown the use of advanced hemodynamic monitoring techniques, such as transpulmonary thermodilution and pulse contour analysis, in managing critically ill patients. These trials demonstrated that these technologies improved fluid management, reduced complications such as pulmonary edema, and shortened ICU length of stay [12, 34].

7. *Controversy: Does personalized hemodynamic management lead to better outcomes than standardized treatment protocols?*

Personalized medicine in neurocritical care involves tailoring hemodynamic targets to the individual patient's physiological status. This approach aims to optimize cerebral perfusion and systemic hemodynamics based on real-time data from multimodal monitoring.

Pressure Reactivity Index (PRx) PRx measures the correlation between slow waves of ICP and arterial BP, providing an assessment of cerebrovascular autoregulation. A negative PRx suggests that the autoregulation is still intact, while impaired autoregulation is indicated by a positive PRx. Studies have shown that PRx-guided management of cerebral perfusion pressure (CPP) can improve outcomes in TBI patients by optimizing CPP based on individual autoregulatory status [35].

Cerebral Oximetry Near-infrared spectroscopy (NIRS) allows for continuous, noninvasive monitoring of cerebral oxygenation. NIRS can detect regional cerebral hypoxia, guiding interventions to optimize cerebral perfusion. Recent evidence suggests that integrating NIRS into multimodal monitoring can improve the detection of cerebral ischemia and guide targeted therapies [36].

Microdialysis Cerebral microdialysis measures extracellular concentrations of metabolites such as glucose, lactate, pyruvate, and glutamate, providing insights into cerebral metabolism. This technique can detect early signs of metabolic distress and guide interventions to prevent secondary brain injury. Microdialysis has been particularly useful in managing patients with severe TBI and SAH, offering a window into the brain's metabolic state [37].

The evolution from general to personalized hemodynamic targets in neurocritical care represents a significant advancement in patient management. The integration of multimodal monitoring techniques provides a comprehensive understanding of the patient's hemodynamic status, enabling tailored interventions that optimize cerebral and systemic perfusion. Recent evidence and clinical trials underscore the benefits of personalized hemodynamic management, highlighting the importance of continuous monitoring and dynamic adjustment of targets based on real-time data. As technology continues to advance, the adoption of personalized approaches in neurocritical care is likely to enhance patient outcomes and set new standards for hemodynamic management.

11.4 Hemodynamic Management

Managing shock in the neuro ICU is critical due to its potential impact on cerebral perfusion and overall patient outcomes.

11.4.1 Goal-Directed Therapy (GDT)

8. *Controversy: What is the role of GDT in the neuro ICU, and how does it impact patient outcomes?*

GDT involves the continuous monitoring of hemodynamic parameters to optimize tissue perfusion and oxygen delivery. It typically includes monitoring cardiac output, stroke volume, and other hemodynamic variables to guide fluid resuscitation, vasopressor use, and other therapeutic interventions.

In general critical care, GDT has been shown to improve outcomes, particularly in septic shock and high-risk surgical patients. It reduces mortality, decreases ICU length of stay, and minimizes complications by optimizing hemodynamic parameters [38].

The specific impact of GDT in neurocritical care is less well-established. Neuro ICU patients have unique pathophysiological considerations, such as maintaining cerebral perfusion pressure (CPP) and managing intracranial pressure (ICP). Recent studies did not show any benefit of GDT in postoperative neurosurgical patients [39]. However, GDT has the potential to be beneficial in this setting by ensuring adequate systemic perfusion and oxygen delivery, which are crucial for brain function.

The landmark Rivers et al. study demonstrated that EGDT significantly improved survival in septic shock patients by optimizing hemodynamic parameters during the initial hours of treatment [40]. While GDT has demonstrated benefits in various critical care settings, its specific role in the neuro ICU requires further investigation. Tailoring GDT protocols to address the unique needs of neurocritical care patients, such as maintaining CPP and managing ICP, is essential for optimizing outcomes.

11.5 Fluid Management

9. *Controversy: What are the best practices for fluid management in neuro ICU patients to balance cerebral perfusion with the risk of edema?*

The debate over the use of crystalloids versus colloids in fluid resuscitation continues. Crystalloids, such as saline and Ringer's lactate, are commonly used due to their low cost and availability. However, they may require larger volumes to achieve the desired hemodynamic effect. Colloids, such as albumin and hydroxyethyl starch, are more effective in expanding plasma volume but are associated with risks such as coagulopathy and renal impairment [41].

Maintaining optimal volume status is essential to prevent both hypovolemia and hypervolemia. Dynamic assessments of fluid responsiveness using techniques such as pulse pressure variation (PPV) and stroke volume variation (SVV) can guide fluid management. Recent guidelines emphasize the importance of individualized fluid therapy based on continuous monitoring [7].

The Saline versus Albumin Fluid Evaluation (SAFE) study compared the effects of saline and albumin in ICU patients. Although no significant difference was observed in mortality between the two groups, the trial highlighted that albumin might be beneficial in specific subgroups, such as patients with traumatic brain injury (TBI) [42]. The CRISTAL trial compared the use of crystalloids and colloids in critically ill patients. It found no significant difference in 28-day mortality but suggested that colloids are associated with a lower risk of renal failure and better fluid balance [43]. The choice between crystalloids and colloids should be individualized based on the patient's condition, the clinical scenario, and potential risks.

Continuous monitoring and dynamic assessment of fluid responsiveness are vital for guiding fluid management in neuro ICU patients.

The choice of fluid in critically ill patients ranges from isotonic and balanced to hypertonic fluids. For volume expansion, the guideline offers conditional recommendations as follows: crystalloids are preferred over albumin for critically ill patients in general (moderate certainty of evidence), those with sepsis (moderate certainty of evidence), patients with acute respiratory failure (very low certainty of evidence), and those in the perioperative period or at risk for bleeding (very low certainty of evidence). It also advises using isotonic saline instead of albumin for patients with traumatic brain injury (very low certainty of evidence) and recommends albumin over crystalloids for patients with cirrhosis (very low certainty of evidence). Furthermore, balanced crystalloids are favored over isotonic saline for critically ill patients overall (low certainty of evidence), for those with sepsis (low certainty of evidence), and for patients with kidney injury (very low certainty of evidence). Lastly, the guideline suggests isotonic saline rather than balanced crystalloids for patients with traumatic brain injury (very low certainty of evidence) and recommends isotonic crystalloids over small-volume hypertonic crystalloids for critically ill patients in general (very low certainty of evidence) [44].

11.6 Transfusion Triggers in Neurocritical Care

10. *Controversy: What are the optimal transfusion thresholds for neurocritical care patients to balance the risk of anemia with the potential for transfusion-related complications?*

Current guidelines recommend restrictive transfusion strategies, with a hemoglobin threshold of 7–8 g/dL for most critically ill patients [45]. However, neurocritical care patients may have different requirements due to their unique pathophysiology. Some studies suggest higher thresholds (9–10 g/dL) to ensure adequate cerebral oxygenation, but the evidence is not conclusive. Maintaining adequate hemoglobin levels is crucial for oxygen delivery to the brain. Anemia can exacerbate cerebral hypoxia and increase the risk of secondary brain injury. Conversely, liberal transfusion strategies can increase the chances of complications such as transfusion-related acute lung injury (TRALI) and infections [46].

In SAH, a higher hemoglobin goal may be targeted in order to prevent secondary brain injury. The Neurocritical Care Society recommends transfusion of packed RBC to maintain hemoglobin levels above 8–10 g/dL, especially in the setting of cerebral vasospasm [47]. Conversely, the approach to anemia in spontaneous intracerebral hemorrhage (ICH) is less studied. Anemia in ICH has been associated with larger hematoma sizes, which significantly contribute to mortality. However, patients with ICH are not particularly at risk for delayed cerebral ischemia secondary to vasospasm, potentially justifying a more conservative transfusion threshold. In traumatic brain injury (TBI), the appropriate transfusion threshold is also controversial. Despite limited evidence, general practice often favors a higher hemoglobin goal to ensure adequate cerebral oxygen delivery during the acute phase of trauma [48].

11. *Controversy: How should coagulopathy be managed in neurocritical care patients to balance the risk of bleeding with the potential for thromboembolic events?*

Coagulopathy in neurocritical care can result from various factors, including traumatic brain injury, intracerebral hemorrhage, and the use of anticoagulant medications. The management involves correcting coagulation deficits to prevent bleeding while minimizing the risk of thromboembolic events. This can include the use of anticoagulants, reversal agents, and transfusion products. The balance between preventing bleeding and avoiding thrombosis is particularly challenging in neurocritical care, where both complications can have severe consequences. Ensuring adequate coagulation while preventing excessive clotting requires careful monitoring and individualized treatment strategies [49].

One of the dreaded consequences of oral anticoagulation therapy is intracerebral hemorrhage (ICH). Stroke prevention in atrial fibrillation, thromboembolic disease, and hypercoagulable states is one of the common indications for OAT. The risk of ICH increases with prolonged anticoagulation and higher international normalized ratio (INR) values. Vitamin K is used to promote the replenishment of coagulation factors, but its effects can take up to 24 hours. Intravenous administration is recommended for rapid reversal in life-threatening hemorrhage. Fresh frozen plasma (FFP) and prothrombin complex concentrate (PCC) are commonly used for emergency OAT reversal.

Effective management of coagulopathy in neurocritical care requires rapid reversal of anticoagulation with agents such as vitamin K, FFP, and PCC. Individualized treatment strategies, based on the severity of hemorrhage, underlying conditions, and risk of thromboembolic events, are crucial for optimizing outcomes [50].

12. *Controversy: When and how should platelet transfusions be administered in neurocritical care to manage thrombocytopenia and platelet dysfunction?*

Patients presenting with significant thrombocytopenia during intracerebral hemorrhage (ICH) should receive platelet transfusion according to the American Heart Association guidelines. Decreased platelet counts are associated with hematoma growth, but platelet counts alone do not account for platelet dysfunction due to systemic illness or medication effects. Platelet dysfunction is common in patients with intracranial bleeding, especially those on antiplatelet medications such as aspirin and clopidogrel. Platelet transfusion for antiplatelet reversal is considered to be an investigational treatment, and there is no strong recommendation for the same [51]. However, in clinical practice, we often transfuse platelets to patients presenting with intracranial hemorrhage with a history of antiplatelet use [52].

The PATCH trial investigated platelet transfusion in patients with spontaneous ICH on antiplatelet therapy, showing no significant improvement in outcomes and suggesting potential harm, leading to cautious use of platelet transfusion in this setting [53].

Platelet transfusion should be considered in patients with ICH and significant thrombocytopenia or platelet dysfunction, particularly those with a history of antiplatelet use. Individualized treatment strategies, based on continuous monitoring and platelet function assays, are essential to balance the risks and benefits of transfusion.

11.7 Inotropes and Vasopressors in Neuro ICU

The use of inotropes and vasopressors in the Neuro ICU is critical for managing patients with hemodynamic instability. These agents are essential for maintaining adequate cerebral perfusion and systemic blood pressure in neurocritical care patients. This section explores the controversies, evidence, and clinical trials related to the use of inotropes and vasopressors in the Neuro ICU.

13. *Controversy: What is the most appropriate vasopressor or inotrope for managing hypotension in neurocritical care patients, considering their effects on cerebral perfusion and ICP?*

Norepinephrine is often preferred due to its balanced α- and β-adrenergic effects, which increase both mean arterial pressure (MAP) and cerebral perfusion pressure (CPP) without significantly raising heart rate. Phenylephrine, with its pure α-adrenergic activity, is another option, but it may reduce cardiac output and worsen cerebral perfusion in some patients [54].

The use of dopamine has declined due to concerns about its arrhythmogenic potential and inconsistent effects on cerebral perfusion. While dopamine can increase cardiac output, it may also raise ICP and exacerbate cerebral edema, making it less favorable in neurocritical care [55]. Epinephrine has strong β-adrenergic effects that can increase heart rate and cardiac output, but its use is often limited by the potential for tachyarrhythmias and increased myocardial oxygen demand. Its role in neurocritical care is less defined compared to norepinephrine. This trial compared the effects of norepinephrine and phenylephrine on cerebral perfusion and ICP in patients with TBI. It found that norepinephrine improved CPP without significantly increasing ICP, while phenylephrine was associated with reduced cardiac output and variable effects on CPP [56]. Norepinephrine is generally favored in neurocritical care due to its balanced hemodynamic effects. However, the choice of vasopressor or inotrope should be individualized based on the patient's hemodynamic profile, underlying condition, and response to therapy. Continuous monitoring of hemodynamic parameters, including CPP and ICP, is essential to guide the choice and dosing of these agents [12].

14. *Controversy: How do vasopressors and inotropes affect cerebral perfusion and intracranial pressure in different neurocritical conditions?*

In AIS, maintaining adequate cerebral perfusion is crucial to support the ischemic penumbra. Norepinephrine is often used to increase systemic blood pressure and CPP, but careful titration is required to avoid excessive hypertension and the risk of hemorrhagic transformation [14]. In ICH, the goal is to prevent hematoma expansion while maintaining cerebral perfusion. Vasopressors like norepinephrine are used to achieve target BP levels, with studies suggesting a systolic BP target of less than 140 mmHg to reduce the risk of rebleeding while ensuring adequate CPP [20]. SAH management often involves preventing and treating cerebral vasospasm. Vasopressors are used to maintain high-normal BP and CPP to prevent delayed cerebral ischemia. However, excessive use of vasopressors often results in problems such as myocardial ischemia and pulmonary edema [22].

The effects of vasopressors and inotropes on cerebral perfusion and ICP vary across different neurocritical conditions. Norepinephrine is commonly preferred for its balanced hemodynamic profile, but individualized therapy based on continuous monitoring and specific patient needs is essential to optimize outcomes [56].

11.8 Advanced Hemodynamic Management Techniques and Emerging Therapies in Neuro ICU

15. *Controversy: Should CPP targets be individualized to optimize cerebral perfusion in patients with traumatic brain injury (TBI)?*

The concept of CPPopt involves tailoring CPP targets based on real-time assessments of cerebrovascular autoregulation. The pressure reactivity index (PRx) is used to determine the optimal CPP range for individual patients. Studies have shown that maintaining CPP within the PRx-determined optimal range can reduce secondary brain injury and improve outcomes in TBI patients. Studies demonstrated that using PRx to determine optimal CPP targets led to better neurological outcomes in TBI patients, highlighting the benefits of individualized CPP management [57].

16. *Controversy: Should hemodynamic management in SAH prioritize pressure targets or flow targets to prevent delayed cerebral ischemia?*

Traditionally, managing SAH has focused on maintaining high-normal blood pressure to prevent vasospasm and delayed cerebral ischemia. However, recent evidence suggests that focusing on cerebral blood flow (CBF) targets may be more effective. Advanced monitoring techniques, such as transcranial Doppler ultrasonography and cerebral perfusion imaging, can help guide therapy based on flow rather than pressure alone [58].

This study compared pressure-targeted versus flow-targeted management in SAH patients, finding that flow-targeted management led to better outcomes in terms of preventing delayed cerebral ischemia [59, 60].

17. *Controversy: What is the role of milrinone in managing cerebral vasospasm and improving outcomes in neurocritical care patients?*

Milrinone, a phosphodiesterase inhibitor with inotropic and vasodilatory effects, has been studied for its potential to manage cerebral vasospasm, particularly in SAH patients. It improves CBF by reducing vasospasm and enhancing cardiac output. However, its use requires careful monitoring due to potential side effects such as hypotension and arrhythmias. Studies have investigated the use of milrinone in SAH patients with cerebral vasospasm, showing that it effectively improved CBF and reduced the incidence of delayed cerebral ischemia [61].

18. *Controversy: Is ECMO beneficial in managing severe neurocritical conditions, and what are the indications and outcomes of its use in the Neuro ICU?*

ECMO provides temporary cardiac and respiratory support in patients with severe cardiopulmonary failure. Its use in neurocritical care is emerging, particularly for patients with severe traumatic brain injury, stroke, or cardiac arrest who develop refractory cardiopulmonary failure. ECMO can stabilize patients hemodynamically, allowing for better cerebral perfusion and potential neurological recovery. There is a lack of practice guidelines or management strategies specifically addressing neurocritical care for patients on ECMO. These patients face significant risks, including hypoxic-ischemic brain injury, intracranial hemorrhage, cerebral edema, and brain death. Enhancing clinical outcomes hinges on a clearer definition of the neurologic complications and the underlying pathophysiology associated with ECMO [62].

19. *Controversy: What are the best practices for hemodynamic management in brain-dead patients to optimize organ perfusion for transplantation?*

Brain death leads to significant hemodynamic instability due to the loss of autonomic regulation, causing hypotension, arrhythmias, and hormonal imbalances. Managing these hemodynamic changes is critical to maintain organ viability for transplantation. Strategies include the use of vasopressors to maintain blood pressure, hormonal therapy (e.g., thyroid hormone, corticosteroids, vasopressin) to stabilize the endocrine environment, and optimizing fluid management to prevent hypovolemia. Studies have investigated various hemodynamic management protocols in brain-dead patients, showing that a combination of vasopressors, hormonal therapy, and careful fluid management significantly improved organ preservation and transplantation outcomes [63].

11.9 Conclusion

In neurocritical care, the utilization of advanced hemodynamic management techniques and emerging therapies is crucial for optimizing patient outcomes. Techniques such as intracranial pressure monitoring, cerebral perfusion pressure optimization, cerebral blood flow assessment, cerebral oxygenation monitoring, and cerebral metabolism analysis are fundamental in providing a comprehensive understanding of a patient's physiological status.

Multimodal neuromonitoring techniques, when integrated effectively, allow for a personalized approach to the complex challenges presented by neurocritical conditions. Real-time data from these monitoring tools enables practitioners to tailor treatments precisely to the individual needs of each patient, enhancing the precision and efficacy of care.

References

1. Prabhakar H, Sandhu K, Bhagat H, Durga P, Chawla R. Current concepts of optimal cerebral perfusion pressure in traumatic brain injury. J Anaesthesiol Clin Pharmacol. 2014;30(3):318–27.
2. Steiner LA, Andrews PJD. Monitoring the injured brain: ICP and CBF. Br J Anaesth. 2006;97(1):26–38.
3. Smith M. Cerebral perfusion pressure. Br J Anaesth. 2015;115(4):488–90.
4. Dietvorst S, Depreitere B, Meyfroidt G. Beyond intracranial pressure: monitoring cerebral perfusion and autoregulation in severe traumatic brain injury. Curr Opin Crit Care. 2023;29(2):85–8.
5. Bernard F. Neurotrauma and intracranial pressure management. Crit Care Clin. 2023;39(1):103–21.
6. Carney N, Totten AM, O'Reilly C, Ullman JS, Hawryluk GWJ, Bell MJ, et al. Guidelines for the management of severe traumatic brain injury. Fourth Edition Neurosurgery. 2017;80(1):6–15.
7. Pinsky MR, Cecconi M, Chew MS, De Backer D, Douglas I, Edwards M, et al. Effective hemodynamic monitoring. Crit Care. 2022;26(1):294.
8. Rajagopalan S, Sarwal A. Neuromonitoring in critically ill patients. Crit Care Med. 2023;51(4):525–42.
9. Chesnut R, Aguilera S, Buki A, Bulger E, Citerio G, Cooper DJ, et al. A management algorithm for adult patients with both brain oxygen and intracranial pressure monitoring: the Seattle international severe traumatic brain injury consensus conference (SIBICC). Intensive Care Med. 2020;46(5):919–29.
10. Le Roux P, Menon DK, Citerio G, Vespa P, Bader MK, Brophy G, et al. The international multidisciplinary consensus conference on multimodality monitoring in Neurocritical care: evidentiary tables: a statement for healthcare professionals from the Neurocritical care society and the European Society of Intensive Care Medicine. Neurocrit Care. 2014;21(S2):297–361.
11. Vitt JR, Loper NE, Mainali S. Multimodal and autoregulation monitoring in the neurointensive care unit. Front Neurol. 2023;14:1155986.
12. Sivakumar S, Taccone FS, Rehman M, Hinson H, Naval N, Lazaridis C. Hemodynamic and neuro-monitoring for neurocritically ill patients: an international survey of intensivists. J Crit Care. 2017;39:40–7.
13. Meyfroidt G, Baguley IJ, Menon DK. Paroxysmal sympathetic hyperactivity: the storm after acute brain injury. Lancet Neurol. 2017;16(9):721–9.
14. Powers WJ, Rabinstein AA, Ackerson T, Adeoye OM, Bambakidis NC, Becker K, et al. Guidelines for the early Management of Patients with acute ischemic stroke: 2019 update

to the 2018 guidelines for the early Management of Acute Ischemic Stroke: a guideline for healthcare professionals from the American Heart Association/American Stroke Association. Stroke. 2019;50(12):e344–418.
15. Anderson CS, Huang Y, Lindley RI, Chen X, Arima H, Chen G, et al. Intensive blood pressure reduction with intravenous thrombolysis therapy for acute ischaemic stroke (ENCHANTED): an international, randomised, open-label, blinded-endpoint, phase 3 trial. Lancet. 2019;393(10174):877–88.
16. Gąsecki D, Kwarciany M, Kowalczyk K, Narkiewicz K, Karaszewski B. Blood pressure management in acute ischemic stroke. Curr Hypertens Rep. 2021;23(1):3.
17. Qureshi AI, Palesch YY, Barsan WG, Hanley DF, Hsu CY, Martin RL, et al. Intensive blood-pressure lowering in patients with acute cerebral Hemorrhage. N Engl J Med. 2016;375(11):1033–43.
18. Anderson CS, Heeley E, Huang Y, Wang J, Stapf C, Delcourt C, et al. Rapid blood-pressure lowering in patients with acute intracerebral hemorrhage. N Engl J Med. 2013;368(25):2355–65.
19. Qureshi AI, Palesch YY, Foster LD, Barsan WG, Goldstein JN, Hanley DF, et al. Blood pressure-attained analysis of ATACH 2 trial. Stroke. 2018;49(6):1412–8.
20. Moullaali TJ, Wang X, Sandset EC, Woodhouse LJ, Law ZK, Arima H, et al. Early lowering of blood pressure after acute intracerebral haemorrhage: a systematic review and meta-analysis of individual patient data. J Neurol Neurosurg Psychiatry. 2022;93(1):6–13.
21. Connolly ES, Rabinstein AA, Carhuapoma JR, Derdeyn CP, Dion J, Higashida RT, et al. Guidelines for the management of aneurysmal subarachnoid hemorrhage: a guideline for healthcare professionals from the American Heart Association/American Stroke Association. Stroke. 2012;43(6):1711–37.
22. Hoh BL, Ko NU, Amin-Hanjani S, Chou SHY, Cruz-Flores S, Dangayach NS, et al. Guideline for the management of patients with aneurysmal subarachnoid hemorrhage: a guideline from the American Heart Association/American Stroke Association. Stroke [Internet]. 2023, 2023 Jul;54(7) [cited 2024 Jul 29]. Available from: https://www.ahajournals.org/doi/10.1161/STR.0000000000000436
23. Toth P, Szarka N, Farkas E, Ezer E, Czeiter E, Amrein K, et al. Traumatic brain injury-induced autoregulatory dysfunction and spreading depression-related neurovascular uncoupling: Pathomechanisms, perspectives, and therapeutic implications. Am J Physiol-Heart Circ Physiol. 2016;311(5):H1118–31.
24. Fehlings MG, Tetreault LA, Wilson JR, Kwon BK, Burns AS, Martin AR, et al. A clinical practice guideline for the management of acute spinal cord injury: introduction, rationale, and scope. Glob Spine J. 2017;7(3 Suppl):84S–94S.
25. Ryken TC, Hurlbert RJ, Hadley MN, Aarabi B, Dhall SS, Gelb DE, et al. The acute cardiopulmonary management of patients with cervical spinal cord injuries. Neurosurgery. 2013;72(suppl 2):84–92.
26. Saadeh YS, Smith BW, Joseph JR, Jaffer SY, Buckingham MJ, Oppenlander ME, et al. The impact of blood pressure management after spinal cord injury: a systematic review of the literature. Neurosurg Focus. 2017;43(5):E20.
27. Evaniew N, Davies B, Farahbakhsh F, Fehlings MG, Ganau M, Graves D, et al. Interventions to optimize spinal cord perfusion in patients with acute traumatic spinal cord injury: an updated systematic review. Glob Spine J. 2024;14(3_suppl):58S–79S.
28. Vincent JL, Rhodes A, Perel A, Martin GS, Rocca G, Vallet B, et al. Clinical review: update on hemodynamic monitoring – a consensus of 16. Crit Care. 2011;15(4):229.
29. Cecconi M, De Backer D, Antonelli M, Beale R, Bakker J, Hofer C, et al. Consensus on circulatory shock and hemodynamic monitoring. Task force of the European Society of Intensive Care Medicine. Intensive Care Med. 2014;40(12):1795–815.
30. Monnet X, Teboul JL. Transpulmonary thermodilution: advantages and limits. Crit Care. 2017;21(1):147.
31. Saugel B, Kouz K, Scheeren TWL, Greiwe G, Hoppe P, Romagnoli S, et al. Cardiac output estimation using pulse wave analysis-physiology, algorithms, and technologies: a narrative review. Br J Anaesth. 2021;126(1):67–76.

32. Kok B, Wolthuis D, Bosch F, Van Der Hoeven H, Blans M. POCUS in dyspnea, nontraumatic hypotension, and shock; a systematic review of existing evidence. Eur J Intern Med. 2022;106:9–38.
33. Deimantavicius M, Chaleckas E, Boere K, Putnynaite V, Tamosuitis T, Tamasauskas A, et al. Feasibility of the optimal cerebral perfusion pressure value identification without a delay that is too long. Sci Rep. 2022;12(1):17724.
34. Huygh J, Peeters Y, Bernards J, Malbrain MLNG. Hemodynamic monitoring in the critically ill: an overview of current cardiac output monitoring methods. F1000Res. 2016;5:2855.
35. Zeiler FA, Ercole A, Beqiri E, Cabeleira M, Thelin EP, Stocchetti N, et al. Association between cerebrovascular reactivity monitoring and mortality is preserved when adjusting for baseline admission characteristics in adult traumatic brain injury: a CENTER-TBI study. J Neurotrauma. 2020;37(10):1233–41.
36. Mathur R, Meyfroidt G, Robba C, Stevens RD. Neuromonitoring in the ICU – what, how and why? Curr Opin Crit Care. 2024;30(2):99–105.
37. Nordström CH. Cerebral energy metabolism and microdialysis in neurocritical care. Childs Nerv Syst. 2010;26(4):465–72.
38. Dunn JOC, Grocott MP, Mythen MMG. The place of goal-directed haemodynamic therapy in the 21st century. BJA Educ. 2016;16(6):179–85.
39. Le Guen M, Le Gall-Salaun A, Josserand J, Gaudin De Vilaine A, Viquesnel S, Muller D, et al. Goal-directed fluid therapy and major postoperative complications in elective craniotomy. A retrospective analysis of a before-after multicentric study. BMC Anesthesiol. 2023;23(1):11.
40. Rivers E, Nguyen B, Havstad S, Ressler J, Muzzin A, Knoblich B, et al. Early goal-directed therapy in the treatment of severe sepsis and septic shock. N Engl J Med. 2001;345(19):1368–77.
41. Lewis SR, Pritchard MW, Evans DJ, Butler AR, Alderson P, Smith AF, et al. Colloids versus crystalloids for fluid resuscitation in critically ill people. Cochrane Database Syst Rev. 2018;8(8):CD000567.
42. SAFE Study Investigators, Australian and New Zealand Intensive Care Society Clinical Trials Group, Australian Red Cross Blood Service, George Institute for International Health, Myburgh J, Cooper DJ, et al. Saline or albumin for fluid resuscitation in patients with traumatic brain injury. N Engl J Med. 2007;357(9):874–84.
43. Annane D, Siami S, Jaber S, Martin C, Elatrous S, Declère AD, et al. Effects of fluid resuscitation with colloids vs crystalloids on mortality in critically ill patients presenting with hypovolemic shock: the CRISTAL randomized trial. JAMA. 2013;310(17):1809–17.
44. Arabi YM, Belley-Cote E, Carsetti A, De Backer D, Donadello K, Juffermans NP, et al. European society of intensive care medicine clinical practice guideline on fluid therapy in adult critically ill patients. Part 1: the choice of resuscitation fluids. Intensive Care Med. 2024;50(6):813–31.
45. Carson JL, Stanworth SJ, Dennis JA, Trivella M, Roubinian N, Fergusson DA, et al. Transfusion thresholds for guiding red blood cell transfusion. Cochrane Database Syst Rev. 2021;12(12):CD002042.
46. Yu Y, Fu Y, Li W, Sun T, Cheng C, Chong Y, et al. Red blood cell transfusion in neurocritical patients: a systematic review and meta-analysis. BMC Anesthesiol. 2024;24(1):106.
47. Terrett LA, McIntyre L, Turgeon AF, English SW. Anemia and red blood cell transfusion in aneurysmal subarachnoid hemorrhage. Neurocrit Care. 2023;39(1):91–103.
48. Vanhala H, Junttila E, Kataja A, Huhtala H, Luostarinen T, Luoto T. Incidence and associated factors of Anemia in patients with acute moderate and severe traumatic brain injury. Neurocrit Care. 2022;37(3):629–37.
49. Helms J, Iba T, Connors JM, Gando S, Levi M, Meziani F, et al. How to manage coagulopathies in critically ill patients. Intensive Care Med. 2023;49(3):273–90.
50. Frontera JA, Lewin JJ, Rabinstein AA, Aisiku IP, Alexandrov AW, Cook AM, et al. Guideline for reversal of Antithrombotics in intracranial Hemorrhage: a statement for healthcare professionals from the Neurocritical care society and society of critical care medicine. Neurocrit Care. 2016;24(1):6–46.

51. Nagalla S, Sarode R. Role of platelet transfusion in the reversal of anti-platelet therapy. Transfus Med Rev. 2019;33(2):92–7.
52. Naidech AM, Liebling SM, Rosenberg NF, Lindholm PF, Bernstein RA, Batjer HH, et al. Early platelet transfusion improves platelet activity and may improve outcomes after intracerebral hemorrhage. Neurocrit Care. 2012;16(1):82–7.
53. Baharoglu MI, Cordonnier C, Al-Shahi Salman R, de Gans K, Koopman MM, Brand A, et al. Platelet transfusion versus standard care after acute stroke due to spontaneous cerebral haemorrhage associated with antiplatelet therapy (PATCH): a randomised, open-label, phase 3 trial. Lancet Lond Engl. 2016;387(10038):2605–13.
54. Bangash MN, Kong ML, Pearse RM. Use of inotropes and vasopressor agents in critically ill patients. Br J Pharmacol. 2012;165(7):2015–33.
55. Johnston AJ, Steiner LA, Chatfield DA, Coles JP, Hutchinson PJ, Al-Rawi PG, et al. Effect of cerebral perfusion pressure augmentation with dopamine and norepinephrine on global and focal brain oxygenation after traumatic brain injury. Intensive Care Med. 2004;30(5):791–7.
56. Salvagno M, Geraldini F, Coppalini G, Robba C, Gouvea Bogossian E, Annoni F, et al. The impact of inotropes and vasopressors on cerebral oxygenation in patients with traumatic brain injury and subarachnoid hemorrhage: a narrative review. Brain Sci. 2024;14(2):117.
57. Kramer AH, Couillard PL, Zygun DA, Aries MJ, Gallagher CN. Continuous assessment of "optimal" cerebral perfusion pressure in traumatic brain injury: a cohort study of feasibility, reliability, and relation to outcome. Neurocrit Care. 2019;30(1):51–61.
58. Bijlenga P, Czosnyka M, Budohoski KP, Soehle M, Pickard JD, Kirkpatrick PJ, et al. "Optimal cerebral perfusion pressure" in poor grade patients after subarachnoid Hemorrhage. Neurocrit Care. 2010;13(1):17–23.
59. Deem S, Diringer M, Livesay S, Treggiari MM. Hemodynamic management in the prevention and treatment of delayed cerebral ischemia after aneurysmal subarachnoid Hemorrhage. Neurocrit Care. 2023;39(1):81–90.
60. Kim DH, Joseph M, Ziadi S, Nates J, Dannenbaum M, Malkoff M. Increases in cardiac output can reverse flow deficits from vasospasm independent of blood pressure: a study using xenon computed tomographic measurement of cerebral blood flow. Neurosurgery. 2003;53(5):1044–52.
61. Lakhal K, Hivert A, Alexandre PL, Fresco M, Robert-Edan V, Rodie-Talbere PA, et al. Intravenous milrinone for cerebral vasospasm in subarachnoid hemorrhage: the MILRISPASM controlled before–after study. Neurocrit Care. 2021;35(3):669–79.
62. Cho SM, Farrokh S, Whitman G, Bleck TP, Geocadin RG. Neurocritical care for extracorporeal membrane oxygenation patients. Crit Care Med. 2019;47(12):1773–81.
63. Lazzeri C, Bonizzoli M, Guetti C, Fulceri GE, Peris A. Hemodynamic management in brain dead donors. World J Transplant. 2021;11(10):410–20.

Fluid Management in Neurocritical Care 12

S. Rakulprasath, Sonia Bansal, and Sriganesh Kamath

Abstract

Fluid management in the neurocritical care unit (NCCU) requires careful consideration of the cerebral physiology and implications in acute brain injury conditions. Crystalloids are recommended as the preferred fluid, and using colloids, glucose-containing solutions, other hypotonic solutions, or albumin for maintenance or resuscitation is discouraged in the setting of acute brain injury in the NCCU. Avoiding both hypovolemia and hypervolemia and targeting normovolemia are beneficial and, therefore, suggested. Monitoring with multiple hemodynamic variables, invasive blood pressure, and fluid balance is recommended during fluid management in the NCCU. Fluid therapy may require alterations in specific conditions of sodium and water disturbances, such as cerebral salt wasting, syndrome of inappropriate anti-diuretic hormone secretion, and diabetes insipidus. Osmotherapy is commonly employed after acute brain injury to reduce intracranial pressure and improve cerebral perfusion and oxygenation. The clinical condition should determine the choice of the hyperosmolar agent rather than drug characteristics, as both are equivalent in terms of effectiveness in reducing intracranial pressure and improving neurological outcomes and side-effect profiles.

Keywords

Goal-directed therapy · Hyponatremia · Osmotherapy · Sodium-water imbalance Intravenous fluids

S. Rakulprasath · S. Bansal · S. Kamath (✉)
Department of Neuroanaesthesia and Neurocritical Care, National Institute of Mental Health and Neurosciences, Bengaluru, Karnataka, India

P. U. Bidkar, M. Krishnakumar (eds.), *Controversies in Neurocritical Care*,
https://doi.org/10.1007/978-981-95-4419-6_12

12.1 Introduction

Administration of intravenous fluids such as crystalloids, colloids, hyperosmotic agents, and albumin is common in the intensive care unit (ICU). They help to maintain organ function and hemodynamic homeostasis. Movement of water from the intravascular to the interstitial compartment can lead to fluid accumulation, with hydrostatic and osmotic pressures governing water transport across capillary membranes.

Fluid therapy in the neurocritical care unit (NCCU) is important as the volume status determines the perfusion, substrate delivery and oxygenation of the brain. The brain and the spinal cord are normally separated from the intravascular compartment by the blood–brain barrier (BBB), which comprises endothelial cells with tight junctions. These tight junctions prevent the diffusion of even small molecules/ions between the intravascular space and the brain. Therefore, the osmolarity determines the movement of water molecules across the intact BBB. However, if the BBB is compromised, secondary to trauma or other pathologies, it becomes permeable to a variety of molecules. Figure 12.1 depicts the structure of the BBB and the blood–cerebrospinal fluid barrier.

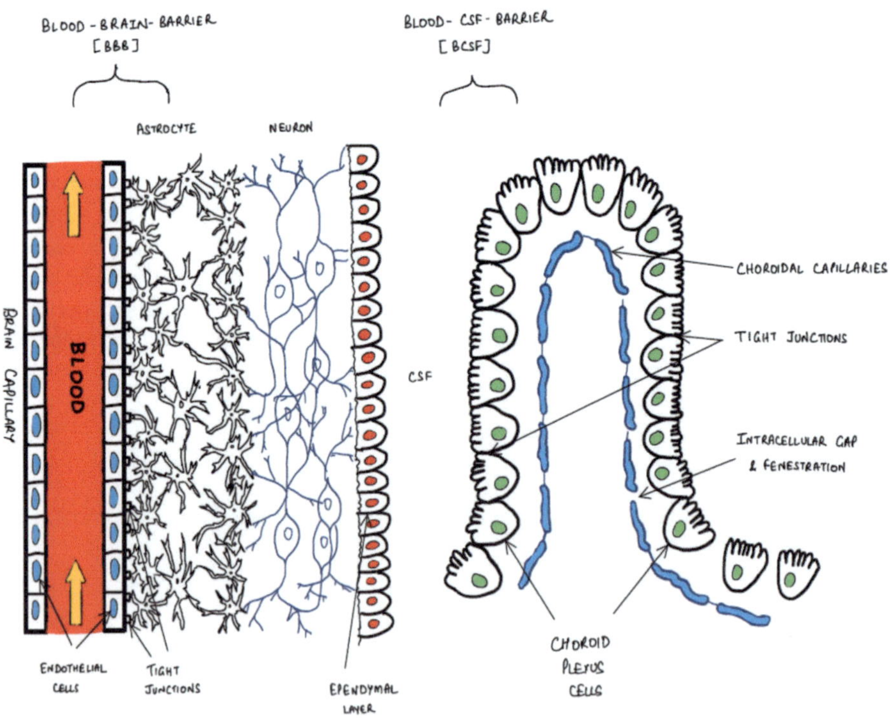

Fig. 12.1 Structure of the BBB and Blood-cerebrospinal fluid barrier

Fluid management in NCCU is more challenging than in a general ICU because tools for monitoring cerebral physiological endpoints of cerebral blood flow (CBF) and cerebral oxygenation are less rigorously implemented than hemodynamic monitoring to guide fluid therapy in routine clinical practice.

12.2 Fluid Balance in NCCU

Fluid therapy in NCCU should aim to maintain CBF and cerebral perfusion pressure (CPP) and reduce intracranial pressure (ICP) and cerebral blood volume (CBV). Maintaining the fluid balance is important as the hypovolemic state can lead to decreased oxygen delivery, and in patients with acute brain injury (ABI), it can lead to secondary injuries. Parameters to guide the assessment of volume status include hemodynamic indicators such as central venous pressure (CVP), stroke volume variation (SVV), and pulse pressure variation (PPV); laboratory markers such as blood urea, hemoglobin, and lactate levels; ultrasonography for evaluation of inferior vena cava distensibility, chest X-ray, etc. Goal-directed therapy (GDT) using cardiac index (CI) or cardiac output (CO) is advocated as it reduces the incidence of complications and length of hospital stay [1]. Conversely, hypervolemia can also have detrimental effects, and patients may require de-resuscitation to restore fluid balance. The negative fluid balance may have beneficial effects in patients with capillary leaks. A restrictive fluid approach is associated with a lower incidence of hypoxemia in aneurysmal subarachnoid hemorrhage (aSAH) on days 3 and 7 without any detrimental effect on renal function or vasospasm [2]. Maintaining euvolemia is the preferred approach while managing patients with ABI. Figure 12.2 depicts the effects of fluid intake on the occurrence of secondary brain insults.

High-quality evidence to guide fluid therapy in NCCU is absent. In this section, we will discuss the evidence about fluid management in the common NCCU diagnoses of traumatic brain injury (TBI), aSAH, acute ischemic stroke (AIS), and intracerebral hemorrhage (ICH).

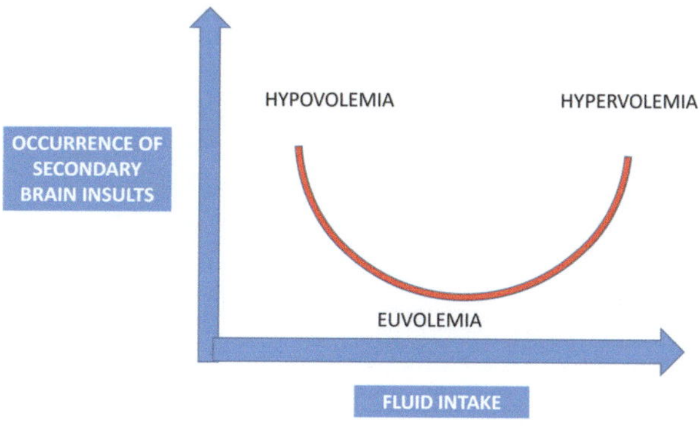

Fig. 12.2 Effects of fluid intake on the occurrence of secondary brain insults

Patients with TBI have compromised cerebral perfusion as a result of cytotoxic and vasogenic edema, vasospasm, and impaired autoregulation. However, substantial variation in the practice of fluid management exists in patients with TBI [3]. Maintaining a neutral balance and avoiding hypervolemia improves outcomes after TBI [4]. The Brain Trauma Foundation (BTF) guidelines do not provide any recommendations on fluid therapy in patients with TBI. However, it recommends maintaining a CPP of 60–70 mmHg for achieving favorable outcomes and suggests against a CPP >70 mmHg with fluids and vasopressors, as it increases the risk of acute respiratory distress syndrome (ARDS) [5]. The Lund concept also proposes avoiding positive fluid balance by administering albumin to maintain colloid osmotic pressure and intravascular volume in patients with severe TBI [6].

In patients with aSAH, the main cause of poor outcomes is delayed cerebral ischemia (DCI), and intravascular volume depletion can worsen the DCI. Conversely, positive fluid balance is associated with a higher probability of developing vasospasm and longer hospital stays, with no differences in mortality or new stroke occurrence in the NCCU [7]. The triple-H therapy does not decrease DCI or increase global end-diastolic volume index (GEDVI), and CO [8]. A positive fluid balance leads to poor functional outcomes on the modified Rankin scale (mRS) and cerebral infarction on imaging [9]. These studies do not mention whether colloids were used to achieve hypervolemia. Other studies have also observed complications of DCI, pulmonary edema, and poor functional outcomes with high fluid input in poor-grade aSAH [10]. Thus, hypervolemia has no benefit in patients with aSAH. No difference in the global CBF or CBV is seen between patients receiving hypervolemia and normovolemia [11]. The current literature also does not support volume expansion therapy in patients with aSAH [12]. The GEDVI is different between patients with and without DCI. The threshold value of GEDVI that best correlates with DCI is <822 mL/m^2, and it has a positive correlation with extravascular lung water and the occurrence of pulmonary edema [13]. Additionally, CI and systemic vascular resistance index during the third to sixth day of aSAH are independently associated with the onset of DCI [14]. However, GDT may be useful only in poor-grade aSAH to improve clinical outcomes [15]. While hypertension increases regional CBF and oxygenation, hypervolemia only slightly increases the CBF with negative effects on oxygenation, questioning the usefulness of triple-H therapy [16]. Infusion of 23.5% hypertonic saline (HTS) augments CBF, CPP, cerebral oxygenation, and metabolic status in patients with poor-grade aSAH [17]. However, expansion of intravascular volume using 5% albumin does not increase the CBF [18].

In patients with AIS, a positive fluid balance of >1650 ml is associated with the development of malignant cerebral edema [19]. Similarly, volume expansion with crystalloids or colloids is associated with decreased odds of favorable outcomes in patients with AIS [20]. Therefore, both hypovolemia and hypervolemia should be avoided in TBI, aSAH, and AIS.

12.3 Type of Fluids

Brain volume regulation in response to changes in osmolarity is critical in the fluid management of patients with intact or disrupted BBB. Table 12.1 depicts the characteristics of the commonly used fluids in the NCCU. Hypotonic and glucose-containing fluids lower the serum osmolarity and contribute to poor outcomes in neurological patients.

In patients with isolated TBI, there is minimal loss of extracellular fluid (ECF). In polytrauma, fluid resuscitation is often needed and can be achieved with 0.9% saline. Balanced salt solutions (BSS) may be associated with better outcomes due to the decreased incidence of hyperchloremia and metabolic acidosis [21, 22]. However, few studies have reported no difference in mortality or acute kidney injury (AKI) between patients receiving saline or BSS [23, 24]. The saline versus albumin fluid evaluation trial (SAFE) study observed higher mortality in TBI patients receiving low-dose albumin compared to patients receiving saline [25]. The findings of this study should be interpreted with caution, as the relative hypotonicity of the 4% albumin solution used or albumin leakage via disrupted BBB could have led to increased cerebral edema. Hypoalbuminemia is correlated with poor outcomes in patients with TBI and stroke [26, 27]. There are studies which support as well as refute improved outcomes with albumin administration [28–30].

In a multicenter randomized clinical trial (RCT) comparing 25% albumin with isotonic saline for 90-day outcomes (mRS/National Institute of Health Stroke Scale [NIHSS]) in patients with AIS (NIHSS >6), no benefit was observed with albumin [31]. Treatment with 25% albumin also increases the risk of pulmonary edema and ICH [32].

Table 12.1 Characteristics of the commonly used fluids

	0.9% Saline	Lactated ringer	Plasmalyte A	DNS	Plasma
Sodium	154	130	140	154	134–145
Potassium		4	5		3.4–5
Chloride	154	109	98	154	98–108
Calcium		2.7			2.25–2.65
Bicarbonate			27 (acetate) 23 (gluconate)		22–32
Lactate		28			
Magnesium			3		0.7–1.1
Dextrose (g/100 ml)				5	
Osmolarity	308	273	294	586	280–295

In patients with aSAH, albumin infusion is associated with better clinical outcomes at 3 months [33]. Albumin at 1.25 g/kg for 7 days is well-tolerated with neuroprotective effects [34]. Infusing isotonic, isoncotic albumin during the initial 5 days of NCCU stay after aSAH reduces the incidence of DCI and hyponatremia and lowers the volume of fluid administration [35]. No difference is noted between patients with aSAH receiving colloids versus crystalloids with respect to delayed ischemic neurological deficit (DIND) or the presence or size of delayed infarcts. However, colloid administration and a positive fluid balance result in poor neurological outcomes on NIHSS and mRS assessments [36]. Colloid fluids (4% gelatin or 6% pentastarch) are associated with poor Glasgow Outcome Scale (GOS) scores at 6 months, while crystalloids reduce the unfavorable outcomes in aSAH [37]. The risk of AKI is also likely with colloids. In an RCT, the saline-based crystalloid-colloid fluid group had a higher incidence of hyperchloremia, hyperosmolality, and positive fluid balance than those who received a BSS-based crystalloid-colloid fluid regimen [38]. Therefore, euvolemia with crystalloids appears to be the appropriate approach for now. Pentastarch administration did not increase mortality in patients with severe TBI [39]. However, this study did not evaluate neurological outcomes or survival rates based on the fluid used.

The European Society of Intensive Care Medicine (ESICM) recommends crystalloids as the preferred fluid and recommends against using colloids, glucose-containing solutions, other hypotonic solutions, or albumin for fluid maintenance or resuscitation in NCCU. The use of high-dose albumin in AIS patients is also not recommended. Targeting normovolemia is suggested. Monitoring multiple hemodynamic variables (and not CVP alone), invasive blood pressure, and fluid balance is recommended to optimize fluid therapy [40]. Overall, there is variability in the practice of fluid therapy, hemodynamic management protocols, and targets embraced while managing patients with cerebrovascular pathology [41]. Routine fluid management is likely to affect outcomes. However, literature regarding fluid therapy is predominantly in patients with aSAH, TBI, and stroke and is scarce in other pathologies in NCCU.

12.4 Hyponatremia in NCCU: Incidence and Causes

Hyponatremia, defined as a serum sodium concentration of <135 mmol/l, is reported in about 50% of critically ill neurological patients [42]. Among the ABI conditions, TBI and aSAH are those with the highest incidence of hyponatremia [43, 44].

Hyponatremia occurs more commonly in high-grade aSAH, especially involving anterior circulation aneurysms and in the presence of hydrocephalus. Cerebral Salt Wasting (CSW) accounts for 22.9%, while the syndrome of inappropriate antidiuretic hormone (SIADH) contributes to 35.4% of hyponatremia [45, 46]. Hyponatremia is associated with the development of cerebral vasospasm [47]. The time to sodium nadir is 9–34 hours of admission after TBI and about 80 hours after aSAH. The time to enter into the cerebral vasospasm window after aSAH mirrors the time to sodium nadir, supporting that some of the pathophysiology of aSAH may contribute to hyponatremia and vice versa [48, 49].

Dysfunction of the hypothalamic-hypophyseal-adrenal axis is noted in TBI, resulting in hyponatremia incidence of 15–68%. SIADH is seen in one-third of TBI patients, predominantly after subdural hematoma and focal contusions, and often manifests during the second week of NCCU admission [50]. Hyponatremia in TBI may also occur after administration of mannitol for ICP control secondary to osmotic diuresis and with carbamazepine and desmopressin used for treating central diabetes insipidus (DI) [51].

Hyponatremia occurs in about 11.6% of patients with the first episode of AIS and results in poor outcomes, including the development of seizures and urinary tract infections [52].

Trans-sphenoidal surgery has also been associated with hyponatremia, manifesting between the fifth and ninth postoperative days with peaking on the seventh day. Such hyponatremia may be early (secondary to axonal degeneration and release of antidiuretic hormone (ADH)) or late (secondary to adrenal insufficiency) [8].

12.5 Management of Hyponatremia

Treatment of hyponatremia in NCCU requires identification of the following: (1) severity of hyponatremia, (2) duration (acute or chronic), (3) patient volume status, and (4) severity of the clinical condition. Figure 12.3 provides an overview of hyponatremia treatment.

Accurate assessment of volume status is important in hyponatremia management. Hypovolemic patients respond better to volume expansion; euvolemic hyponatremia is usually managed with fluid restriction, and hypervolemic patients may

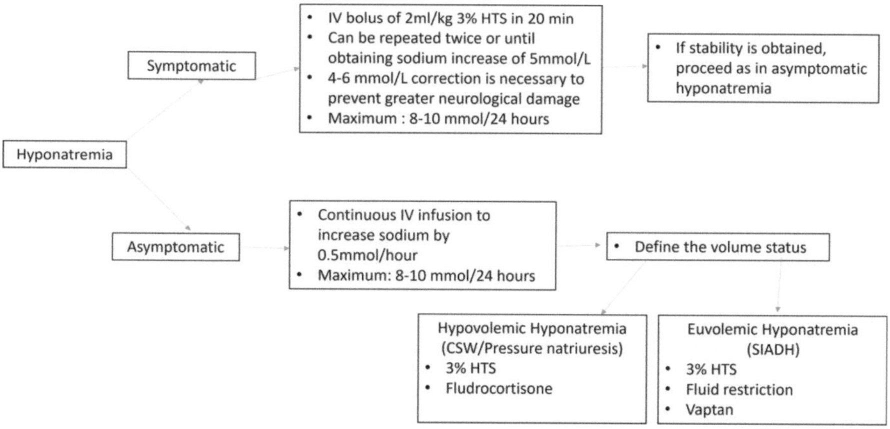

Fig. 12.3 Overview of hyponatremia treatment

require diuretics or ultrafiltration in addition to identifying and addressing the underlying cause. It is generally advised not to restrict to only the clinical criteria for evaluating the total body water (TBW) and extracellular volume (ECV), in critically ill patients, while differentiating normovolemia from hypovolemia [53]. Various methods for the evaluation of volume status can be combined—Non-Instrumental: Clinical history, Physical examination; Static Instrumental: Bioimpedance, Ultrasound (Inferior vena cava diameter, E/e' ratio, E/A ratio), CVP, GEDVI; Dynamic Instrumental: SVV, PPV, and Passive Leg Raise test. Guidelines for hyponatremia management are provided by European (2014) and American groups (2013), with American guidelines being simpler than the comprehensive European guidelines. Table 12.2 shows American guidelines for hyponatremia management, and Figs. 12.4, 12.5, and 12.6 demonstrate the approach to hyponatremia management as in European guidelines. The clinical advice in the management of patients with hyponatremia in European guidelines includes—weight-based (2 mL/kg) not fixed 150 mL infusion in case of obviously deviant body composition; Correction of hypokalemia if present, to increase serum sodium concentration; expect increase in sodium levels more than calculated when Adrogue´-Madias formula is used; acute increase in urine output more than 100 mL/h increases the possibility of sudden rise in serum sodium levels and to measure the serum sodium concentration every 2–4 hours.

Table 12.2 American guidelines for hyponatremia management

Type	American guidelines
Acute/symptomatic hyponatremia	Severe symptoms: IV Bolus of 3% HTS (100 ml over 10 minutes—can be repeated 3 times as needed) Moderate symptoms: 0.5–2 ml/kg/h continuous infusion of 3% HTS
Chronic hyponatremia	SIADH: first line: Fluid restriction, second line: vaptan, demeclocycline, urea Hypovolemic hyponatremia: Isotonic Saline Hypervolemic hyponatremia: fluid restriction, vaptan

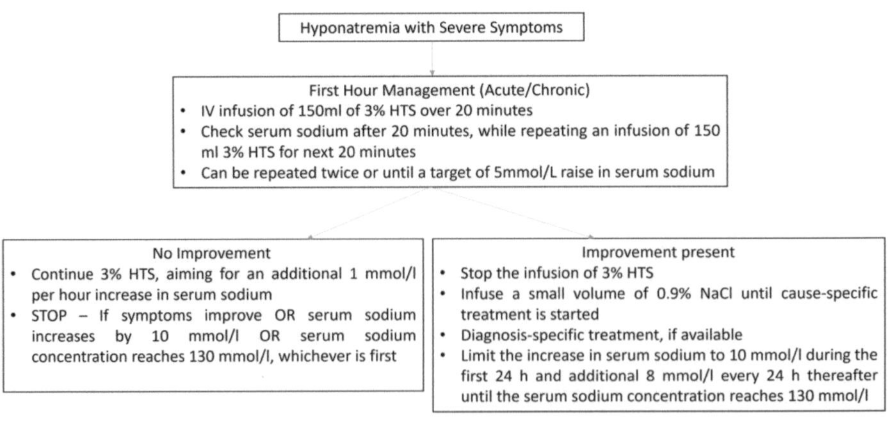

Fig. 12.4 Approach to Severe Hyponatremia

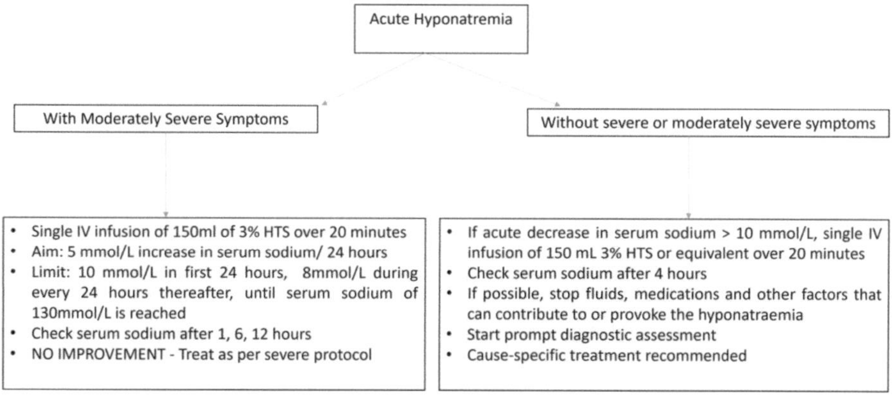

Fig. 12.5 Approach to Moderate Hyponatremia

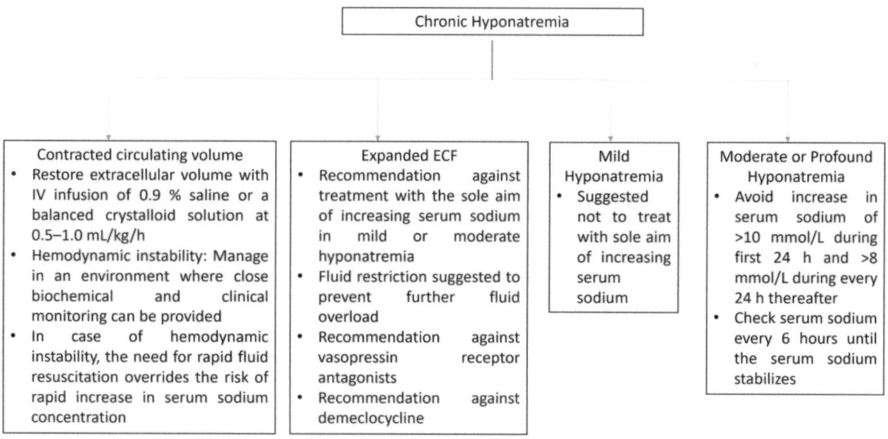

Fig. 12.6 Approach to Chronic Hyponatremia

The frequent causes of hyponatremia in TBI are CSW, SIADH, hypopituitarism, and insufficient dietary salt intake. Biochemical evaluation of pituitary hormones helps rule out hypopituitarism, and inadequate salt intake can be diagnosed if the urine spot sodium is low (<20–40 mEq/L). After excluding these causes, the clinician is left with CSW and SIADH, both manifesting as hyponatremia and natriuresis (urine spot sodium >40 mEq/L). The result is a clinical dilemma, considering the different fluid management strategies in CSW and SIADH. Fluid restriction is a suboptimal option, considering the clinical consequences of dehydrating a TBI patient. Therefore, serum sodium should be corrected with dietary salt supplementation and hydration with appropriate fluid. Hyponatremia associated with TBI usually responds to salt-retaining therapy in the setting of natriuresis [54].

Hyponatremia following aSAH is most commonly associated with SIADH, followed by acute cortisol insufficiency, CSW, excessive fluid therapy and/or diuretic

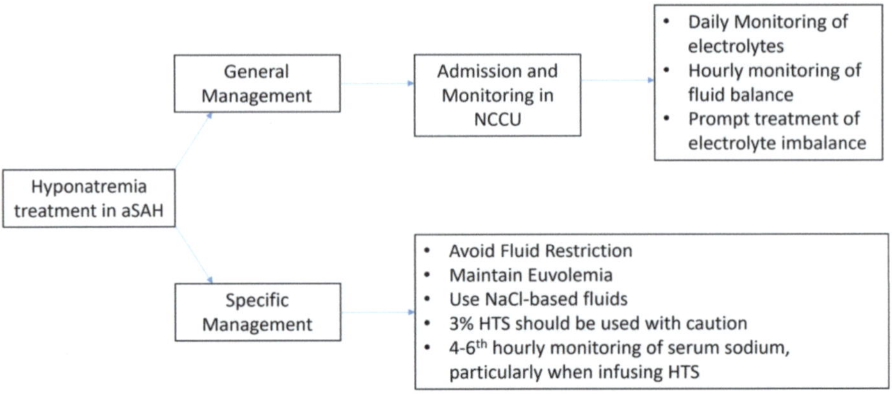

Fig. 12.7 Treatment algorithm in the management of hyponatremia in aSAH

therapy. Because hyponatremia is associated with poor outcomes after aSAH, proper anticipation, prompt identification, and suitable treatment are needed to improve outcomes. Due to hyponatremia, there is transport of water from the extracellular to intracellular space, which can worsen brain edema and ICP after aSAH, further increasing the risk of seizures and neurological injury. Volume contraction is associated with symptomatic vasospasm, while hyponatremia and fluid restriction contribute to DIND. Figure 12.7 depicts the treatment algorithm in the management of hyponatremia in aSAH. Any change in mental status, major variation in fluid balance and/or polyuria should elicit an immediate evaluation of serum sodium concentration. The current guidelines of the Neurocritical Care Society recommend avoiding increased intake of free water and abstaining from restriction of fluid to treat hyponatremia [55]. Additionally, the guidelines from the American Heart Association recommend treating volume contraction with isotonic fluids and avoiding large volumes of hypotonic fluids in aSAH [56]. Use of BSS in the initial period of aSAH may prevent dyselectrolytemia that can be associated with saline-based fluids. Although SIADH is best managed with fluid restriction to <500 mL/day, it may not be possible in aSAH patients, as patients may not be fully conscious, requiring feeding through an enteral tube, with fluid intake of 1–2 L/day. Fluid restriction resulting in hypovolemia increases the risk of the occurrence of vasospasm and cerebral ischemia.

Alternative therapies have been tried, which include HTS and albumin. HTS, administered as 2–3% solutions, can rapidly and efficiently increase plasma sodium, thereby increasing the blood volume. This may result in increased risk of pulmonary edema and cardiac failure, which eventually leads to potential neurological complications [57]. The effects of HTS are usually temporary, as the physiological stimuli for retention of water and secondary natriuresis are present. With its mineralocorticoid action, fludrocortisone may enhance sodium retention, but many studies have suggested that the use of fludrocortisone in correcting hyponatremia is limited and can be associated with fluid overload [58]. Alternatively, vasopressin receptor antagonists (e.g., conivaptan, tolvaptan) have been tried in many studies. A single dose of conivaptan increased plasma sodium by 4 mEq/L in one study and sustained the sodium improvement for 3 days. However, efficacy and safety profiles remain contentious as 1/3rd of the study patients became hyponatremic after its discontinuation [59]. Urea has also been tried, which induces water elimination by osmosis and promotes passive resorption of sodium in the ascending limb of the loop of Henle of the nephron [60]. Hydrocortisone use in aSAH may prevent excess natriuresis and decrease cerebral vasospasm, but its efficacy is yet to be established.

Sodium disturbances are now well recognized as significant prognostic markers in neurocritical care. Their evaluation demands a thorough appraisal of intravascular volume status alongside key biochemical parameters to arrive at the correct diagnosis. This distinction is particularly vital when differentiating the syndrome of inappropriate anti-diuretic hormone secretion (SIADH) from cerebral salt wasting (CSW), since the therapeutic approach to each is diametrically opposed [50, 53].

In addressing either hyponatremia or hypernatremia, clinicians must weigh the rapidity of onset, clinical severity, and the burden of prior neurological injury. Excessively rapid sodium correction carries the danger of osmotic demyelination in the setting of hyponatremia, whereas abrupt reduction of hypernatremia may precipitate cerebral edema. Careful, individualized adjustment of serum sodium, therefore, remains essential to optimize outcomes in the neurocritical care unit [50, 53].

12.6 Role of Osmotherapy: Mannitol Versus Hypertonic Saline

Osmotherapy is a standard treatment to manage raised ICP and cerebral edema after ABI in NCCU. The two most common agents used are mannitol and HTS. Controversy exists regarding the timing, dose, concentration, method, duration, ICP-guided or fixed schedule, monitoring, and superiority of one over the other. We discuss the evidence on osmotherapy in ABI, mainly related to TBI, and, where available, in other ABI conditions.

12.7 The Drug

Mannitol has been used for ICP reduction in ABI for several decades and is considered a gold standard osmotherapeutic agent in clinical practice. However, concerns about hypotension, rebound intracranial hypertension after discontinuation, and AKI from increased serum osmolarity necessitated the exploration of safe and efficacious alternatives. Initial data showed that HTS reduces ICP and improves outcomes after ABI [61]. However, urinary loss of sodium and the inability to sustain a hyperosmolar intravascular state were observed after HTS administration [62]. The debate regarding which (mannitol or HTS) is better in ABI is unsettled despite RCTs studying the efficacy of mannitol and HTS [63, 64]. Systematic reviews of clinical studies in the last decade showed HTS to be equivalent to mannitol for ICP reduction and clinical outcomes [65–67]. One review involving 12 RCTs with 464 patients found lower ICP and higher CPP with HTS than mannitol in TBI [68]. Considering the superior effect of HTS on ICP and CPP, many reviews concluded that HTS may be preferred in TBI [69–73]. In children, contrasting findings were noted, with some observing lower ICP and higher CPP with HTS, while others observed no difference in ICP or neurological outcomes [74–76]. A recent guideline suggests using HTS rather than mannitol in the management of raised ICP or cerebral edema in TBI in the initial period, but does not recommend them for improving neurological outcomes. Mannitol is recommended when HTS administration is not feasible [77]. A survey of neuro-intensivists observed a greater preference for HTS (55%) over mannitol [78].

12.8 Dose, Concentration, and Mechanisms

Mannitol concentration varies from 5% to 25%, with 20% being most used in ABI [79, 80]. The dose of 20% mannitol is 0.25–1 g/kg bolus, repeated every 2–8 hours or based on ICP when monitored. The ICP reduction starts within 5 minutes, and the peak effect is seen between 20 and 60 minutes [81]. Benefits of mannitol include osmotic diuretic properties by drawing edema fluid from the brain parenchyma and decreasing cerebral water content, reducing ICP by altering blood rheology and promoting cerebral vasoconstriction, increasing plasma volume and improving CBF and oxygen delivery by decreasing hematocrit and blood viscosity.

HTS is available at concentrations of 3%, 5%, 7.5%, and 23.4%, with the commonly used 3% HTS administered at 1–4 mL/kg bolus every 4–6 hours or continuous infusion at a rate to achieve and maintain a serum sodium concentration between 145 and 155 mEq/L or achieve ICP below the targeted threshold. When the BBB is intact, HTS draws water from the interstitial spaces of the brain into the intravascular compartment through its osmotic effect and causes cerebral vasoconstriction, which lowers the CBV and ICP. Because of the lack of diuretic effect and plasma expansion from the redistribution of fluid from the extravascular space, hemodynamic stability and CPP are maintained. It has immune-modulatory and anti-inflammatory effects, which might be beneficial in ABI [70, 82].A retrospective study comparing 3% with 23.4% HTS found similar mortality after TBI. However, 23.4% HTS resulted in faster achievement of targeted serum sodium and osmolarity, but the incidence of severe hypernatremia was higher [83]. A review comparing studies using different concentrations of HTS and mannitol concluded that 5% HTS was associated with the lowest mortality, and 10% and 15% HTS solutions decreased ICP the most [84]. However, a recent review observed 3% HTS as the optimal concentration at 1.4–2.5 mL/kg bolus dose [72].

12.9 Method of Administration

Bolus 3% HTS was associated with a reduced time to targeted serum sodium levels, less HTS volume, fewer central venous catheters (CVC), and a similar safety profile compared to infusion in TBI [85]. Another study also found bolus to be better than infusion for target serum sodium and ICP reduction [86]. In contrast, another study found that the infusion method achieved faster target serum sodium concentration and lower neurosurgery requirements [87]. A recent RCT did not find an outcome benefit with additional continuous HTS infusion over standard care as per BTF guidelines [88].

12.10 Route of Administration

Osmotherapeutic agents can irritate peripheral veins with prolonged administration and higher concentrations. Hence, they should preferably be administered through CVC when available [89]. Mannitol is safely administered in a peripheral intravenous line [79]. Peripheral administration of 3% HTS is also safe, considering treatment benefits in ABI and the potential risks with CVC [90].

12.11 Side Effects

The choice of osmotherapy should also take into consideration its adverse effects [91]. The side effects of mannitol include dehydration, hypovolemia, hyperosmolarity, and AKI, which become evident when serum osmolarity exceeds 320 mOsm. It can temporarily increase plasma volume and precipitate heart failure or pulmonary edema in susceptible patients. Other side effects include electrolyte abnormalities, acidosis, and injection site reactions. A longer duration of continuous HTS infusion has more adverse effects than limited boluses. HTS can cause hypernatremia, hyperchloremic metabolic acidosis, osmotic demyelination syndrome, altered mentation, coagulopathy, hypervolemia and volume overload from plasma volume expansion, and thrombophlebitis and extravasation with peripheral vein administration [79]. Both agents should be used with caution in pregnancy and renal failure [89].

12.12 Initiation and Discontinuation

Osmotherapy should be considered for reducing ICP and cerebral edema in ABI. The BTF recommends osmotherapy guided by ICP monitoring and restricting its prior use in the setting of herniation or neurological deterioration [92]. The osmotic reflection coefficient of HTS is higher than that of mannitol (1 versus 0.9); hence, it does not penetrate the BBB. Therefore, no rebound effect should be seen after its discontinuation [93]. Mannitol should be gradually tapered before stopping. However, in the presence of hypernatremia, slow discontinuation of HTS is warranted to minimize acute changes in serum sodium concentration and its consequences, such as seizures and changes in mental functions. This approach is contested by an alternate theory. The brain tries to compensate for the osmotic gradient by forming osmotically active radiogenic osmoles when either agent is used for a prolonged period. Hence, their gradual weaning is suggested as abrupt discontinuation will cause gradient reversal and rebound ICP increase. Also, BBB disruption can accumulate osmotically active molecules, leading to local edema and elevating ICP [94].

A review involving 175 patients with aSAH found ICP reduction with HTS [95]. However, no RCTs compare mannitol with HTS for ICP reduction after aSAH. A symptom-based bolus dose of HTS rather than a sodium target-based dose is recommended for treating raised ICP or cerebral edema [76].

Both HTS and mannitol are recommended for treating raised ICP or cerebral edema, but not for improving neurological outcomes after AIS. The choice of HTS or mannitol should be based on clinical conditions. Mannitol may be preferred if the risk of pulmonary edema exists in elderly patients and those with congestive heart failure, while HTS is prudent in the presence of hypotension and hypovolemia [76, 96]. Mannitol insignificantly increases CBF in the non-ischemic hemisphere without any difference in other cerebral physiological parameters [97].

In patients with ICH, hyperosmolar therapy did not improve neurological outcomes. Osmotherapy is more likely required in patients with significant edema and herniation [98]. Recent guidelines suggest using HTS over mannitol for managing ICP or cerebral edema, considering the recognized benefits of HTS in fluid resuscitation and cerebral perfusion [76, 95].

There is insufficient evidence to suggest HTS or mannitol for reducing ICP or cerebral edema in patients with bacterial meningitis [76]. Only glycerol has been studied in meningitis, and no outcome benefit was noted [99]. However, in children with central nervous system (CNS) infection, ICP reduction was higher with 3% HTS than with 20% mannitol [100].

Recent guidelines suggest using either HTS or mannitol for reducing ICP or cerebral edema (not neurological outcomes) in patients with hepatic encephalopathy [76].

There are no studies comparing mannitol with HTS for ICP management or neurological outcomes in patients with cerebral venous thrombosis, although osmotherapy is widely used to reduce ICP in this setting. Similarly, there are no studies to guide osmotherapy in status epilepticus-induced cerebral edema and raised ICP.

12.13 Monitoring During Osmotherapy

Recent guidelines suggest using an osmolar gap (insufficient evidence to recommend a cutoff value, though 20 mOsm is used in clinical settings) over osmolarity of serum thresholds during administration of mannitol to monitor for the risk of AKI. Severe hypernatremia (155–160 mEq/L) and hyperchloremia (110–115 mEq/L) should be avoided during HTS therapy to decrease the risk of AKI. It is a good practice to monitor renal function and serum sodium and chloride parameters during osmotherapy [76, 95].

Available evidence suggests that osmotherapy with mannitol and HTS is beneficial in reducing ICP and cerebral edema in patients with TBI, aSAH, AIS, ICH, and hepatic encephalopathy in the NCCU. When used appropriately in these settings, the benefits of osmotherapy outweigh the potential risks, as adverse events associated with its use are few. Osmotherapy has mechanisms other than lowering ICP, which may help improve outcomes after ABI. Currently, there appears to be no difference in the effects of mannitol and HTS on ICP reduction and neurological outcomes. However, other physiological properties of blood rheology, inflammation, neurochemistry, and hemodynamic regulation make HTS preferable over mannitol in most settings.

Conflict of Interests None for any of the authors.

References

1. Corcoran T, Rhodes JE, Clarke S, Myles PS, Ho KM. Perioperative fluid management strategies in major surgery: a stratified meta-analysis. Anesth Analg. 2012;114(3):640–51.
2. Drevet CM, Opprecht N, Nadji A, et al. Impact of restrictive fluid protocol on hypoxemia after aneurysmal subarachnoid hemorrhage. J Crit Care. 2017;42:152–6.
3. Clifton GL, Miller ER, Choi SC, Levin HS. Fluid thresholds and outcome from severe brain injury. Crit Care Med. 2002;30:739–45.
4. Wiegers EJA, Lingsma HF, Huijben JA, et al. Fluid balance and outcome in critically ill patients with traumatic brain injury (CENTER-TBI and OzENTER-TBI): a prospective, multicentre, comparative effectiveness study. Lancet Neurol. 2021;20(8):627–38.
5. Robertson CS, Valadka AB, Hannay HJ, et al. Prevention of secondary ischemic insults after severe head injury. Crit Care Med. 1999;27:2086–95.
6. Grande PO. The "Lund concept" for treatment of severe head trauma—physiological principles and clinical applications. Intensive Care Med. 2006;17:561–2.
7. Martini RP, Deem S, Brown M, et al. The association between fluid balance and outcomes after subarachnoid hemorrhage. Neurocrit Care. 2012;17(2):191–8.
8. Tagami T, Kuwamoto K, Watanabe A, et al. Effect of triple-h prophylaxis on global end-diastolic volume and clinical outcomes in patients with aneurysmal subarachnoid hemorrhage. Neurocrit Care. 2014;21(3):462–9.
9. Kissoon NR, Mandrekar JN, Fugate JE, Lanzino G, Wijdicks EF, Rabinstein AA. Positive fluid balance is associated with poor outcomes in subarachnoid Hemorrhage. J Stroke Cerebrovasc Dis. 2015;24(10):2245–51.
10. Rass V, Gaasch M, Kofler M, Schiefecker AJ, Ianosi BA, Steinkohl F, Beer R, Pfausler B, Gizewski ER, Thomé C, Schmutzhard E, Helbok R. Fluid intake but not fluid balance is associated with poor outcome in nontraumatic subarachnoid Hemorrhage patients. Crit Care Med. 2019;47(7):e555–62.
11. Lennihan L, Mayer SA, Fink ME, Beckford A, Paik MC, Zhang H, Wu YC, Klebanoff LM, Raps EC, Solomon RA. Effect of hypervolemic therapy on cerebral blood flow after subarachnoid hemorrhage: a randomized controlled trial. Stroke. 2000;31(2):383–91.
12. Rinkel GJ, Feigin VL, Algra A, van Gijn J. Circulatory volume expansion therapy for aneurysmal subarachnoid haemorrhage. Cochrane Database Syst Rev. 2004;2004(4):CD000483.
13. Tagami T, Kuwamoto K, Watanabe A, Unemoto K, Yokobori S, Matsumoto G, Yokota H, SAH PiCCO Study Group. Optimal range of global end-diastolic volume for fluid management after aneurysmal subarachnoid hemorrhage: a multicenter prospective cohort study. Crit Care Med. 2014;42(6):1348–56.
14. Yoneda H, Nakamura T, Shirao S, Tanaka N, Ishihara H, Suehiro E, Koizumi H, Isotani E, Suzuki M, SAH PiCCO Study Group. Multicenter prospective cohort study on volume management after subarachnoid hemorrhage: hemodynamic changes according to severity of subarachnoid hemorrhage and cerebral vasospasm. Stroke. 2013;44(8):2155–61.

15. Mutoh T, Kazumata K, Terasaka S, Taki Y, Suzuki A, Ishikawa T. Early intensive versus minimally invasive approach to postoperative hemodynamic management after subarachnoid hemorrhage. Stroke. 2014;45(5):1280–4.
16. Muench E, Horn P, Bauhuf C, Roth H, Philipps M, Hermann P, Quintel M, Schmiedek P, Vajkoczy P. Effects of hypervolemia and hypertension on regional cerebral blood flow, intracranial pressure, and brain tissue oxygenation after subarachnoid hemorrhage. Crit Care Med. 2007;35(8):1844–51.
17. Tseng MY, Al-Rawi PG, Pickard JD, Rasulo FA, Kirkpatrick PJ. Effect of hypertonic saline on cerebral blood flow in poor-grade patients with subarachnoid hemorrhage. Stroke. 2003;34(6):1389–96.
18. Yamakami I, Isobe K, Yamaura A. Effects of intravascular volume expansion on cerebral blood flow in patients with ruptured cerebral aneurysms. Neurosurgery. 1987;21(3):303–9.
19. Dharmasaroja PA. Fluid intake related to brain Edema in acute middle cerebral artery infarction. Transl Stroke Res. 2016;7(1):49–53.
20. Miller JB, Lewandowski C, Wira CR, Taylor A, Burmeister C, Welch R. Volume of plasma expansion and functional outcomes in stroke. Neurocrit Care. 2017;26(2):191–5.
21. Semler MW, Self WH, Wanderer JP, et al. Balanced crystalloids versus saline in critically ill adults. N Engl J Med. 2018;378:829–39.
22. Yunos NM, Bellomo R, Hegarty C, Story D, Ho L, Bailey M. Association between a chloride-liberal vs chloride-restrictive intravenous fluid administration strategy and kidney injury in critically ill adults. JAMA. 2012;308(15):1566–72.
23. Semler MW, Wanderer JP, Ehrenfeld JM, et al. Balanced crystalloids versus saline in the intensive care unit. The SALT randomized trial. Am J Respir Crit Care Med. 2017;195:1362–72.
24. Young P, Bailey M, Beasley R, et al.. SPLIT Investigators, ANZICS CTGEffect of a buffered crystalloid solution vs saline on acute kidney injury among patients in the intensive care unit: the SPLIT randomized clinical trial. JAMA. 2015;314:1701–10.
25. SAFE Study Investigators, Australian and New Zealand Intensive Care Society Clinical Trials Group, Australian Red Cross Blood Service, George Institute for International Health, Myburgh J, Cooper DJ, Finfer S, Bellomo R, Norton R, et al. Saline or albumin for fuid resuscitation in patients with traumatic brain injury. N Engl J Med. 2007;357(9):874–84.
26. Schirmer-Mikalsen K, Vik A, Gisvold SE, Skandsen T, Hynne H, Klepstad P. Severe head injury: control of physiological variables, organ failure and complications in the intensive care unit. Acta Anaesthesiol Scand. 2007;51:1194–201.
27. Famakin B, Weiss P, Hertzberg V, et al. Hypoalbuminemia predicts acute stroke mortality: Paul Coverdell Georgia stroke registry. J Stroke Cerebrovasc Dis. 2010;19:17–22.
28. Tone O, Ito U, Tomita H, Masaoka H, Tominaga B. High colloid oncotic therapy for brain edema with cerebral hemorrhage. Acta Neurochir Suppl (Wien). 1994;60:568–70.
29. Tomita H, Ito U, Tone O, Masaoka H, Tominaga B. High colloid oncotic therapy for contusional brain edema. Acta NeurochirSuppl (Wien). 1994;60:547–9.
30. Cochrane Injuries Group Albumin Reviewers. Human albumin administration in critically ill patients: systematic review of randomised controlled trials. BMJ. 1998;317(7153):235–40.
31. Ginsberg MD, Palesch YY, Hill MD, et al. High-dose albumin treatment for acute ischaemic stroke (ALIAS) part 2: a randomised, double-blind, phase 3, placebo-controlled trial. Lancet Neurol. 2013;12(11):1049–58.
32. Martin RH, Yeatts SD, Hill MD, Moy CS, Ginsberg MD, Palesch YY, ALIAS Parts 1 and 2 and NETT Investigators. ALIAS (albumin in acute ischemic stroke) trials: analysis of the combined data from parts 1 and 2. Stroke. 2016;47(9):2355–9.
33. Suarez JI, Shannon L, Zaidat OO, et al. Effect of human albumin administration on clinical outcome and hospital cost in patients with subarachnoid hemorrhage. J Neurosurg. 2004;100(4):585–90.
34. Suarez JI, Martin RH, Calvillo E, Dillon C, Bershad EM, Macdonald RL, Wong J, Harbaugh R, Investigators ALISAH. The albumin in subarachnoid Hemorrhage (ALISAH) multicenter pilot clinical trial: safety and neurologic outcomes. Stroke. 2012;43(3):683–90. https://doi.org/10.1161/STROKEAHA.111.633958.

35. Gempeler A, Gaviria L, Ortiz A, Jaramillo N, Beltrán L, Escobar S, Rondón M, Rosselli D, Martinez-Buitrago JE, Mejía-Mantilla JH. Effect of an albumin infusion treatment protocol on delayed cerebral ischemia and relevant outcomes in patients with subarachnoid Hemorrhage. Neurocrit Care. 2023;39(1):180–90.
36. Ibrahim GM, Macdonald RL. The effects of fluid balance and colloid administration on outcomes in patients with aneurysmal subarachnoid hemorrhage: a propensity score-matched analysis. Neurocrit Care. 2013;19(2):140–9.
37. Tseng MY, Hutchinson PJ, Kirkpatrick PJ. Effects of fluid therapy following aneurysmal subarachnoid haemorrhage: a prospective clinical study. Br J Neurosurg. 2008;22(2):257–68.
38. Lehmann L, Bendel S, Uehlinger DE, et al. Randomized, double-blind trial of the effect of fluid composition on electrolyte, acid-base, and fluid homeostasis in patients early after subarachnoid hemorrhage. Neurocrit Care. 2013;18(1):5–12.
39. Sekhon MS, Dhingra VK, Sekhon IS, Henderson WR, McLean N, Griesdale DE. The safety of synthetic colloid in critically ill patients with severe traumatic brain injuries. J Crit Care. 2011;26(4):357–62.
40. Oddo M, Poole D, Helbok R, et al. Fluid therapy in neurointensive care patients: ESICM consensus and clinical practice recommendations. Intensive Care Med. 2018;44(4):449–63.
41. Messina A, Villa F, Lionetti G, et al. Hemodynamic management of acute brain injury caused by cerebrovascular diseases: a survey of the European Society of Intensive Care Medicine. Intensive Care Med Exp. 2022;10:42.
42. Funk GC, Lindner G, Druml W, Metnitz B, Schwarz C, Bauer P, et al. Incidence and prognosis of dysnatremias present on ICU admission. Intensive Care Med. 2010;36:304–11.
43. Kirkman MA. Managing hyponatremia in neurosurgical patients. Minerva Endocrinol. 2014;39:13–26.
44. Sherlock M, O'Sullivan E, Agha A, Behan LA, Rawluk D, Brennan P, et al. The incidence and pathophysiology of hyponatraemia after subarachnoid haemorrhage. Clin Endocrinol. 2006;64:250–4.
45. Kao L, Al-Lawati Z, Vavao J, Steinberg GK, Katznelson L. Prevalence and clinical demographics of cerebral salt wasting in patients with aneurysmal subarachnoid hemorrhage. Pituitary. 2009;12:347–51.
46. Hannon MJ, Behan LA, O'Brien MMC, Tormey W, Ball SG, Javadpour M, et al. Hyponatremia following mild/moderate subarachnoid hemorrhage is due to SIAD and glucocorticoid deficiency and not cerebral salt wasting. J Clin Endocrinol Metab. 2014;99:291–8.
47. Nakagawa I, Hironaka Y, Nishimura F, Takeshima Y, Matsuda R, Yamada S, et al. Early inhibition of natriuresis suppresses symptomatic cerebral vasospasm in patients with aneurysmal subarachnoid hemorrhage. Cerebrovasc Dis. 2013;35:131–7.
48. Lerner DP, Shepherd SA, Batra A. Hyponatremia in the neurologically ill patient: a review. Neurohospitalist. 2020;10:208–16.
49. Sterns RH, Rondon-Berrios H, Adrogué HJ, Berl T, Burst V, Cohen DM, et al. Treatment guidelines for hyponatremia: stay the course. Clin J Am Soc Nephrol. 2024;19:129.
50. Hwang JJ, Hwang DY. Treatment of endocrine disorders in the neuroscience intensive care unit. Curr Treat Options Neurol. 2014;16:271.
51. Moro N, Katayama Y, Igarashi T, Mori T, Kawamata T, Kojima J. Hyponatremia in patients with traumatic brain injury: incidence, mechanism, and response to sodium supplementation or retention therapy with hydrocortisone. Surg Neurol. 2007;68:387–93.
52. Wang G, Jia H, Chen C, Lang S, Liu X, Xia C, et al. Analysis of risk factors for first seizure after stroke in Chinese patients. Biomed Res Int. 2013;2013:702871.
53. Broch Porcar MJ, Rodríguez Cubillo B, Domínguez-Roldán JM, Álvarez Rocha L, Ballesteros Sanz MÁ, Cervera Montes M, et al. Practical document on the management of hyponatremia in critically ill patients. Medicina Intensiva (English Edition). 2019;43:302–16.
54. Rajagopal R, Swaminathan G, Nair S, Joseph M. Hyponatremia in traumatic brain injury: a practical management protocol. World Neurosurg. 2017;108:529–33.
55. Diringer MN, Bleck TP, Claude Hemphill J, Menon D, Shutter L, Vespa P, et al. Critical care management of patients following aneurysmal subarachnoid hemorrhage: recommenda-

tions from the Neurocritical care society's multidisciplinary consensus conference. Neurocrit Care. 2011;15:211–40.
56. Hoh BL, Ko NU, Amin-Hanjani S, et al. 2023 Guideline for the Management of Patients With Aneurysmal Subarachnoid Hemorrhage: A Guideline From the American Heart Association/ American Stroke Association. Stroke. 2023;54(7):e314–70.
57. Decaux G, Musch W, Soupart A. Management of Hypotonic Hyponatremia. Acta Clin Belg. 2010;65:437–45.
58. Mori T, Katayama Y, Kawamata T, Hirayama T. Improved efficiency of hypervolemic therapy with inhibition of natriuresis by fludrocortisone in patients with aneurysmal subarachnoid hemorrhage. J Neurosurg. 1999;91:947–52.
59. Wright WL, Asbury WH, Gilmore JL, Samuels OB. Conivaptan for hyponatremia in the neurocritical care unit. Neurocrit Care. 2009;11:6–13.
60. Pierrakos C, Taccone FS, Decaux G, Vincent JL, Brimioulle S. Urea for treatment of acute SIADH in patients with subarachnoid hemorrhage: a single-center experience. Ann Intensive Care. 2012;2:13.
61. Ziai WC, Toung TJ, Bhardwaj A. Hypertonic saline: first-line therapy for cerebral edema? J Neurol Sci. 2007;261(1–2):157–66.
62. Jagannatha AT, Sriganesh K, Devi BI, Umamaheswara Rao GS. Urinary sodium loss following hypertonic saline administration curtails its superior Osmolar effect in comparison to mannitol in severe traumatic brain injury: a secondary analysis of a randomized controlled trial. J Neuroanaesthesiol Crit Care. 2018;5(3):164–7.
63. Patil H, Gupta R. A comparative study of bolus dose of hypertonic saline, mannitol, and mannitol plus glycerol combination in patients with severe traumatic brain injury. World Neurosurg. 2019;125:e221–8.
64. Jagannatha AT, Sriganesh K, Devi BI, Rao GS. An equiosmolar study on early intracranial physiology and long-term outcome in severe traumatic brain injury comparing mannitol and hypertonic saline. J Clin Neurosci. 2016;27:68–73.
65. Bernhardt K, McClune W, Rowland MJ, Shah A. Hypertonic saline versus other intracranial-pressure-lowering agents for patients with acute traumatic brain injury: a systematic review and meta-analysis. Neurocrit Care. 2024;40(2):769–84.
66. Iqbal U, Kumar A, Arsal SA, et al. Efficacy of hypertonic saline and mannitol in patients with traumatic brain injury and cerebral edema: a systematic review and meta-analysis. Egypt J Neurosurg. 2023;38:54.
67. Cai L, He W. Effectiveness of hypertonic saline infusion in management of traumatic brain injury: an updated systematic review and meta-analysis of randomized controlled trials. Brain Inj. Published online 2024.
68. Schwimmbeck F, Voellger B, Chappell D, Eberhart L. Hypertonic saline versus mannitol for traumatic brain injury: a systematic review and meta-analysis with trial sequential analysis. J Neurosurg Anesthesiol. 2021;33(1):10–20.
69. Shi J, Tan L, Ye J, Hu L. Hypertonic saline and mannitol in patients with traumatic brain injury: a systematic and meta-analysis. Medicine (Baltimore). 2020;99(35):e21655.
70. Gu J, Huang H, Huang Y, Sun H, Xu H. Hypertonic saline or mannitol for treating elevated intracranial pressure in traumatic brain injury: a meta-analysis of randomized controlled trials. Neurosurg Rev. 2019;42(2):499–509.
71. Gharizadeh N, Ghojazadeh M, Naseri A, Dolati S, Tarighat F, Soleimanpour H. Hypertonic saline for traumatic brain injury: a systematic review and meta-analysis. Eur J Med Res. 2022;27(1):254.
72. Karamian A, Seifi A, Lucke-Wold B. Comparing the effects of mannitol and hypertonic saline in severe traumatic brain injury patients with elevated intracranial pressure: a systematic review and meta-analysis. Neurol Res. Published online, 2024.
73. Susanto M, Riantri I. Optimal dose and concentration of hypertonic saline in traumatic brain injury: a systematic review. Medeni Med J. 2022;37(2):203–11.

74. Kumar SA, Devi BI, Reddy M, Shukla D. Comparison of equiosmolar dose of hyperosmolar agents in reducing intracranial pressure-a randomized control study in pediatric traumatic brain injury. Childs Nerv Syst. 2019;35(6):999–1005.
75. Kochanek PM, Adelson PD, Rosario BL, et al. Comparison of intracranial pressure measurements before and after hypertonic saline or mannitol treatment in children with severe traumatic brain injury. JAMA Netw Open. 2022;5(3):e220891.
76. Mishra NR, Agrawal A, Das RR. Hypertonic saline vs. mannitol in Management of Elevated Intracranial Pressure in children: a meta-analysis. Indian J Pediatr. 2023;90(9):899–906.
77. Cook AM, Morgan Jones G, Hawryluk GWJ, Mailloux P, McLaughlin D, Papangelou A, Samuel S, Tokumaru S, Venkatasubramanian C, Zacko C, Zimmermann LL, Hirsch K, Shutter L. Guidelines for the acute treatment of cerebral Edema in Neurocritical care patients. Neurocrit Care. 2020;32(3):647–66.
78. Hays AN, Lazaridis C, Neyens R, Nicholas J, Gay S, Chalela JA. Osmotherapy: use among neurointensivists. Neurocrit Care. 2011;14:222–8.
79. Peters NA, Farrell LB, Smith JP. Hyperosmolar therapy for the treatment of cerebral Edema. US Pharm. 2018;43(1):HS-8–HS-11.
80. Mason A, Malik A, Ginglen JG. Hypertonic fluids. [Updated 2023 Apr 17]. In: StatPearls [Internet]. Treasure Island (FL): StatPearls Publishing; 2024 Jan. Available from: https://www.ncbi.nlm.nih.gov/books/NBK542194/].
81. Rangel-Castilla L, Gopinath S, Robertson CS. Management of intracranial hypertension. Neurol Clin. 2008;26:521–41.
82. Chen H, Song Z, Dennis JA. Hypertonic saline versus other intracranial pressure–lowering agents for people with acute traumatic brain injury. Cochrane Database Syst Rev. 2020;(1):CD010904.
83. Traficante D, Galaktionova D, Marseille U, et al. Comparison of 3% vs. 23.4% hypertonic saline in traumatic brain injury. Journal of. Curr Surg. 2019;9(4):39–44.
84. Wang X, He Q, Ma L, You C. Comparison of different concentrations of hypertonic saline in patients with traumatic brain injury: evidence from direct and indirect comparisons. Injury. 2022;53(11):3729–35.
85. Daley M, Cox E, Schroeder J, et al. 636: getting salty: infusion vs bolus dosing of hypertonic saline in patients with traumatic brain injury. Crit Care Med. 2024;52(1):S291.
86. Wahdan AS, Al-Madawi AA, El-Shafey KA, Othman SH. Comparison of intermittent versus continuous infusion of 3% hypertonic saline on intracranial pressure in traumatic brain injury using ultrasound assessment of optic nerve sheath. Egyptian Journal of Anaesthesia. 2022;38(1):291–9.
87. Parizh D, Parizh I, Kuwata C, et al. Traumatic brain injury: bolus versus continuous infusion of 3% hypertonic saline. Int Surg. 2016;101:361–6.
88. Roquilly A, Moyer JD, Huet O, et al. Effect of continuous infusion of hypertonic saline vs standard care on 6-month neurological outcomes in patients with traumatic brain injury: the COBI randomized clinical trial. JAMA. 2021;325(20):2056–66.
89. Holden DN, Mucksavage JJ, Cokley JA, et al. Hypertonic saline use in neurocritical care for treating cerebral edema: a review of optimal formulation, dosing, safety, administration and storage. Am J Health Syst Pharm. 2023;80(6):331–42.
90. Khasiyev F, Hakoun A, Christopher K, Braun J, Wang F. Safety and effect on intracranial pressure of 3% hypertonic saline bolus via peripheral intravenous catheter for neurological emergencies. Neurocrit Care. Published online 2024.
91. Freeman N, Welbourne J. Osmotherapy: science and evidence-based practice. BJA Educ. 2018;18(9):284–90.
92. Carney N, Totten AM, O'Reilly C, et al. Guidelines for the management of severe traumatic brain injury. Neurosurgery. 2017;80(1):6–15.
93. Kim JH, Jeong H, Choo YH, Kim M, Ha EJ, Oh J, Shim Y, Kim SB, Jung HG, Park SH, Kim JO, Kim J, Kim HS, Lee S. Optimizing mannitol use in managing increased intracra-

nial pressure: a comprehensive review of recent research and clinical experiences. Korean J Neurotrauma. 2023;19(2):162–76.

94. Boone MD, Oren-Grinberg A, Robinson TM, Chen CC, Kasper EM. Mannitol or hypertonic saline in the setting of traumatic brain injury: what have we learned? Surg Neurol Int. 2015;6:177.
95. Pasarikovski CR, Alotaibi NM, Al-Mufti F, Macdonald RL. Hypertonic saline for increased intracranial pressure after aneurysmal subarachnoid Hemorrhage: a systematic review. World Neurosurg. 2017;105:1–6.
96. Mohney N, Alkhatib O, Koch S, O'Phelan K, Merenda A. What is the role of hyperosmolar therapy in hemispheric stroke patients? Neurocrit Care. 2020;32:609–19.
97. Diringer MN, Scalfani MT, Zazulia AR, Videen TO, Dhar R. Cerebral hemodynamic and metabolic effects of equi-osmolar doses mannitol and 23.4% saline in patients with edema following large ischemic stroke. Neurocrit Care. 2011;14(1):11–7.
98. Shah M, Birnbaum L, Rasmussen J, et al. Effect of hyperosmolar therapy on outcome following spontaneous intracerebral Hemorrhage: ethnic/racial variations of intracerebral Hemorrhage (ERICH) study. J Stroke Cerebrovasc Dis. 2018;27(4):1061–7.
99. Wall EC, Ajdukiewicz KM, Bergman H, Heyderman RS, Garner P. Osmotic therapies added to antibiotics for acute bacterial meningitis. Cochrane Database Syst Rev. 2018;2(2):CD008806.
100. Rameshkumar R, Bansal A, Singhi S, Singhi P, Jayashree M. Randomized clinical trial of 20% mannitol versus 3% hypertonic saline in children with raised intracranial pressure due to acute CNS infections. Pediatr Crit Care Med. 2020;21(12):1071–80.

Ventilatory Strategies in Neurocritical Care Patients

13

Nitasha Mishra and Prasanna Udupi Bidkar

Abstract

This chapter aims to explore the multifaceted of mechanical ventilation (MV) in neurocritical care, identifying the controversies that arise when managing patients with neurological injuries. Key topics that are discussed include the following:

Lung-protective vs. neuroprotective ventilation strategies
Advanced ventilatory techniques: alveolar recruitment maneuvers (RMs), modes, and extracorporeal membrane oxygenation (ECMO)
Extubation criteria
Timing of tracheostomy
Ventilator-associated pneumonia: the role of VAP bundles, prophylactic antibiotics, and inhaled antibiotics

Through a comprehensive review of these topics, this chapter will provide clinicians with critical insights into the effective management of mechanical ventilation in neurocritical care settings. The aim is to enhance patient outcomes, facilitate neurological recovery, and address the complex interplay between neurological injury and respiratory failure.

N. Mishra (✉)
Department of Anesthesiology and Critical Care, AIIMS, Bhubaneshwar, Odisha, India

P. U. Bidkar
JIPMER, Puducherry, India

P. U. Bidkar, M. Krishnakumar (eds.), *Controversies in Neurocritical Care*,
https://doi.org/10.1007/978-981-95-4419-6_13

Keywords

Lung protective ventilation · Brain Protective ventilation · Extubation Criteria Ventilator-associated pneumonia · Tracheostomy

13.1 Introduction

Mechanical ventilation (MV) is a vital intervention in neurocritical care, with neurological conditions accounting for the need for MV in approximately 20% of general intensive care unit (ICU) patients, a figure that rises to 80% in specialized neurocritical care units (NCCUs). This highlights its pivotal role in managing patients with acute brain injuries (ABIs). Unlike typical ICU cases, patients with ABIs often require mechanical support not due to lung disease but because of compromised airway protection and impaired respiratory function.

These patients are at a heightened risk for pulmonary complications linked to their neurological condition. Common issues include aspiration pneumonia, neurogenic pulmonary edema, and pulmonary embolism, stemming from impaired airway reflexes; reduced consciousness; and limited mobility. Ventilator-associated pneumonia (VAP), with reported incidences of up to 36–57% in neurocritical care, is a significant complication that poses considerable challenges. It not only increases the duration of mechanical ventilation but also prolongs ICU stays and adversely impacts patient outcomes.

(A) *Oxygen Targets*: Although the primary goal is to avoid hypoxia in critically ill patients, the optimal oxygenation targets in brain-injured cohorts remain uncertain. Latest research also brings forth the evidence of toxicity of hyperoxemia, revealing its association with oxidative stress and worsened outcomes in neurocritical care patients. The CENTER-TBI and Oz-CENTER-TBI studies, large European and Australian cohort analyses, respectively, demonstrated that higher arterial oxygen levels lead to an increased risk of mortality at 6 months. In the CENTER-TBI study, the median highest PaO_2 was reported to be 134 mmHg in the first week of ICU admission, and higher maximal PaO_2 levels were associated with unfavorable neurological outcomes or death at 6 months, and this finding was not altered by the severity of the injury. However, this study did not provide a safe upper limit of PaO_2 [1]. In contrast, some studies have reported no significant differences in outcomes across PaO_2 levels ranging from 60 to over 300 mmHg [2, 3], with others suggesting beneficial neurological outcomes with levels between 150 and 200 mm of Hg [4]. While a meta-analysis of observational studies found that hyperoxemia ($PaO_2 > 200$ mmHg) is associated with poor neurological outcomes [5], particularly in patients with subarachnoid hemorrhage and ischemic stroke, randomized trials in ICU settings have not confirmed this [6]. Another recent meta-analysis also could not provide a safe upper limit for PaO_2 [7].

A recent study using machine learning models from the pragmatic investigation of optimal oxygen targets (PILOT) and intensive care unit randomized trial comparing two approaches to oxygen therapy (ICU-ROX) studies predicted that treatment with a lower SpO_2 target could benefit by providing a 27% absolute risk reduction in 28-day mortality, while a higher $SpOO_2$ target could lead to a 34% absolute increase in mortality [8]. Patients with isolated brain injuries may benefit from lower oxygen targets, whereas those predicted to benefit from higher SpO_2 targets often have a higher prevalence of sepsis and abnormal vitals.

Therefore, an individualized approach using machine learning models should be used when deciding the ideal oxygen targets. Monitoring cerebral oxygen supply using brain tissue oxygen monitoring can help identify impending cerebral hypoxia. Ongoing studies are evaluating the effectiveness of targeting oxygen levels based on continuous brain tissue oxygen monitoring.

In conclusion, the potential risks of excessive hyperoxemia are not fully understood, and avoiding it seems prudent, especially in patients with purely brain injury without any multiorgan dysfunction or reduced perfusion. Current recommendations suggest maintaining a target PaO_2 of 80–120 mmHg in patients, regardless of whether intracranial pressure (ICP) is elevated. Key points in the context of oxygen targets are enumerated in Table 13.1.

(B) *Carbon Dioxide Levels*: Hypocapnia is often employed to control acute bursts of high intracranial pressure (ICP). Due to the potential risk of cerebral ischemia, extreme hypocapnia (defined as a $PaCO_2 < 30$ mmHg) should be avoided or employed only for short periods in emergency situations, particularly when intracranial hypertension is present, and may be used along with monitoring of cerebral oxygenation [9].

Theoretically, carbon dioxide levels >45 mm of Hg should also be avoided as it causes deranged cerebral compliance because of its vasodilatory properties. Interestingly, in cases of hypoxic encephalopathy, levels of $PaCO_2$ of up to 52 mmHg did not cause any increase in mortality rates, provided the pH remained within the normal range [10]. Recent animal studies have also investigated the potential neuroprotective effects of hypercapnia [11]. Further research is warranted to explore the neuroprotective role of hypercapnia.

Table 13.1 Key points in oxygen targets

1.	Both hypoxemia and hyperoxemia should be avoided.
2.	Among mechanically ventilated patients, a target saturation level of 91–96% may be adequate under most clinical circumstances.
3.	Hyperoxemia >200 mm of hg should be avoided in purely brain-injured patients without any signs of organ perfusion/sepsis.
4.	The safe limits of oxygen therapy remain unclear. The range of safety may vary depending on the underlying condition. Hypoxic–ischemic encephalopathy may exacerbate the vulnerability to the adverse effects of excessive oxygen.
5.	Brain oxygen monitoring may be utilized for patients needing titration of oxygen levels.
6.	Both hypocapnia and hypercapnia should be avoided. If hypercapnia occurs due to a lung-protective ventilation (LPV) strategy, normal pH should be ensured to avoid increases in ICP.

(C) *Lung-Protective vs. Neuroprotective Ventilation Strategy*: There is no one-size-fits-all mechanical ventilation approach for neurocritical care patients. The optimal ventilation parameters should be individualized based on each patient's unique cerebral pathophysiology and the underlying mechanism of lung injury, aiming to minimize additional brain and lung damage.

Protective tidal volumes of 6–8 ml/kg and plateau pressures below 30 cm H_2O have been recommended as ideal strategies in patients with brain injury with a PaO_2/FiO_2 ratio above 150 [12]. In contrast, tidal volumes of 4–6 ml/kg are usually recommended when the PaO_2/FiO_2 ratio < 150 [13]. Interestingly, in patients with acute brain injury (ABI), tidal volumes greater than 9 ml/kg have been identified as a risk factor for acute respiratory distress syndrome (ARDS) [14]. However, other studies did not confirm this association but did find that high driving pressures were linked to the development of ARDS [15].

In the BIVILI study, a ventilation strategy with tidal volume <8 ml/kg, positive end-expiratory pressure (PEEP) of 6–8 mmHg, and early extubation reduced the duration of MV and mortality in neuro-ICU patients [16]. A recent meta-analysis also found that low tidal volume (<8 ml/kg) and moderate-to-high PEEP (>5 cm H_2O) did not increase the incidence of ARDS or mortality in neuro-ICU patients undergoing mechanical ventilation while improving oxygenation and being safely applicable in this setting [17].

Another important aspect of LPV, which is to be considered in ABI, is the PEEP, with high levels (PEEP ≥15 cm H_2O) being recommended only in cases of moderate-to-severe ARDS [18]. In a study of brain-injured patients requiring MV with PEEP increments, an improvement in brain oxygenation was seen without any dangerous rises in ICP [13]. However, another study found contradictory results, showing that PEEP increments led to dangerously high levels of ICP, which necessitated interruptions of interventions, and that higher PEEP levels could benefit patients with lower brain tissue oxygen levels [19].

To summarize, a personalized approach should be employed to select the right ventilation strategy for patients with ABI, depending on whether the patient has a significantly high intracranial pressure (ICP) or acute respiratory distress syndrome (ARDS) and its severity. The recent european society of intensive care medicine (ESCIM) consensus recommends the following strategy in patients with ABI.

(i) *Patients Without Significant High ICP*: For patients on mechanical ventilation without significant high ICP, lung-protective ventilation may be recommended for patients with ARDS using low tidal volumes (6–8 ml/kg predicted body weight (PBW)) and ensuring that plateau pressures remain below 30 cm H_2O to minimize the risk of ventilator-induced lung injury (VILI).

(ii) *Patients with Significant High ICP*: The implementation of a lung-protective ventilation (LPV) strategy must consider the primary brain injury, the patient's clinical status, current brain imaging findings, and the presence of intracranial monitoring. While the benefits of LPV remain debated in the absence of lung injury, cerebral physiology often guides management. This approach becomes particularly challenging when acute respiratory distress syndrome (ARDS) coexists. Continuous monitoring of ICP and cerebral perfusion pressure (CPP)

Table 13.2 Key points in lung-protective ventilation

LPV strategy with TV of 6–8 ml/kg should be used in patients with ARDS without raised ICP.
The effect of ICP and CPP of LPV in patients with raised ICP is not clear. LPV can be utilized on a case-to-case basis with the monitoring of ICP and CPP.
Systemic hemodynamics must be maintained throughout.
No benefit of LPV in patients without ARDS.

is advisable in such cases, where mechanical ventilation may exacerbate cerebral compliance issues. Permissive hypercapnia can be considered if intracranial pressure (ICP) is managed with external ventricular drainage (EVD). Alternatively, increasing the respiratory rate up to the limit of auto-PEEP or plateau pressure might be necessary. However, since respiratory rate contributes to mechanical power (MP), merely increasing the rate to compensate for low tidal volumes (TV) may not be an effective solution for regulating $PaCO_2$ in ABI patients [14]. The key points in LPV are listed in Table 13.2.

(D) *Ventilatory Modes*: Two randomized controlled trials (RCTs) comparing different MV settings in Traumatic brain injury (TBI) patients found that pressure-regulated volume control (PRVC) modes had a lesser impact on intracranial compliance compared to pressure-controlled modes [20, 21].

(E) *Prone Position*: Prone positioning (PP) has demonstrated benefits in patients with severe ARDS [18]; however, evidence in those with deranged cerebral physiology is limited, as these patients have been excluded from most trials. A single-center study found that while the prone position prevented the worsening of respiratory parameters, it could still result in elevated ICP [22]. Therefore, in the absence of robust evidence in favor of PP, it should be considered in cases of refractory hypoxia.

(F) *Alveolar Recruitment Maneuvers*: Similarly, the use of recruitment maneuvers (RMs) in patients with ABI remains unvalidated for those with ARDS, with studies indicating a negative impact on survival [23], though some subgroups may benefit. Consequently, recruitment maneuvers should be performed under continuous neuromonitoring, with careful consideration of the benefit-to-risk ratio.

(G) *Extracorporeal Membrane Oxygenation*: Veno-venous extracorporeal membrane oxygenation (VV-ECMO) may have a role in managing severe ARDS; however, there is currently no evidence supporting its effectiveness in patients with acute brain injury (ABI). The use of ECMO in this population is particularly challenging due to the heightened risk of intracerebral hemorrhage associated with anticoagulation therapy. Further research is needed to evaluate the safety and efficacy of ECMO in the neurocritical care setting, focusing on balancing improved oxygenation with potential cerebral risks.

(H) *Advanced Modes of Ventilation in the NCCU*:

Airway pressure release ventilation (APRV) is an alternative strategy to inverse-ratio, pressure-controlled mode with a higher mean airway pressure as compared to LPV, which could be beneficial in neurologically ill patients with improved systemic and cerebral hemodynamics and reduced sedation requirements [24].

High-frequency oscillatory ventilation (HFOV) has been investigated as a potential salvage approach for adult brain-injured patients with acute lung injury (ALI) and acute respiratory distress syndrome (ARDS). However,

Table 13.3 Key points in advanced modes of ventilation in the NCCU

PRVC would be a safer option as compared to SIMV/VCV with respect to the maintenance of stable ICP and hemodynamics.
Prone positioning can be used in cases of refractory hypoxia.
Safety of ARM and ECMO has not been established in ABI.
APRV may be used as a rescue mode without increases in ICP. However, in deranged cerebral dynamics, it is best to do so under multimodal neuromonitoring.

SIMV synchronized intermittent mandatory ventilation, *VCV* volume-controlled ventilation, *ARM* alveolar recruitment maneuver

current evidence does not show a mortality benefit of HFOV in ARDS patients, and data, specifically for brain-injured patients, are insufficient to draw definitive conclusions. More research is needed to determine its safety and efficacy in this population. The key points in advanced ventilatory modes are enumerated in Table 13.3.

13.2 Extubation and Weaning in the NCCU

One of the major controversies in the intensive care management of neurocritical care population is the high extubation failure rate—reported to be as high as 15%—which has been associated with increased rates of VAP, prolonged ICU stays, and higher mortality [25, 26].

The most common reasons for delays in extubation are that either the underlying condition requiring mechanical ventilation has not been resolved or the assessment of the state of consciousness and readiness for extubation is variable. Regarding the second aspect, while some studies have found a Glasgow Coma Scale (GCS) score greater than 8 to be predictive of successful extubation [27], others have not found an association between GCS [28] or the full outline of unresponsiveness (FOUR) score [29, 30] and successful weaning from mechanical ventilation.

The VISAGE score, developed by Asehnoune et al., is a tool designed specifically for this population to predict successful extubation [31]. It includes four variables significantly associated with extubation success: visual pursuit, swallowing attempts, age under 40 years, and a GCS score greater than 10 points. A VISAGE score of ≥3 points predicts extubation success with a fair sensitivity and specificity.

Similarly, Cinotti et al. developed the extubation strategies in neuro-intensive care unit patients and associations with outcomes (ENIO) score [32] that included seven key predictors for successful extubation: traumatic brain injury diagnosis, vigorous cough, gag reflex, swallowing attempts, endotracheal suctioning frequency ≤ 2 hours, a GCS motor score of 6, and body temperature for extubation success in these subsets of patients.

13.3 Timing of Tracheostomy

The optimal timing of tracheostomy in ICU patients has been the subject of long-standing debates, with no firm evidence supporting early tracheostomy. The decision regarding the timing of tracheostomy varies significantly across different

Table 13.4 Key points in the setting of weaning in the NCCU

The VISAGE score and ENIO score are valid prediction scores to be used for extubation success in the NCCU.
Optimal timing of tracheostomy is still inconclusive and would depend on local policies.
Overall, early tracheostomy has no benefits in terms of the duration of MV, VAP, or mortality.

countries and institutes, often depending on local practices and policies. Therefore, reaching a consensus on the optimal timing of tracheostomy remains challenging. The international consensus statement was unable to provide a recommendation regarding the optimal timing of tracheostomy in patients with acute brain injury (ABI) due to contradictory low-quality evidence. Future studies with an aim to focus on reducing sedation and early weaning of patients with severe ABI to better determine the timing and potential benefits of tracheostomy are warranted. The key points in the area of weaning in the NCCU are listed in Table 13.4.

13.4 Ventilator-Associated Pneumonia (VAP) in Neurocritical Care

VAP is the most common nosocomial infection in the intensive care unit (ICU), with a notable impact on patients requiring invasive mechanical ventilation (IMV). In neurocritical care, the incidence of VAP is approximately 39%, as per the ENIO study [32].

Several risk factors contribute to the development of VAP in neurocritical care. Impaired consciousness due to ABI significantly increases the risk of aspiration, a major contributor to VAP. Additional risk factors include male gender, smoking habits, the use of intraparenchymal probes (IPs), external ventricular drains (EVDs), and therapeutic hypothermia. Sedation, often necessary for neurocritical care, further compromises airway protection, while tracheobronchitis during the ICU stay also poses a significant risk.

The controversies revolving around VAP are discussed below and are also listed in Table 13.5.

1. *Diagnosis of VAP*: Diagnosing VAP remains a challenge due to the lack of a universally accepted definition. In the neurocritical care population, diagnosing VAP is particularly problematic because clinical signs such as fever, leukocytosis, and altered mental status (all components of VAP definitions) are common in acute neurological diseases, regardless of infection. As per a study by Kalanuria et al. [33], only 31.3% of treated VAP cases had a diagnosis as per the centers for disease control (CDC) criteria, and the remaining 70% were solely based on clinical judgment, with the latter also receiving antibiotic treatment for a higher number of days.

Table 13.5 Key points regarding VAP

Aggressive threshold for diagnosis and proactive therapeutic approach to VAP exists in neurocritical care.
Sedation vacations and mobilization may be attempted safely when the primary lesion and ICP are stable.
Early mobilization(<24 hours) has been seen to be harmful in patients with stroke.
Selective digestive tract decontamination may be more beneficial in neurocritical care patients.
A single dose of ceftriaxone was seen to prevent VAP in TBI patients.
No role of inhaled antibiotics in preventing VAP. Can be used for treating VAP in combination with systemic regimens.

Therefore, in neurocritical patients, the intensivist must be aware of the lower threshold for diagnosing and treating VAP based on clinical criteria alone, which may lead to higher costs and more antibiotic resistance.

2. *VAP Prevention Bundles*: Various interventions, including the elevation of the head of the bed, daily sedation vacation and assessment of readiness to extubate, the use of subglottic secretion drainage, avoiding frequent ventilator circuit changes, oral hygiene, and stress ulcer prophylaxis, have been recommended in the literature as a bundle for prevention of VAP. Selective oropharyngeal decontamination (SOD) of the digestive tract is also a recommended protocol, with a 70% decrease in the incidence of VAP rates [21].

Although not much has been evaluated for VAP bundles in neurocritical care per se, many of the components could be difficult to implement in the NCCU, like daily sedation vacation, Spontaneous breathing trial (SBT), early mobilization, and deep vein thrombosis (DVT) prophylaxis, because of inherent issues in this population.

Sedation vacation and *early mobility*, although beneficial in the general critical care population [33, 34], with a significant reduction in hospital acquired pneumonia (HAP) and VAP rates [35], can be implemented for neurocritical care patients once the primary brain insult is stable.

Whereas there are concerns of these protocols with respect to alterations in cerebral physiology [36] in the neuro-ICU, it has been found to be feasible and safe, with reductions in VAP rates and the length of stay in the ICU [37, 38].

Selective decontamination of the digestive tract (SDD): which involves the application of topical, nonabsorbable antibiotics to the mouth and digestive tract, often combined with a short intravenous course of antibiotics lacking an anaerobic spectrum, is frequently debated for adoption in ICUs, primarily due to concerns over the potential for antimicrobial resistance (AMR). Whereas the SuDDICU trial [39], conducted in the low-AMR ICUs of Australia and New Zealand, did not show a significant mortality benefit from SDD, a post hoc analysis in the same trial revealed a 90-day mortality benefit of around 6% in a brain-injured cohort. A systematic review and meta-analysis incorporating this trial and 29 previous RCTs (including 24,034 adult ICU patients) found a 99% probability of reduction of mortality using SDD.

The use of *stress ulcer prophylaxis* in both general and neurocritical care studies has shown a potential risk of pneumonia with proton pump inhibitor (PPI) use compared to histamine-2 receptor antagonist (H2RA)s or no acid-suppressive therapy. While large RCTs and meta-analyses in general critical care show mixed results, large epidemiological studies often suggest an increased risk associated with PPIs. In neurocritical care, particularly among stroke patients, similar trends are observed, with PPIs posing a higher risk of pneumonia. However, the evidence is not entirely consistent, and further studies, particularly high-quality RCTs, are necessary to establish definitive conclusions.

Similarly, the benefit of *short-term antibiotic prophylaxis* for the prevention of VAP remains debated. In a recent multicenter study done at eight intensive care units in France (the PROPHYVAP study) in patients with acute brain injury, a single ceftriaxone dose decreased the risk of early VAP.

3. *Role of Aerosolized Antibiotic Therapy in the Prevention and Treatment of VAP.*

The ongoing debate regarding the evidence for inhaled antibiotics is supported by animal studies showing significantly higher pulmonary concentrations in the lungs compared to parenteral injections [3]. Additionally, since systemic absorption is limited, plasma levels remain much lower than expected with intravenous administration [4]. These low systemic concentrations may reduce overall antibiotic exposure and may counterintuitively increase AMR [5]. Currently, the Infectious Diseases Society of America and the American Thoracic Society recommend the use of inhaled antibiotics solely as a last resort to treat refractory VAP unresponsive to conventional systemic antibiotic therapy [8].

The quality of evidence in comatose patients is even lower, and all the studies in this population were done more than 2 decades ago using endotracheal instillation, which is again an unreliable method for the delivery of antibiotics as compared to nebulization, either by ultrasonic or mesh nebulizers.

13.5 Conclusion

To conclude, mechanical ventilation in neurocritical care is a delicate balancing act, requiring individualized strategies based on the patient's neurological condition and overall hemodynamic status. Close monitoring and tailored interventions are essential to minimize secondary brain injury and improve patient outcomes. Most of the evidence directly stems from the general critical care population, which may have a varying effect in this subset, leaving room for future research to explore the specific impact of mechanical ventilation in neurocritical care patients. Further studies are needed to refine ventilation strategies and improve management protocols for this unique group.

References

1. Asehnoune K, Roquilly A, Cinotti R. Respiratory management in patients with severe brain injury. Crit Care. 2018;22:76.
2. Rezoagli E, Petrosino M, Rebora P, CENTER-TBI, OzENTER-TBI Participants and Investigators, et al. High arterial oxygen levels and supplemental oxygen administration in traumatic brain injury: insights from CENTER-TBI and OzENTER-TBI. Intensive Care Med. 2022;48(12):1709–25.
3. Okonkwo DO, Shutter LA, Moore C, et al. Brain oxygen optimization in severe traumatic brain injury phase-II: a phase II randomized trial. Crit Care Med. 2017;45(11):1907–14.
4. Lång M, Skrifvars MB, Siironen J, et al. A pilot study of hyperoxemia on neurological injury, inflammation and oxidative stress. Acta Anaesthesiol Scand. 2018;62(6):801–10.
5. Janz DR, Hollenbeck RD, Pollock JS, et al. Hyperoxia is associated with increased mortality in patients treated with mild therapeutic hypothermia after sudden cardiac arrest. Crit Care Med. 2012;40:3135–9.
6. Hirunpattarasilp C, Shiina H, Na-Ek N, et al. The effect of hyperoxemia on neurological outcomes of adult patients: a systematic review and meta-analysis. Neurocrit Care. 2022;36(3):1027–43.
7. Semler MW, Casey JD, Lloyd BD, et al. Oxygen-saturation targets for critically ill adults receiving mechanical ventilation. N Engl J Med. 2022;387(19):1759–69.
8. Klitgaard TL, Schjørring OL, Nielsen FM, et al. Higher versus lower fractions of inspired oxygen or targets of arterial oxygenation for adults admitted to the intensive care unit. Cochrane Database Syst Rev. 2023;9(9):CD012631.
9. Robba C, Poole D, McNett M, et al. Mechanical ventilation in patients with acute brain injury: recommendations of the European society of intensive care medicine consensus. Intensive Care Med. 2020;46(12):2397–410.
10. van den Brink WA, van Santbrink H, Steyerberg EW, et al. Brain oxygen tension in severe head injury. Neurosurgery. 2000;46:868–76.
11. Tiruvoipati R, Pilcher D, Botha J, et al. Association of hypercapnia and hypercapnic acidosis with clinical outcomes in mechanically ventilated patients with cerebral injury. JAMA Neurol. 2018;75:818–26.
12. Deng RM, Liu YC, Li JQ, et al. The role of carbon dioxide in acute brain injury. Med Gas Res. 2020;10(2):81–4.
13. Fan E, Del Sorbo L, Goligher EC, et al. An official American thoracic society/European society of intensive care medicine/society of critical care medicine clinical practice guideline: mechanical ventilation in adult patients with acute respiratory distress syndrome. Am J Respir Crit Care Med. 2017;195:1253–63.
14. Picetti E, Pelosi P, Taccone FS, et al. On the behalf of the ESICM NIC/ARF sections. VENTILatOry strategies in patients with severe traumatic brain injury: the VENTILO survey of the European Society of Intensive Care Medicine (ESICM). Crit Care. 2020;24(1):158.
15. Mascia L, Zavala E, Bosma K, et al. High tidal volume is associated with the development of acute lung injury after severe brain injury: an international observational study. Crit Care Med. 2007;35:1815–20.
16. Tejerina E, Pelosi P, Muriel A, et al. Association between ventilatory settings and development of acute respiratory distress syndrome in mechanically ventilated patients due to brain injury. J Crit Care. 2017;38:341–5.
17. Asehnoune K, Mrozek S, Perrigault PF, et al. A multi-faceted strategy to reduce ventilation-associated mortality in brain-injured patients. The BI-VILI project: a nationwide quality improvement project. Intensive Care Med. 2017;43:957–70.

18. Asehnoune K, Rooze P, Robba C, et al. Mechanical ventilation in patients with acute brain injury: a systematic review with meta-analysis. Crit Care. 2023;27(1):221.
19. Gouvea Bogossian E, Cantos J, Farinella A, et al. The effect of increased positive end expiratory pressure on brain tissue oxygenation and intracranial pressure in acute brain injury patients. Sci Rep. 2023;13(1):16657.
20. Beqiri E, Smielewski P, Guérin C, et al. Neurological and respiratory effects of lung protective ventilation in acute brain injury patients without lung injury: brain vent, a single centre randomized interventional study. Crit Care. 2023;27(1):115.
21. Aghadavoudi O, Alikiaii B, Sadeghi F. Comparison of respiratory and hemodynamic stability in patients with traumatic brain injury ventilated by two ventilator modes: pressure regulated volume control versus synchronized intermittent mechanical ventilation. Adv Biomed Res. 2016;5:175.
22. Schirmer-Mikalsen K, Vik A, Skogvoll E, et al. Intracranial pressure during pressure control and pressure-regulated volume control ventilation in patients with traumatic brain injury: a randomized crossover trial. Neurocrit Care. 2016;24(3):332–41.
23. Beuret P, Carton MJ, Nourdine K, et al. Prone position as prevention of lung injury in comatose patients: a prospective, randomized, controlled study. Intensive Care Med. 2002;28:564–9.
24. Cavalcanti AB, Suzumura EA, Laranjeira LN, et al. Effect of lung recruitment and titrated positive end-expiratory pressure (PEEP) vs low peep on mortality in patients with acute respiratory distress syndrome: a randomized clinical trial. JAMA. 2017;318:1335–45.
25. Edgerton CA, Leon SM, Hite MA, et al. Airway pressure release ventilation does not increase intracranial pressure in patients with traumatic brain injury with poor lung compliance. J Crit Care. 2019;50:118–21.
26. Karanjia N, Nordquist D, Stevens R, et al. A clinical description of extubation failure in patients with primary brain injury. Neurocrit Care. 2011;15(1):4–12.
27. Coplin WM, Pierson DJ, Cooley KD, et al. Implications of extubation delay in brain-injured patients meeting standard weaning criteria. Am J Respir Crit Care Med. 2000;161(5):1530–6.
28. Namen AM, Ely EW, Tatter SB, et al. Predictors of successful extubation in neurosurgical patients. Am J Respir Crit Care Med. 2001;163(3 Pt 1):658–64.
29. Mahanes D, Lewis R. Weaning of the neurologically impaired patient. Crit Care Nurs Clin North Am. 2004;16(3):387–93.
30. Ko R, Ramos L, Chalela JA. Conventional weaning parameters do not predict extubation failure in neurocritical care patients. Neurocrit Care. 2009;10(3):269–73.
31. Asehnoune K, Seguin P, Lasocki S, ATLANREA group, et al. Extubation success prediction in a multicentric cohort of patients with severe brain injury. Anesthesiology. 2017;127(2):338–46.
32. Cinotti R, Mijangos JC, Pelosi P, ENIO Study Group, the PROtective VENTilation Network, the European Society of Intensive Care Medicine, the Colegio Mexicano de Medicina Critica, the Atlanréa group and the Société Française d'Anesthésie-Réanimation–SFAR Research Network, et al. Extubation in neurocritical care patients: the ENIO international prospective study. Intensive Care Med. 2022;48(11):1539–50.
33. Moscote-Salazar LR, Florez-Perdomo WA, Janjua T. Sedation vacation in neurocritical care: a proposal algorithm. Indian J Neurotrauma. 2023;21(01):87–90.
34. Bailey P, Thomsen GE, Spuhler VJ, et al. Early activity is feasible and safe in respiratory failure patients. Crit Care Med. 2007;35(1):139–45.
35. Morris PE, Goad A, Thompson C, et al. Early intensive care unit mobility therapy in the treatment of acute respiratory failure. Crit Care Med. 2008;36(8):2238–43.
36. Qi W, Murphy TE, Doyle MM, et al. Association between daily average of mobility achieved during physical therapy sessions and hospital-acquired or ventilator-associated pneumonia among critically ill patients. J Intensive Care Med. 2023;38(5):418–24.

37. Bartolo M, Bargellesi S, Castioni CA, et al. Intensive care and neurorehabilitation Italian study group; early rehabilitation for severe acquired brain injury in intensive care unit: multicenter observational study. Eur J Phys Rehabil Med. 2016;52(1):90–100.
38. Titsworth WL, Hester J, Correia T, et al. The effect of increased mobility on morbidity in the neurointensive care unit. J Neurosurg. 2012;116(6):1379–88.
39. SuDDICU Investigators for the Australian and New Zealand Intensive Care Society Clinical Trials Group, Myburgh JA, Seppelt IM, Goodman F, et al. Effect of selective decontamination of the digestive tract on hospital mortality in critically ill patients receiving mechanical ventilation: a randomized clinical trial. JAMA. 2022;328(19):1911–21.

Multimodal Monitoring in Neurocritical Care

14

Hirok Roy and Ashish Bindra

Abstract

Cerebral multimodal monitoring (MMM) offers diverse cerebral monitoring techniques, providing a vital and dynamic evaluation of brain function. It marks a considerable stride in neurocritical care. It enhances the precision of diagnosis, treatment, and prognosis in patients with acute neurological conditions and provides detailed insights into brain function and dynamics. It integrates several monitoring modalities of cerebral hemodynamics, oxygenation, and metabolism. The commonly used techniques include those measuring intracranial pressure (ICP), brain tissue oxygenation ($PbtO_2$), transcranial Doppler (TCD), continuous electroencephalography (cEEG), and near-infrared spectroscopy (NIRS). These techniques can be used individually or combined using an advanced interface. Advancements in multimodality monitoring have paved the way from fixed therapeutic targets toward a patient-specific approach. However, the literature is still evolving regarding therapeutic endpoints to be chased. Therefore, a know-how of the strengths and limitations of each monitoring system is of paramount importance. Implementing various monitoring systems can complicate data interpretation and increase both manpower and costs. Data is still evolving, and a clear benefit of MMM in outcomes remains to be established by robust research.

Keywords

Cerebral multimodal monitoring · Intracranial pressure · Brain tissue oxygenation · Transcranial Doppler · Continuous EEG · Near-infrared spectroscopy

H. Roy · A. Bindra (✉)
Neuroanaesthesiology and Critical Care, AIIMS, New Delhi, India

P. U. Bidkar, M. Krishnakumar (eds.), *Controversies in Neurocritical Care*,
https://doi.org/10.1007/978-981-95-4419-6_14

14.1 Introduction

The human brain is an intricate organ accountable for overseeing numerous bodily functions, including cognition, movement, and sensory perception. Cerebral pathophysiology delves into the detailed mechanisms underlying brain dysfunction, encompassing a wide range of neurological disorders, injuries, and diseases. An in-depth understanding of cerebral pathophysiology is crucial for clinicians to diagnose, treat, and manage conditions affecting the brain. The delicate pathophysiology of an acutely injured brain encompasses primary and secondary events working in tandem. The initial cerebral insult at the moment of impact constitutes the primary event, and the subsequent phenomenon resulting from ischemia and neurochemical pathways is described as the secondary event [1].

The concept of multimodal monitoring (MMM) was developed in the 1990s to provide a comprehensive real-time assessment of cerebral function [2]. In monitoring brain-injured patients, the importance of clinical examination cannot be overstated. Traditionally, monitoring relied on reactive measures, such as responding to a rise in intracranial pressure (ICP) and treating it accordingly. However, over time, management is shifting to a more proactive approach, addressing potential issues during the period before significant clinical deterioration occurs. Cerebral microdialysis (CMD) can predict cerebral ischemia before explicit clinical signs and symptoms appear. Clinical signs of neurological deterioration may evolve at a very late stage, leading to futile efforts to negate the secondary cerebral insults. This approach aims to capture the complex and dynamic nature of brain injury and enable the early detection of secondary insult before irreversible damage occurs.

Various neuromonitors proposed in neurocritical care track cerebral physiology, including hemodynamics, oxygenation, metabolism, and electrophysiology. However, no single monitoring modality is sufficient on its own; effective patient management relies on the interplay of various pathophysiological parameters. The integration of data from various monitoring systems offers a panoramic view of cerebral pathophysiology.

Instead of overwhelming intensivists with new variables, MMM integrates data from various sources to create an individualized "injury profile" for effective management. Given the complexity of the data and variables, it is crucial to aggregate and analyze this information in a clinician-friendly manner.

Although many monitors are well-established in the market, some are still finding their role in patient management, and others are currently being developed. In this chapter, we will discuss the role of commonly used bedside monitors in patient management.

14.2 Clinical Applications

MMM provides a detailed and real-time overview of cerebral physiology, facilitating timely and appropriate interventions to prevent secondary brain injury. It can be used for personalized targeted therapy following acute brain injury and also aids in prognostication. Table 14.1 defines the indication, range, and therapeutic targets of commonly used devices for neuromonitoring.

Table 14.1 Various cerebral monitoring modalities and their clinical applications

Modality	Pathological conditions	Normal value	Applications	Limitations
Transcranial Doppler (TCD) ultrasound [CBF monitor]	Vascular diseases (aSAH, TBI, stroke)	MCA: 55 ± 12 cm/s (toward the probe) ACA: 50 ± 11 cm/s (away from the probe) PCA 1: 39 ± 11 cm/s (toward the probe) PCA2: 40 ± 10 cm/s (away from the probe) BA: 41 ± 10 cm/s (away from the probe) VA: 38 ± 10 cm/s (away from the probe)	Noninvasive, repeatable, episodic/continuous measurements. Detects early signs of vasospasm and delayed cerebral ischemia (DCI). Noninvasive intracranial pressure. Cerebral autoregulation. Ancillary test for the determination of brain death.	Operator-dependent, absent bone acoustic window
Established monitor				
Near-infrared spectroscopy (NIRS) [cerebral oxygenation monitor]	Regional cerebral oxygenation in TBI, aSAH, stroke, carotid vessel disease. Cerebral autoregulation	Normal values: 60–80% Threshold not clearly defined; a decrease of 20% from baseline is suggestive of ischemia	Noninvasive, continuous. Regional cerebral oxygenation. Intracranial pressure. Pressure reactivity index.	Focal area is monitored, scalp injury, hematoma limits its efficacy
Evolving monitor				
qEEG [cerebral electrical activity, indirect monitor of cerebral metabolism monitor]	Primarily epileptic disorders, vascular diseases, TBI	NA	Continuous, noninvasive. Seizures. Nonconvulsive status. Depth of sedation. Prognostic tool after ischemic insult (HIBI). Ancillary test for brain death.	Possibility of misinterpretation
EEG is established, data evolving on qEEG				
Invasive intracranial pressure (ICP) [cerebral hemodynamics monitor]	TBI, aSAH, tumors, stroke, hepatic encephalopathy	Number and waveform analysis Threshold for intervention: *Number* Adults ≥22 mm Hg Children ≥20 mm Hg Infants ≥15 mm Hg *Waveform* P2 > P1	Continuous. Intracranial compliance, reactivity index.	Invasive Errors due to lack of recalibration and zero drift Infection

(continued)

Table 14.1 (continued)

Modality	Pathological conditions	Normal value	Applications	Limitations
Established monitor				
Brain tissue oxygenation ($PbtO_2$) [cerebral oxygenation monitor]	TBI, aSAH	Normal values: 35–50 mm Hg Threshold for intervention: Adults: ≤ 15–20 mm Hg Pediatric: ≤ 10 mm Hg	Continuous monitoring. Focal cerebral oxygenation, temperature. Useful to monitor the effects of therapeutic interventions.	Invasive, focal measurements
Established monitor				
Cerebral microdialysis (CMD) [cerebral metabolism monitor]	TBI, aSAH	Threshold for intervention: Glucose ≤0.7–1.0 mmol/L LPR ≥ 40 Normal value: Glucose: 1.7–2.1 mmol/L Lactate: 2.9–3.1 mmol/L Pyruvate: 151–166 μmol/L LPR 19–23 Glycerol: 50–100 μmol/L Glutamate: 14–16 μmol/L	Direct measurement of metabolites in the brain	Invasive limited data available
Evolving monitor				
Cranial ultrasound Optic nerve sheath diameter (ONSD) [ICP monitor]	TBI, malignant infarct, tumor	ONSD more than 55 mm corresponds to an elevated ICP	Noninvasive. Rapid screening for raised ICP, midline shift, hematoma or tumor volume, lateral ventricle, midbrain.	Operator-dependent, poor acoustic window, ONSD cannot be used for guiding therapy, lack of data

Abbreviations: *ACA*, anterior cerebral artery, *BA* basilar artery, *CA* cerebral autoregulation, *cEEG* continuous EEG, *CMD* cerebral microdialysis, *qEEG* quantitative electroencephalography, *HIBI* hypoxic ischemic brain injury, *ICP* intracranial pressure, *MCA* middle cerebral artery, *NA* not applicable, *NCSE* nonconvulsive status epilepticus, *NIRS* near-infrared spectroscopy, *PCA* posterior cerebral artery, $PbtO_2$ brain tissue oxygen partial pressure, *TCD* transcranial Doppler, *VA* vertebral artery

14.3 Modalities

14.3.1 Transcranial Doppler Ultrasound

Transcranial Doppler (TCD) ultrasonography is used to study the intracranial blood flow, especially in the circle of Willis and carotid vessels. TCD-derived parameters, along with diagnostic imaging modalities, provide a holistic overview of cerebral blood flow dynamics. The core principle of insonating cerebral arteries is to measure parameters related to cerebral blood flow using the Doppler effect [3]. Traversing red blood cells in the blood vessels reflect the ultrasound (US) waves emitted by the probe, creating a Doppler shift. By analyzing these frequency changes of ultrasound waves reflected by the moving red blood cells, we can measure the blood flow velocity [4]. The parameters measured are average velocity (Vmean), peak systolic velocity (PSV), end-diastolic velocity (EDV), Gosling index/pulsatility index (PI), and Pourcelot index/resistance index (RI) [5]. A 2-MHz ultrasound probe is commonly used for intracranial vessels' examination, and a 4-MHz ultrasound probe is used for extracranial vessels' examination.

TCD parameters can be extrapolated to evaluate cerebral autoregulation (CA), cerebral perfusion pressure (CPP), and noninvasive ICP via advanced model-based algorithms.

TCD has been particularly utilized in the therapeutic management of subarachnoid hemorrhage (vasospasm), traumatic brain injury (TBI) (autoregulation and ICP), acute ischemic stroke, detection of cerebral microemboli, sickle cell disease (SCD), and carotid artery disease and as an ancillary tool in determining brain death. Vasospasm of the middle cerebral artery (MCA) and basilar artery (BA) can be detected with high specificity and sensitivity by TCD examination [6]. A Vmean >120 cm/s of MCA suggests mild vasospasm, whereas mean velocities higher than 200 cm/s are suggestive of severe vasospasm. Likewise, BA flow velocities exceeding 85 cm/s indicate moderate-to-severe vasospasm [7]. The ratio of the Vmean of the MCA to the ipsilateral extracranial internal carotid artery (ICA) is described as the Lindegaard ratio (LR). LR can be used to differentiate vasospasm from hyperemia, which can depict elevated mean flow velocities. An LR below 3 suggests hyperemia, whereas an LR above 3 is more suggestive of vasospasm [8]. Similarly, the Sviri ratio, derived by dividing the Vmean of the BA by that of the vertebral artery (extracranial), is utilized for identifying vasospasm in posterior circulation vessels [7].

TCD can be utilized to measure ICP noninvasively by deriving it from the blood flow velocities and pulsatility index (PI) [9]. Noninvasive ICP can be predicted using the equation, $ICP = (10.93 \times PI) - 1.28$, exhibiting an 89% sensitivity and a 92% specificity [10].

TCD can be used for the management of stroke and microemboli detection. TCD can be used to detect recanalization and evaluate the efficacy of therapeutic intervention by using the thrombolysis in brain ischemia (TIBI) score, post-thrombolysis in acute ischemic stroke [11]. The occurrence of microemboli leads to momentary interruptions in the TCD waves, giving rise to high-intensity transient signals

(HITS). TCD can be used in the management of patients with sickle cell anemia. Sickle-shaped red blood cells have a tendency to adhere to the endothelium, causing accumulation, which causes narrowing or blockage of blood vessels. A Vmean in ICA or MCA exceeding 200 cm/s is linked to a higher likelihood of ischemic stroke in individuals having SCD [12].

14.3.1.1 Pitfalls

Transcranial Doppler (TCD) is an effective tool and a key component of cerebral MMM, but it does have limitations. TCD provides a snapshot view of cerebrovascular anatomy and is highly dependent on the operator's skill. The incident angle of ultrasound waves in relation to the blood vessel should be less than 30 degrees; otherwise, it results in spurious flow velocities. In 10% of the general population, the absence of an acoustic window can impede TCD examination [13]. Several physiological factors can influence cerebral blood flow velocities, including factors such as age, gender, levels of carbon dioxide (CO_2) or oxygen (O_2) partial pressure, blood pressure, hematocrit levels, and pregnancy [5]. Furthermore, measurements of flow velocities in other cerebral vessels, excluding MCA and distal vessels, were found to be less sensitive and specific for detecting vasospasm.

14.3.2 Near-Infrared Spectroscopy

Near-infrared spectroscopy (NIRS) is a noninvasive method for the assessment of regional brain oxygenation. It is also an indirect indicator of cerebral perfusion and correlates well with other established techniques [14–16]. It assesses the regional tissue oxygenation by calculating the ratio of oxyhemoglobin (O_2Hb) concentration to the combined amount of O_2Hb and reduced hemoglobin [17]. The principle behind NIRS lies in near-infrared wavelengths (700–1000 nm) being capable of penetrating the skin and subcutaneous tissue, cranium, and brain to a certain distance. Based on the modified Beer–Lambert law, reflectance spectroscopy is used to determine the optical attenuation. Optodes are positioned on one side of the forehead with a distance between them of 4–7 cm, allowing for the estimation of oxygen levels in all vascular components, including arterial, capillary, and venous compartments [18]. Typical values of regional Oxygen Saturation (rSO_2) are in the range of 60–80%. A decrease of 20% or more in rSO_2 values from the baseline is indicative of an ischemic event [18]. NIRS is valuable for monitoring the "watershed" area of the brain that receives blood supply from the anterior cerebral artery (ACA) and middle cerebral artery (MCA) territories. This creates a distinctive scenario where ACA–MCA vasospasm can be monitored, and it is advantageous over TCD since the latter is less sensitive for detecting ACA vasospasm [19]. NIRS can be useful for the management of blood transfusion strategy, especially in the critically ill [20]. NIRS can be utilized to guide therapy in TBI and intracerebral hemorrhage (ICH), as well as in individuals undergoing carotid endarterectomy.

14.3.2.1 Pitfalls

NIRS may not be a reliable tool in patients having underlying cerebral hematoma, scalp lacerations, and calvarial implants and during the administration of certain contrast agents. rSO_2 values are to be interpreted on the basis of emerging trends rather than the absolute value at any single point of time. Studies are lacking regarding NIRS-based management and its effect on outcomes.

14.3.3 Brain Tissue Oxygenation ($PbtO_2$)

$PbtO_2$ is a monitor of brain tissue oxygenation. Ensuring adequate oxygen supply to the brain is crucial in managing acute brain injuries, making $PbtO_2$ monitoring essential, alongside other MMM techniques. Increased ICP can disrupt diffusion, leading to ischemic risks in TBI. $PbtO_2$ monitoring confers a more accurate assessment of tissue oxygenation and correlates more directly with neurological outcomes than ICP values alone. Two probes commonly used for invasive brain tissue oxygen monitoring are the Licox (Integra LifeSciences, Plainsboro, NJ) and Neurovent-PTO systems(Raumedic multiparameter sensor, Munchberg, Germany) [21]. These systems also include ICP and temperature monitors, along with the probe. Normal $PbtO_2$ values range from 25 to 50 mm Hg. Values of $PbtO_2 < 10$ mm Hg are suggestive of severe brain ischemia, and values <5 mm Hg indicate cell death [22].

$PbtO_2$ has shown promising results with numerous studies showing the correlation between decreased $PbtO_2$ and worse neurological prognosis after TBI, independent of ICP and CPP [23, 24]. In TBI, it is recommended to maintain $PbtO_2 > 20$ mm Hg [25]. The BOOST-II trial compared ICP-guided with both ICP and $PbtO_2$–guided management of patients with severe TBI. The combination of $PbtO_2$ and ICP monitoring resulted in more favorable outcomes, decreased brain tissue oxygenation, and reduced mortality in comparison to stand-alone ICP monitoring [26]. The BOOST-III trial will further assess the effect of this MMM on neurological outcomes [27].

The recent French OXY-TC trial found that combined ICP and $PbtO_2$–guided management did not reduce the incidence of adverse neurological outcomes [28]. Various trials, viz. BOOST-III and the Brain Oxygen Neuromonitoring in Australia and New Zealand Assessment (BONANZA) trial (ACTRN12619001328167), are underway to assess the efficacy of tiered algorithms using combined ICP and $PbtO_2$ measurements [27, 29].

14.3.3.1 Pitfalls

Although invasive $PbtO_2$ monitoring is corroborated by extensive literature, it has its inherent limitations. As an invasive procedure, it carries a risk of hemorrhage and infection, though these complications occur in less than 1% of cases [30]. The device measures around 15 mm^2 near the catheter tip, providing a focal rather than a global assessment of brain tissue oxygenation [21]. Other drawbacks include the risk of hyperoxia from overzealous treatment and possible catheter and device malfunctions.

14.3.4 Intracranial Pressure (ICP)

Despite various ongoing debates regarding the utility of ICP monitoring, ICP is a key element in guiding therapy for acutely injured brain, particularly TBI [31]. On the basis of the Monro–Kellie doctrine, elevated ICP can lead to herniation syndromes or secondary injuries due to reduced CPP. Continuous ICP monitoring is proposed for severe TBI, tumors, malignant ischemic strokes, intracerebral hemorrhage, or aneurysmal subarachnoid hemorrhage (aSAH). ICP can be measured invasively with external ventricular drains (EVDs) or monitoring devices implanted in the intraparenchymal, epidural, subdural, or subarachnoid spaces. Commonly used methods are intraventricular catheters and intraparenchymal microtransducer sensors, such as the Codman microsensor (Johnson and Johnson Professional Inc., Raynham, Mass.) or the Integra Camino sensor (Camino Laboratories, San Diego, Calif.). Monitoring techniques like TCD, pupillometry, and optic nerve sheath diameter (ONSD) can be employed to estimate ICP noninvasively.

Furthermore, ICP monitoring enables the computation of CPP and the evaluation of cerebral compliance, cerebrovascular reactivity, and autoregulatory function. The Brain Trauma Foundation (BTF) guidelines (4e) recommend the utility of monitoring of ICP, which will be beneficial to decrease the mortality of patients during hospital stay and within 2 weeks of injury [25]. It is crucial to not only monitor the absolute ICP value but also simultaneously analyze the accompanying waveforms. ICP waveforms can reveal deteriorating pressure dynamics, such as the presence of pathological Lundberg waves.

14.3.5 Recent Trends in ICP Monitoring: ICP Burden, Waveform Analysis, and the Use of Brain Models

Assessing the total duration and magnitude of increased ICP has a better prognostic value than a single, episodic rise in ICP [32]. However, such values are only possible with minute-to-minute recording of ICP and other hemodynamic parameters to obtain color-coded plots and thus require additional software and monitoring logistics. Likewise, a multicenter study by the BrainIT group showcased that a machine learning model could accurately forecast ICP elevations 30 min in advance by analyzing ICP and mean arterial pressure (MAP) data from the previous 5 h [33]. A multimodal approach that integrates metrics like brain autoregulation and oxygenation would be ideal. This requires advancements in hardware to support integrated sensors and in computational algorithms to process and analyze multiple continuous neuromonitoring data streams. Furthermore, the ongoing development of noninvasive ICP sensors holds promise for reducing the need for invasive interventions in various patient populations.

It is advisable to utilize ICP and CPP adjusted to the patient's autoregulation, which ensures individualized optimal ICP and CPP targets on the basis of pressure reactivity index [34]. Individual-specific ICP targets can be more effective predictors of poorer outcomes compared to the predetermined ICP target of 20–25 mm Hg.

14.3.5.1 Pitfalls

Epidural, subdural, or subarachnoid bolt devices have demonstrated lower accuracy and are consequently infrequently employed. Although intraparenchymal sensors offer dependable ICP values, certain models have recalibration issues, making them more susceptible to zero drift over extended periods of use. Furthermore, in a scenario of a focal lesion, there is a likelihood that pressure values may depict an interhemispheric ICP gradient rather than an absolute ICP value. The lack of cerebrospinal fluid (CSF) drainage capabilities and expense further restrict the utilization.

Noninvasive ICP monitoring methods have advantages of a reduced risk of complications, continuous monitoring capabilities, cost-effectiveness compared to invasive methods, and potential for early intervention based on ICP trends. However, they are highly operator-dependent and may affect the accuracy and reliability when compared to invasive techniques.

14.3.6 Cerebral Metabolism Monitoring

Cerebral microdialysis (CMD) evaluates brain metabolism by analyzing compounds of energy metabolism like glucose, lactate, pyruvate, glycerol, and glutamate [35]. A CMD catheter contains a semipermeable membrane, usually of 20 kDa, placed in the area of interest of the cerebral parenchyma. A CSF-like solution is continuously flushed through the catheter, which allows periodic sampling of the brain extracellular fluid for analysis. Catheter placement depends on cerebral pathology, perilesional for focal lesions, diffuse injury requires placement in right frontal lobe, and vasospastic territory for aSAH. Interventions are needed if glucose levels fall below 0.8 mM or if the lactate-to-pyruvate ratio (LPR) exceeds 40. Studies have shown that increased LPR occurs 11–13 h before the onset of clinical delayed cerebral ischemia (DCI) in patients with aSAH [36]. The utility of CMD has been confirmed in various conditions, viz. TBI, aSAH, epilepsy, ischemic stroke, and tumors, and in the context of neurosurgical procedures [37]. Clinical applications of CMD, investigating various biomarkers, glycemic status, and their interaction within cerebral metabolic homeostasis, are being undertaken and will strengthen the efficacy of CMD-guided interventions [38].

14.3.6.1 Pitfalls

Besides being expensive, invasive, and labor-intensive, the supporting evidence of using CMD in relation to favorable neurological outcomes is scarce [39, 40]. The placement position of the catheter needs to be checked by computed tomography (CT) scan. The position of the catheter tip can affect the value of biochemical substrates. A significant drawback of this method is the lack of continuous monitoring, as existing devices necessitate hourly analyses of the dialysate.

14.3.7 Quantitative EEG (qEEG)

In critically ill patients, various types of seizure disorders are encountered, with incidences occurring in up to 40% of cases [41]. Abnormal motor activities are often encountered, but they may be due to non-epileptogenic causes. However, convulsive seizures can still occur, alongside these non-epileptic movements. qEEG provides continuous real-time monitoring (Fig. 14.1). Indications include identifying non-convulsive seizures, characterizing seizures, guiding therapy, detecting ischemia, and assessing prognosis following events like cardiac arrest or brain injury [42–45].

14.3.7.1 Pitfalls

Using qEEG as the exclusive method for EEG interpretation is not recommended, and raw EEG readings must be interpreted with electrographic correlation. There is a risk of misinterpreting rhythmic or periodic EEG patterns as an indication of seizure activity or potentially obscuring the progression of seizures in qEEG-automated seizure detection.

14.3.8 Brain Ultrasound (US) in Neurocritical Care

Brain US is a noninvasive modality that is used to see the brain structure, vascular anatomy, and optic nerve sheath diameter. US is increasingly used to determine the

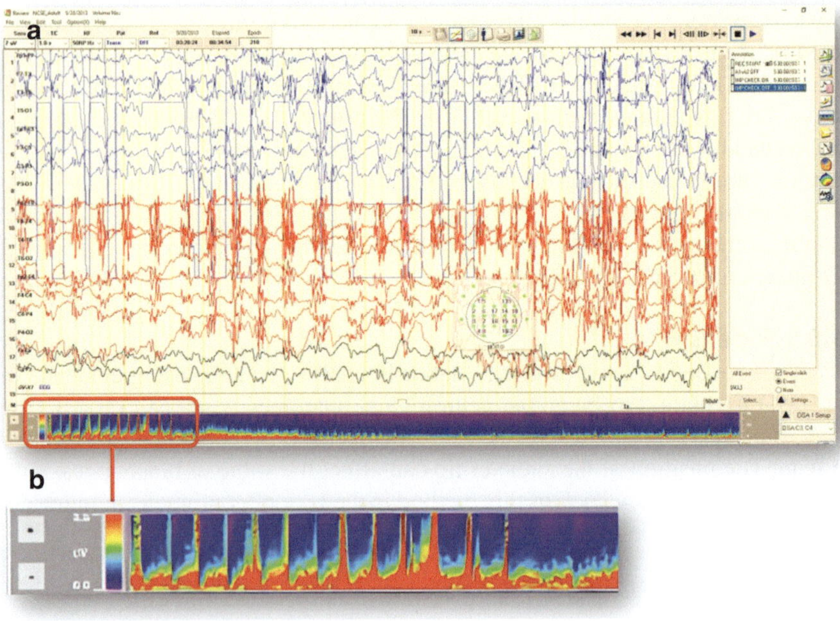

Fig. 14.1 qEEG recordings in critically ill patients with seizure: (**a**) EEG waveform showing convulsive activity and (**b**) qEEG spectrogram showing flame pattern, indicative of seizure activity

intracranial hematoma volume, identify the third ventricle dilatation, and determine the midline shift [46].

Anatomically, a dural sheath encases the optic nerve while it traverses down to the orbit. Increased ICP can cause the optic nerve sheath to expand, which can be assessed by trans-ocular ultrasound (Fig. 14.2). Studies show a strong correlation between invasive ICP measurements and ONSD via ultrasound, with 90% sensitivity and 85% specificity [47]. ONSD measuring 5.6 mm can be considered a cut-off for detecting raised ICP in adults [48]. The value may vary depending upon age, gender, ethnicity, and ultrasound technique.

14.3.9 Emerging Trends in ONSD

Ophthalmic ultrasound is being explored for new insights, with optical coherence tomography (OCT) showing promise in assessing ICP in children [49]. Some research suggests that the ONSD/eye transverse diameter (ETD) ratio may offer a better predictive value than ONSD alone, though further study is needed [50]. Additionally, the deformability index (DI), a new ultrasound-based optic nerve sheath parameter, shows potential for noninvasively assessing ICP [51].

14.3.9.1 Pitfalls

ONSD measurements are not suitable in a scenario of facial or globe injury or any medical conditions that may impact ONSD, such as Graves' disease or sarcoidosis. Its specificity is reported to decline in response to acute variations in ICP. ONSD measurements may serve as a valuable preliminary tool for assessing ICP in scenarios where immediate invasive ICP monitoring is not feasible.

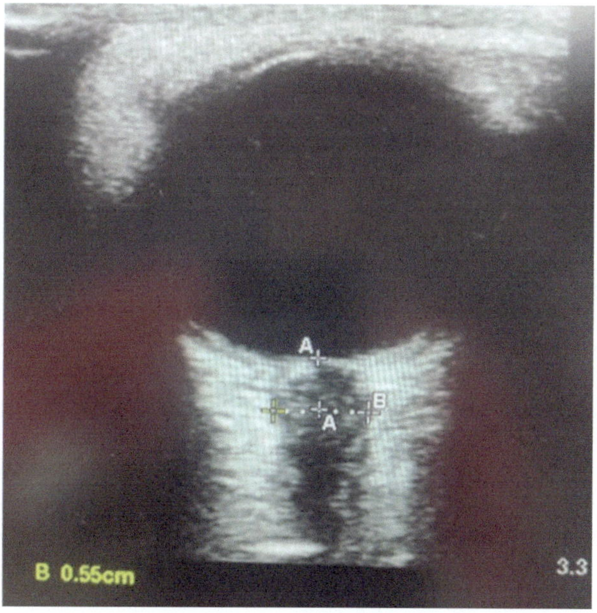

Fig. 14.2 Ultrasound showing ONSD measurement

14.3.10 Pupilometer

A pupillometer is a handheld device used to measure the pupillary size and reactivity to light with high precision and objectivity. Unlike manual pupil assessments, pupillometers provide quantitative measurements of pupil size and reactivity and reduce interobserver variability. Neurological Pupil Index (NPi), a quantitative measurement derived from pupillometry, can assess the pupillary light reflex (PLR). It is a composite score ranging from 0 to 5, with higher values indicating normal pupillary function and lower values suggesting impairment. Mobile-based pupillometry applications are also being developed as technology advances [52].

The subtle changes in pupil dynamics indicate rising intracranial pressure, brainstem dysfunction, or other neurological deteriorations. It can be used as a modality for detecting raised ICP. Numerous studies have explored the relationship between pupillometry and elevated ICP [53]. Noninvasive techniques like optic nerve sheath diameter and pupillometry are being studied as effective supplementary screening tools for severe TBI [54]. The prognosis and survival of the patient following brain injury can be accurately predicted by PLR [55].

14.3.10.1 Pitfalls

While there is growing evidence supporting its usage, much of it comes from small studies. However, the initial pupil size and reflexes may differ among individuals. Various aspects like the type of device, exposure duration and intensity of light source, and the patient's physical status also vary across trials. Furthermore, the use of several variables, including NPi, dilatation velocity, constriction velocity, and latency, complicates data interpretation and cross-study comparisons. However, automated pupillometry holds potential in clinical practice.

14.3.11 Controversies in MMM

14.3.11.1 Continuous Versus Episodic Monitoring Strategies

The choice between continuous versus episodic monitoring strategies has the potential to impact patient outcomes. Each strategy has its advantages and challenges, and the best option typically resides in the specific clinical context, available resources, and specific patient needs.

Continuous cerebral MMM involves the uninterrupted collection and analysis of physiological data over an extended period, often critical for capturing dynamic changes in brain function in real time. The advantages include real-time and immediate detection of variables being monitored like ICP, CPP, and $PbtO_2$, which allows for proactive management. It enables early detection of secondary insults like seizures and ischemic events. Proactive management of critical thresholds has the potential to mitigate secondary brain injury and improve long-term outcomes. Continuous data collection supports the refinement of therapeutic strategies, including ventilation adjustments, osmotherapy, and perfusion management [56].

However, such a strategy is resource-intensive and needs dedicated personnel to interpret the data and respond promptly, resulting in increased cost and the need for specialized training. Continuous data streams can lead to information overload, demanding sophisticated integration systems and analytics to differentiate between actionable changes and normal variability. Prolonged use of invasive monitoring devices increases the risk of infections.

Two common clinical scenarios for continuous MMM include TBI, where ICP, CPP, and $PbtO_2$ are monitored for managing secondary injuries, and aSAH, where continuous TCD and EEG allow prompt detection of vasospasm and delayed cerebral ischemia [57]. The Seattle International Severe Traumatic Brain Injury Consensus Conference (SIBICC) suggested a tiered protocol using ICP and PbtO2 monitoring for severe TBI [58].

Episodic cerebral MMM involves the periodic assessment of physiological parameters, relying on scheduled or clinically indicated intervals rather than continuous data collection. It is resource-efficient and provides targeted data that can be sufficient for making clinical decisions. However, episodic monitoring can miss transient or rapidly evolving events like sudden increases in ICP, hypoxic episodes, or seizure activity, resulting in a delay in intervention. So it tends to be reactive rather than proactive, often intervening after significant changes have already occurred.

The choice between continuous and episodic monitoring should be individualized based on patient needs, clinical settings, available resources, and the specific neurological condition being managed. The integration of both strategies in a flexible manner, adapting to the evolving clinical context, can optimize the care and outcomes for neurocritical care patients (Fig. 14.3).

14.3.12 Role of Patient-Specific Thresholds Versus Standard Protocols

Standard protocols refer to predefined clinical guidelines based on population-level evidence and expert consensus. These protocols provide general thresholds and management strategies that are widely accepted in clinical practice. They provide a reliable framework for managing common neurocritical care scenarios and ensure a consistent approach across different healthcare providers and institutions. As they provide clear, actionable guidelines, they can be readily applied in various clinical settings and reduce complexity and decision-making burden on clinicians. At the same time, these protocols are not individualized to patient pathophysiology and do not adjust for dynamic changes in patient condition.

Patient-specific thresholds involve tailoring monitoring and management strategies to the unique physiological and clinical characteristics of an individual patient. They have the potential to lead to more precise and effective interventions, improving patient outcomes [59, 60]. Continuous monitoring of data facilitates real-time adjustments to the changing dynamics of the patient. However, it is complex and

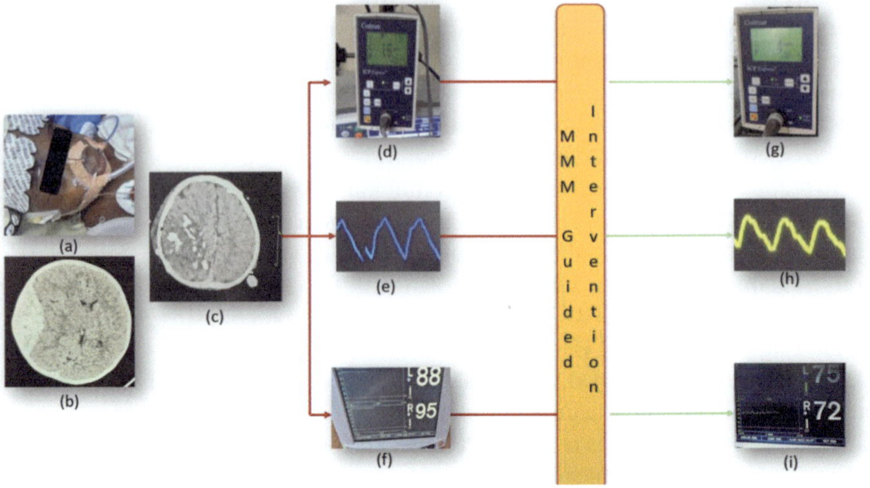

Fig. 14.3 Case scenario: (**a**) A 3-year-old child with a history of fall from height came with severe TBI; (**b**) initial computed tomography (CT) scan revealed a right parietal extradural hematoma, which was surgically evacuated; (**c**) the patient developed right parieto-occipital venous infarct with hemorrhagic transformation on postoperative day 1. Multimodal neuromonitoring was done with (**d**) Codman ICP monitor, with (**e**) waveform analysis and (**f**) NIRS oximetry showing an elevated ICP with P2 > P1 waves and elevated rSO_2 values. MMM-guided therapy was instituted, resulting in (**g**) a decrease in ICP, with (**h**) the normalizing of ICP waveforms (P1 > P2), and (**i**) normal rSO_2 values

costly and needs trained manpower. It increases the cognitive load on clinicians to continuously interpret data to make individualized decisions. A high degree of variability in patient-specific thresholds may lead to inconsistencies in care if not managed appropriately. The potential for errors or misjudgments is high.

Optimal cerebral MMM involves a harmonious integration of standard protocols with patient-specific thresholds. This blended approach capitalizes on the strengths of each method, ensuring both evidence-based consistency and personalized precision in patient care. Standard protocols can be used for initial management and stabilization. As continuous monitoring data is collected, clinicians can adjust thresholds and interventions to better suit individual patient needs. Advanced analytics and decision support systems can aid in identifying appropriate patient-specific adjustments.

14.3.13 Integration of Multimodal Monitoring: Role of Artificial Intelligence

Artificial intelligence (AI) has transformed healthcare by improving data analysis and clinical decision-making. In MMM, AI processes and integrates data from various devices for a comprehensive brain function assessment [61]. Utilizing machine learning, deep learning, and advanced techniques, AI helps manage information overload and ensures timely interventions. AI is increasingly applied for triage, diagnosis, and management, with platforms like ICM+ (https://icmplus.neurosurg.cam.ac.uk) from the University of Cambridge and the Moberg (Moberg Solutions, Inc.; Ambler, PA) monitor integrating data from multiple systems. These innovations have significant potential to revolutionize neurological monitoring and treatment.

Applications of artificial intelligence in MMM are numerous and include the following:

Data integration and fusion: AI algorithms can merge data from different monitoring modalities such as EEG, NIRS, TCD, and ICP sensors to create a unified picture of cerebral function and hemodynamics.

Predictive analytics: AI models can potentially forecast neurological outcomes, predict trends in intracranial dynamics, and alert clinicians to impending changes in cerebral physiology before clinical symptoms manifest.

Decision support systems: AI-driven algorithm tools can aid health professionals in analyzing intricate monitoring data, suggesting treatment options, and enhancing patient management strategies in neurocritical care environments.

Personalized management: By analyzing individual patient data and adapting to unique physiological responses, AI technologies enable personalized treatment plans tailored to the specific needs of each patient undergoing multimodal neuromonitoring (Fig. 14.4).

However, there is a need for conducting robust clinical validation studies and real-world trials to demonstrate the efficacy, safety, and impact of AI-enhanced multimodal neuromonitoring on patient outcomes. It is of paramount importance to lay down regulatory usage guidelines, robust protection against any data/privacy breach, and a clear foundation of ethical use.

14.3.14 Current Scenario

However, the questions that need clear answers are the following: What should be monitored? How extensively should it be monitored? Should patient-specific thresholds or standard protocols be used for management? While using these combined modalities of neuromonitoring and MMM-driven interventions, multiple factors should be taken into account. Most of the indices of various monitoring modalities are from a small regional area of the brain, which may not be reflective of dynamic changes occurring elsewhere. During any cerebral insult, there may be diverse and opposing physiologies occurring simultaneously [62]. The feasibility of catching these variations over time requires high-frequency data acquisition, which is lacking at this juncture in certain neuromonitoring modalities. Hence, compilation of data from such devices with that from other data sources may lead to misinterpretation of the actual pathophysiology and misguided therapeutic interventions.

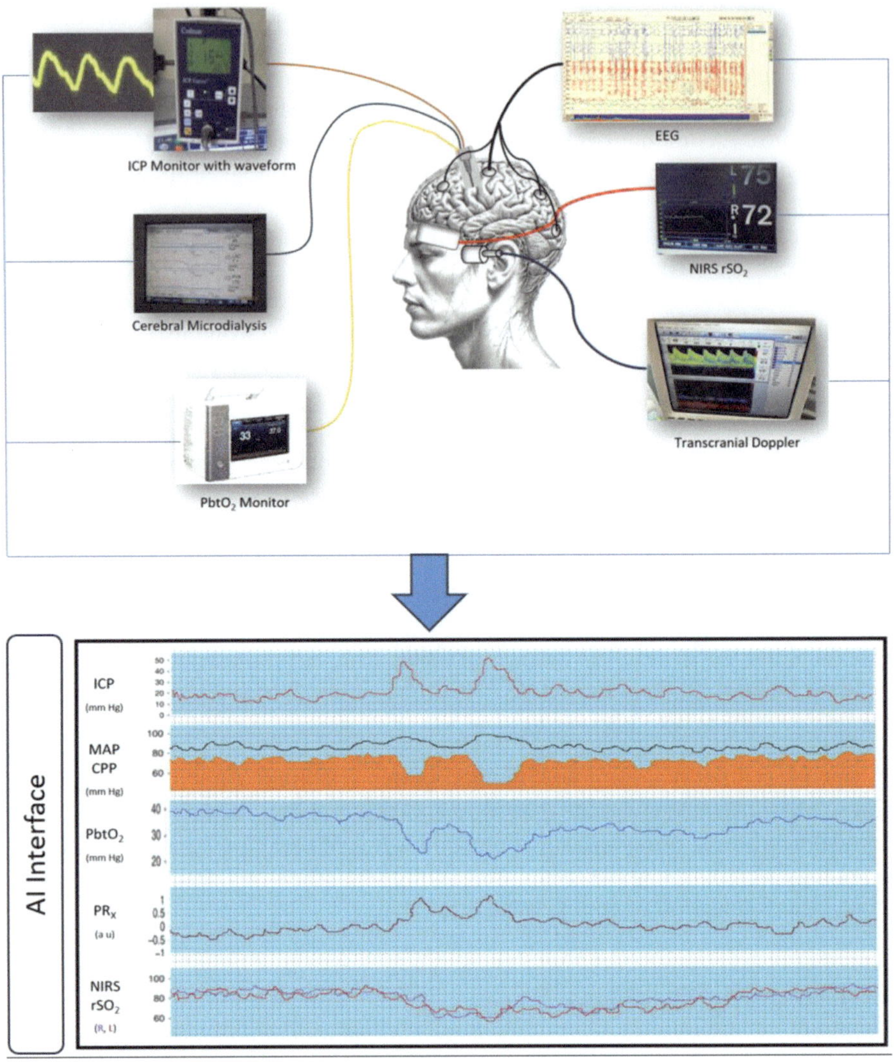

Fig. 14.4 Schematic diagram showing various cerebral multimodal monitoring devices and data integration using AI interface in a simplified single-display unit

Majority of the evidence regarding the use of MMM depicts the use of ICP and $PbtO_2$ in combination. ICP monitoring is the most commonly used system, in conjunction with other modalities of monitoring, followed by $PbtO_2$ monitoring. The duration of monitoring needs to be defined. A lesser duration of monitoring may result in skipping of a critical event, while a longer duration of monitoring may lead to infection and increased cost burden. Most of the studies evaluated the patients for at least 24 h [57]. Also, the MMM-guided intervention should take into account the time frame of the disease process. The evidence to support the use of MMM to guide intervention and clinical outcomes is scarce. A paradox was encountered with the results of the BEST-TRIP trial, which concluded that therapeutic intervention guided by ICP monitoring was not more effective than neurological examinations and serial imaging for immediate and lasting recovery in cases of severe TBI [63]. Therefore, the importance of a thorough neurological examination cannot be overstated.

14.4 Conclusion

The primary goal of cerebral MMM is to establish guidelines and treatment thresholds that correlate with improved patient outcomes. Ample evidence supports the utility of MMM systems over isolated single monitors. However, there is still a paucity of evidence demonstrating additional benefits of such MMM in terms of neurological outcomes. The ongoing evolution of monitoring technologies and data integration systems promises to enhance the effectiveness of MMM, solidifying its role as a cornerstone of advanced neurocritical care. With technological advancements and further robust trials, MMM systems will illuminate the pathophysiology of acute brain trauma and facilitate targeted therapeutic interventions.

References

1. Reilly PL. Brain injury: the pathophysiology of the first hours. 'Talk and Die revisited'. J Clin Neurosci Off J Neurosurg Soc Australas. 2001;8(5):398–403. https://doi.org/10.1054/jocn.2001.0916.
2. De Georgia MA. Multimodal monitoring in neurocritical care. Cleve Clin J Med. 2004;71(Suppl 1):S16–7. https://doi.org/10.3949/ccjm.71.suppl_1.s16.
3. Purkayastha S, Sorond F. Transcranial Doppler ultrasound: technique and application. Semin Neurol. 2012;32(4):411–20. https://doi.org/10.1055/s-0032-1331812.
4. RBC motion and the basis of ultrasound Doppler instrumentation – Uppal – 2010 – Australas J Ultrasound Med – Wiley Online Library. Accessed July 24, 2024. https://onlinelibrary.wiley.com/doi/full/10.1002/j.2205-0140.2010.tb00216.x.
5. Sharma D, Prabhakar H. Chapter 5 – Transcranial Doppler ultrasonography. In: Prabhakar H, editor. Neuromonitoring techniques. Academic; 2018. p. 113–45. https://doi.org/10.1016/B978-0-12-809915-5.00005-X.
6. Aaslid R, Huber P, Nornes H. A transcranial Doppler method in the evaluation of cerebrovascular spasm. Neuroradiology. 1986;28(1):11–6. https://doi.org/10.1007/BF00341759.
7. Sviri GE, Ghodke B, Britz GW, et al. Transcranial Doppler grading criteria for basilar artery vasospasm. Neurosurgery. 2006;59(2):360–6; discussion 360–6. https://doi.org/10.1227/01.NEU.0000223502.93013.6E.
8. Naqvi J, Yap KH, Ahmad G, Ghosh J. Transcranial Doppler ultrasound: a review of the physical principles and major applications in critical care. Int J Vasc Med. 2013;2013:629378. https://doi.org/10.1155/2013/629378.
9. Lau VI, Arntfield RT. Point-of-care transcranial Doppler by intensivists. Crit Ultrasound J. 2017;9(1):21. https://doi.org/10.1186/s13089-017-0077-9.
10. Bellner J, Romner B, Reinstrup P, Kristiansson KA, Ryding E, Brandt L. Transcranial Doppler sonography pulsatility index (PI) reflects intracranial pressure (ICP). Surg Neurol. 2004;62(1):45–51. https://doi.org/10.1016/j.surneu.2003.12.007.

11. Demchuk AM, Burgin WS, Christou I, et al. Thrombolysis in brain ischemia (TIBI) transcranial Doppler flow grades predict clinical severity, early recovery, and mortality in patients treated with intravenous tissue plasminogen activator. Stroke. 2001;32(1):89–93. https://doi.org/10.1161/01.str.32.1.89.
12. Adams RJ, McKie VC, Hsu L, et al. Prevention of a first stroke by transfusions in children with sickle cell anemia and abnormal results on transcranial Doppler ultrasonography. N Engl J Med. 1998;339(1):5–11. https://doi.org/10.1056/NEJM199807023390102.
13. Alexander TH, Hennigan A, Harrison P, Plotkin G. Transcranial Doppler: the fifth decade. J Vasc Ultrasound. 2021;45(1):15–24. https://doi.org/10.1177/1544316720976210.
14. AD ML, Igielman F, Elwell C, Cope M, Smith M. Measuring cerebral oxygenation during normobaric hyperoxia: a comparison of tissue microprobes, near-infrared spectroscopy, and jugular venous oximetry in head injury. Anesth Analg. 2003:851–6. https://doi.org/10.1213/01.ANE.0000072541.57132.BA.
15. Bendahan N, Neal O, Ross-White A, Muscedere J, Boyd JG. Relationship between near-infrared spectroscopy-derived cerebral oxygenation and delirium in critically ill patients: a systematic review. J Intensive Care Med. 2019;34(6):514–20. https://doi.org/10.1177/0885066618807399.
16. Rivera-Lara L, Geocadin R, Zorrilla-Vaca A, et al. Validation of near-infrared spectroscopy for monitoring cerebral autoregulation in comatose patients. Neurocrit Care. 2017;27(3):362–9. https://doi.org/10.1007/s12028-017-0421-8.
17. Pisano A, Di Fraja D, Palmieri C. Monitoring cerebral oximetry by near-infrared spectroscopy (NIRS) in anesthesia and critical care: progress and perspectives. In: Cascella M, editor. General anesthesia research, Neuromethods, vol. 150. Springer US; 2020. p. 75–96. https://doi.org/10.1007/978-1-4939-9891-3_4.
18. Bhatia A, Gupta AK. Neuromonitoring in the intensive care unit. II. Cerebral oxygenation monitoring and microdialysis. Intensive Care Med. 2007;33(8):1322–8. https://doi.org/10.1007/s00134-007-0660-9.
19. Wozniak MA, Sloan MA, Rothman MI, et al. Detection of vasospasm by transcranial Doppler sonography. The challenges of the anterior and posterior cerebral arteries. J Neuroimaging Off J Am Soc Neuroimaging. 1996;6(2):87–93. https://doi.org/10.1111/jon19966287.
20. Chan YL, Han ST, Li CH, Wu CC, Chen KF. Transfusion of red blood cells to patients with sepsis. Int J Mol Sci. 2017;18(9):1946. https://doi.org/10.3390/ijms18091946.
21. Ristic A, Sutter R, Steiner L. Current neuromonitoring techniques in critical care. J Neuroanaesth Crit Care. 2015;02(02):097–103. https://doi.org/10.4103/2348-0548.154234.
22. Oddo M, Le Roux P. Brain oxygen. In: Monitoring in neurocritical care. 1st ed. Elsevier; 2013. p. 348–55.
23. Oddo M, Levine JM, Mackenzie L, et al. Brain hypoxia is associated with short-term outcome after severe traumatic brain injury independently of intracranial hypertension and low cerebral perfusion pressure. Neurosurgery. 2011;69(5):1037–45; discussion 1045. https://doi.org/10.1227/NEU.0b013e3182287ca7.
24. Narotam PK, Morrison JF, Nathoo N. Brain tissue oxygen monitoring in traumatic brain injury and major trauma: outcome analysis of a brain tissue oxygen-directed therapy. J Neurosurg. 2009;111(4):672–82. https://doi.org/10.3171/2009.4.JNS081150.
25. Carney N, Totten AM, O'Reilly C, et al. Guidelines for the management of severe traumatic brain injury, fourth edition. Neurosurgery. 2017;80(1):6–15. https://doi.org/10.1227/NEU.0000000000001432.
26. Okonkwo DO, Shutter LA, Moore C, et al. Brain oxygen optimization in severe traumatic brain injury phase-II: a phase II randomized trial. Crit Care Med. 2017;45(11):1907–14. https://doi.org/10.1097/CCM.0000000000002619.
27. Bernard F, Barsan W, Diaz-Arrastia R, Merck LH, Yeatts S, Shutter LA. Brain oxygen optimization in severe traumatic brain injury (BOOST-3): a multicentre, randomised, blinded-endpoint, comparative effectiveness study of brain tissue oxygen and intracranial pressure monitoring versus intracranial pressure alone. BMJ Open. 2022;12(3):e060188. https://doi.org/10.1136/bmjopen-2021-060188.

28. Payen JF, Richard M, Francony G, et al. Comparison of strategies for monitoring and treating patients at the early phase of severe traumatic brain injury: the multicentre randomised controlled OXY-TC trial study protocol. BMJ Open. 2020;10(8):e040550. https://doi.org/10.1136/bmjopen-2020-040550.
29. Udy, Andrew. Brain oxygen neuromonitoring in Australia and New Zealand assessment trial. 12619001328167p [Internet]. Published online 2021. https://www.anzics.com.au/current-active-endorsed-research/bonanza/.
30. Maloney-Wilensky E, Le Roux P. The physiology behind direct brain oxygen monitors and practical aspects of their use. Childs Nerv Syst. 2010;26(4):419–30. https://doi.org/10.1007/s00381-009-1037-x.
31. Cnossen MC, Huijben JA, van der Jagt M, et al. Variation in monitoring and treatment policies for intracranial hypertension in traumatic brain injury: a survey in 66 neurotrauma centers participating in the CENTER-TBI study. Crit Care Lond Engl. 2017;21(1):233. https://doi.org/10.1186/s13054-017-1816-9.
32. Güiza F, Depreitere B, Piper I, et al. Visualizing the pressure and time burden of intracranial hypertension in adult and paediatric traumatic brain injury. Intensive Care Med. 2015;41(6):1067–76. https://doi.org/10.1007/s00134-015-3806-1.
33. Lazaridis C, DeSantis SM, Smielewski P, et al. Patient-specific thresholds of intracranial pressure in severe traumatic brain injury. J Neurosurg. 2014;120(4):893–900. https://doi.org/10.3171/2014.1.JNS131292.
34. Tas J, Beqiri E, van Kaam RC, et al. Targeting autoregulation-guided cerebral perfusion pressure after traumatic brain injury (COGiTATE): a feasibility randomized controlled clinical trial. J Neurotrauma. 2021;38(20):2790–800. https://doi.org/10.1089/neu.2021.0197.
35. Bellander BM, Cantais E, Enblad P, et al. Consensus meeting on microdialysis in neurointensive care. Intensive Care Med. 2004;30(12):2166–9. https://doi.org/10.1007/s00134-004-2461-8.
36. Timofeev I, Carpenter KLH, Nortje J, et al. Cerebral extracellular chemistry and outcome following traumatic brain injury: a microdialysis study of 223 patients. Brain J Neurol. 2011;134(Pt 2):484–94. https://doi.org/10.1093/brain/awq353.
37. Winberg J, Holm I, Cederberg D, Rundgren M, Kronvall E, Marklund N. Cerebral microdialysis-based interventions targeting delayed cerebral ischemia following aneurysmal subarachnoid hemorrhage. Neurocrit Care. 2022;37(1):255–66. https://doi.org/10.1007/s12028-022-01492-5.
38. Kurtz P, Rocha EEM. Nutrition therapy, glucose control, and brain metabolism in traumatic brain injury: a multimodal monitoring approach. Front Neurosci. 2020;14:190. https://doi.org/10.3389/fnins.2020.00190.
39. Mishra RK, Bindra A, Khandelwal A, et al. Brain regional energy metabolism in patients with traumatic brain injury: a cerebral microdialysis guided study. Neurol India. 2024;72(1):78–82. https://doi.org/10.4103/neuroindia.NI_37_21.
40. Gupta DK, Singla R, Kale SS, Sharma BS. Intracerebral hypoglycemia and its clinical relevance as a prognostic indicator in severe traumatic brain injury: a cerebral microdialysis study from India. Neurol India. 2016;64(2):259–64. https://doi.org/10.4103/0028-3886.177617.
41. Koubeissi M, Alshekhlee A. In-hospital mortality of generalized convulsive status epilepticus: a large US sample. Neurology. 2007;69(9):886–93. https://doi.org/10.1212/01.wnl.0000269791.96189.70.
42. Szurhaj W, Lamblin MD, Kaminska A, Sediri H, Société de Neurophysiologie Clinique de Langue Française. EEG guidelines in the diagnosis of brain death. Neurophysiol Clin Neurophysiol. 2015;45(1):97–104. https://doi.org/10.1016/j.neucli.2014.11.005.
43. Claassen J, Mayer SA, Kowalski RG, Emerson RG, Hirsch LJ. Detection of electrographic seizures with continuous EEG monitoring in critically ill patients. Neurology. 2004;62(10):1743–8. https://doi.org/10.1212/01.WNL.0000125184.88797.62.
44. Hartings JA, Andaluz N, Bullock MR, et al. Prognostic value of spreading Depolarizations in patients with severe traumatic brain injury. JAMA Neurol. 2020;77(4):489–99. https://doi.org/10.1001/jamaneurol.2019.4476.

45. Fergusson NA, Hoiland RL, Thiara S, et al. Goal-directed care using invasive neuromonitoring versus standard of care after cardiac arrest: a matched cohort study. Crit Care Med. 2021;49(8):1333–46. https://doi.org/10.1097/CCM.0000000000004945.
46. Robba C, Goffi A, Geeraerts T, et al. Brain ultrasonography: methodology, basic and advanced principles and clinical applications. A narrative review. Intensive Care Med. 2019;45(7):913–27. https://doi.org/10.1007/s00134-019-05610-4.
47. Aletreby W, Alharthy A, Brindley PG, et al. Optic nerve sheath diameter ultrasound for raised intracranial pressure: a literature review and meta-analysis of its diagnostic accuracy. J Ultrasound Med. 2022;41(3):585–95. https://doi.org/10.1002/jum.15732.
48. Jeon JP, Lee SU, Kim SE, et al. Correlation of optic nerve sheath diameter with directly measured intracranial pressure in Korean adults using bedside ultrasonography. PLoS One. 2017;12(9):e0183170. https://doi.org/10.1371/journal.pone.0183170.
49. Swanson JW, Aleman TS, Xu W, et al. Evaluation of optical coherence tomography to detect elevated intracranial pressure in children. JAMA Ophthalmol. 2017;135(4):320–8. https://doi.org/10.1001/jamaophthalmol.2017.0025.
50. Zhu S, Cheng C, Zhao D, Zhao Y, Liu X, Zhang J. The clinical and prognostic values of optic nerve sheath diameter and optic nerve sheath diameter/eyeball transverse diameter ratio in comatose patients with supratentorial lesions. BMC Neurol. 2021;21:259. https://doi.org/10.1186/s12883-021-02285-7.
51. Netteland DF, Aarhus M, Sandset EC, Padayachy L, Helseth E, Brekken R. Noninvasive assessment of intracranial pressure: deformability index as an adjunct to optic nerve sheath diameter to increase diagnostic ability. Neurocrit Care. 2024; https://doi.org/10.1007/s12028-024-01955-x.
52. Hsu CH, Kuo LT. Application of pupillometry in neurocritical patients. J Pers Med. 2023;13(7):1100. https://doi.org/10.3390/jpm13071100.
53. Stevens AR, Su Z, Toman E, Belli A, Davies D. Optical pupillometry in traumatic brain injury: neurological pupil index and its relationship with intracranial pressure through significant event analysis. Brain Inj. 2019;33(8):1032–8. https://doi.org/10.1080/02699052.2019.1605621.
54. Singer KE, Wallen TE, Jalbert T, et al. Efficacy of noninvasive technologies in triaging traumatic brain injury and correlating with intracranial pressure: a prospective study. J Surg Res. 2021;262:27–37. https://doi.org/10.1016/j.jss.2020.12.042.
55. Oddo M, Taccone FS, Petrosino M, et al. The neurological pupil index for outcome prognostication in people with acute brain injury (ORANGE): a prospective, observational, multicentre cohort study. Lancet Neurol. 2023;22(10):925–33. https://doi.org/10.1016/S1474-4422(23)00271-5.
56. Al-Mufti F, Lander M, Smith B, et al. Multimodality monitoring in neurocritical care: decision-making utilizing direct and indirect surrogate markers. J Intensive Care Med. 2019;34(6):449–63. https://doi.org/10.1177/0885066618788022.
57. Tas J, Czosnyka M, van der Horst ICC, et al. Cerebral multimodality monitoring in adult neurocritical care patients with acute brain injury: a narrative review. Front Physiol. 2022;13:1071161. https://doi.org/10.3389/fphys.2022.1071161.
58. Hawryluk GWJ, Aguilera S, Buki A, et al. A management algorithm for patients with intracranial pressure monitoring: the Seattle international severe traumatic brain injury consensus conference (SIBICC). Intensive Care Med. 2019;45(12):1783–94. https://doi.org/10.1007/s00134-019-05805-9.
59. Makarenko S, Griesdale DE, Gooderham P, Sekhon MS. Multimodal neuromonitoring for traumatic brain injury: a shift towards individualized therapy. J Clin Neurosci Off J Neurosurg Soc Australas. 2016;26:8–13. https://doi.org/10.1016/j.jocn.2015.05.065.
60. Tisdall MM, Smith M. Multimodal monitoring in traumatic brain injury: current status and future directions. Br J Anaesth. 2007;99(1):61–7. https://doi.org/10.1093/bja/aem143.

61. Schmidt JM, De Georgia M, Participants in the International Multidisciplinary Consensus Conference on Multimodality Monitoring. Multimodality monitoring: informatics, integration data display and analysis. Neurocrit Care. 2014;21(Suppl 2):S229–38. https://doi.org/10.1007/s12028-014-0037-1.
62. Launey Y, Fryer TD, Hong YT, et al. Spatial and temporal pattern of ischemia and abnormal vascular function following traumatic brain injury. JAMA Neurol. 2020;77(3):339. https://doi.org/10.1001/jamaneurol.2019.3854.
63. Chesnut RM, Temkin N, Carney N, et al. A trial of intracranial-pressure monitoring in traumatic brain injury. N Engl J Med. 2012;367(26):2471–81. https://doi.org/10.1056/NEJMoa1207363.

Sedation Practices in Neurocritical Care 15

Geetha Lakshminarasimhaiah and Pramod Kalgudi

Abstract

Neurocritical care unit (NCCU) population requires a targeted approach to sedation and analgesia. Sedo-analgesia facilitates the management of acute neurological insult by positively affecting the intracranial hemodynamics, in addition to improving conditions for intubation and mechanical ventilation (MV). The significance of sedation and analgesia is recognized by widely adopted recommendations. However, many randomized trials evaluating the optimal sedation management have excluded critically ill neurological patients; hence, controversies exist in this area. Here, we will review the controversies in sedation practices, highlighting the rationale for the use of sedo-analgesia, the advantages and disadvantages of various agents, clinical pitfalls, evidence-based practices, and emerging evidence, which will facilitate clinical decision-making in neurocritical care.

Keywords

Analgosedation · Paroxysmal Sympathetic Hyperactivity · Sedation withdrawal Ketofol · Agitation in NCC · Neuromuscular blockers in NCC

15.1 Introduction

Critically ill patients with neurological injury require a specialized approach to sedation and analgesia. Sedo-analgesia in such patients not only improves tolerance to intubation and mechanical ventilation (MV) but also facilitates the management

G. Lakshminarasimhaiah (✉) · P. Kalgudi
Neuroanaesthesia, M. S. Ramaiah Medical College, Bengaluru, Karnataka, India

P. U. Bidkar, M. Krishnakumar (eds.), *Controversies in Neurocritical Care*,
https://doi.org/10.1007/978-981-95-4419-6_15

of acute neurological insult. Sedative agents cross the blood-brain barrier and alter cerebral hemodynamics [1]. Hence, sedation plays a key role in controlling intracranial pressure (ICP) and seizures and increasing the neurological threshold to develop ischemic injury by reducing the cerebral metabolic rate of oxygen ($CMRO_2$), cerebral blood flow (CBF), and cerebral blood volume (CBV). It becomes imperative to choose sedation agents with a favorable profile on cerebral hemodynamics in patients with neurological insult and also having a rapid offset to facilitate timely neurological examination. The significance of sedation in the management of traumatic brain injury (TBI) has been recognized in multiple widely adopted recommendations [2].

Most of the randomized trials evaluating the optimal sedation management have systematically excluded critically ill patients with brain insult; hence, controversies persist in this arena. [3] Even the recent guidelines for sedation in critically ill patients have factored out neurological patients, and the Brain Trauma Foundation guidelines do not recommend any specific pharmacological agent due to a lack of studies and substantial scientific evidence [2, 3].

Despite the understanding of the importance of sedation in the neurocritical care unit (NCCU), disputes exist with regard to choosing the ideal agent for sedation in neurocritical unit patients. In this chapter, we will review the controversies in sedation practices, highlighting the rationale for the use of sedo-analgesia in neurocritical care, the advantages and disadvantages of various agents, clinical pitfalls, evidence-based practices, emerging evidence, areas needing further research, and the landmark studies in this area.

15.2 Rationale for the Use of Sedo-Analgesia in Neurocritical Care

In patients with acute neurological insult, sedation brings in specific cerebral protective effects, which can be outlined as follows.

1. *Effects on the cerebral metabolic rate of oxygen consumption*: Sedative therapies in patients with brain injuries act by decreasing the cerebral metabolic rate of oxygen ($CMRO_2$), enhancing cerebral tolerance to ischemia, and mitigating supply–demand discrepancies in situations of compromised autoregulation [4]. Sedatives typically reduce $CMRO_2$ metabolically in a dose-dependent manner until the EEG is isoelectric. Cerebral oxygen consumption cannot be further suppressed beyond isoelectricity, but limited consumption for cellular homeostasis continues [5, 6].
2. *Effects on CBF*: The intravenous sedative agents cause a dose-dependent decrease in CBF [4–7], although CBF reductions are variable with different agents. The coupled CBF/$CMRO_2$ reduction with sedative agents also induces a fall in mean arterial pressure (MAP) due to myocardial depression and peripheral vasodilatation. Whether the autoregulation is preserved or impaired, the reduction in MAP causes secondary brain injury by increasing the ICP and

through a critical drop in cerebral perfusion pressure (CPP), respectively [4]. To minimize the risk of hypotension and fall in CPP, it is important to attain normovolemia and preload, especially in those with preexisting heart disease [8].

3. *Control of ICP*: Initially, sedo-analgesics lower $CMRO_2$ and, consequently, CBF, which, in turn, lowers the cerebral blood volume accordingly. A decrease in intracranial capacity and, consequently, ICP results from this decrease in cerebral blood volume. These medications' effects on lowering ICP also result from their ability to reduce agitation and discomfort, which can lead to arterial hypertension and an ICP spike. Last but not least, analgesia promotes endotracheal tube tolerance and prevents intrathoracic pressure rises, which can lower jugular venous outflow and raise ICP, by lowering agitation and coughing.
4. *Inhibition of seizures*: Cerebral metabolism rises during seizures, and there may be a discrepancy between oxygen delivery and metabolism. Sedatives, when used with antiepileptic medications, lessen seizure episodes in the NCCU [9]. Propofol can be used to treat status epilepticus and as an anticonvulsant. Because they are γ-aminobutyric acid (GABA) receptor agonists, benzodiazepines, propofol, and barbiturates can be used to treat refractory status epilepticus and lower the risk of secondary seizures in individuals with acute brain injury (ABI). In this context, ketamine, an N-methyl-D-aspartate (NMDA) receptor antagonist, serves as a substitute or supplement to conventional GABA receptor agonists [10].
5. *Control of spreading depression*: Lesion enlargement in traumatic brain injury, intracranial hemorrhage, and other types of ABI can result from cortical spreading depolarization (CSD), sometimes referred to as spreading depression, a type of abnormal brain electrical activity that deteriorates energy balance [11]. Local neuronal dysfunction is the outcome of this event, which starts at the lesion core and gradually extends through the surrounding cortex, upsetting the electrochemical gradients. A few sedatives can alter the frequency and severity of spreading depolarizations, which are known to be related to the outcome following brain injury. According to a recent study, ketamine sedation was linked to the lowest incidence of spreading depolarizations when compared to opioids, midazolam, and propofol [10].

15.3 Choice of Sedative Agents in Neurocritical Care: The Debate

In the neurocritical care unit, sedative agents are used for specific therapeutic indications. Though randomized controlled trials (RCTs) have demonstrated the short-term benefits of sedation policy, including the reduced intensive care unit (ICU) length of stay (LOS) and a shorter duration of mechanical ventilation, it interferes with the clinical neurological assessment of the patient [12–14]. Hence, the agents for this purpose are to be tailor-made for patients with neurological disorders. Currently, propofol and dexmedetomidine are the most commonly used sedative agents in the NCCU. In this section, we describe the most commonly used agents with clinical evidence, followed by the second line of drugs.

15.4 Propofol vs. Dexmedetomidine in the NCCU

Traditionally, propofol is used as the standard of care for sedation management in neurological patients, especially in traumatic brain injury (TBI). It is one of the first-line sedatives to use in patients with raised ICP due to its rapid onset of action (30 s to 2 min) and can last up to 15 min, facilitating neurological examination once sedation is turned off [12–14].

Though propofol is effective in reducing ICP, it may lead to cerebral vasoconstriction and dose-dependent reduction in CBF and oxygenation, particularly compared to sevoflurane and isoflurane [15, 16].

Further studies using invasive brain monitoring have proved the beneficial effects of propofol in reducing ICP and mortality in TBI patients despite reducing MAP and CPP [17]. Caution must be exercised when using propofol, as it can lead to systemic vasodilation and negative inotropy, causing a reduction in MAP and deranged cerebral autoregulation. Among the other side effects of propofol, propofol infusion syndrome is considered serious if long-term sedation is needed [12].

There are no substantial RCTs evaluating light vs. deep sedation using propofol with neurological patients. Recently, studies conducted in acute ischemic stroke (AIS) receiving general anesthesia (GA) vs. conscious sedation (CS) using propofol for endovascular treatment (EVT), looking at neurological outcomes, are noteworthy. Three months after the stroke, there was no discernible difference in the neurological results of the 90-patient general anesthesia (GA) vs. conscious sedation (CS) for EVT of AIS (AnSTROKE) experiment conducted in 2017 [18]. In 2018, another RCT with 128 patients examined infarct growth and the impact of GA and CS during EVT on infarct growth and clinical outcomes in AIS (GOLIATH). A low-dose propofol infusion was administered after a fentanyl bolus to induce conscious sedation. A larger dose of propofol infusion and remifentanil drip were used to sedate the general anesthesia arm. The researchers discovered that, while there was no statistically significant difference in the infarct volume between the groups, the GA group's modified Rankin scale score differed significantly from the CS group's [19]. A meta-analysis of the GOLIATH, AnSTROKE, and SIESTA trials was conducted in 2019 to assess the outcomes at 3 months for patients who received CS as opposed to GA during thrombectomy. The authors of this meta-analysis came to the conclusion that the GA group had a lower three-month disability rate [20]. According to these studies, patients who receive deeper sedation during endovascular treatment for acute ischemic strokes may benefit slightly; the exact mechanism of this benefit is unknown, but it could be due to either the sedatives' direct cerebral metabolic effects or different reperfusion rates.

However, the most recent Brain Trauma Foundation guidelines (2017) recommending propofol usage for the management of elevated ICP reiterate caution against the use of high doses of propofol, given the known morbidity.

Dexmedetomidine, a centrally acting alpha-2 ($\alpha 2$) adrenergic receptor agonist [21], has anesthetic, analgesic, and sedative properties, leading to a lesser requirement of other anesthetics/opioids, without causing respiratory depression [17, 22]. These characteristics make it helpful since low-to-moderate dosages allow a patient to stay awake during a neurological evaluation. [23] According to a study, TBI patients' agitation decreased within 96 h of taking dexmedetomidine [24]. Although dexmedetomidine has little influence on cerebral hemodynamics, it may lower the intracranial pressure (ICP) due to its moderate effects on cerebral vasoconstriction, cerebral blood volume (CBV), and cerebral metabolic rate [12, 25–27]. According to a recent study, dexmedetomidine infusion was linked to a lower requirement for rescue hypertonic therapy in the TBI group, suggesting that it may lower ICP [28]. Dexmedetomidine has been shown to cause clinically significant bradycardia and hypotension, which is consistent across all the ICUs, and a higher incidence of hypotension compared to propofol [21, 29, 30]. When weaning off long-duration dexmedetomidine infusion, clonidine (also a centrally acting α2 agonist), either orally or transdermally, is a useful technique because patients may have rebound effects such as tachycardia, hypertension, and a possible reemergence of agitation [31].

15.5 Alternative Sedative Agents: Advantages and Limitations

15.5.1 Benzodiazepines

The benzodiazepine (BZD) that is most commonly used, midazolam, works by altering GABA receptors in the central nervous system to lessen neuronal excitement and perhaps lower cerebral metabolism. [32, 33] Intravenous midazolam typically reaches peak concentration in less than 5 min and has a half-life of around 1.5–3.5 h [32]. More than two-thirds of patients with severe TBI had their ICP managed by sedation with midazolam, according to a prospective study that evaluated 96 patients with severe TBI [34]. However, due to the greater incidence of delirium and the longer period of mechanical ventilation and ICU hospitalization, BZDs are less desirable than other drugs for both sedation and ICP control [34–36]. They may be preferred over propofol in the setting of propofol infusion syndrome [34].

15.5.2 Ketamine

Ketamine operates on muscarinic, nicotinic, and mu-opioid receptors, in addition to reducing the excitatory effects of glutamate by antagonistically binding to NMDA receptors. High-dose ketamine has been shown in recent studies to provide both sedative and analgesic properties while maintaining MAP, CPP, and ICP and, in some cases, lowering ICP [8, 38, 39] despite the fact that it was not previously preferred in ABI patients for causing surges in ICP through sympathetic stimulation [37]. It may also contribute to neuroprotection by lowering excitotoxicity, cortical spreading depolarization (CSD), and microglial activation, among other ways [40]. In addition to providing drowsiness and analgesia, ketamine may be helpful in ABI patients because it maintains MAP, even at larger dosages.

15.5.3 Ketofol

Ketofol, a novel method for conscious procedural sedation, was created by mixing ketamine and propofol. However, certain prospective experiments suggest that this combination can be well-tolerated and may result in a more stable sedative state. [41, 42] There is no obvious clinical advantage over propofol alone, according to other research, and there may be a larger risk of hypotension and other side effects [43]. Therefore, additional RCTs are necessary to demonstrate the advantages of this combined approach in the NCCU.

15.5.4 Barbiturates

In the current day NCCU practice, the use of barbiturates is restricted to refractory elevated ICP but not as first-line agents for sedation. They increase the duration of chloride channel opening, which further enhances GABA-induced postsynaptic inhibition [44]. In patients with refractory intracranial hypertension, barbiturates (phenobarbital or pentobarbital) dramatically reduce cerebral metabolism by inducing coma [45]. Reducing CBF, cerebral oxygen consumption and metabolism, and neuro-excitotoxicity through a decrease in brain glutamate and aspartate release is the mechanism that lowers ICP [46, 47]. Barbiturate coma was shown to double the likelihood of stabilizing ICP in patients with resistant ICP crises in a randomized multicenter experiment [48]. Although the results are limited, a small experiment conducted in 2021 assessed a unique step-down infusion approach of barbiturate therapy and found promising results on the safety and effectiveness of using barbiturates to reduce ICP. Barbiturates can cause severe acute hypokalemia and a reduction in heart function [49]. Long-term use of medium-acting pentobarbital infusions (half-life: 24–96 h) can make it impossible to perform a timely neurological examination for a long time, while long-acting barbiturates (half-life: 20–45 h) can also significantly delay elimination [45].

15.6 Opioids: Balancing Analgesia and Neurological Assessment

A combination of analgesia and sedation (“analgo-sedation”) is mostly beneficial in a critical care setting, depending on painful interventions, the presence of brain injury, and the degree of ventilator synchrony. Currently, there are no pain scales available specific to patients with neurological insult, but a few objectively assessed scales, namely the Critical Care Pain Observation Tool (CPOT) or Behavioral Pain Scale (BPS), can be used [50]. In many intensive care units, opioids are used as the primary analgesic, especially for patients who have an endotracheal tube, which may cause direct tracheal stimulation or the cough reflex. According to studies, using opioids reduces ventilator asynchrony when compared to sedation alone [51]. Although morphine and hydromorphone are also used, fentanyl and remifentanil, which have short half-lives of about 2 h and 10 min, respectively, are frequently chosen drugs. The longer-acting medications, however, can lengthen the ventilator time and make routine neurological examinations more difficult [52]. Pain treatment in the NCCU should always follow a multimodal approach combining moderate doses of both opioids and non-opioids (paracetamol, nonsteroidal anti-inflammatory drugs (NSAIDs), ketamine, neuropathic pain agents, etc.), aiming toward avoiding toxicity and creating synergism. Typical non-opioid pharmacologic agents include NSAIDs, acetaminophen, ketamine, and neuropathic pain agents, among others [53]. Although opioids typically have minimal impact on cerebral hemodynamics, bolus dosage may cause MAP as well as CPP to drop [54]. The use of morphine and hydromorphone metabolites (morphine-3-glucuronide and hydromorphone-3-glucuronide) is discouraged in patients with acute brain injury and renal impairment because they have been associated with neurotoxicity, which includes seizures, tremors, and myoclonus, especially when taken in large quantities and for an extended period of time [55].

15.7 Volatile Anesthetics: Revival or Risk?

Volatile anesthetics have the potential benefits of rapid onset, bronchodilation, a decreased $CMRO_2$, and easy titration through end-tidal gas monitoring, and with the advent of anesthetic reflectors "AnaConDa" and "Mirus" have revived interest for sedation in the ICU [56]. When administered for a long time, volatile agents also improved sedation stability with fewer dose adjustments [56, 57]. Significantly shorter awakening and extubation times were observed with volatile anesthetics vs. propofol and midazolam, according to a recent meta-analysis, with no difference in LOS [58]. Nonetheless, these agents are still not routinely used in the NCCU because of the risk of ICP elevations due to a rise in CBF, even though one study by Villa et al. [59] showed no difference in ICP levels compared to propofol. Some of the concerns about sedation with volatile agents include environmental contamination (need for scavenging) and a strong association with long-term cognitive deficits, particularly in children [60–62]. These potential neurotoxic effects preclude their use in the NCCU, even though a study on rats in 2014 showed a decrease in CSD when using isoflurane compared to propofol. [63]

15.7.1 PSH Management with Sedatives

One specific instance where sedatives may be used to reduce excessive autonomic activation and motor hyperactivity is paroxysmal sympathetic activity (PSH) [64]. In the prospective study by Tang et al. [65], 50 postoperative patients with severe TBI who received dexmedetomidine infusions were assessed for PSH; the participants received a loading dexmedetomidine dose of 0.8 μg/kg over 10 min, followed by a continuous infusion of 0.25–0.75 μg/kg/h. Compared with controls who received a standard sedation regimen of propofol and midazolam, PSH assessment measurement scores were significantly lower in those receiving dexmedetomidine (5.26 ± 4.66 vs. 8.58 ± 8.09, respectively; P = 0.017); however, there was no difference in mortality or outcome (assessed by the Glasgow Outcome Scale score) at discharge or 3 months.

15.8 Sedation Withdrawal in Neurocritical Care: Timing and Risks

Evidence from the early twenty-first century presented that withdrawing sedation or everyday alternation between sedation and awakening reduces the patients' period on mechanical ventilation and the duration of stay in patients admitted to the general ICU. Withholding sedation every day in neurocritical care patients not only facilitates neurological examination but also helps shorten the duration of invasive ventilation and the necessity for tracheostomy. The drawback of sedation on cerebral hemodynamics, specifically in the early phases following brain injury, offsets these possible advantages.

Withdrawing sedation in patients with acute brain injury led to consistent variations in brain metabolism. Lower cerebral perfusion pressure and higher ICP have been linked to withdrawing sedation. Although the ICP response to sedation withdrawal varied widely in these studies, in certain patients, concurrent reductions in CPP occurred, and the ICP increased to dangerous levels (>40 mmHg). ICP spikes peaked during the initial days of acute brain injury, and the effects of sedation withdrawal on ICP were only moderate after 4 or 5 days. Sedation withdrawal also led to an increase in the levels of stress hormones, catecholamines, and cortisol [66–69].

Helbok et al. noticed that 34 percent of trials about sedation withdrawal were halted due to a substantial surge in ICP, along with an equivalent decrease in cerebral perfusion pressure. Twenty percent of trials had to be stopped because brain tissue PO_2 had significantly dropped below the critical thresholds of cerebral hypoxia [66]. Furthermore, in a very small proportion of wake-up tests performed in this investigation, new neurological deficits were observed. An additional significant advantage of sedation following an acute brain injury is the avoidance of shivering in the course of targeted temperature management [70]. In such circumstances, sedation should not be stopped until normal temperature has reverted. Prolonged sedation in pathologies with relevant ICP elevation is often discontinued only after several days due to neurointensivists' reluctance to implement spontaneous breathing trials and daily sedation withdrawal. Confusion and uneven treatment result from a lack of knowledge regarding when to intervene most effectively and clinical biomarkers that can forecast unfavorable outcomes in the intensive care unit following prolonged sedation [71, 72]. Moritz et al., in their recent study, explored frequency, risks, and outcomes of sedation withdrawal among patients having aneurysmal subarachnoid hemorrhage (aSAH). In patients with good-grade SAH, sedation was withdrawn within the first 5 days after disease onset, whereas in poor-grade SAH patients, it was done by 10 days after ictus. The major culprit for neurological adverse effects that occurred in 60% of patients with aSAH was the duration of ICP >20 mmHg before commencing sedation withdrawal. Patients with a prolonged duration of disease since ictus and high oxygen saturation and those who had craniotomy were deemed to be protected from neurological adverse events following sedation withdrawal [73]. Among the pediatric population with severe TBI, the primary reason for not doing the neurological wake-up test was intracranial hypertension, whereas non-arousal or severe agitation were the main causes for the failure of the neurological wake-up test [74].

In summary, all patients in the NCCU should be evaluated for daily sedation break and weaning but only after cerebral physiology has reverted to normal or when ICP and brain tissue PO_2 are no longer targeted for therapy. In general, this transpires after 5–7 days.

15.9 Agitation, Delirium, and Sedation: The Controversial Interplay

In the NCCU, agitation and delirium frequently cause problems, but it can be tricky to differentiate between the two. An injury to the brain may be the cause of agitation, whereas long-term sedation and ICU interventions are the leading causes of delirium. In patients hospitalized in the neuro-ICU, delirium represents an extremely difficult condition to handle. In the NCCU, patients are usually admitted because of neurological diseases, like brain trauma, stroke, and neuromuscular disease, which cause neurological dysfunction. Due to the fact that delirium itself is an acute brain dysfunction, diagnosing whether a patient's behavior is due to a primary neurological disease or if it is a separate new-onset brain dysfunction can be difficult. The incidence rates of delirium in the neuro-ICU vary from 19% to 70% [75–77]. The PRE-DELIRIC scale having ten risk elements (Acute Physiology And Chronic Health Evaluation (APACHE)-II score, age of the patient, admission group, underlying infection, coma, use of sedatives and morphine, metabolic acidosis, concentration of urea, and needing urgent admission) has been used in a small group of neuro-ICU patients to foresee the possibility of developing delirium [78]. Using this scale before sedation withdrawal in the neuro-ICU needs to be investigated for the prediction of delirium on sedation withdrawal. Using midazolam alone or in combination with propofol increases the risk of developing delirium during the sedation withdrawal period in the ICU compared to using propofol alone [79].

Delirium may develop as a consequence of either poorly managed or overtreated analgesia. Whenever there is a possibility that pain is causing delirium, the Behavioral Pain Scale and Critical Care Pain Observation Tool (Annexure) must be utilized to judge the need for analgesics.

One of the hallmarks of delirium is an altered mental state. A patient may be experiencing delirium if there is an inexplicable change in their mental state. It has been demonstrated that daily sedation breaks, combined with the use of validated sedation–agitation tools, for instance Richmond Agitation-Sedation Scale (RASS) and Riker Sedation-Agitation Scale (SAS), reduce the amount and extent of sedative medication use in intensive care units (Annexure).

The PRE-DELIRIC model was able to predict the patients' delirium within a day of their admission into the general ICU [80]. But there are no neuro-ICU patient population–specific scales apart from the Confusion Assessment Method for ICU [CAM-ICU] (Annexure), which has been authenticated in patients with intracranial bleeding and acute ischemic stroke, for the assessment of delirium and its severity [81]. The Braden score could be an easy-to-use screening tool for determining patients' risk of delirium following an ischemic stroke [82]. Larsen et al. proposed that CAM-ICU is less suitable for identifying delirium in patients having ABI secondary to TBI, ischemic stroke, or hemorrhagic stroke than the Intensive Care Delirium Screening Checklist [83]. The meta-analysis and systematic review revealed that the ABCDEF bundle approach (Assess, prevent, manage pain; Both spontaneous awakening, spontaneous breathing trials; Choice of analgesia, sedation; Delirium: assess, prevent, manage; Early mobility, exercise; Family engagement, empowerment) significantly reduced the duration of intensive care unit delirium [84].

There are numerous non-pharmacological and pharmacological treatments to manage delirium in the ICUs. A systematic review and network meta-analysis revealed that early mobilization and family participation were more effective in lowering the incidence of ICU delirium among the multicomponent strategies for non-pharmacological therapies [85]. ICU delirium is treated with a wide variety of medications. In the neuro-ICU, we typically use benzodiazepines, antipsychotics, and alpha-2 agonists. Benzodiazepines are routinely used among patients with alcohol withdrawal–related delirium. Research on the impact of antipsychotics on cerebral hemodynamics has mainly focused on risperidone and haloperidol in patients diagnosed with schizophrenia. When compared to risperidone, haloperidol increases global [86] and regional [87] CBF; however, it is unclear if these differences are clinically significant or have an impact on ICP. Clonidine and dexmedetomidine are chosen for patients with benzodiazepine and alcohol withdrawal–related delirium. Although bradycardia and hypotension are common side effects of these medications, dexmedetomidine does not seem to have caused severe, uncompensated systemic or cerebral hemodynamic disturbances [88]. Dexmedetomidine infusion in the neuro-ICU also lowered the delirium rate in patients with TBI who went to general wards after craniotomy surgeries [89].

15.10 Neuromuscular Blockers in Neurocritical Care: Necessary or Overused?

The use of neuromuscular blockers (NMBs), in conjunction with sedatives, is advantageous in the neurocritical care population. They facilitate intubation and ventilator compliance. An NMB is used to treat refractory ICP crises; however, there is no high-quality evidence supporting this practice [90]. Succinylcholine, the widely used depolarizing group of NMB agents, is ideal for rapid sequence intubation due to its rapid onset and offset, especially in the NCCU [91]. However, succinylcholine has a number of known side effects, particularly in NCCUs. These include hypersensitivity, malignant hyperthermia, and a brief rise in potassium levels. Nicotinic acetylcholine receptors in weakened musculature may upregulate compensatorily in patients with neurological conditions that cause paralysis, spinal cord injury, demyelinating disorders, and prolonged immobility; succinylcholine use in these patients may result in prolonged paralysis, and non-depolarizing agents are preferred [92]. Since succinylcholine might result in deadly hyperkalemia, it is obviously contraindicated in Guillain–Barré syndrome, according to numerous case reports [93–95]. Previously hypothesized depolarization-induced muscle fasciculations, causing a transient rise in ICP, have little importance, as a meta-analysis conducted failed to prove so [96].

15.11 Critical Illness Myopathy: A Hidden Consequence of Prolonged Sedation

Neurological patients are often mechanically ventilated for prolonged periods and, therefore, at a higher risk of developing conditions called critical illness polyneuropathy (CIP) and/or critical illness myopathy (CIM), which often coexist many a time and result in prolonged weaning and weakness. [97] The infusion of NMBs may not play a certain role in CIP/CIM, as before [98]. With the development of CIP/CIM, the weaning period multiplies by two- to sevenfold in the general ICU population, [99] and such data are lacking in neurological patients due to their exclusion from RCTs on weaning strategies. [100] Caution should be exercised while considering NMB for mechanically ventilated neurological patients for prolonged periods since the link between NMB and CIP/CIM is not clear. A negative impact on weaning, in turn, would delay the rehabilitation process and affect neurological recovery [101]. Besides, a severe CIP/CIM may also result in false-negative prognostication of NCCU patients. These data suggest that it is wiser to avoid prolonged usage of NMBs in NCCU.

Strategies for avoiding NMB-induced weakness include the following:

1. Avoid unindicated usage of NMB infusions when mandates prefer shorter-acting agents.
2. Frequent interruption of sedation/NMB infusions to perform neurological examination (neurological wake-up tests).
3. Use of quantitative monitoring (Electromyography /Train-of-Four (EMG/TOF)) to assess the NMB degree.

15.12 Challenges in Sedating Patients with Nonconvulsive Status Epilepticus (NCSE)

NCSE is a diagnosis based on clinical suspicion in patients having a wide range of symptoms varying from a little confusion to coma, based on the type of NCSE, either absent or complex partial SE [102]. Sedating these patients is even more challenging, let alone treating them. The diagnosis and treatment of NCSE is by continuous EEG monitoring to attain therapeutic endpoints on similar lines to convulsive status epilepticus [103]. Though there is not much literature regarding sedation in such patients, it is advisable to sedate the ones who are confused, psychotic, having gross body movements, or experiencing myoclonus to prevent them from inflicting self-injury. Sedating those who are comatose should be strictly based on continuous EEG monitoring and also should be individualized based on the severity of acute brain injury, taking into account the cerebral hemodynamics using multimodal monitoring in the NCCU.

15.13 Landmark Trials and Emerging Evidence in Sedation Practices

15.13.1 NONSEDA: Non-sedation or Light Sedation in Critically Ill, Mechanically Ventilated Patients [104]

This multicenter RCT was conducted in eight Scandinavian ICU patients aged ≥18 years, intubated <24 h prior and expected to be ventilated ≥24 h, to assess whether a strategy of non-sedation compared to one of light sedation (with daily interruption of sedation) would impact the 90-day mortality. The patients in the non-sedation group received no routine sedation apart from bolus doses of morphine for analgesia. The control group that was under light sedation received continuous sedation, aiming for a Richmond Agitation-Sedation Scale (RASS) score of −2 to −3, with propofol for the first 48 h, which was then swapped to midazolam; the daily sedation breaks were given every morning, aiming to get them to full wakefulness. There was no appreciable difference in the 90-day mortality between light and non-sedation techniques, according to this study. While there were fewer deep vein thrombosis (DVT)/ Pulmonary edema (PE) episodes in the non-sedation group, there were also more inadvertent extubations and removals of arterial and nasogastric tube (NGT) lines. Targeting light sedation (RASS: −2–1), in conjunction with daily sedation breaks, is advised, being cautious not to over-sedate during ventilation. The mortality point estimate supports light sedation and raises questions about the safety of a non-sedation strategy. Further studies in this area should assess the psychological effects of not using sedation on patients, the amount of work that nurses have to do, and whether this is feasible in a neuro–intensive care unit.

15.13.2 SLEAP: Daily Sedation Interruption in Mechanically Ventilated Critically Ill Patients Cared for with a Sedation Protocol—A Randomized Controlled Trial [105]

The RCT was conducted in Canadian intensive care units to evaluate whether everyday breaks in sedation with opioids and/or benzodiazepines shorten the time until extubation in patients, apart from the ones who had cardiac arrest or traumatic brain injury or in whom neuromuscular blockers were administered, expected to require at least 48 h of mechanical ventilation. The authors found no variance in median time for successful extubation (1.08 h, CI: 0.86–1.35; $P = 0.52$), and median days to extubation were 7 days in both groups. The reintubation rates were 5.6% and 7.7%; the tracheostomy rates were 23.2% and 26.3%. Hence, daily interruptions are not helpful while using a sedation protocol in an ICU to target a light plane of sedation. They are also challenging to carry out effectively and may add to the nurses' workload. Propofol was not used for sedation, which is more often used in the neuro-ICU, and hence, the study is less generalizable to neuro-ICU settings.

15.13.3 SPICE III: Early Sedation with Dexmedetomidine in Critically Ill Patients [106]

This multicenter randomized controlled trial assessed whether using dexmedetomidine as the principal sedative instead of more common sedatives affected the 90-day mortality rate in critically ill, ventilated patients. Dexmedetomidine (1 μg/kg/hr) was infused continuously without a loading dose to sedate ICU patients who were under the age of 18 and in need of ventilation for more than 12 h prior to enrollment. These patients did not have an acute primary brain injury and were anticipated to stay in the ICU till at least the day after the next. The dose was adjusted to 1.5 μg/kg/hr., as needed. A difference was observed in the median days free from coma to day 28 (24 vs. 23; 95% CI 0.5–1.5) and median ventilator-free days at day 28 (23 vs. 22; 95% CI 0.4–1.6). However, there was no difference in the 90-day mortality rates between dexmedetomidine and usual care, 29.1% (566/1848) and 29.1% (569/1956) [95% CI -2.9–2.8, P = 0.98]. Bradycardia and hypotension were more common in the dexmedetomidine group. Thus, there was no reduction in the 90-day mortality when dexmedetomidine was used as the only or primary sedative in ventilated ICU patients. Although those who used it experienced fewer days in coma and delirium, as well as one less day on the ventilator, these results were not corrected for multiple comparisons.

15.13.4 DahLIA: Effect of Dexmedetomidine Added to Standard Care on Ventilator-Free Time in Patients with Agitated Delirium—A Randomized Clinical Trial [107]

This trial examined whether dexmedetomidine is useful in lowering the incidence of agitated delirium and the number of days on a ventilator. This multicenter RCT included adult ICU patients whose grade of agitation was deemed to be so severe that the risk of decreasing their sedation and extubation was considered unsafe. They excluded the ones who were pregnant, breastfeeding, having dementia, requiring specialized nursing care, or having an altered mental status secondary to head injury. Dexmedetomidine was started for the patients at a rate of 0.5ug /kg/hr. and titrated to a range of 0–1.5ug/kg/hr. to achieve a score of 0 on RASS or as directed by the doctor. The researchers found that the dexmedetomidine group had a statistically significant increase in median hours free from ventilation at 7 days (144.8 vs. 127.5 h, $P = 0.01$) and a decrease in median hours until the bedside nurse considered the patient ready for extubation. According to this underpowered study, using dexmedetomidine alongside standard care for ventilated patients with agitated delirium, who are otherwise prepared for extubation, might be advantageous. Specifically, there was a slight decrease in the amount of time needed to be weaned off from the ventilator, a quicker resolution of delirium, and opioid sparing effects of sedation..

15.14 Conclusion

The current approach to sedation and analgesia in the neuro–intensive care population is advancing, incorporating generalized data from all ICU units and tailoring it to the specific needs of these patients with an understanding of neurophysiology. While the principal goal remains adequate sedation, close neuromonitoring and maintaining cerebral hemodynamics are indispensable. Meticulous selection of drugs (**Annexure**), active monitoring, and adjustments as per the requirements are cornerstones to attaining these goals.

References

1. Oddo M, Crippa IA, Mehta S, et al. Optimizing sedation in patients with acute brain injury. Crit Care. 2016;20:128. https://doi.org/10.1186/s13054-016-1294-5.
2. Carney N, Totten AM, O'Reilly C, et al. Guidelines for the management of severe traumatic brain injury, Fourth Edition. Neurosurgery. 2017;80:6–15. https://doi.org/10.1227/NEU.0000000000001432.
3. Devlin JW, Skrobik Y, Gélinas C, et al. Clinical practice guidelines for the prevention and management of pain, agitation/sedation, delirium, immobility, and sleep disruption in adult patients in the ICU. Crit Care Med. 2018;46:e825–73.
4. Oddo M, Crippa IA, Mehta S, Menon D, Payen J-F, Taccone FS, Citerio G. Optimizing sedation in patients with acute brain injury. Crit Care. 2016;20:128.
5. Adembri C, Venturi L, Pellegrini-Giampietro DE. Neuroprotective effects of propofol in acute cerebral injury. CNS Drug Rev. 2007;13:333–51.
6. Urwin SC, Menon DK. Comparative tolerability of sedative agents in head-injured adults. Drug Saf. 2004;27:107–33.
7. Fodale V, Schifilliti D, Pratico C, Santamaria LB. Remifentanil and the brain. Acta Anaesthesiol Scand. 2008;52:319–26.
8. Roberts DJ, Hall RI, Kramer AH, Robertson HL, Gallagher CN, Zygun DA. Sedation for critically ill adults with severe traumatic brain injury: a systematic review of randomized controlled trials. Crit Care Med. 2011;39:2743–51.
9. Brophy GM, Bell R, Claassen J, Alldredge B, Bleck TP, Glauser T, et al. Guidelines for the evaluation and management of status epilepticus. Neurocrit Care. 2012;17:3–23.
10. Fang Y, Wang X. Ketamine for the treatment of refractory status epilepticus. Seizure. 2015;30:14–20.
11. Meierkord H, Boon P, Engelsen B, Gocke K, Shorvon S, Tinuper P, et al. EFNS guideline on the management of status epilepticus in adults. Eur J Neurol. 2010;17:348–55.

12. Ramineni A, Roberts EA, Vora M, Mahboobi SK, Nozari A. Anesthesia considerations in neurological emergencies. Neurol Clin. 2021;39(2):319–32.
13. Schizodimos T, Soulountsi V, Iasonidou C, Kapravelos N. An overview of management of intracranial hypertension in the intensive care unit. J Anesth. 2020;34(5):741–57.
14. Wu M, Yin X, Chen M, Liu Y, Zhang X, Li T, et al. Effects of propofol on intracranial pressure and prognosis in patients with severe brain diseases undergoing endotracheal suctioning. BMC Neurol. 2020;20(1):394.
15. Preethi J, Bidkar PU, Cherian A, Dey A, Srinivasan S, Adinarayanan S, et al. Comparison of total intravenous anesthesia vs inhalational anesthesia on brain relaxation, intracranial pressure, and hemodynamics in patients with acute subdural hematoma undergoing emergency craniotomy: a randomized control trial. Eur J Trauma Emerg Surg. 2021;47(3):831–7.
16. Vimala S, Arulvelan A, Chandy VG. Comparison of the effects of propofol and sevoflurane induced burst suppression on cerebral blood flow and oxygenation: a prospective, randomised, double-blinded study. World Neurosurg. 2020;135:e427–34.
17. Jeffcote T, Weir T, Anstey J, Mcnamara R, Bellomo R, Udy A. The impact of sedative choice on intracranial and systemic physiology in moderate to severe traumatic brain injury: a scoping review. J Neurosurg Anesthesiol. 2022;35:265–73.
18. Lowhagen Henden P, Rentzos A, Karlsson JE, Rosengren L, Leiram B, Sundeman H, et al. General anesthesia versus conscious sedation for endovascular treatment of acute ischemic stroke: the AnStroke trial (anesthesia during stroke). Stroke. 2017;48(6):1601–7.
19. Simonsen CZ, Yoo AJ, Sorensen LH, Juul N, Johnsen SP, Andersen G, et al. Effect of general anesthesia and conscious sedation during endovascular therapy on infarct growth and clinical outcomes in acute ischemic stroke: a randomized clinical trial. JAMA Neurol. 2018;75(4):470–7.
20. Schonenberger S, Henden PL, Simonsen CZ, Uhlmann L, Klose C, Pfaff JAR, et al. Association of general anesthesia vs procedural sedation with functional outcome among patients with acute ischemic stroke undergoing thrombectomy: a systematic review and meta-analysis. JAMA. 2019;322(13):1283–93.
21. Pertzov B, Krasulya B, Azem K, Shostak Y, Izhakian S, Rosengarten D, Kharchenko S, Kramer MR. Dexmedetomidine versus propofol sedation in flexible bronchoscopy: a randomized controlled trial. BMC Pulm Med. 2022;22(1):87.
22. Liu X, Li Y, Kang L, Wang Q. Recent advances in the clinical value and potential of dexmedetomidine. J Inflamm Res. 2021;14:7507.
23. Kallioinen M, Posti JP, Rahi M, Sharma D, Katila A, Gronlund J, et al. Cerebral autoregulation after aneurysmal subarachnoid haemorrhage. A preliminary study comparing dexmedetomidine to propofol and/or midazolam. Acta Anaesthesiol Scand Wiley-Blackwell; 2020. p. 1278–86, 64.
24. Bilodeau V, Saavedra-Mitjans M, Frenette AJ, et al. Safety of dexmedetomidine for thecontrol of agitation in critically ill traumatic brain injury patients: a descriptive study. J Clin Pharm Ther. 2021;46(4):1020–6.
25. Khallaf M, Thabet AM, Ali M, Sharkawy E, Abdel-rehim S. The effect of dexmedetomidine versus propofol in traumatic brain injury: evaluation of some hemodynamic and intracranial pressure changes. Egypt J Neurosurg. 2019;34(1):17.
26. James ML, Olson DM, Graffagnino C. A pilot study of cerebral and haemodynamic physiological changes during sedation with dexmedetomidine or propofol in patients with acute brain injury. Anaesth Intensive Care. 2012;40(6):949–57.
27. Oddo M, Crippa IA, Mehta S, Menon D, Payen JF, Taccone FS, et al. Optimizing sedation in patients with acute brain injury. Crit Care. 2016;20(1):128.
28. Schomer KJ, Sebat CM, Adams JY, Duby JJ, Shahlaie K, Louie EL. Dexmedetomidine for refractory intracranial hypertension. J Intensive Care Med. 2019;34(1):62–6.
29. Abowali HA, Paganini M, Enten G, Elbadawi A, Camporesi EM. Critical review and meta-analysis of postoperative sedation after adult cardiac surgery: dexmedetomidine versus propofol. J Cardiothorac Vasc Anesth. 2021;35(4):1134–42.

30. Xiao Z, He T, Jiang X, Xie F, Xia L, Zhou H. Effect of dexmedetomidine and propofol sedation on the prognosis of children with severe respiratory failure: a systematic review and metaanalysis. Transl Pediatr. 2022;11(2):260–9.
31. Glaess SS, Attridge RL, Christina GG. Clonidine as a strategy for discontinuing dexmedetomidine sedation in critically ill patients:a narrative review. Am J Health-Syst Pharm. 2020;77(7):515–22.
32. Kienitz R, Kay L, Beuchat I, Gelhard S, von Brauchitsch S, Mann C, et al. Benzodiazepines in the management of seizures and status epilepticus: a review of routes of delivery, pharmacokinetics, efficacy, and tolerability. CNS Drugs. 2022;36(9):951–75.
33. Weiss B, Hilfrich D, Vorderwulbecke G, Heinrich M, Grunow JJ, Paul N, et al. Outcomes in critically ill patients sedated with intravenous lormetazepam or midazolam: a retrospective cohort study. J Clin Med. 2021;10(18):4091.
34. George S, Mathew J. Midazolam is effective in controlling intracranial pressure in severe traumatic brain injury. CHRISMED J Health Res. 2019;6(4):242–7.
35. Garcia R, Salluh JIF, Andrade TR, Farah D, da Silva PSL, Bastos DF, et al. A systematic review and meta-analysis of propofol versus midazolam sedation in adult intensive care (ICU) patients. J Crit Care. 2021;64:91–9.
36. Pandharipande PP, Pun BT, Herr DL, Maze M, Girard TD, Miller RR, et al. Effect of sedation with dexmedetomidine vs lorazepam on acute brain dysfunction in mechanically ventilated patients: the MENDS randomized controlled trial. JAMA. 2007;298(22):2644–53.
37. Zanza C, Piccolella F, Racca F, Romenskaya T, Longhitano Y, Franceschi F, et al. Ketamine in acute brain injury: currentopinion following cerebral circulation and electrical activity. Healthcare (Basel). 2022;10(3):566.
38. Zeiler FA, Teitelbaum J, West M, Gillman LM. The ketamine effect on intracranial pressure in nontraumatic neurological illness. J Crit Care. 2014;29(6):1096–106.
39. Gregers MCT, Mikkelsen S, Lindvig KP, Brochner AC. Ketamine as an anesthetic for patients with acute brain injury: a systematic review. Neurocrit Care. 2020;33(1):273–82.
40. Pribish A, Wood N, Kalava A. A review of nonanesthetic uses of ketamine. Anesthesiol Res Pract. 2020;2020:5798285.
41. Andolfatto G, Abu-Laban RB, Zed PJ, Staniforth SM, Stackhouse S, Moadebi S, et al. Ketamine-propofol combination (ketofol) versus propofol alone for emergency department procedural sedation and analgesia: a randomized double-blind trial. Ann Emerg Med. 2012;59(6):504–12.e1–2.
42. Walravens S, Buylaert W, Steen E, De Paepe P. Implementation of a protocol using ketamine-propofol ('ketofol') in a 1 to 4 ratio for procedural sedation in adults at a university hospital emergency department – report on safety and effectiveness. Acta Clin Belg. 2021;76(5):359–64.
43. Ferguson I, Bell A, Treston G, New L, Ding M, Holdgate A. Propofol or ketofol for procedural sedation and analgesia in emergency medicine-the POKER study: a randomized doubleblind clinical trial. Ann Emerg Med. 2016;68(5):574–82 e1.
44. Murala S, Yelam A, Ismail MM, Bollu PCGABA. In: Bollu PC, editor. Neurochemistry in clinical practice. Cham: Springer International Publishing; 2022. p. 73–89.
45. Mathur M, Malik MT. Benzodiazepines and barbiturates. In: Kamat PP, Berkenbosch JW, editors. Sedation and analgesia for the pediatric intensivist: a clinical guide. Cham: Springer International Publishing; 2021. p. 401–10.
46. Bernstein JE, Ghanchi H, Kashyap S, Podkovik S, Miulli DE, Wacker MR, et al. Pentobarbital coma with therapeutic hypothermia for treatment of refractory intracranial hypertension in traumatic brain injury patients: a single institution experience. Cureus. 2020;12(9):e10591.
47. Navarro JC, Kofke WA. Chapter 24: Perioperative management of acute centralnervous system injury. In: Perioperative Medicine. 2nd ed; 2022. p. 355–409.
48. Aisiku IP. Chapter 387: Critical care management of traumatic brain injury. In: Youmansand Winn neurological surgery. 8th ed. Philadelphia, PA: Elsevier, Inc.; 2023. p. 3003–26.

49. Yamakawa Y, Morioka M, Negoto T, Orito K, Yoshitomi M, Nakamura Y, et al. A novel step-down infusion method of barbiturate therapy: its safety and effectiveness for intracranial pressure control. Pharmacol Res Perspect. 2021;9(2):e00719.
50. Severgnini P, Pelosi P, Contino E, Serafinelli E, Novario R, Chiaranda M. Accuracy of critical care pain observation tool and behavioral pain scale to assess pain in critically ill conscious and unconscious patients: prospective, observational study. J Intensive Care. 2016;4:68.
51. de Haro C, Magrans R, Lopez-Aguilar J, Montanya J, Lena E, Subira C, et al. Effects of sedatives and opioids on trigger and cycling asynchronies throughout mechanical ventilation: an observational study in a large dataset from critically ill patients. Crit Care. 2019;23(1):245.
52. Casamento AJ, Serpa Neto A, Young M, Lawrence M, Taplin C, Eastwood GM, et al. A phase II cluster-crossover randomized trial of fentanyl versus morphine for analgosedation in mechanically ventilated patients. Am J Respir Crit Care Med. 2021;204(11):1286–94.
53. Devlin JW, Skrobik Y, Gelinas C, Needham DM, Slooter AJC, Pandharipande PP, et al. Clinical practice guidelines for the prevention and management of pain, agitation/sedation, delirium, immobility, and sleep disruption in adult patients in the ICU. Crit Care Med. 2018;46(9):e825–73.
54. Wiener J, McIntyre A, Janzen S, Mirkowski M, MacKenzie HM, Teasell R. Opioids and cerebral physiology in the acute management of traumatic brain injury: a systematic review. Brain Inj. 2019;33(5):559–66.
55. Lee KA, Ganta N, Horton JR, Chai E. Evidence for neurotoxicity due to morphine or hydromorphone use in renal impairment: a systematic review. J Palliat Med. 2016;19(11):1179–87. https://doi.org/10.1089/jpm.2016.0101. Epub 2016 Jul 11. PMID: 27399959.
56. Laferriere-Langlois P, d'Aragon F, Manzanares W. Halogenated volatile anesthetics the intensive care unit: current knowledge on an upcoming practice. Minerva Anesthesiologica. 2017;83:737–48.
57. Kim HY, Lee JE, Kim HY, Kim J. Volatile sedation in the intensive care unit. Medicine. 2017;96:e8976.
58. Jerath A, Panckhurst J, Parotto M, et al. Safety and efficacy of volatile anesthetic agents compared with standard intravenous midazolam/propofol sedation in ventilated critical care patients: a meta-analysis and systematic review of prospective trials. Anesth Analg. 2017;124:1190–9.
59. Villa F, Iacca C, Molinari AF, et al. Inhalation versus endovenous sedation in subarachnoid hemorrhage patients: effects on regional cerebral blood flow. Crit Care Med. 2012;40:2797–804.
60. Jerath A, Wąsowicz M. In reply: anesthesia scavenging in critical care areas:beware of possible hazards and questionable efficacy. Can J Anesth. 2017;64:98–9.
61. Manatpon P, Kofke WA. Toxicity of inhaled agents after prolonged administration. J Clin Monit Comput. 2018;32:651–66.
62. Ing C, Hegarty MK, Perkins JW, et al. Duration of general anaesthetic exposure in early childhood and long-term language and cognitive ability. Br J Anaesth. 2017;119:532–40.
63. Takagaki M, Feuerstein D, Kumagai T, et al. Isoflurane suppresses cortical spreading depolarizations compared to propofol - implications for sedation of neurocritical care patients. Exp Neurol. 2014;252:12–7.
64. Perkes I, Baguley IJ, Nott MT, Menon DK. A review of paroxysmal sympathetic hyperactivity after acquired brain injury. Ann Neurol. 2010;68:126–35.
65. Tang Q, Wu X, Weng W, Li H, Feng J, Mao Q, Gao G, Jiang J. The preventive effect of dexmedetomidine on paroxysmal sympathetic hyperactivity in severe traumatic brain injury patients who have undergone surgery: a retrospective study. PeerJ. 2017;5:e2986. https://doi.org/10.7717/peerj.2986. PMID: 28229021; PMCID: PMC5314954.
66. Helbok R, Kurtz P, Schmidt MJ, Stuart MR, Fernandez L, Connolly SE, et al. Effects of the neurological wake-up test on clinical examination, intracranial pressure, brain metabolism and brain tissue oxygenation in severely brain-injured patients. Crit Care. 2012;16:R226. https://doi.org/10.1186/cc11880.

67. Skoglund K, Enblad P, Marklund N. Effects of the neurological wake-up test on intracranial pressure and cerebral perfusion pressure in brain-injured patients. Neurocrit Care. 2009;11:135–42. https://doi.org/10.1007/s12028-009-9255-3.
68. Skoglund K, Enblad P, Hillered L, Marklund N. The neurological wake-up test increases stress hormone levels in patients with severe traumatic brain injury. Crit Care Med. 2012;40:216–22. https://doi.org/10.1097/CCM.0b013e31822d7dbd.
69. Skoglund K, Hillered L, Purins K, Tsitsopoulos PP, Flygt J, Engquist H, et al. The neurological wake-up test does not alter cerebral energy metabolism and oxygenation in patients with severe traumatic brain injury. Neurocrit Care. 2014;20:413–26. https://doi.org/10.1007/s12028-013-9876-4.
70. Oddo M, Frangos S, Maloney-Wilensky E, Andrew Kofke W, Le Roux PD, Levine JM. Effect of shivering on brain tissue oxygenation during induced normothermia in patients with severe brain injury. Neurocrit Care. 2010;12(1):10–6. https://doi.org/10.1007/s12028-009-9280-2.
71. Schmidbauer ML, Lanz H, Maskos A, Putz T, Kunst S, Dimitriadis K. Sedation protocols in non-traumatic SAH (SPRINT-SAH): a cross-sectional survey among German-speaking neurointensivists. Front Neurol. 2023;14:1058804. https://doi.org/10.3389/fneur.2023.1058804.
72. Dolmans RGF, Nahed BV, Robertson FC, Peul WC, Rosenthal ES, Broekman MLD. Practice-pattern variation in sedation of neurotrauma patients in the intensive care unit: an international survey. J Intensive Care Med. 2023;38:1143–50. https://doi.org/10.1177/08850666231186563.
73. Schmidbauer ML, Läufer S, Maskos A, Dimitriadis K. Risk factors and outcomes after interruption of sedation in subarachnoid hemorrhage (ROUTINE-SAH)-a retrospective cohort study. Front Neurol. 2024;15:1363107. https://doi.org/10.3389/fneur.2024.1363107. PMID: 38545282; PMCID: PMC10965800.
74. Mulder HD, Helfferich J, MCJ K. The neurological wake-up test in severe pediatric traumatic brain injury: a long term, single-center experience. Front Pediatr. 2024;12:1367337. https://doi.org/10.3389/fped.2024.1367337. PMID: 38464893; PMCID: PMC10920253.
75. Bhalerao SU, Geurtjens C, Thomas GR, et al. Understanding the neuropsychiatric consequences associated with significant traumatic brain injury. Brain Inj. 2013;27(7–8):767–74.
76. Carin-Levy G, Mead GE, Nicol K, et al. Delirium in acute stroke: screening tools,incidence rates and predictors: a systematic review. J Neurol. 2012;259(8):1590–9.
77. Salluh JI, Wang H, Schneider EB, et al. Outcome of delirium in critically ill patients:systematic review and meta-analysis. BMJ. 2015;350:h2538.
78. van den Boogaard M, Schoonhoven L, Maseda E, et al. Recalibration of the delirium prediction model for ICU patients (PRE-DELIRIC): a multinational observational study. Intensive Care Med. 2014;40(3):361–9.
79. van Gelder TG, van Diem-Zaal IJ, SMA D-K, de Mul N, Lalmohamed A, AJC S. The risk of delirium after sedation with propofol or midazolam in intensive care unit patients. Br J Clin Pharmacol. 2024;90(6):1471–9. https://doi.org/10.1111/bcp.16031. Epub 2024 Mar 14. PMID: 38482541.
80. Linkaitė G, Riauka M, Bunevičiūtė I, Vosylius S. Evaluation of PRE-DELIRIC (PREdiction of DELIRium in ICu patients) delirium prediction model for the patients in the intensive care unit. Acta Med Litu. 2018;25:14–22. https://doi.org/10.6001/actamedica.v25i1.3699.
81. Mitasova A, Kostalova M, Bednarik J, et al. Post stroke delirium incidence and outcomes: validation of the confusion assessment method for the intensive care unit (CAM-ICU). Crit Care Med. 2012;40(2):484–90.
82. Cheng H, Ling Y, Li Q, Tang Y, Li X, Liang X, Huang X, Su L, Lyu J. ICU admission Braden score independently predicts delirium in critically ill patients with ischemic stroke. Intensive Crit Care Nurs. 2024;82:103626. https://doi.org/10.1016/j.iccn.2024.103626. Epub 2024 Jan 13. PMID: 38219301.
83. Larsen LK, Frøkjaer VG, Nielsen JS, Skrobik Y, Winkler Y, Møller K, Petersen M, Egerod I. Delirium assessment in neuro-critically ill patients: a validation study. Acta Anaesthesiol Scand. 2019;63(3):352–9. https://doi.org/10.1111/aas.13270. Epub 2018 Oct 16. PMID: 30324653.

84. Sosnowski K, Lin F, Chaboyer W, Ranse K, Heffernan A, Mitchell M. The effect of the ABCDE/ABCDEF bundle on delirium, functional outcomes, and quality of life in critically ill patients: a systematic review and meta-analysis. Int J Nurs Stud. 2023;138:104410. https://doi.org/10.1016/j.ijnurstu.2022.104410. Epub 2022 Nov 29. PMID: 36577261.
85. Chen TJ, Traynor V, Wang AY, Shih CY, Tu MC, Chuang CH, Chiu HY, Chang HR. Comparative effectiveness of non-pharmacological interventions for preventing delirium in critically ill adults: a systematic review and network meta-analysis. Int J Nurs Stud. 2022;131:104239. https://doi.org/10.1016/j.ijnurstu.2022.104239. Epub 2022 Mar 28. PMID: 35468538.
86. Lee SM, Chou YH, Li MH, Wan FJ, Yen MH. Effects of haloperidol and risperidone on cerebrohemodynamics in drug-naive schizophrenic patients. J Psychiatr Res. 2008;42(4):328–35. https://doi.org/10.1016/j.jpsychires.2007.02.007. Epub 2007 Apr 6. PMID: 17412363.
87. Miller DD, Andreasen NC, O'Leary DS, Watkins GL, Boles Ponto LL, Hichwa RD. Comparison of the effects of risperidone and haloperidol on regional cerebral blood flow in schizophrenia. Biol Psychiatry. 2001;49(8):704–15. https://doi.org/10.1016/s0006-3223(00)01001-5. PMID: 11313038.
88. Tran A, Blinder H, Hutton B, English SW. A systematic review of Alpha-2 agonists for sedation in mechanically ventilated Neurocritical care patients. Neurocrit Care. 2018;28(1):12–25. https://doi.org/10.1007/s12028-017-0388-5. PMID: 28547318.
89. Deng Z, Gu Y, Luo L, Deng L, Li Y, Huang W. The effect of dexmedetomidine on the postoperative recovery of patients with severe traumatic brain injury undergoing craniotomy treatment: a retrospective study. Eur J Med Res. 2024;29(1):256. https://doi.org/10.1186/s40001-024-01861-0. PMID: 38689332; PMCID: PMC11059576.
90. Sanfilippo F, Santonocito C, Veenith T, Astuto M, Maybauer MO. The role of neuromuscular blockade in patients with traumatic brain injury: a systematic review. Neurocrit Care. 2015;22(2):325–34.
91. Lee S-J, Sung T-Y, Cho C-K. Comparison of emergence agitation between succinylcholine and rocuronium-sugammadex in adults following closed reduction of a nasal bone fracture: a prospective randomized controlled trial. BMC Anesthesiol. 2019;19(1):228.
92. Renew JR, Ratzlaff R, Hernandez-Torres V, Brull SJ, Prielipp RC. Neuromuscular blockade management in the critically ill patient. J Intensive Care. 2020;8(1):37.
93. Feldman JM. Cardiac arrest after succinylcholine administration in a pregnant patient recovered from Guillain-Barre syndrome. Anesthesiology. 1990;72(5):942–4.
94. Reilly M, Hutchinson M. Suxamethonium is contraindicated in the Guillain-Barre syndrome. J Neurol Neurosurg Psychiatry. 1991;54(11):1018–9.
95. Hor JY. Cardiac arrhythmia after succinylcholine administration in a patient with Guillain-Barre syndrome–a case report. Middle East J Anaesthesiol. 2010;20(6):881–3.
96. Kramer N, Lebowitz D, Walsh M, Ganti L. Rapid sequence intubation in traumatic brain-injured adults. Cureus. 2018;10(4):e2530.
97. Latronico N, Bolton CF. Critical illness polyneuropathy and myopathy: a major cause of muscle weakness and paralysis. Lancet Neurol. 2011;10:931–41.
98. Stevens RD, Dowdy DW, Michaels RK, Mendez-Tellez PA, Pronovost PJ, Needham DM. Neuromuscular dysfunction acquired in critical illness: a systematic review. Intensive Care Med. 2007;33:1876–91.
99. Latronico N, Shehu I, Seghelini E. Neuromuscular sequelae of critical illness. Curr Opin Crit Care. 2005;11:381–90.
100. Lazaridis C, DeSantis SM, McLawhorn M, Krishna V. Liberation of neurosurgical patients from mechanical ventilation and tracheostomy in neurocritical care. J Crit Care. 2012;27(417):e1–8.
101. Andelic N, Bautz-Holter E, Ronning P, et al. Does an early onset and continuous chain of rehabilitation improve the long-term functional outcome of patients with severe traumatic brain injury? J Neurotrauma. 2012;29:66–74.
102. Chang AK, Shinnar S. Nonconvulsive status epilepticus. Emerg Med Clin North Am. 2011;29(1):65–72. https://doi.org/10.1016/j.emc.2010.08.006. PMID: 21109103.

103. Ilhan Algın D, Uncu G, Ozbabalık Adapınar D, Osman Erdinç O. Nonconvulsive status epilepticus and coma [Internet]. In: Disorders of consciousness – a review of important issues. IntechOpen; 2020. https://doi.org/10.5772/intechopen.89428.
104. Olsen HT, Nedergaard HK, Strøm T, Oxlund J, Wian KA, Ytrebø LM, Kroken BA, Chew M, Korkmaz S, Lauridsen JT, Toft P. Nonsedation or light sedation in critically ill, mechanically ventilated patients. N Engl J Med. 2020;382(12):1103–11. https://doi.org/10.1056/NEJMoa1906759. Epub 2020 Feb 16. PMID: 32068366.
105. Mehta S, Burry L, Cook D, Fergusson D, Steinberg M, Granton J, Herridge M, Ferguson N, Devlin J, Tanios M, Dodek P, Fowler R, Burns K, Jacka M, Olafson K, Skrobik Y, Hébert P, Sabri E, Meade M, SLEAP Investigators; Canadian Critical Care Trials Group. Daily sedation interruption in mechanically ventilated critically ill patients cared for with a sedation protocol: a randomized controlled trial. JAMA. 2012;308(19):1985–92. https://doi.org/10.1001/jama.2012.13872. Erratum in: JAMA. 2013;309(3):237. PMID: 23180503.
106. Shehabi Y, Howe BD, Bellomo R, Arabi YM, Bailey M, Bass FE, Bin Kadiman S, McArthur CJ, Murray L, Reade MC, Seppelt IM, Takala J, Wise MP, Webb SA, ANZICS Clinical Trials Group and the SPICE III Investigators. Early sedation with Dexmedetomidine in critically ill patients. N Engl J Med. 2019;380(26):2506–17. https://doi.org/10.1056/NEJMoa1904710. Epub 2019 May 19. PMID: 31112380.
107. Reade MC, Eastwood GM, Bellomo R, Bailey M, Bersten A, Cheung B, Davies A, Delaney A, Ghosh A, van Haren F, Harley N, Knight D, McGuiness S, Mulder J, O'Donoghue S, Simpson N, Young P, DahLIA Investigators, Australian and New Zealand Intensive Care Society Clinical Trials Group. Effect of Dexmedetomidine added to standard care on ventilator-free time in patients with agitated delirium: a randomized clinical trial. JAMA. 2016;315(14):1460–8. https://doi.org/10.1001/jama.2016.2707. Erratum in: JAMA. 2016;316(7):775. https://doi.org/10.1001/jama.2016.9458. PMID: 26975647.

Controversies in Diagnostic Modalities in Neurocritical Care

16

Ajay Prasad Hrishi, Aswin Ram SPS, and Rahul Belgaonkar

Abstract

The combination of repeated neurological assessments with neuroimaging is paramount to contemporary neurocritical care. While alternative neuromonitoring methods are gaining importance, the skill to swiftly and accurately analyze images within the patient's clinical context remains crucial for neurocritical care specialists. Computed tomography (CT) stands out as the most valuable neuroimaging modality for intensive care unit (ICU) patients due to its rapid imaging speed and effectiveness in identifying conditions like intracerebral hemorrhage (ICH) and cerebral edema. Head CT scans are essential for making time-sensitive decisions in the neurological ICU (NICU). They play an important role in the evaluation of neurological disorders like traumatic brain injury (TBI) and subarachnoid hemorrhage (SAH). Magnetic resonance imaging (MRI) offers detailed images beneficial for detecting conditions like ischemia and aids in neuroprognostication, particularly for patients stable enough to undergo the procedure. Nuclear medicine imaging techniques, commonly used in neurocritical care research, have clinical utility in supplementary brain death evaluations. Furthermore, point-of-care ultrasound studies are increasingly employed in the NICU setting, enhancing the neurointensivist's diagnostic capabilities and patient care quality during transportation for radiological assessments.

Keywords

Stroke imaging · CT ASPECS · Fisher grading · Stroke MRI protocol · POCUS

A. P. Hrishi (✉) · A. R. SPS · R. Belgaonkar
Neuroanesthesia and Critical Care, Sree Chitra Tirunal Institute for Medical Sciences and Technology, Trivandrum, Kerala, India
e-mail: drajay@sctimst.ac.in

P. U. Bidkar, M. Krishnakumar (eds.), *Controversies in Neurocritical Care*, https://doi.org/10.1007/978-981-95-4419-6_16

16.1 Introduction

Neuroimaging is a vital component of the neuro–intensive care unit (ICU). With many imaging modalities available, we will go over each of them in brief. This article aims to provide the reader with information to arm themselves regarding the imaging of patients with acute stroke. Also, the imaging of patients with traumatic brain injury (TBI) and their prognostication aided by such imaging techniques will be touched upon. With ultrasonography (USG) becoming an essential tool in ICUs, we will also learn the role of point-of-care ultrasound in the neuro-ICU.

16.2 Stroke Imaging: When, What, and How?

There are two types of acute stroke:

I. Acute hemorrhagic stroke
II. Acute ischemic stroke

The treatment approach differs for each type, making an accurate diagnosis essential before initiating treatment. Clinically, both types of strokes can present with similar signs and symptoms, which necessitates the use of imaging to distinguish between them. Non-contrast computed tomography (NCCT) scans are particularly valuable in this context, as they provide a rapid means of differentiating between hemorrhagic and ischemic strokes. Therefore, it is recommended to perform an NCCT scan whenever a patient presents to the hospital with symptoms of an acute stroke. Below are some images illustrating acute stroke cases.

16.3 Stroke Imaging: When to Image

The American Stroke Association/American Heart Association (ASA/AHA) guidelines state that brain imaging should be performed urgently for all patients suspected of acute stroke on arrival at the hospital. NCCT or magnetic resonance imaging (MRI) can be used to rule out intracerebral hemorrhage (ICH) before the administration of alteplase. However, systems should ensure that the imaging process is streamlined so that it does not delay the initiation of treatment [1]. Gradient-echo MRI sequences can diagnose hyperacute (<6 h) intraparenchymal hemorrhage. In patients who woke up with a stroke or those with an ill-defined time of onset >4.5 h from the last time of having been seen normal, MRI fluid attenuation and inverse recovery (FLAIR) can be used to identify those who will benefit from alteplase [1]. The American College of Radiology (ACR) practice parameters recommend using CT angiography (CTA) to visualize the occluded vasculature. CT perfusion imaging can also help identify the infarct core and the penumbra. It can help rule out large irreversible infarcts that are not amenable to endovascular procedures.

16.4 Acute Ischemic Stroke: CT ASPECTS and the Implications

The Alberta Stroke Program Early CT Score (ASPECTS) [2] is a ten-point scale used to assess the extent of ischemic changes to the middle cerebral artery (MCA) territory on CT scans of stroke patients. To determine the ASPECTS score, you examine ten specific regions within the MCA territory and subtract 1 point for each region showing early ischemic signs, such as hypodensity or swelling. The ten regions are as follows (Fig. 16.1):

1. Caudate nucleus
2. Internal capsule
3. Lentiform nucleus
4. Insular cortex
5. Anterior MCA cortex (M1)
6. Lateral MCA cortex (M2)
7. Posterior MCA cortex (M3)
8. Anterior cortex above M1 (M4)
9. Lateral cortex above M2 (M5)
10. Posterior cortex above M3 (M6)

The ASPECTS score has a range of 0–10, with higher scores indicating less ischemic damage. A score of 10 indicates no ischemic changes, while a score of 0 means diffuse ischemia across the entire MCA territory. An ASPECTS score of 7 or lower is associated with poorer functional outcomes and a higher risk of hemorrhagic transformation following thrombolysis.

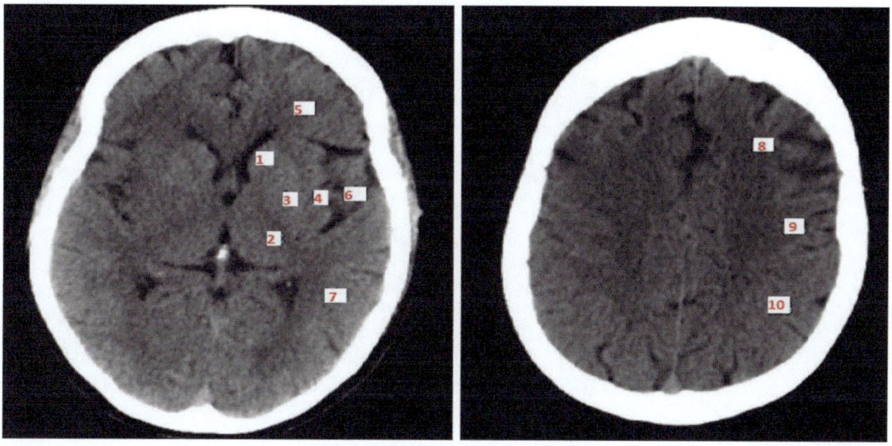

Fig. 16.1 Axial non-contrast CT of the brain showing regions numbered from 1 to 10. 1: caudate nucleus, 2: internal capsule, 3: lentiform nucleus, 4: insular cortex, 5: anterior MCA cortex (M1), 6: lateral MCA cortex (M2), 7: posterior MCA cortex (M3), 8: anterior cortex above M1 (M4), 9: lateral cortex above M2 (M5), and 10: posterior cortex above M3 (M6)

16.5 The Middle Cerebral Artery Dense Sign: A Reliable Early Indicator?

The term "dense sign" in brain imaging refers to the increased radiodensity of an artery or vein on a non-contrast CT scan, indicating the presence of a thrombus or a clot [3]. The dense sign can be observed in various locations, such as the following:

- *Middle cerebral artery (MCA)*, known as the hyperdense MCA sign or the Gács sign: This is among the earliest indicators of MCA infarction. It appears within 90 min after the event. The hyperdense MCA sign, also known as the Gács sign, is a type of hyperdense vessel sign indicating hyperdensity of the middle cerebral artery (MCA) on an NCCT scan. [4] (Figs. 16.2 and 16.3).
- This sign results from an embolic red blood clot originating from the heart or arteries. The high attenuation is primarily due to the elevated globin concentration in the clot. Typically, the clot lodges in the proximal MCA (Fig. 16.20). Sensitivity is 30%, and specificity is 90% [5].
- *Basilar artery*, known as the hyperdense basilar tip sign: This indicates basilar artery occlusion and is associated with a poor prognosis [6].
- *Cerebral veins or sinuses*, known as the dense clot sign: This suggests cerebral venous sinus thrombosis and is visible in about one-third of the cases.

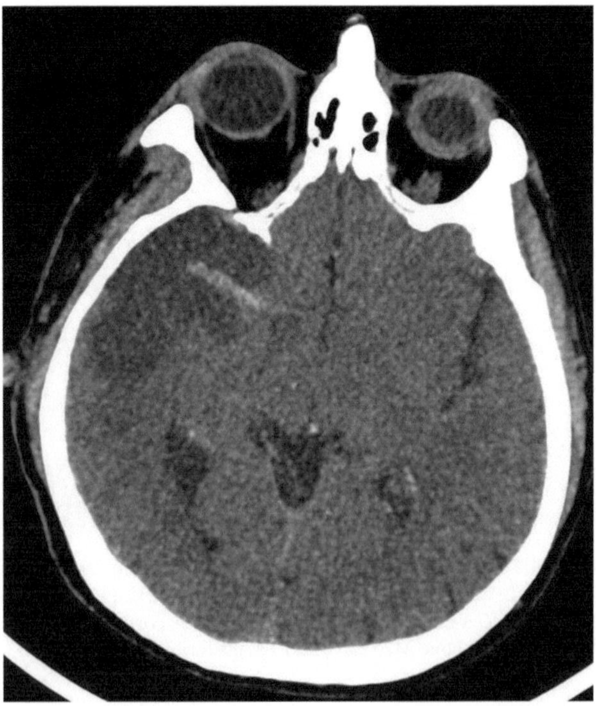

Fig. 16.2 Axial non-contrast CT of the head showing the right MCA infarct, appearing as a hypodensity in the image

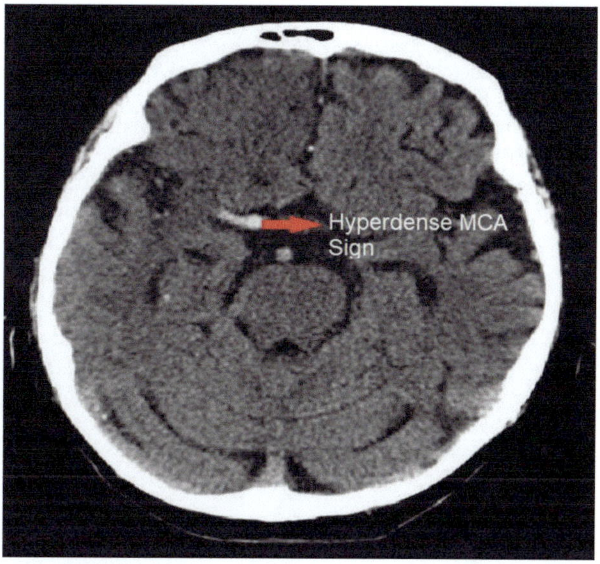

Fig. 16.3 Axial non-contrast CT of the head showing the right MCA hyperdense sign

16.6 Acute Hemorrhagic Stroke: How and Why to Measure Hematoma Volume

The volume of a hematoma in cases of intracerebral hemorrhage (ICH) is typically measured using the *ABC*/2 formula. This assumes the hematoma is an ellipsoid [7]. To apply this formula, you need to measure the following dimensions on CT images:

- *A*: The longest diameter of the hematoma in the axial plane (Fig. 16.4)
- *B*: The diameter perpendicular to *A* in the axial plane (Fig. 16.4)
- *C*: The craniocaudal diameter of the hematoma, calculated by multiplying the number of hematoma slices by the slice thickness or by using multi-planar reformats (Fig. 16.5)

The volume of the hematoma is then calculated by multiplying *A*, *B*, and *C* and dividing the result by 2 [8].

Larger hematomas tend to cause more severe neurological damage, leading to poorer functional outcomes. Additionally, while the exact role of hematoma expansion in increasing hematoma volume is not fully understood, it is believed to occur during the acute phase. This expansion can be exacerbated by existing health conditions and medications. So an intervention aims to reduce neurological damage [9].

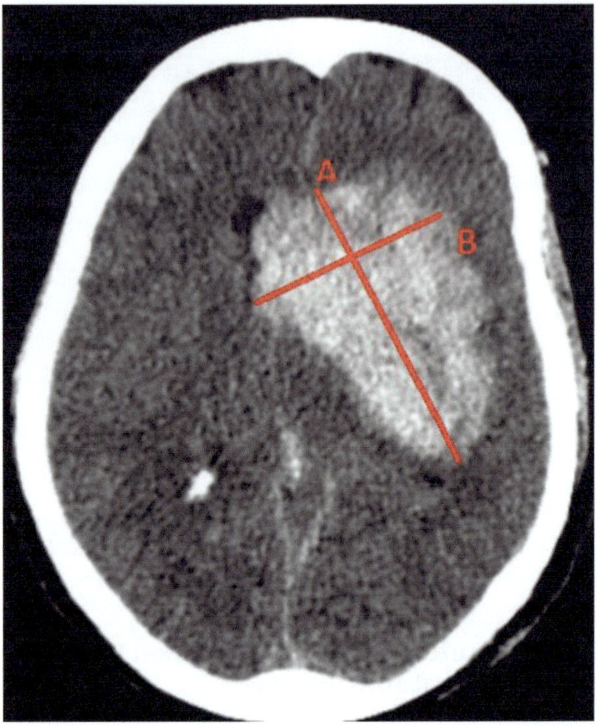

Fig. 16.4 Axial non-contrast CT of the head with an intraparenchymal hematoma. First, measure the maximum diameter of the hematoma as *A* and the length perpendicular to it as *B* in the axial plane

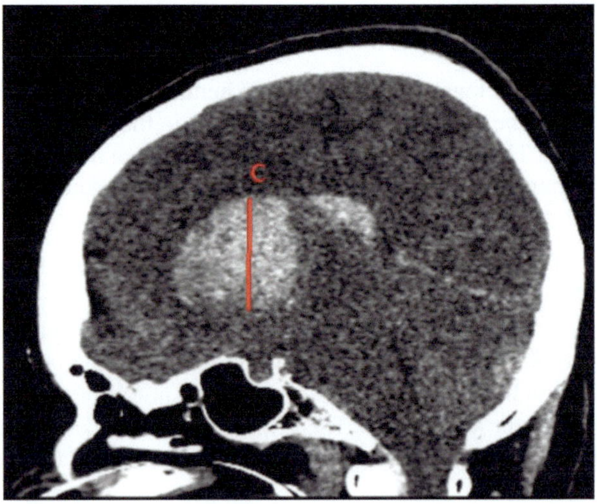

Fig. 16.5 Sagittal non-contrast CT of the head. Measure *C*, the craniocaudal diameter, in the sagittal plane

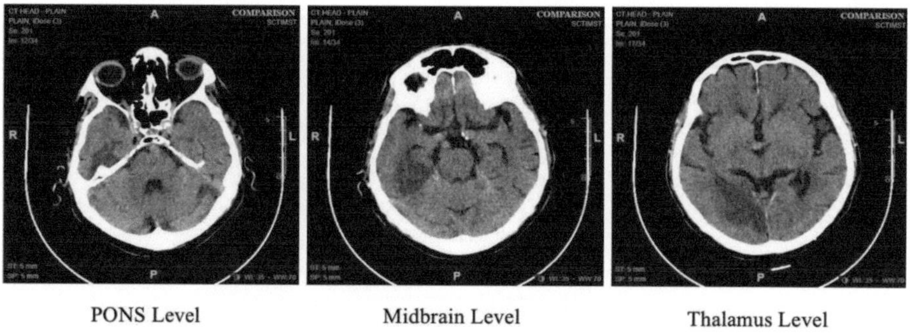

Fig. 16.6 The Posterior Circulation Alberta Stroke Program Early CT Score (PC-ASPECTS). This image shows an infarct in the left occipital lobe. The areas to look for are labeled as follows: T thalamus, OL occipital lobe, M midbrain, P pons, and C cerebellum

16.7 Posterior Circulation Stroke and PC-ASPECTS Implications (Fig. 16.6)

A meta analysis of retrospective studies found a significant link between low baseline PC-ASPECTS score and unfavorable functional outcomes (UFOs). A PC-ASPECTS score below 7 was identified as the most effective threshold for predicting a UFO. The variability in imaging modalities and recanalization treatments contributed to the heterogeneity observed in the analysis. Additionally, even a single-point reduction in PC-ASPECTS will impact the outcomes [10].

16.8 Imaging Modality in Posterior Fossa Bleeding: Which Is the Imaging Modality?

The posterior cranial fossa (PCF) is the deepest and most confined area of the skull, with a limited capacity to accommodate any expansion of its contents. It encompasses 6.3%–16.4% of all intracranial hemorrhages, seen more commonly in middle-aged and elderly patients. Despite various treatment approaches, the mortality rates for posterior fossa bleeding range from 20% to 75%, with total surgical mortality rates between 20% and 50% [11, 12] (Fig. 16.7).

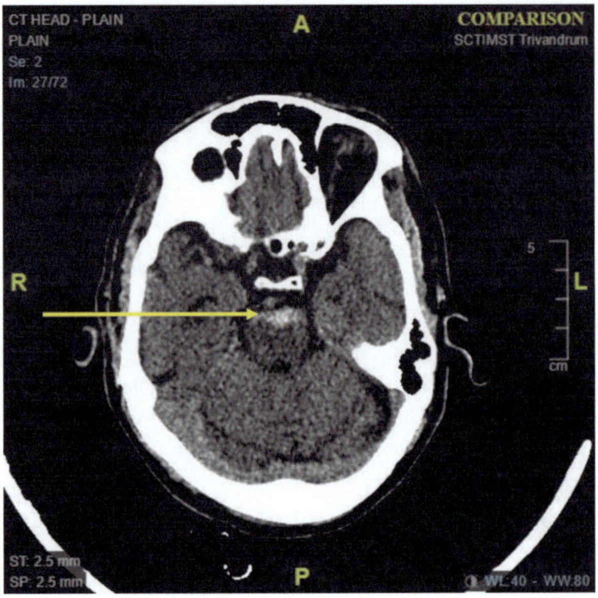

Fig. 16.7 Axial non-contrast CT of the head showing a pontine hemorrhage, appearing as a hyperdensity

16.9 Why to Use CT Contrast in Intracranial Hematoma: The Spot Sign

The spot sign is seen with CTA. It represents the pooling, accumulation, or extravasation of contrast material within the hematoma. It is critical to identify this sign during the evaluation of acute cerebral hemorrhage, as it increases the likelihood of the hematoma expanding [13].

It is a region of contrast enhancement seen within a hematoma compared to the rest of it. It can be of various shapes, ranging from spherical or branching to linear [14] (Fig. 16.8).

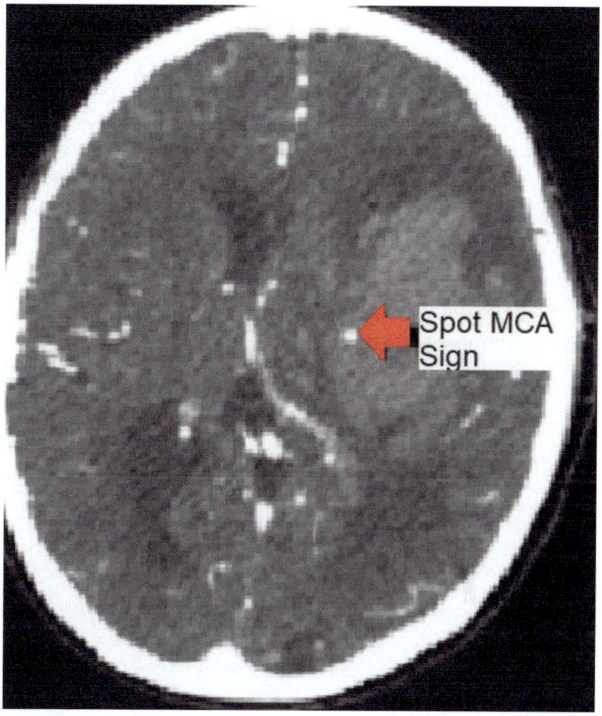

Fig. 16.8 Axial contrast-enhanced CT of the head showing the spot sign, as shown by an arrow

16.10 MRI Stroke Protocol: A Useful Tool for Acute Strokes

The MRI protocol for stroke assessment includes a series of MRI sequences designed to investigate brain ischemia accurately. The protocol typically consists of the following sequences:

- *T1-Weighted Sequence*: Provides anatomical evaluation.
- *T2-Weighted Axial Sequence*: Signal void loss in large arteries may be visible immediately. After 6–12 h, infarcted tissue appears as a high signal. Within a few days, sulcal effacement and mass effect develop, which can be picked up.
- *FLAIR Sequence*: Infarcted tissue shows high signal after 6–12 h.
- *Diffusion-Weighted Imaging (DWI)*: Enables early identification of ischemic stroke.
- *Susceptibility-Weighted Imaging (SWI)*: Ideal for detecting hemorrhage due to its high sensitivity; T2-weighted imaging (T2WI) can also be used.
- *MR Angiography (MRA)*: Time-of-flight (TOF) angiography can be used to assess the diameter of vessels and identify any occlusions.

This comprehensive protocol ensures a thorough assessment of stroke, enabling accurate diagnosis and timely intervention.

16.11 Application of SWI

SWI is a 3D, high-spatial-resolution, fully velocity-corrected gradient-echo MRI sequence. In contrast to usual conventional sequences, SWI utilizes both phase and magnitude effects. Compounds with paramagnetic, diamagnetic, or ferromagnetic properties interact with the local magnetic field, producing distortions that alter the phase of nearby tissues and consequently change the signal [15].

SWI is used to detect even small amounts of hemorrhage, blood products, or calcium, which may not be visible on other sequences. Also, it is an ideal technique to evaluate veins. The deoxyhemoglobin causes both a reduction in signal magnitude and a phase shift [15] (See Fig. 16.9).

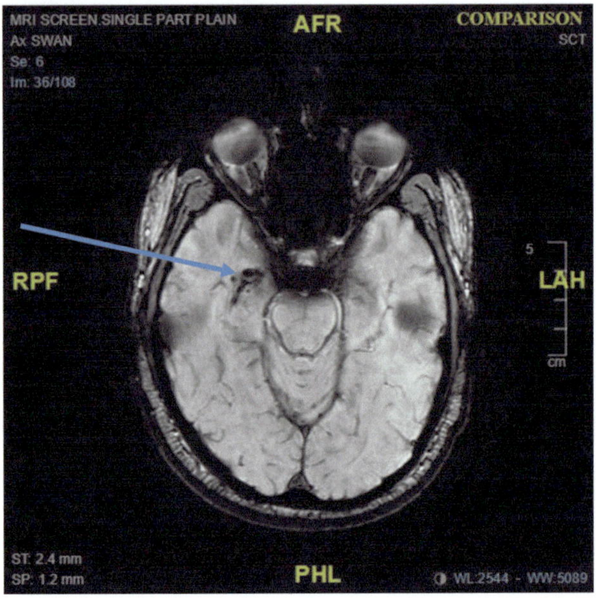

Fig. 16.9 Axial MRI of the head showing the SWI sequence, showing the appearance of a hemorrhage in the right hippocampus

16.12 Need for Advanced Sequences: DWI and ADC

The most sensitive sequence for stroke imaging is DWI. It detects the restricted Brownian motion of extracellular water, which occurs due to cytotoxic edema. Normally, water protons can diffuse extracellularly, resulting in signal loss. However, a high intensity on DWI indicates restricted diffusion of water protons in the extracellular space [16] (Fig. 16.10).

DWI is negative only in a small percentage of cases (~6.8%) [17].

Apparent diffusion coefficient (ADC) is a measure of the magnitude of diffusion of water molecules within tissues. It is calculated with DWI [18] (Fig. 16.5).

The appearance of DWI/ADC depends on the timing.

1. Acute (0–7 days): The ADC value decreases, with maximal signal reduction at 1–4 days.
2. Subacute (1–3 weeks): ADC values rise and return to baseline (pseudo-normalization).
3. Chronic (>3 weeks): ADC values increase.

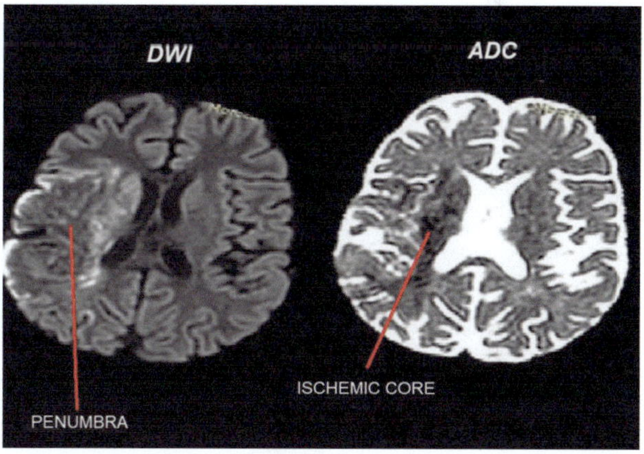

Fig. 16.10 Axial MRI of the head showing both the DWI and ADC sequences. The ischemic core in the ADC sequence and the penumbra in the DWI sequence are marked

16.13 Subarachnoid Hemorrhage (SAH): The Applications of Grading

The Fischer grading system is used to classify subarachnoid hemorrhage(SAH) based on the quantity and distribution of blood on non-contrast CT scans of the brain [19]. This classification is helpful in predicting the likelihood and severity of cerebral vasospasm, a common complication of SAH. The Fischer grading system includes four grades:

- *Grade 1*: No SAH detected
- *Grade 2*: Diffuse, thin SAH (<1 mm) with no clots
- *Grade 3*: Localized clots and/or layers of blood >1 mm in thickness, without intraventricular hemorrhage (IVH)
- *Grade 4*: Diffuse or no SAH, with IVH or intracerebral hemorrhage (ICH) present

This grading helps in assessing the risk of vasospasm and guiding the management of patients with SAH (Figs. 16.11, 16.12, and 16.13). Higher Fischer grades are associated with an increased risk of vasospasm.

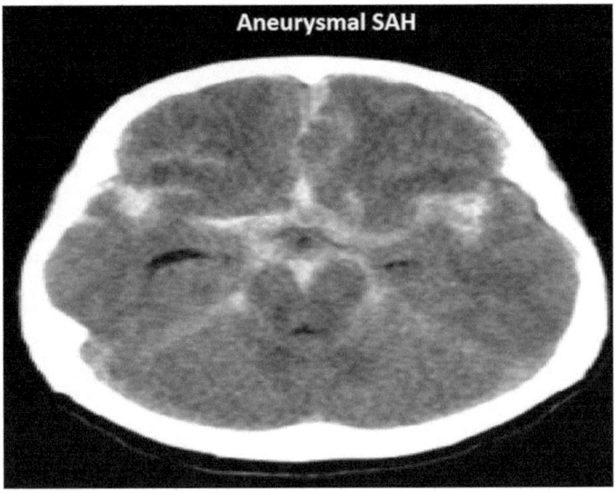

Fig. 16.11 Axial non-contrast CT of the head showing subarachnoid hemorrhage

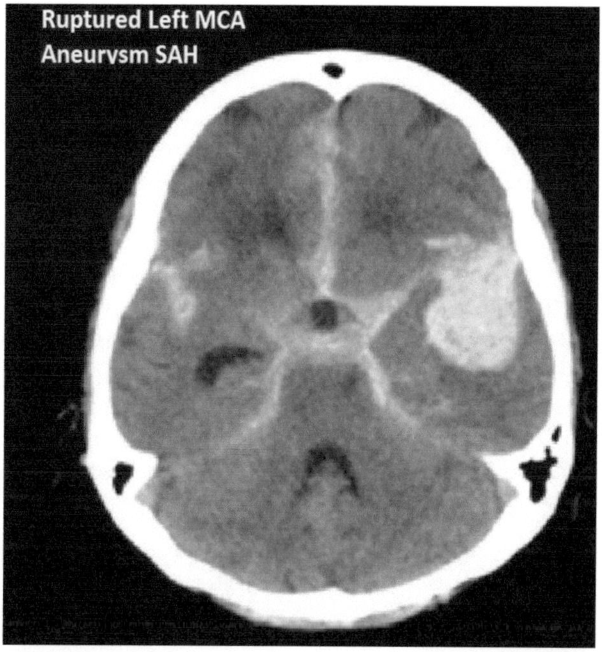

Fig. 16.12 Axial non-contrast CT of the head showing subarachnoid hemorrhage

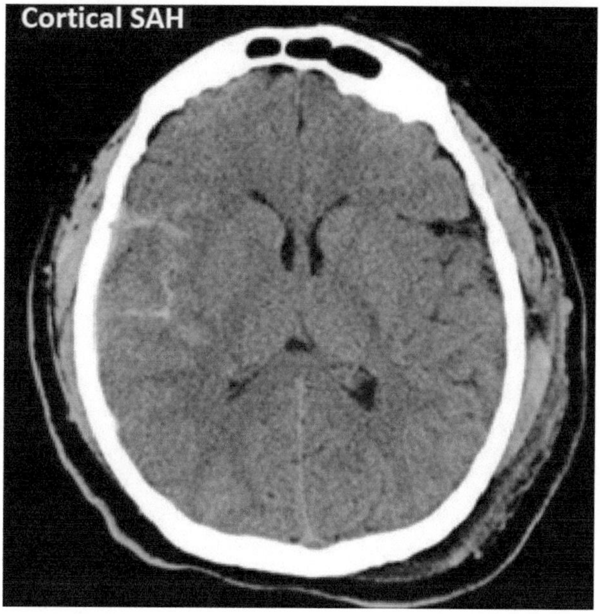

Fig. 16.13 Axial non-contrast CT of the head showing a cortical SAH

16.14 Vasospasm: Digital Subtraction Angiography (DSA) and Its Use

Cerebral vasospasm is defined as a narrowing of a cerebral blood vessel, causing a reduction in distal blood flow [20]. Seventy percent of aneurysmal subarachnoid hemorrhage (aSAH) patients develop angiographic vasospasm, but only 30% progress to developing neurological deficits [21] (Fig. 16.14).

Vasospasm of the cerebral blood vessels is a common complication of aneurysmal subarachnoid hemorrhage (aSAH), which can cause delayed cerebral ischemia (DCI) and worsening of the patient's outcome [22].

Early suspicion and detection of vasospasm can help initiate interventions to prevent the development of DCI and improve survival.

The criterion for diagnosing severe vasospasm is a reduction in vessel caliber >50%. Moderate vasospasm is diagnosed if the reduction in vessel caliber is between 25% and 50%, and mild vasospasm is diagnosed if it is <25% [23].

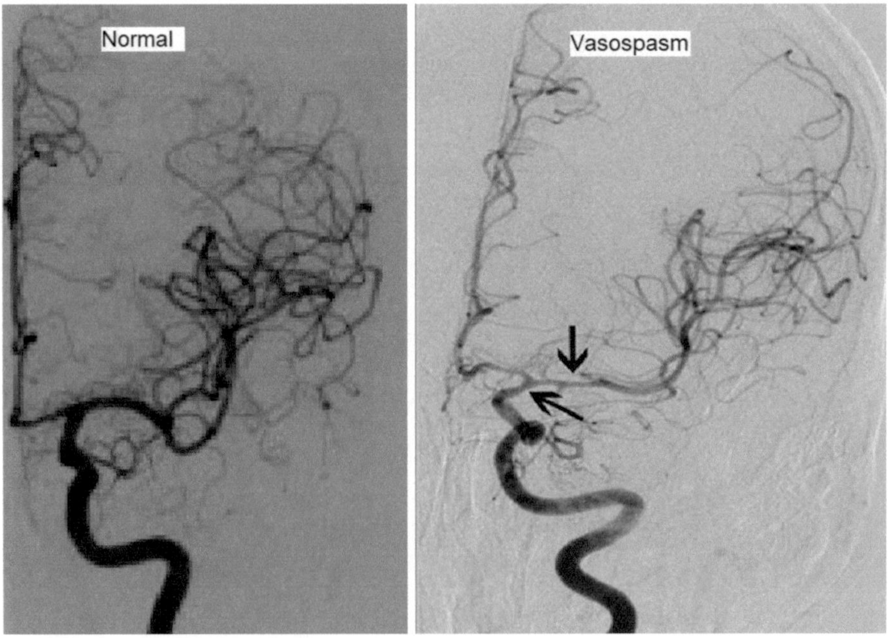

Fig. 16.14 Digital subtraction angiography image of the internal carotid artery and its terminal branches, showing normal angiogram on the left and vasospasm on the right, as evidenced by the reduced vessel diameter

16.15 CT Angiography vs. DSA to Diagnose SAH: Which Is Better?

CT angiography is a class I recommendation according to the ASA/AHA guidelines for detecting aneurysmal SAH. The same guideline also says that in the event that CT angiography is inconclusive, DSA can be used to diagnose aneurysmal SAH [24].

DSA is, however, considered the gold standard to diagnose ruptured aneurysms. Certain anatomic variants are better diagnosed in DSA compared to CT angiography. CT angiography is less effective for diagnosing finer vessel details, collateral circulation, and direction of flow. It is poor at detecting aneurysms closely associated with bony structures [25].

According to Philipp et al., they found CT angiography to be less sensitive in picking up aneurysms less than 5 mm in size. Their study states that CTA failed to detect 67.5% of ruptured aneurysms between 0 and 3 mm, 6% of those between 3 and 5 mm, and 10.9% of those between 5 and 10 mm [25].

However, when all factors are taken into consideration, CT angiography is still an effective, economical, and quick way to diagnose most of the bled aneurysms. It is good enough in most cases. Most studies that compared CTA and DSA conclude that any uncertainty in diagnosing aneurysmal SAH requires DSA. DSA continues to be the gold standard.

16.16 Hydrocephalus: The Need for Serial Imaging

Hydrocephalus assessment is done using the Evans Index [26].

- It is a measure of the ratio of the maximum width of the frontal horns of the lateral ventricles to the maximum inner skull diameter (Fig. 16.15).
- It is used as an indirect indicator of ventriculomegaly, which is the enlargement of the ventricles due to excess cerebrospinal fluid (CSF).
- The normal value of the Evans Index is between 0.20 and 0.25, while a value above 0.30 suggests ventriculomegaly.

Serial imaging is crucial for diagnosing and monitoring hydrocephalus. Here are some key imaging techniques used:

1. Computed Tomography (CT): Often used initially to diagnose hydrocephalus, CT scans can quickly show ventricular enlargement and help identify the cause, such as a mass or a hemorrhage [27].
2. Magnetic Resonance Imaging (MRI): It gives detailed images of brain structures and is useful for assessing the underlying cause of hydrocephalus. MRI can also help differentiate between types of hydrocephalus (e.g., obstructive vs. communicating) and monitor changes over time.

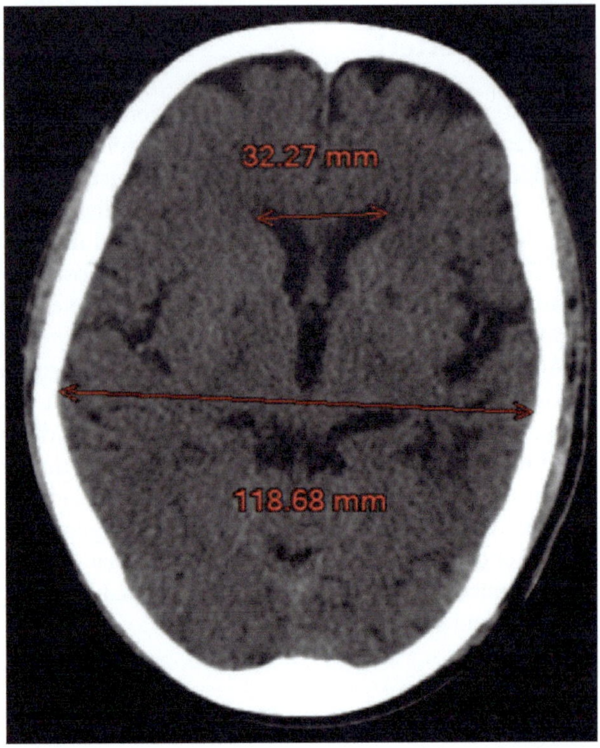

Fig. 16.15 Axial non-contrast CT of the head showing the measurement of the Evans Index. Two diameters, the inner skull diameter and the maximum frontal horn width, are mentioned

3. Ultrasonography: Primarily used in infants with open fontanelles, it allows for a noninvasive monitoring of the ventricular size and progression of hydrocephalus [28].
4. Phase-Contrast Imaging: This MRI technique can measure CSF flow dynamics, helping pinpoint the location of CSF obstruction and differentiate between communicating and noncommunicating hydrocephalus.
5. Diffusion Tensor Imaging (DTI): DTI is a newer, more advanced MRI technique that assesses white matter integrity and detects subtle changes in brain tissue due to hydrocephalus.

Regular imaging helps track the effectiveness of treatments, such as shunt placement or endoscopic third ventriculostomy (ETV), and detect any complications early.

16.17 Cerebral Venous Thrombosis: Which Modality to Use?

Cerebral venous thrombosis (CVT) is the occlusion of venous channels, including cortical venous thrombosis, dural venous thrombosis, and deep cerebral vein thrombosis [29].

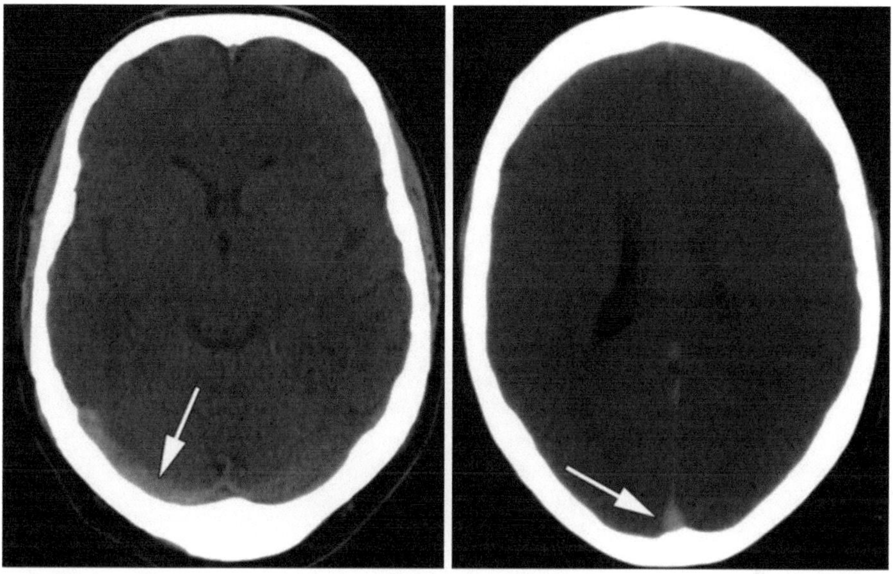

Fig. 16.16 Axial non-contrast CT of the head showing the right transverse sinus and the inferior sagittal sinus thrombosis, seen as a hyperdensity, marked by the arrow

NCCT is the first imaging modality. There is abnormal hyperattenuation of the cortical venous sinuses.

Abnormal hyperattenuation in the right transverse sinus and superior sagittal sinus (Fig. 16.16).

CT venography can help identify any occlusion in the dural venous sinus. The delta sign (Fig. 16.17) is classically seen in superior sagittal sinus CVT, where there is contrast enhancement around a triangular hypoattenuating area [30].

Compared to CT, MRI is more sensitive for detecting CVT in the venous sinuses. Acute CVT will appear isointense on T1 and hypointense on T2. A subacute CVT will appear hyperintense on T2. MR venography will show an absence of flow. Contrast MR venography is better than TOF MRI in diagnosing it. Of all the MRI sequences, MR venography is the best to diagnose CVT [30].

DSA used to be the gold standard before to diagnose CVT. However, with advances in MRI and CT imaging and due to the invasive nature of DSA, its use has declined significantly as the first imaging modality.

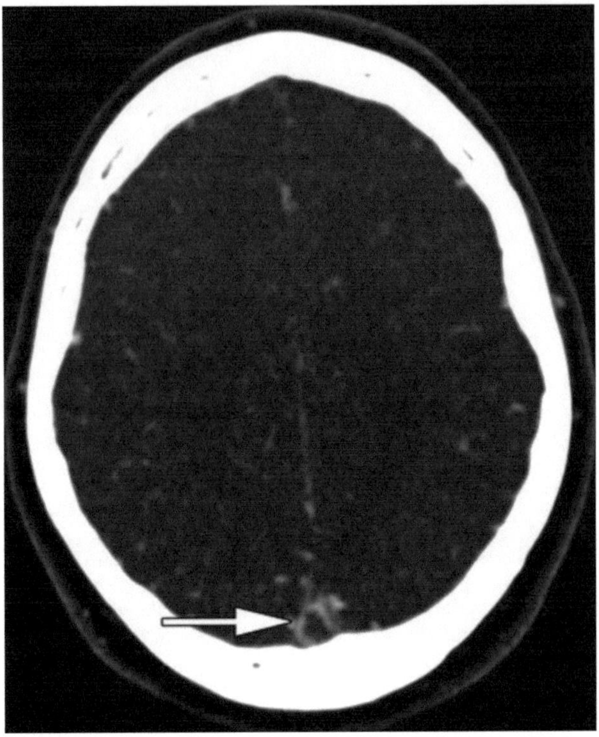

Fig. 16.17 Axial non-contrast CT of the head showing the delta sign

16.18 Marshall Classification for TBI: Why Do We Need to Know It?

The Marshall classification of traumatic brain injury is a CT-based metric. It uses only a few features and is capable of predicting outcomes in patients with TBI.

It was published in 1992 based on the findings of a large cohort of TBI patients in 1990. It is commonly used to grade acute TBI [31].

The Marshall classification distributes patients into six categories (I–VI). The severity of injury increases progressively at higher levels. Higher categories have worse prognosis and survival.

Classification:

Diffuse injury I	No visible intracranial pathology
Diffuse injury II	Midline shift of 0–5 mm Basal cisterns remain visible No high- or mixed-density lesions >25 cm^3
Diffuse injury III	Midline shift of 0–5 mm Basal cisterns compressed or completely effaced No high- or mixed-density lesions >25 cm^3

Diffuse injury IV	Midline shift >5 mm No high- or mixed-density lesions >25 cm^3
Evacuated mass lesion V	Any lesion evacuated surgically
Non-evacuated mass lesion VI	High- or mixed-density lesions >25 cm^3 Not surgically evacuated

The Marshall classification is associated with increased odds of mortality in adult patients with TBI. Grades less than 4 are associated with increased survival [32].

16.19 Traumatic Brain Injury: Imaging-Based Prognostication

The common modalities used in TBI include non-contrast CT and basic MRI sequences.

The American College of Radiology (ACR) Appropriateness Criteria, in their 2021 update, mention that MRI is not indicated in acute TBI.

For patients with chronic or subacute trauma, especially for people like sports personnel or boxers, MRI is the best initial modality to find any small contusions or microbleeds. T1 and T2 weighted imaging, along with DWI, can be used. Chronic sequelae of previous acute TBI can manifest as encephalomalacia, which can be picked up by SWI. In patients with acute TBI, with unchanged neurologic status and unremarkable initial imaging, MRI can be used for short-term follow-up (<7 days). MRI is more sensitive than CT for diagnosing small cortical contusions and subdural hematomas. It is also more sensitive for detecting small white matter lesions. Only 10% of diffuse axonal injury (DAI) is seen on CT [33].

In patients with acute TBI but unremarkable CT, MRI can reveal underlying findings. In one study, 27% of patients of mild TBI with normal CT but with abnormalities in early MRI, showed that these findings are important for prognostication at 3 months. It showed that these people were associated with worse outcomes compared to those with normal MRI [34].

Studies in which MRI was done in the acute phase reveal greater sensitivity in diagnosing subtle shearing injuries, small contusions, and extra-axial hematomas. However, this extra information did not affect treatment in the acute phase [35].

Axial T2 FLAIR images showing punctate hyperintensities in the right subcortical white matter and the splenium of the corpus callosum (Fig. 16.18).

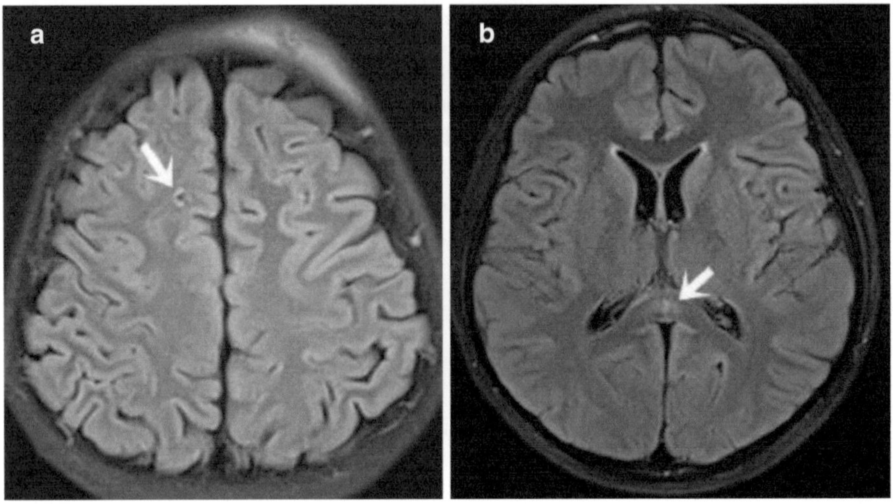

Fig. 16.18 Axial MRI T2 FLAIR sequence of the head showing punctate hyperintensities in the right subcortical white matter (**a**) and the corpus callosum (**b**), as marked by the arrows. This is a case of traumatic brain injury

16.20 Advanced MRI for Brain Tumors: The Need in Certain Situations

For many years, conventional MRI has been the primary method for diagnosing and locating brain tumors, performing stereotactic biopsies, planning surgical resections, and distinguishing between posttreatment changes and recurrent tumors. Perfusion imaging, which relies on cerebral microvascular perfusion, has had a great impact on the diagnosis, treatment, and monitoring of central nervous system (CNS) tumors. The techniques are dynamic susceptibility contrast (DSC) MRI, dynamic contrast-enhanced (DCE) MRI, and arterial spin labeling (ASL) MRI [36]. DSC-MRI can help distinguish a tumor from a pseudo-mass (e.g., abscess). It can also determine tumor vascularity. It can help define the fractional tumor burden (FTB) (Fig. 16.19) by measuring the regional cerebral blood volume. This can help identify the extent of tumor recurrence. Gliomas can be differentiated from lymphomas as gliomas have increased vascularity, as evidenced by increased relative Cerebral Blood Volumer (rCBV) [37]. DCE MRI can help determine the transfer constant. This is a measure of capillary permeability, denoted as K^{trans}. This

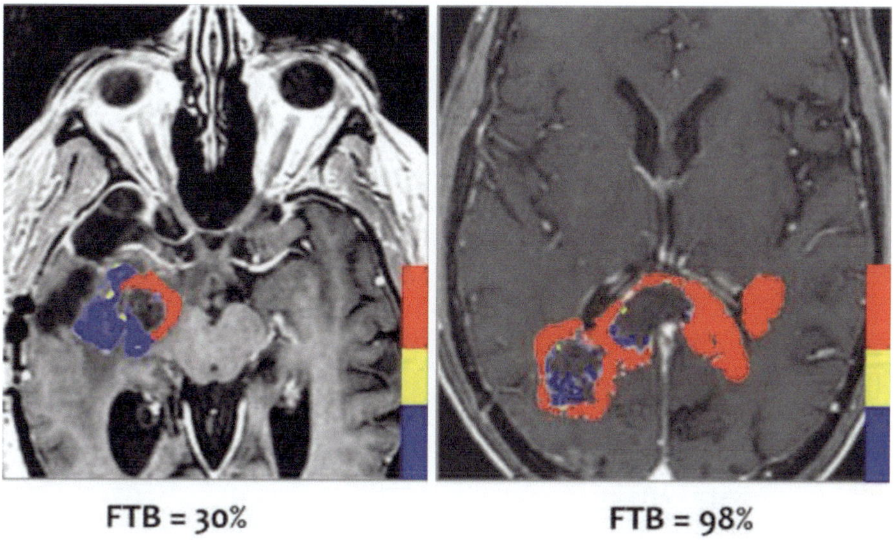

Fig. 16.19 Axial MRI of the head with dynamic susceptibility contrast, with fractional tumor burden (FTB) mapping. The red area denotes the tumor area, whereas blue denotes no tumor

correlates well with the tumor grade of gliomas. It can also distinguish between radiation necrosis and recurrence, as a recurrent tumor will have a high K^{trans} [36]. With ASL, Cerebral blood flow (CBF) can be measured. This helps in tumor grading, follow-up, and treatment [38]. Diffusion-weighted imaging (DWI) shows diffusion restriction in highly cellular tumors. The apparent diffusion coefficient (ADC) obtained from DWI can help identify tumor grades. Low ADC corresponds to high tumor grade [39]. Diffusion tensor imaging (DTI) can help identify if a tumor is invading the white matter fiber tracts. This can help during tumor resection [40]. MR spectroscopy (Fig. 16.20) can help identify the type of chemical compounds present within a tumor and aid in diagnosis. The most commonly studied ones are the following:

1. N-acetyl aspartate (NAA): A marker of neuronal viability.
2. Creatine: A marker of cellular metabolism.
3. Cho: A marker of cell membrane turnover.
4. Myoinositol: A marker of cell membrane integrity [41].

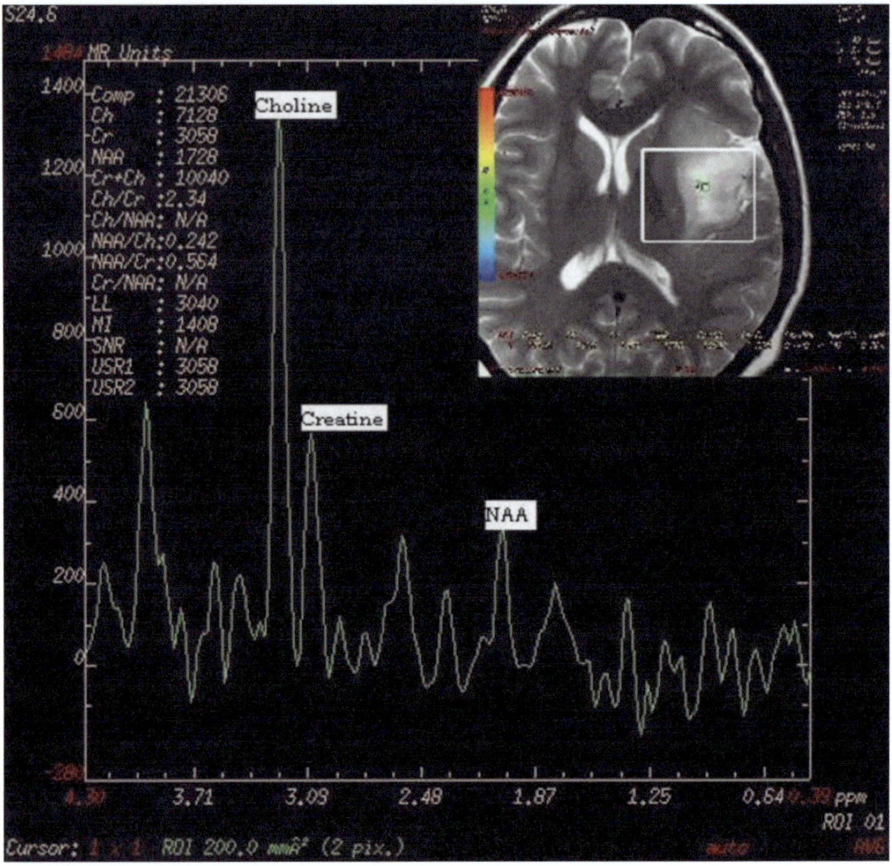

Fig. 16.20 MR spectroscopy of a glioma showing increased choline and decreased NAA levels

16.21 Neuroimaging in Status Epilepticus: Which Is the Modality, and What Is to Be Looked For?

Neuroimaging is recommended for all patients with status epilepticus (SE) and all known patients with epilepsy presenting with SE for the first time. CT scans are the most readily available. CT generally shows edema of the brain. However, MRI provides the highest diagnostic yield. Depending on the clinical presentation, MRI can be opted for if the patient is stable. The most common findings seen in MR images are the following (Fig. 16.21):

- Increased T2/FLAIR signal.
- Diffusion restriction.
- DWI and ADC can reveal local edema caused by status epilepticus.
- Increased signal intensity is usually seen in subcortical areas like the basal ganglia, thalamus, hippocampus, and cerebellum [42].

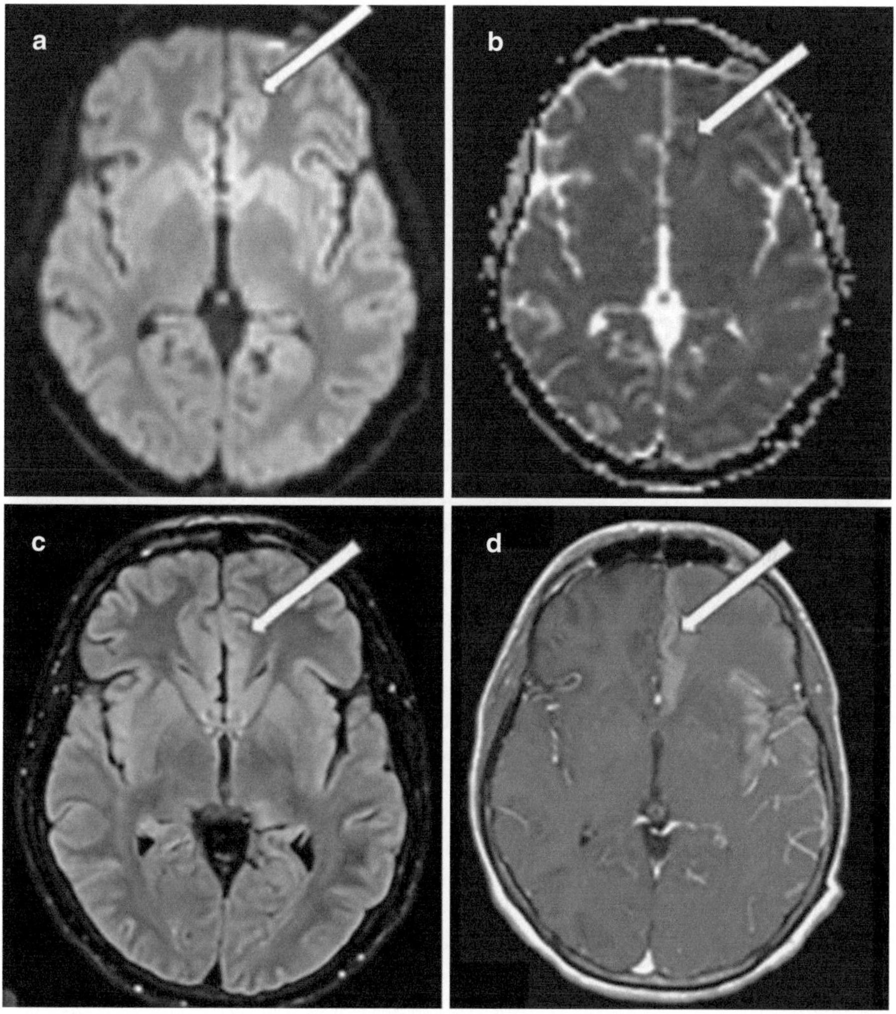

Fig. 16.21 (**a**) Axial MRI diffusion-weighted imaging (DWI) sequence of the head showing increased intensity in the left insula and the frontal cortex, as marked by the arrow. (**b**) Axial MRI apparent diffusion coefficient (ADC) sequence showing reduced ADC, as marked by the arrow. (**c**) Axial MRI fluid attenuation and inverse recovery (FLAIR) sequence showing increased intensity, as marked by the arrow. (**d**) Axial MRI T1 contrast sequence showing increased enhancement, as marked by the arrow

16.22 Spinal Cord Injury: Which Imaging Modalities Work Best?

Spinal trauma can cause severe spinal column or cord injuries, leading to paraplegia, quadriplegia, or death. The most common cause is blunt trauma from motor vehicle accidents, followed by falls, assaults, and sports injuries. Imaging is crucial in the initial assessment of spinal trauma. Based on clinical presentation and availability, the imaging modality is chosen. CT and MRI are the most commonly used, with newer technologies like advanced CT, DTI, fMRI, and perfusion imaging also being utilized [43]. The American College of Radiology recommends using CT as the first imaging method for spinal trauma in adults and children over 14 years of age. CT offers detailed views of bone anatomy and can detect issues like traumatic disk herniations and epidural or subdural hematomas. For patients with abnormal anatomy, whether congenital or iatrogenic, CT is crucial for surgical planning. In conditions like ankylosing spondylitis (AS) or diffuse idiopathic skeletal hyperostosis (DISH), CT provides detailed images of bony fusion, surpassing X-ray or MRI. Similarly, for patients with metallic spinal implants and suspected trauma, CT is the best method to assess the injury and the implant itself [33, 44].

MRI is the gold standard for evaluating spinal cord injuries and trauma due to its high-contrast resolution and multi-planar capabilities. It effectively identifies spinal cord compression, ligamentous instability, disk herniation, contusion, hemorrhage, and injuries to vertebral bodies and paraspinal tissues. A review by Sliker et al. found that MRI detected ligamentous injuries in 22.7% of blunt trauma cases, with 80.8% requiring treatment. Despite the time required, MRI is recommended pre- and postoperatively when feasible, as it is safe and significantly influences surgical decisions [45].

Conventional MRI, including T1- and T2-weighted imaging, has less prognostic value. However, T2-weighted and short tau inversion recovery (STIR) sequences are crucial in acute spinal cord injury because of their high sensitivity to intramedullary pathology and acute injury/edema. STIR images are good at detecting edema in the spinal cord, surrounding soft tissue, and ligaments. It gives more consistent fat suppression than fat-suppressed T2WI. The presence of STIR signals, combined with acute neurological deficits and potential bony or ligamentous injuries, helps guide the spine surgeons' decisions [46].

T2-weighted MRI has an interaction with the iron in blood products. Intramedullary hemorrhage appears as hypointense areas, which has prognostic implications. T2W and susceptibility-weighted (SWI) imaging sequences are also used to detect intramedullary hemorrhage. The main drawback of MRI is the lengthy scan time. However, protocols can help mitigate this. Performing a T2 sagittal survey first, followed by targeted sequences at the identified level of interest, has significantly reduced scan times in many centers (Fig. 16.22).

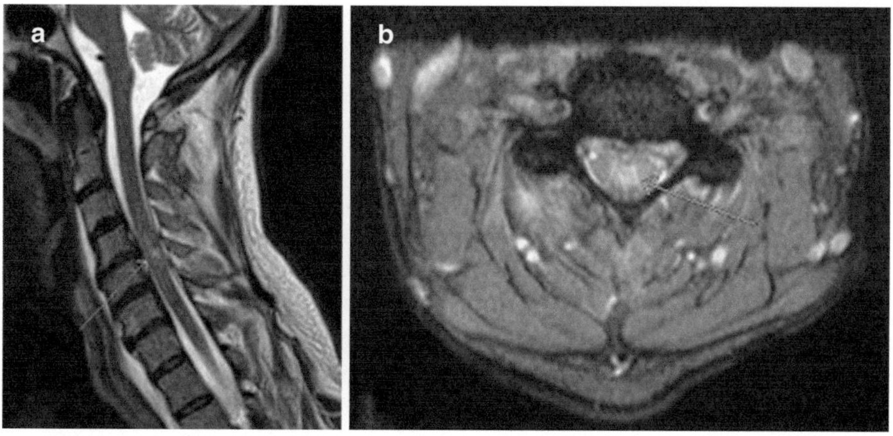

Fig. 16.22 MRI T2-weighted sagittal (**a**) and axial (**b**) images showing spinal cord contusion (arrows)

16.23 Meningitis Neuroimaging Before Lumbar Puncture: Is It Necessary?

Neuroimaging is often done before a lumbar puncture to rule out other diagnoses or check for high intracranial pressure. However, doing this for all suspected bacterial meningitis cases can delay the lumbar puncture and the collection of cerebrospinal fluid (CSF) needed for crucial diagnostic tests. This delay can also postpone effective treatment and management (Fig. 16.23).

The National Institute for Health and Care Excellence (NICE) guidelines released in March 2024 reviewed the evidence pertaining to lumbar puncture before and after CT. The committee found that in adults with bacterial meningitis, performing a lumbar puncture without prior CT was associated with lower mortality rates, reduced long-term neurological and hearing impairments, faster antibiotic treatment (within 1 or 2 h), and a higher rate of individuals without functional impairment. However, there was no significant difference in long-term neurological deficits like cranial nerve palsy and arm/leg drift. The evidence for these outcomes is highly inaccurate, except for the absence of functional impairment, so these results should not be considered definitive proof of association or a lack thereof [47].

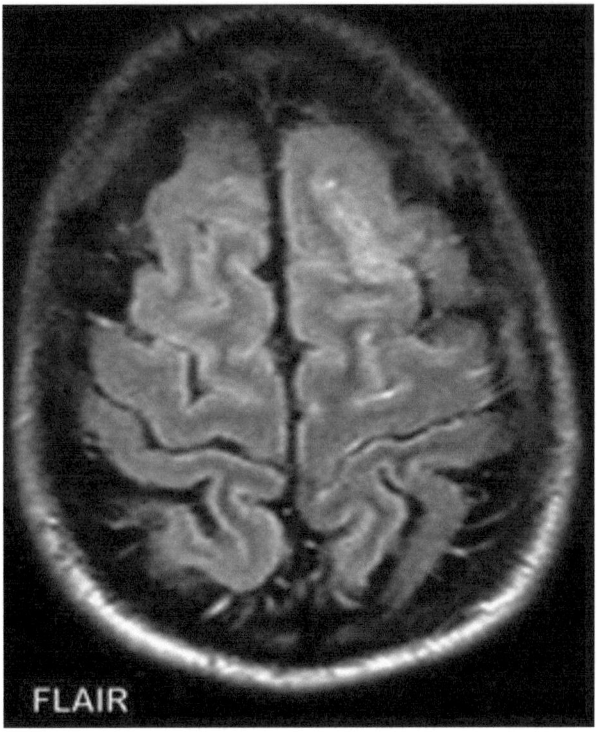

Fig. 16.23 Axial MRI of the head FLAIR sequence showing hyperintensities in the left frontal and subarachnoid space, consistent with meningitis

References

1. Powers WJ, Rabinstein AA, Ackerson T, et al. Guidelines for the early management of patients with Acute Ischemic Stroke: 2019 update to the 2018 guidelines for the early management of Acute Ischemic Stroke: a guideline for healthcare professionals from the American Heart Association/American Stroke Association. Stroke. 2019;50 https://doi.org/10.1161/STR.0000000000000211. Epub ahead of print December.
2. Barber PA, Demchuk AM, Zhang J, et al. Validity and reliability of a quantitative computed tomography score in predicting outcome of hyperacute stroke before thrombolytic therapy. Lancet. 2000;355:1670–4.
3. Chavhan GB, Shroff MM. Twenty classic signs in neuroradiology: a pictorial essay. Indian J Radiol Imag. 2009;19:135–45.
4. Tomsick T, Brott T, Barsan W, et al. Prognostic value of the hyperdense middle cerebral artery sign and stroke scale score before ultraearly thrombolytic therapy. AJNR Am J Neuroradiol. 1996;17:79–85.
5. Jensen-Kondering U. Hyperdense artery sign on computed tomography in acute ischemic stroke. WJR. 2010;2:354.
6. Goldmakher GV, Camargo ECS, Furie KL, et al. Hyperdense basilar artery sign on unenhanced CT predicts thrombus and outcome in acute posterior circulation stroke. Stroke. 2009; https://doi.org/10.1161/STROKEAHA.108.516690. Epub ahead of print 1 January.
7. Kothari RU, Brott T, Broderick JP, et al. The ABCs of measuring intracerebral hemorrhage volumes. Stroke. 1996; https://doi.org/10.1161/01.STR.27.8.1304. Epub ahead of print August.

8. Huttner HB, Steiner T, Hartmann M, et al. Comparison of ABC/2 estimation technique to computer-assisted Planimetric analysis in warfarin-related intracerebral parenchymal hemorrhage. Stroke. 2006; https://doi.org/10.1161/01.STR.0000198806.67472.5c. Epub ahead of print 1 February.
9. LoPresti MA, Bruce SS, Camacho E, et al. Hematoma volume as the major determinant of outcomes after intracerebral hemorrhage. J Neurol Sci. 2014;345:3–7.
10. Lu W-Z, Lin H-A, Bai C-H, et al. Posterior circulation acute stroke prognosis early CT scores in predicting functional outcomes: a meta-analysis. PLoS One. 2021;16:e0246906.
11. Patel VD, Garcia RM, Swor DE, et al. Natural history of Infratentorial intracerebral hemorrhages: two subgroups with distinct presentations and outcomes. J Stroke Cerebrovasc Dis. 2020;29:104920.
12. Hill MD, Silver FL. Epidemiologic predictors of 30-day survival in cerebellar hemorrhage. J Stroke Cerebrovasc Dis. 2001;10:118–21.
13. Peng W-J, Reis C, Reis H, et al. Predictive value of CTA spot sign on hematoma expansion in intracerebral hemorrhage patients. Biomed Res Int. 2017;2017:1–9.
14. Kim H, Goo JH, Kwak HS, et al. Correlation between spot sign and intracranial hemorrhage expansion on dual-phase CT angiography. Diagnostics (Basel). 2019;9:215.
15. Halefoglu AM, Yousem DM. Susceptibility weighted imaging: clinical applications and future directions. WJR. 2018;10:30–45.
16. Clinical applications of diffusion-weighted sequence in brain imaging: beyond stroke – PubMed. https://pubmed.ncbi.nlm.nih.gov/34596716/. Accessed 17 July 2024.
17. Edlow BL, Hurwitz S, Edlow JA. Diagnosis of DWI-negative acute ischemic stroke. Neurology. 2017;89:256–62.
18. Sener RN. Diffusion MRI: apparent diffusion coefficient (ADC) values in the normal brain and a classification of brain disorders based on ADC values. Comput Med Imaging Graph. 2001;25:299–326.
19. Fisher M, editor. Stroke. Edinburgh/New York: Elsevier; 2009.
20. Lindbohm JV, Kaprio J, Jousilahti P, et al. Sex, smoking, and risk for subarachnoid hemorrhage. Stroke. 2016;47:1975–81.
21. Rumalla K, Smith KA, Arnold PM, et al. Subarachnoid hemorrhage and readmissions: National Rates, causes, risk factors, and outcomes in 16,001 hospitalized patients. World Neurosurg. 2018;110:e100–11.
22. Nassar HGE, Ghali AA, Bahnasy WS, et al. Vasospasm following aneurysmal subarachnoid hemorrhage: prediction, detection, and intervention. Egypt J Neurol Psychiatr Neurosurg. 2019;55:3.
23. Janjua N, Mayer SA. Cerebral vasospasm after subarachnoid hemorrhage. Curr Opin Crit Care. 2003;9:113–9.
24. 2023 guideline for the management of patients with aneurysmal subarachnoid hemorrhage: a guideline from the American Heart Association/American Stroke Association. Stroke. https://www.ahajournals.org/doi/10.1161/STR.0000000000000436. Accessed 21 Aug 2024.
25. Philipp LR, McCracken DJ, McCracken CE, et al. Comparison between CTA and digital subtraction angiography in the diagnosis of ruptured aneurysms. Neurosurgery. 2017;80:769.
26. Runge VM, Smoker WRK, Valavanis A. Neuroradiology: the essentials with MR and CT. Thieme; 2014.
27. Blitz AM, Nayate AP, Higginbotham A, et al. Hydrocephalus Imaging. In: Faro SH, Mohamed FB, editors. Functional neuroradiology: principles and clinical applications. Cham: Springer International Publishing. p. 1439–54.
28. Brant WE, Helms CA. Fundamentals of diagnostic radiology. Lippincott Williams & Wilkins; 2007.
29. Rodallec MH, Krainik A, Feydy A, et al. Cerebral venous thrombosis and multidetector CT angiography: tips and tricks. RadioGraphics. 2006; https://doi.org/10.1148/rg.26si065505. Epub ahead of print 1 October 2006.

30. Canedo-Antelo M, Baleato-González S, Mosqueira AJ, et al. Radiologic clues to cerebral venous thrombosis. Radiographics. 2019; https://doi.org/10.1148/rg.2019190015. Epub ahead of print 7 October.
31. Marshall LF, Marshall SB, Klauber MR, et al. The diagnosis of head injury requires a classification based on computed axial tomography. J Neurotrauma. 1992;9(Suppl 1):S287–92.
32. Elkbuli A, Shaikh S, McKenney K, et al. Utility of the Marshall & Rotterdam Classification Scores in predicting outcomes in trauma patients. J Surg Res. 2021;264:194–8.
33. Shih RY, Burns J, Ajam AA, et al. ACR appropriateness criteria® head trauma: 2021 update. J Am Coll Radiol. 2021;18:S13–36.
34. Yuh EL, Mukherjee P, Lingsma HF, et al. Magnetic resonance imaging improves 3-month outcome prediction in mild traumatic brain injury. Ann Neurol. 2013;73:224–35.
35. Manolakaki D, Velmahos GC, Spaniolas K, et al. Early magnetic resonance imaging is unnecessary in patients with traumatic brain injury. J Trauma. 2009;66:1008–12; discussion 1012–4.
36. Geer CP, Simonds J, Anvery A, et al. Does MR perfusion imaging impact management decisions for patients with brain tumors? A prospective study. AJNR Am J Neuroradiol. 2012;33:556–62.
37. Floriano VH, Torres US, Spotti AR, et al. The role of dynamic susceptibility contrast-enhanced perfusion MR imaging in differentiating between infectious and neoplastic focal brain lesions: results from a cohort of 100 consecutive patients. PLoS One. 8 https://doi.org/10.1371/journal.pone.0081509. Epub ahead of print 2013.
38. Lehmann P, Monet P, De Marco G, et al. A comparative study of perfusion measurement in brain tumours at 3 tesla MR: arterial spin labeling versus dynamic susceptibility contrast-enhanced MRI. Eur Neurol. 2010;64:21–6.
39. Advanced MR Imaging Techniques in the Diagnosis of Intraaxial Brain Tumors in Adults. RadioGraphics. https://pubs.rsna.org/doi/10.1148/rg.26si065513?url_ver=Z39.88-2003&rfr_id=ori:rid:crossref.org&rfr_dat=cr_pub%20%200pubmed. Accessed 22 Aug 2024.
40. Yan J-L, Van Der Hoorn A, Larkin TJ, et al. Extent of resection of peritumoral diffusion tensor imaging–detected abnormality as a predictor of survival in adult glioblastoma patients. JNS. 2017;126:234–41.
41. Thieme E-Journals – Seminars in Neurology/Abstract. https://www.thieme-connect.com/products/ejournals/abstract/10.1055/s-0032-1331814. Accessed 22 Aug 2024.
42. Meletti S, Monti G, Mirandola L, et al. Neuroimaging of status epilepticus. Epilepsia. 2018;59:113–9.
43. van Den Hauwe L, Sundgren PC, Flanders AE. Spinal trauma and spinal cord injury (SCI). In: Hodler J, Kubik-Huch RA, von Schulthess GK (eds) Diseases of the brain, head and neck, spine 2020–2023: diagnostic Imaging. Cham: Springer; 2020. http://www.ncbi.nlm.nih.gov/books/NBK554330/. Accessed 23 Aug 2024.
44. Shabani S, Kaushal M, Hesham MS, et al. AOSpine global survey: international trends in utilization of magnetic resonance imaging/computed tomography for spinal trauma and spinal cord injury across AO regions. J Neurotrauma https://doi.org/10.1089/neu.2019.6464. Epub ahead of print 2 December 2019.
45. Fehlings MG, Rao SC, Tator CH, et al. The optimal radiologic method for assessing Spinal Canal compromise and cord compression in patients with cervical spinal cord injury: part II: results of a multicenter study. Spine. 1999;24:605.
46. Ghaffari-Rafi A, Peterson C, Leon-Rojas JE, et al. The role of magnetic resonance imaging to inform clinical decision-making in acute spinal cord injury: a systematic review and meta-analysis. J Clin Med. 2021;10:4948.
47. Evidence review for role of neuroimaging prior to lumbar puncture: meningitis (bacterial) and meningococcal disease: recognition, diagnosis and management: evidence review B5. 2024. London: National Institute for Health and Care Excellence (NICE). http://www.ncbi.nlm.nih.gov/books/NBK604145/. Accessed 23 Aug 2024.

Neuroprotection: Quest for the Holy Grail

17

Joseph Nascimento Monteiro, Joslita Rebello, and Nimisha Thakur

Medicine is a science of uncertainty and an art of probability—William Osler

Abstract

Neuroprotection remains a critical yet contentious area in neurological research, with ongoing debates about the efficacy and timing of various interventions.

Targeted temperature management (TTM), the use of corticosteroids in traumatic brain injury (TBI), the choice of hypertonic saline (HS) vs. mannitol, the management of blood pressure (BP) targets, and neuroprotection in stroke are some of the ongoing and evolving practices that are being refined into recommendations and guidelines.

Prophylactic anticonvulsant use, the role of statins in acute brain injury, glycemic control, depth of anesthesia, remote ischemic preconditioning, the use of biomarkers, the role of sedatives and anesthetic agents, pediatric TBI neuroprotection, timing, duration, and combination therapy in neuroprotection highlight the complexity and the iterative progress of neuroprotection being translated into clinical practice.

Neuroprotection holds significant promise, yet addressing these issues requires a multifaceted approach, including rigorous clinical trials, advanced biomarker research, and a deeper understanding of pathophysiological mechanisms. Only through such comprehensive efforts can we hope to unlock the full potential of neuroprotective therapies and improve outcomes for patients with neurological conditions.

J. N. Monteiro (✉) · J. Rebello · N. Thakur
Division of Neuroanesthesia and Neurocritical Care, Department of Anesthesiology, PD Hinduja Hospital and Medical Research Centre, Mumbai, India

P. U. Bidkar, M. Krishnakumar (eds.), *Controversies in Neurocritical Care*,
https://doi.org/10.1007/978-981-95-4419-6_17

Keywords

Neuroprotection · Targeted temperature management · Statins · Brain biomarkers
Remote ischemic conditioning

17.1 Introduction

Neuroprotection is defined as a treatment initiated before the onset of ischemia, intended to modify intra-ischemic cellular and vascular biological responses to the deprivation of energy supply to increase tissue tolerance to ischemia, resulting in improved outcomes [1]. Neuroresuscitation, in contrast, implies treatment begun after the ischemic insult has occurred, which is intended to optimize reperfusion.

Neuroprotective strategies are limited; however, the capacity to exacerbate cerebral ischemia is infinite. Outcomes of such events range from subclinical neurocognitive deficits to catastrophic neurological morbidity and death. This has led to efforts and interest in reducing the neuronal vulnerability to ischemia.

The goal of neuroprotection is to reduce the clinical effects of cerebral damage, essentially through two primary mechanisms: increasing the tolerance of neurological tissue to ischemia and changing the intracellular response to energy supply deprivation [2].

Neuroprotection holds significant promise, which requires a multifaceted approach, including rigorous clinical trials, advanced biomarker research, and a deeper understanding of pathophysiological mechanisms.

Neuroprotection Controversies in Neurocritical Care The ongoing debates on neuroprotection in neurocritical care highlight the complexity and the iterative progress of neuroprotection being translated into clinical practice.

Targeted Temperature Management There is an ongoing debate surrounding the ideal temperature (32–34 °C or 36 °C) and duration for therapeutic hypothermia in cardiac arrest and traumatic brain injury (TBI) patients. Targeted temperature management (TTM) is often used in neurocritical care to minimize secondary neurological injury and improve outcomes.

Therapeutic hypothermia, controlled normothermia, and fever management are all essential parts of TTM. The strongest evidence of TTM comes from out-of-hospital cardiac arrest and hypoxic–ischemic encephalopathy in neonates. It has further been studied in patients with hemorrhagic or nonhemorrhagic stroke and traumatic brain injury. The clinical application of TTM must be meticulous, with continuous patient monitoring and means to manage shivering. Cooling must be done at an appropriate rate using safe and effective cooling techniques [3].

TTM may aid in improving the long-term recovery of neurocritical care patients by reducing secondary cerebral injury. Benefits of early initiation of TTM, preferably within 6 h of the neurological insult, are seen in preclinical literature. Other studies, where TTM was initiated after a longer period of time following the insult, showed lesser benefits of therapeutic hypothermia (TH). These investigations unequivocally show a relationship between the final TTM duration needed and the rate at which cooling is started [4]. The current evidence fails to demonstrate a clear benefit of TTM with respect to intracranial pressure (ICP), neurological recovery, and length of ICU/hospital stay. Hence, no recommendations currently exist for the timing of TTM initiation.

Sustained fever after injury, refractory to the usual treatment, may call for controlled normothermia to prevent the related complications. Temperature-modulating devices with servo-control mechanisms are superior to their conventional counterparts. The maintenance phase of TTM can be enhanced by intravascular and gel pad surface devices that effectively reduce the temperature variation [5]. The data lacks in providing evidence of the best interventions to reduce shivering. Nonetheless, it is vital to monitor and quantify shivering response with the bedside shivering assessment scale (BSAS) [6].

Controlled prospective studies regarding the practical application of TTM are lacking and present a potential area for future research. Many crucial problems pertaining to the application of TTM are still poorly understood.

On the bright side, none of the large randomized controlled trials (RCTs) so far demonstrate any significant complication rate with TTM, including renal, gastric, or cardiovascular complications; seizures; deep venous thrombosis (DVT) risk; or increased duration of mechanical ventilation [7].

There is a dearth of high-quality data on the ideal site for temperature monitoring, the duration of TTM in different conditions, and the use of pharmacological drugs during cooling.

Recommendations must be tailored to the needs of the system and each patient. Further studies are likely to enable more definitive standards of patient care and recommendations of higher levels of evidence.

Corticosteroids in Traumatic Brain Injury The debate about the use of corticosteroids to reduce intracranial pressure and improve outcomes is ongoing despite conflicting evidence. The results of the large CRASH trial suggest that steroids should not be used in head injury, as they appear to increase mortality. Despite the heterogeneity, the results of this trial are the most relevant to current practice and should be the basis for clinical decisions, rather than any of the earlier trials or their meta-analysis [8].

Hypertonic Saline vs. Mannitol The deliberation about the optimal agent for managing elevated intracranial pressure and, thus, providing neuroprotection continues, with varying opinions on efficacy and safety. Mannitol and hypertonic saline (HS) are both hyperosmolar agents, each with distinct physiological properties affecting blood rheology, inflammation, neurochemistry, and hemodynamic regulation. While the idea of a universally applicable, single optimal agent is appealing, it is more plausible that different hyperosmolar agents may exert optimal therapeutic effects in diverse clinical contexts. For example, the relative merit of using HS, which expands systemic volume status, vs. mannitol, which depletes it, needs exploration in patients with congestive heart failure, experiencing elevated intracranial hypertension. Trials should consider testing equimolar agents infused over the same period to mitigate the effects of molarity and infusion time, a consideration often absent in existing literature. An analysis of individual clinical scenarios and a patient-specific, individualized tailored approach is recommended [9].

Blood Pressure (BP) Management Most of the cases presenting to the neurocritical care setting with hypertensive emergencies are ischemic strokes and intracranial hemorrhages (ICHs).

Controversies exist in the blood pressure management means and targets in this as well as related patient populations, including TBI, subarachnoid hemorrhage (SAH), and traumatic spinalcord injury (TSI).

Acute Ischemic Stroke (AIS) Different targets for blood pressure management are described in patients with acute ischemic stroke. It depends on the patient's comorbid status, presenting BP, and the means of treatment that is planned.

The Enhanced Control of Hypertension and Thrombolysis in Stroke Study (ENCHANTED) is a phase III clinical trial that studied the effect of rigorous BP lowering to 140 mmHg SBP in patients eligible for endovascular thrombolysis. The results showed a reduction in ICH in the intervention group; however, no outcome benefit in terms of mortality or independence was noted [10]. This study had several limitations. The exact BP at which the risk of hemorrhage is reduced could not be discerned. Among the study population, only 1.9% of patients underwent endovascular treatment. Further, the study failed to weigh in on the revascularization status. It also failed to show an effective correlation of adjusting the dose of alteplase based on the BP achieved with long-term outcome.

For patients who are not candidates for IV thrombolysis, it may be reasonable to lower BP, only if it is greater than 220/110 mmHg [11]. However, patients with accelerated hypertension, with BP >220/120, have been excluded from most of the studies; hence, the reliability of these findings cannot be left unquestioned.

The REVASCAT and SWIFT trials, which studied different modalities of endovascular treatment, including the STENT RETRIEVER and SOLITAIRE FR devices, included patients with BP <185/110 mmHg, thus studying outcome benefit only in this controlled patient population [12, 13].

The DAWN trial demonstrated that, in patients presenting 6–24 hours after stroke onset with a mismatch between clinical deficits and infarct volume, mechanical thrombectomy significantly improved 90-day disability and functional independence outcomes compared with standard care. In the control group, the BP target was <185/110 mmHg pre-thrombolysis, <180/105 mmHg post-thrombolysis, and <220/110 in non-thrombolysis candidates. In the intervention group, similar targets were used in patients with thrombolysis in cerebral infarction (TICI) IIa or lesser (i.e., poor perfusion) post-thrombectomy, and a reduction of BP to 140 mmHg SBP was targeted in patients with successful thrombectomy (TICI IIb or III) [14].

Table 17.1 ACC/AHA recommendations for practice guidelines for the early management of patients with acute ischemic stroke [16]

Sr. No.	Recommendation	COR	LOE
1.	Hypotension and hypovolemia should be corrected to maintain systemic perfusion levels necessary to support organ function	I	C
2.	Patients eligible for IV alteplase: before thrombolysis; BP, if elevated: to be reduced to SBP <185 mmHg and DBP <110 mmHg	I	B
3.	BP <180/105 mmHg after IV alteplase treatment for 24 h: immediate posttreatment	I	B
3.	In patients planned for mechanical thrombectomy, who have not received IV thrombolysis, it may be reasonable to maintain BP <185/110 mmHg before the procedure	IIa	B
4.	The usefulness of drug-induced hypertension in patients with AIS is not well-established	IIb	B

COR class of recommendation, *LOE* level of evidence

Similar targets were identified in the DEFUSE III trial, which also concluded with lower rates of disability and better 90-day functional outcome with endovascular treatment, along with medical therapy [15].

Some smaller studies show the correlation of BP with the outcome to follow a U-shaped curve. BP variability has also been shown to correlate with the outcome, a higher variability being associated with a poorer outcome.

The current practice is to follow the 2018 American College of Cardiology/American Heart Association (ACC/AHA) guidelines [16] (Table 17.1). However, the only class I recommendations are to correct hypotension and hypovolemia to maintain organ perfusion and maintain a BP target of 185/110 mmHg before IV fibrinolytic therapy. Even among these, the former has only a class C level of evidence.

BP management forms a crucial part of the medical management of patients with AIS, as the cerebral perfusion is pressure-passive in the face of possible failing autoregulation, and more robust data is needed to back the available guidelines.

Intracranial Hemorrhage Of the stroke patients presenting to the neurocritical care setup, 10–20% are diagnosed with intracranial hemorrhage. Hypertension is present in the majority of these patients, most likely as a result of a preexisting chronic hypertensive state. Accelerated hypertension is associated with side effects such as rebleeding, hematoma expansion, and perihematomal edema. However, as much as the control of hypertension is crucial for a good outcome, hypotension can potentially cause cerebral ischemia, especially in the perihematomal region.

Two milestone trials exist that form the basis of the current practice guidelines (Table 17.2).

The Invasive Blood Pressure Reduction in Acute Cerebral Hemorrhage-2 (INTERACT-2) trial studied patients with BP between 150 and 220 mmHg within 6 h of ICH and analyzed the effect of rigorous vs. standard practice of BP reduction on neurological outcome. Despite a nonsignificant difference between the modified

Table 17.2 Differences in methodologies and findings between the INTERACT2 and ATACH2 trials [17, 18]

Sr. No.	Parameter	INTERACT-2	ATACH-2
1.	Time to start antihypertensives	Within 6 h of ICH	Within 4.5 h of ICH
2.	Target BP in the control group	<180 mmHg	140–179 mmHg
3.	Target BP in the treatment group	<140 mmHg	110–139 mmHg
4.	Mean minimum SBP in the first 2 h	141.1 mmHg	128.9 mmHg
5.	Difference in the 3-month mRS of the two groups	Nonsignificant ($p = 0.06$)	Nonsignificant ($p = 0.72$)
6.	Difference in functional outcomes and quality of life of the two groups	Better in the treatment group	No difference
7.	Adverse effects of organ ischemia	None in either group	Higher in the treatment group

Rankin Scale (mRS) scores of the two groups, the rigorous BP reduction group had better physical and mental health–related quality of life. This group had no major events of organ dysfunction. Thus, the study concluded that rigorous BP reduction to an SBP of 140 mmHg was safe and associated with better functional outcomes [17].

A similar methodology and analysis were done in the Antihypertensive Treatment for Acute Cerebral Hemorrhage-2 (ATACH-2) trial. However, this study went one step further in the BP reduction protocol used. The standard treatment was to maintain BP in the 140–179 mmHg range, while rigorous BP reduction involved reducing it to the 110–139 mmHg range [18]. The BP reduction was more rapid in this study (within 4.5 h of ICH). The trial was terminated after the interim analysis showed no effect on the functional outcomes of the two groups and higher renal complications in the intense BP reduction group, thus pointing out the adverse effects of rapid and intense BP reduction in patients with ICH.

The current practice of acute BP lowering in patients with ICH follows the 2022 ACC/AHA guidelines [19]:

1. Careful titration to ensure continuous, smooth, and sustained control of BP, avoiding large variability in SBP [COR IIa; LOE B-NR].
2. Initiating BP lowering within 2 h of ICH onset and reaching the target within 1 h [COR IIa; LOE C-LD].
3. In patients with spontaneous ICH with an SBP of 150–220 mmHg, acute BP lowering to a target of 140 mmHg and maintaining a range of 130–150 mmHg may be safe and reasonable [COR IIb; LOE B-R].
4. In patients with severe ICH or those requiring surgical decompression, the safety and efficacy of BP lowering is not established [COR IIb; LOE c-LD].
5. In patients with mild-to-moderate ICH with SBP >150 mmHg, lowering it to <130 mmHg is potentially harmful [COR III; LOE B-R].

As can be seen, none of the guidelines have a class I recommendation, and the level of evidence backing them is only moderate.

The only definitive practice is to limit the intensity of BP lowering. Owing to these lacunae in the guidelines, it is crucial to consider the physiological status of other organ systems and the comorbid status and individualize the BP management protocol accordingly.

Prophylactic Anticonvulsants Post-traumatic seizures (PTSs) or early seizures after head injuries are a common occurrence, with 2–17% overall occurrence (being more common in children than adults) and higher (10–15% for adults; 30–35% for children) after severe head injuries [20].

Prophylactic treatment of PTS has stood the test of time despite the several controversies surrounding it owing to the significant risk of developing epilepsy following head trauma. Studies done on antiepileptic drugs do not show any evidence of such treatment preventing the development of seizure foci. Further, the prevention of early seizures firsthand does not translate into better neurological outcomes. Thus, it is safe to conclude that prophylactic medications for early PTS are optional [21].

Secondary prophylaxis after one episode of early PTS is another area to explore. Sparse high-quality evidence exists to provide therapeutic guidance. Early PTS episode is not associated with such a high risk of recurrence to transform into pulmonary thromboembolism (PTE). However, it is common practice to administer antiepileptic drugs after one episode for several weeks to several months and taper off slowly if no late PTS is noted.

Neuroprotection in Stroke The treatment of acute ischemic stroke (AIS) has seen a transition over the years, especially with the advent of endovascular thrombectomy (EVT). However, despite the recanalization rate being much larger, intravenous thrombolysis and endovascular thrombectomy remain the two principal reperfusion therapies [22]. For almost a quarter of a century, alteplase was the thrombolytic in use. Recently, after trial results showing non-inferiority against alteplase, tenecteplase has been popularized as a suitable alternative [1]. Despite improved functional outcomes seen with reperfusion therapies, nearly half of the patients end up with neurological impairments or complications like intracranial hemorrhage. To mitigate such complications and achieve better neurological recovery, adjunctive therapies are needed. Thrombo-inflammation, impaired microcirculatory reperfusion, and blood-brain barrier breakdown are potential targets to develop effective supportive therapies [23].

Adjunctive drugs that can see promising development are oxidative and nitrosative stress inhibitors and neurogenesis/regeneration and recovery promoters. Drugs that target systemic hemodynamics and N-methyl-D-aspartate (NMDA) and α-amino-3-hydroxy-5-methyl-4-isoxazolepropionic acid (AMPA) receptor blockers seem to have the least hope for further research, partly because they are more harmful than the rest. The development of these therapeutic adjuncts paved the way to further trials that need to be more standardized in approach with respect to the initiation and duration of treatment and the combination of thrombolysis/thrombectomy with additional drugs to intervene with detrimental ischemia-related pathways and stimulate regenerating pathways. With the superiority of endovascular thrombectomy over standard medical care [24], new possibilities are making way. Trials should be designed to revolve around the principle that for the drug to reach the areas of interest (the penumbra and the core), reperfusion in a primary prerequisite.

Timing and Duration of Neuroprotection There is an ongoing debate about the optimal timing and duration of neuroprotective interventions. The concept of a critical window of opportunity for neuroprotection is widely accepted, yet identifying this optimal timing remains elusive. Early intervention is often emphasized, but the precise timing of the intervention in the ideal therapeutic window and the duration of the intervention vary across different neurological conditions, complicating clinical applications.

Combination Therapy for Neuroprotection There is a controversy surrounding the use of combination therapy for neuroprotection, including the potential for synergistic effects. Each of the various neuroprotective agents, along with tissue plasminogen activator (tPA), has seen improvements via studies, which have translated into clinical application. The effective recanalization achieved by edaravone, when given early after tPA-induced recanalization, was revealed in a multicenter, single-blind, randomized, open-label study [25]. Another randomized double-blind clinical trial [26] showed the inhibition of lipid peroxidation and the prevention of early fall of serum uric acid, with the co-administration of uric acid and tPA. Additionally, when statins and tPA were combined in stroke patients, neurological injury was significantly reduced [27]. This approach of combination therapy is seeing promising results in studies and is gradually entering clinical practice.

The pathophysiology of TBI is heterogeneous; thus, the inclination toward combination therapies over the current single-agent interventions is not unjustified.

Having established that combination therapy is the way forward, several steps have been identified for advancing its research. Developing therapies that target multiple complementary mechanisms, supporting therapy development at every stage with valid surrogate markers to monitor the cerebral effects (injury and recovery) of the targeted treatment, developing multiple laboratories (in vitro, animal, and clinical) for coordinated research, and recruiting efficient data analysis tools are among the potential steps forward. A uniform standard of care adopted in clinical trials and mimicked in preclinical studies is essential to develop a shared database of reproducible and reliable data of positive and negative results [28].

Statins in Acute Brain Injury Similar to the effects of physical activity, steroid hormones, and nutrients, endothelial nitric oxide (NO), selectively augmented by statins and other modalities, reduces injury in animal models of cerebral ischemia. Endothelial nitric oxide synthase (eNOS) is an attractive target for preventive and therapeutic drug development for stroke despite its considerable pros and cons, including eNOS uncoupling and the dual role that NO plays in ischemic injury [29]. The cholesterol-independent protective effects of statins can be attributed to their NO-mediated effects. The earliest action of statins includes endothelial function improvement, an effect that precedes its cholesterol-lowering action. Indeed, the protective effects of statins are apparent within days and weeks [30]. If evidence is obtained of the cholesterol-independent properties of statins being clinically important, the double-fold action of this class of drugs can make them indispensable in the management of various cerebrovascular diseases in patients with or without hypercholesterolemia. This calls for further research to explore preliminary observations suggesting the neuroprotective properties of statins by developing investigation tools that employ neuroimaging and serial cognitive evaluation.

Glycemic Control Despite several efforts to resolve the conflict between strict and liberal glucose control, the optimal glycemic target range remains uncertain among TBI patients. Cerebral micro-dialysis is a neurochemical research tool in neuro–intensive care that can be effectively employed to identify a safe glycemic target range. It monitors the metabolic state of the injured brain and identifies metabolic crises displayed as low/high glucose level or high lactate/pyruvate ratio [31, 32]. While hyperglycemia is convincingly detrimental in TBI, intensive insulin therapy (IIT) remains controversial to date due to the associated increased risk of hypoglycemia (glucose <2.2 mmol/L). During the clinical course, close monitoring of blood glucose and frequent adjustment of insulin are strongly recommended [33]. Safe and effective implementation of IIT without the risk of its secondary complications, including hypoglycemia, must be the goal, going forward.

Biomarkers are crucial in predicting and guiding treatment decisions for numerous neurological conditions. S100 and neuron-specific enolase (NSE) are particularly noteworthy for their important roles in clinical practice. S100 proteins, especially S100B, are calcium-binding proteins primarily located in the glial and Schwann cells. They have been widely researched for their involvement in neurological disorders. Normal values range from 0.1 to 0.5 μg/L. Elevated S100B levels in the blood signal brain damage and serve as a biomarker for traumatic brain injury (TBI), stroke, and other neurodegenerative conditions [34]. In TBI, levels above 0.1 μg/L are often used to decide whether a CT scan is necessary, while levels above 0.5 μg/L are associated with more severe injuries and poorer outcomes [35]. Recent research has underscored the prognostic significance of S100B in stroke patients, where high levels are associated with poor outcomes and increased mortality. In ischemic stroke, elevated S100B levels above 0.2 μg/L are linked to larger infarct sizes and poorer clinical outcomes. In hemorrhagic stroke, higher S100B levels exceeding 0.5 μg/L can signify more extensive brain damage [36].

Neuron-specific enolase (NSE) is found in neurons and neuroendocrine cells. Normal values range from 12 to 20 ng/mL. Its elevated blood levels can signal neuronal damage. NSE is especially valuable in cases of TBI and cardiac arrest, where it helps predict the extent of brain injury and the chances of recovery. For TBI, NSE levels above 20 ng/mL indicate more severe injury, whereas levels exceeding 40 ng/mL are strongly associated with severe brain injury. In cardiac arrest, NSE levels above 33 ng/mL post-resuscitation predict poor outcomes, with levels above 69.3 ng/mL for shockable rhythms and 102.7 ng/mL for non-shockable rhythms indicating a worse prognosis. In stroke, NSE levels above 14.2 ng/mL at admission and 26.3 ng/mL at 48 h are linked to larger infarct sizes and poorer outcomes, with higher levels in hemorrhagic stroke associated with increased mortality [37, 38].

Glial fibrillary acidic protein (GFAP), a protein produced by astrocytes in the central nervous system, is released into the bloodstream when astrocytes are damaged, making it a dependable biomarker for brain injuries. Recent studies have demonstrated that GFAP levels increase significantly in the early stages of stroke, offering an opportunity for early intervention [1]. Ubiquitin C-terminal hydrolase (UCH-L1), a neuronal biomarker, is involved in the degradation of ubiquitinated proteins and is highly expressed in neurons, indicating TBI and neuronal injury through elevated blood levels [39].

Neuroprotective Effects of Anesthetic Agents and Sedatives Anesthetics are believed to offer neuroprotection by reducing the brain's metabolic rate, thereby increasing its tolerance to ischemic insults. Isoflurane and xenon have shown promise in experimental models by suppressing excitatory neurotransmission and enhancing inhibitory activity [40]. However, translating these findings into clinical practice has proven challenging. A significant controversy in this field revolves around the optimal depth of anesthesia required for neuroprotection. The study by Warner et al. suggests that deeper levels of anesthesia may provide greater neuroprotective benefits by more effectively reducing metabolic demand and preventing excitotoxicity. However, the research by Tu, Z., Zhang, Y., Lv, X. et al. indicates that excessively deep anesthesia can lead to adverse outcomes, such as postoperative cognitive dysfunction and an increased risk of complications [41]. This has led to ongoing debates about the balance between achieving sufficient neuroprotection and avoiding potential neurotoxicity. Another area of contention is the variability in patient responses to anesthetic agents. Factors such as age, underlying health conditions, and genetic predispositions can influence how individuals respond to anesthesia, making it difficult to establish standardized protocols [42]. This variability underscores the need for personalized approaches to anesthesia management, tailored to the specific needs and characteristics of each patient. The introduction of advanced monitoring techniques, such as electroencephalogram (EEG) monitoring, has provided new insights into the relationship between anesthesia depth and neuroprotection. These technologies allow for a more precise assessment of anesthesia depth and its effects on brain activity, potentially improving the ability to optimize anesthetic management. However, the implementation of these techniques in clinical practice remains limited, and further research is needed to validate their effectiveness. Despite the potential benefits of anesthetic neuroprotection, some studies have raised concerns about the consistency and reproducibility of these effects in clinical settings. The discrepancy between experimental and clinical findings suggests that additional factors, such as the timing and duration of anesthesia, may play a critical role in determining its neuroprotective efficacy [42]. This highlights the importance of continued research to better understand the underlying mechanisms and develop evidence-based guidelines for clinical practice.

Remote Ischemic Conditioning The ongoing debate about the effectiveness of remote ischemic conditioning (RIC) in reducing ischemic brain injury is complex and multifaceted. Recent studies have yielded mixed results, highlighting both the potential benefits and limitations of this intervention. A study published by Chen H et al. found that RIC could improve neurological outcomes in patients with acute moderate ischemic stroke, as evidenced by significant improvements in the modified Rankin Scale scores. However, the study also noted that the benefits might be influenced by the timing and frequency of the conditioning sessions [43]. Similarly, a review by Saccaro, L. F., et al. discussed the challenges of translating RIC's promising results in reducing biomarkers of ischemic injury into clinical practice, emphasizing the need for standardized protocols and further research [44]. A systematic review by Purroy, F., et al. focused on the neuroprotective effects of remote ischemic preconditioning (RIPreC) during the acute phase of ischemic stroke, concluding that, while RIPreC is safe and feasible, the heterogeneity of clinical trial designs and outcomes makes it difficult to draw definitive conclusions about its efficacy [45]. Despite these promising findings,

Table 17.3 The level of evidence and recommendations for the various contentious issues

Sr. No.	Therapeutic interventions	Recommendation	Trials/evidence
1.	*Therapeutic hypothermia*		
	Timing of TTM initiation	No recommendation	
	Ideal site for temperature monitoring	Lack of high-quality evidence	
	Pharmacotherapy during cooling	Lack of high-quality evidence	
2.	*Steroids in head injury*	Increased mortality	CRASH trial
3.	*Mannitol vs. hypertonic saline*	Patient-specific approach recommended	
4.	*Blood pressure targets in AIS*		
	No benefit of enhanced BP control on outcome	Strong recommendation	ENCHANTED III trial
	Avoid hypotension and hypovolemia; BP <185/110 pre-thrombolysis and <180/105 post-thrombolysis	Strong recommendation	ACC/AHA guidelines
	BP <185/110 in patients planned for mechanical thrombectomy; no use of drug-induced hypertension	Intermediate recommendation	

(continued)

Table 17.3 (continued)

Sr. No.	Therapeutic interventions	Recommendation	Trials/evidence
5.	*Blood pressure targets in ICH*		
	Smooth and sustained BP control with minimum variability; within 2 h; target achieved within 1 h; range 130–150 mmHg SBP	Intermediate recommendation	ACC/AHA guidelines
	BP lowering in severe ICH requiring decompression	No evidence of safety and efficacy	
6.	*Post-traumatic epilepsy*		
	Prophylaxis for early PTS	No benefit on neurological outcome	
	Starting antiepileptic drug (AED) after one episode of early PTS	Lack of high-quality evidence	Most patients receive AEDs for several weeks to months, tapered off slowly
7.	*Acute ischemic stroke (AIS)*		
	Image-guided IV thrombolysis	Can extend the efficacy of IV-tPA to 9 h	EXTEND trial
	Alteplase vs. tenecteplase	Better functional outcomes with alteplase	EXTENT-IA-TNK trial
	Combination therapies	Strong rationale but low-quality evidence	
8.	*Statins in AIS*	Low-quality evidence of its benefit	
9.	*Intensive insulin therapy (IIT) in TBI*		
	Close monitoring of glucose and frequent adjustment of insulin	Strong recommendation	
10.	*Biomarkers*		
	S100B	Good biomarker for TBI	Quantitative marker of brain damage
	NSE	Good biomarker for TBI and brain damage	Prognostic marker for cardiac arrest (post-resuscitation) and stroke
	GFAP	Dependable marker of brain injury	Early biomarker in stroke
11.	*Anesthetic agents*	Lack of specific recommendations	
12.	*Remote ischemic preconditioning*	Safe and effective	Heterogeneity of clinical trials, controversial results, lack of reproducibility of results, and poor understanding of the theory behind RIPreC hamper its practical use

some studies have raised concerns about the consistency and reproducibility of RIC's benefits, highlighting the variability in patient populations, conditioning protocols, and outcome measures. Additionally, the mechanisms underlying RIC's neuroprotective effects are not fully understood, further complicating its application in clinical settings.

A summary of various recommendations for the various contentious issues and their respective studies and level of evidence is listed in Table 17.3.

17.2 Conclusion

Despite the relentless pursuit of the proverbial magic bullet for neuroprotection in the form of several anesthetics, experimental drugs, adjuvants, and therapies, the translation of beneficial experimental results into clinical success remains an unachieved objective.

Brain protection from injuries, not limited to the primary trauma, has proven to be an ambitious goal. The literature is studded with trial failures, especially for pharmacologic protection after TBI. These could be attributable, in part, to flawed methodologies, substandard quality of models, and an incomplete understanding of cerebral pharmacokinetics and action mechanisms in the area of interest.

The maintenance of physiological homeostasis over pharmacological neuroprotection has never lost focus.

Though a "standard-of-care" neuroprotection has not yet arrived, closer collaborations between preclinical investigators and clinical counterparts will be key to improving methodologies in both settings to offer some hope, if not promise, for the future.

References

1. Fukuda S, Warner DS. Cerebral protection. Br J Anaesth. 2007;99(1):10–7. https://doi.org/10.1093/bja/aem140.
2. Bilotta F, Stazi E, Zlotnik A, Gruenbaum SE, Rosa G. Neuroprotective effects of intravenous anesthetics: a new critical perspective. Curr Pharm Des. 2014;20(34):5469–75. https://doi.org/10.2174/1381612820666140325110113. PMID: 24669972; PMCID: PMC4388052.
3. Madden LK, Hill M, May TL, Human T, Guanci MM, Jacobi J, Moreda MV, Badjatia N. The implementation of targeted temperature management: an evidence-based guideline from the neurocritical care society. Neurocrit Care. 2017;27:468–87.
4. MacLellan CL, Clark DL, Silasi G, Colbourne F. Use of prolonged hypothermia to treat ischemic and hemorrhagic stroke. J Neurotrauma. 2009;26(3):313–23.
5. Cariou A, Payen JF, Asehnoune K, Audibert G, Botte A, Brissaud O, Debaty G, Deltour S, Deye N, Engrand N, Francony G, Legriel S, Levy B, Meyer P, Orban JC, Renolleau S, Vigue B, De Saint Blanquat L, Mathien C, Velly L, Société de Réanimation de Langue Française (SRLF) and the Société Française d'Anesthésie et de Réanimation (SFAR) In conjunction with the Association de Neuro Anesthésie Réanimation de Langue Française (ANARLF), the Groupe Francophone de Réanimation et Urgences Pédiatriques (GFRUP), the Société Française de Médecine d'Urgence (SFMU), and the Société Française Neuro-Vasculaire (SFNV). Targeted temperature management in the ICU: guidelines from a French expert panel. Ann Intensive

Care. 2017;7(1):70. https://doi.org/10.1186/s13613-017-0294-1. Epub 2017 Jun 19. PMID: 28631089; PMCID: PMC5476556.

6. Omairi AM, Pandey S. Targeted temperature management. [Updated 2023 Jun 25]. In: StatPearls [Internet]. Treasure Island (FL): StatPearls Publishing; 2024. Available from: https://www.ncbi.nlm.nih.gov/books/NBK556124.
7. Susantitaphong P, Alfayez M, Cohen-Bucay A, et al. Therapeutic hypothermia and prevention of acute kidney injury: a meta-analysis of randomized controlled trials. 2012. In: Database of abstracts of reviews of effects (DARE): quality-assessed reviews [Internet]. York (UK): Centre for Reviews and Dissemination (UK); 1995. Available from: https://www.ncbi.nlm.nih.gov/books/NBK91569/.
8. Alderson P, Roberts I. Corticosteroids for acute traumatic brain injury. Cochrane Database Syst Rev. 2005;2005(1):CD000196. https://doi.org/10.1002/14651858.CD000196.pub2. PMID: 15674869; PMCID: PMC7043302.
9. Nagaraju K, Lobo L, Sharma M. Comparative efficacy analysis of mannitol and hypertonic saline in the management of traumatic brain injury: a scientific exploration of neuroprotective strategies. Emerg Care J. 2024;20(2) https://doi.org/10.4081/ecj.2024.12310
10. Anderson CS, Huang Y, Lindley RI, Chen X, Arima H, Chen G, Li Q, Billot L, Delcourt C, Bath PM, Broderick JP, Demchuk AM, Donnan GA, Durham AC, Lavados PM, Lee TH, Levi C, Martins SO, Olavarria VV, Pandian JD, Parsons MW, Pontes-Neto OM, Ricci S, Sato S, Sharma VK, Silva F, Song L, Thang NH, Wardlaw JM, Wang JG, Wang X, Woodward M, Chalmers J, Robinson TG, ENCHANTED Investigators and Coordinators. Intensive blood pressure reduction with intravenous thrombolysis therapy for acute ischaemic stroke (ENCHANTED): an international, randomised, open-label, blinded-endpoint, phase 3 trial. Lancet. 2019;393(10174):877–88. https://doi.org/10.1016/S0140-6736(19)30038-8. Epub 2019 Feb 7.
11. Der-Nigoghossian C, Levasseur-Franklin K, Makii J. Acute blood pressure management in neurocritically ill patients. Pharmacotherapy. 2019;39(3):335–45. https://doi.org/10.1002/phar.2233. Epub 2019 Mar 11.
12. Molina CA, Chamorro A, Rovira À, de Miquel A, Serena J, Roman LS, Jovin TG, Davalos A, Cobo E. REVASCAT: a randomized trial of revascularization with SOLITAIRE FR device vs. best medical therapy in the treatment of acute stroke due to anterior circulation large vessel occlusion presenting within eight-hours of symptom onset. Int J Stroke. 2015;10(4):619–26. https://doi.org/10.1111/ijs.12157. Epub 2013 Nov 10.
13. Saver JL, Goyal M, Bonafe A, Diener HC, Levy EI, Pereira VM, Albers GW, Cognard C, Cohen DJ, Hacke W, Jansen O, Jovin TG, Mattle HP, Nogueira RG, Siddiqui AH, Yavagal DR, Baxter BW, Devlin TG, Lopes DK, Reddy VK, du Mesnil de Rochemont R, Singer OC, Jahan R, SWIFT PRIME Investigators. Stent-retriever thrombectomy after intravenous t-PA vs. t-PA alone in stroke. N Engl J Med. 2015;372(24):2285–95. https://doi.org/10.1056/NEJMoa1415061. Epub 2015 Apr 17.
14. Nogueira RG, Jadhav AP, Haussen DC, Bonafe A, Budzik RF, Bhuva P, Yavagal DR, Ribo M, Cognard C, Hanel RA, Sila CA, Hassan AE, Millan M, Levy EI, Mitchell P, Chen M, English JD, Shah QA, Silver FL, Pereira VM, Mehta BP, Baxter BW, Abraham MG, Cardona P, Veznedaroglu E, Hellinger FR, Feng L, Kirmani JF, Lopes DK, Jankowitz BT, Frankel MR, Costalat V, Vora NA, Yoo AJ, Malik AM, Furlan AJ, Rubiera M, Aghaebrahim A, Olivot JM, Tekle WG, Shields R, Graves T, Lewis RJ, Smith WS, Liebeskind DS, Saver JL, Jovin TG, DAWN Trial Investigators. Thrombectomy 6 to 24 hours after stroke with a mismatch between deficit and infarct. N Engl J Med. 2018;378(1):11–21. https://doi.org/10.1056/NEJMoa1706442. Epub 2017 Nov 11.
15. Albers GW, Marks MP, Kemp S, Christensen S, Tsai JP, Ortega-Gutierrez S, McTaggart RA, Torbey MT, Kim-Tenser M, Leslie-Mazwi T, Sarraj A, Kasner SE, Ansari SA, Yeatts SD, Hamilton S, Mlynash M, Heit JJ, Zaharchuk G, Kim S, Carrozzella J, Palesch YY, Demchuk AM, Bammer R, Lavori PW, Broderick JP, Lansberg MG, DEFUSE 3 Investigators. Thrombectomy for stroke at 6 to 16 hours with selection by perfusion imaging. N Engl J Med.

2018;378(8):708–18. https://doi.org/10.1056/NEJMoa1713973. Epub 2018 Jan 24. PMID: 29364767; PMCID: PMC6590673.

16. Powers WJ, Rabinstein AA, Ackerson T, Adeoye OM, Bambakidis NC, Becker K, Biller J, Brown M, Demaerschalk BM, Hoh B, Jauch EC, Kidwell CS, Leslie-Mazwi TM, Ovbiagele B, Scott PA, Sheth KN, Southerland AM, Summers DV, Tirschwell DL. Guidelines for the early management of patients with Acute Ischemic Stroke: 2019 update to the 2018 guidelines for the early management of Acute Ischemic Stroke: a guideline for healthcare professionals from the American Heart Association/American Stroke Association. Stroke. 2019;50(12):e344–418. https://doi.org/10.1161/STR.0000000000000211. Epub 2019 Oct 30. Erratum in: Stroke. 2019 Dec;50(12):e440–1. https://doi.org/10.1161/STR.0000000000000215.
17. Anderson CS, Heeley E, Huang Y, Wang J, Stapf C, Delcourt C, Lindley R, Robinson T, Lavados P, Neal B, Hata J, Arima H, Parsons M, Li Y, Wang J, Heritier S, Li Q, Woodward M, Simes RJ, Davis SM, Chalmers J, INTERACT2 Investigators. Rapid blood-pressure lowering in patients with acute intracerebral hemorrhage. N Engl J Med. 2013;368(25):2355–65. https://doi.org/10.1056/NEJMoa1214609. Epub 2013 May 29.
18. Qureshi AI, Palesch YY, Barsan WG, Hanley DF, Hsu CY, Martin RL, Moy CS, Silbergleit R, Steiner T, Suarez JI, Toyoda K, Wang Y, Yamamoto H, Yoon BW, ATACH-2 Trial Investigators and the Neurological Emergency Treatment Trials Network. Intensive blood-pressure lowering in patients with acute cerebral hemorrhage. N Engl J Med. 2016;375(11):1033–43. https://doi.org/10.1056/NEJMoa1603460. Epub 2016 Jun 8. PMID: 27276234; PMCID: PMC5345109.
19. Greenberg SM, Ziai WC, Cordonnier C, Dowlatshahi D, Francis B, Goldstein JN, Claude Hemphill J III, Johnson R, Keigher KM, Mack WJ, Mocco J, Newton EJ, Ruff IM, Sansing LH, Schulman S, Selim MH, Sheth KN, Sprigg N, Sunnerhagen KS, On behalf of the American Heart Association/American Stroke Association. Guideline for the management of patients with spontaneous intracerebral hemorrhage: a guideline from the American Heart Association/American Stroke Association. Stroke. 2022;53(7) https://doi.org/10.1161/STR.0000000000000407.
20. Teasell R, et al. Post-traumatic seizure disorder following acquired brain injury. Brain Inj. 2007;21:201–14.
21. Ding K, Gupta PK, Diaz-Arrastia R. Epilepsy after traumatic brain injury. In: Laskowitz D, Grant G, editors. Translational research in traumatic brain injury. Boca Raton (FL): CRC Press/Taylor and Francis Group; 2016. Chapter 14. Available from: https://www.ncbi.nlm.nih.gov/books/NBK326716/.
22. Mulder IA, van Bavel ET, de Vries HE, et al. Adjunctive cytoprotective therapies in acute ischemic stroke: a systematic review. Fluids Barriers CNS. 2021;18:46. https://doi.org/10.1186/s12987-021-00280-1.
23. Goyal M, Rinkel LA, Ospel JM. A review on adjunctive therapies for endovascular treatment in Acute Ischemic Stroke. J Neuroendovasc Ther. 2023;17(11):263–71. https://doi.org/10.5797/jnet.ra.2023-0035. Epub 2023 Jul 12. PMID: 38025256; PMCID: PMC10657729.
24. Goyal M, Menon BK, van Zwam WH, Dippel DW, Mitchell PJ, Demchuk AM, et al. Endovascular thrombectomy after large-vessel ischaemic stroke: a meta-analysis of individual patient data from five randomised trials. Lancet. 2016;387:1723–31.
25. Kimura K, Aoki J, Sakamoto Y, Kobayashi K, Sakai K, Inoue T, Iguchi Y, Shibazaki K. Administration of edaravone, a free radical scavenger, during t-PA infusion can enhance early recanalization in acute stroke patients–a preliminary study. J Neurol Sci. 2012;313:132–6.
26. Amaro S, Soy D, Obach V, Cervera Á, Planas AM, Chamorro Á. A pilot study of dual treatment with recombinant tissue plasminogen activator and uric acid in acute ischemic stroke. Stroke. 2007;38:2173–5.
27. Alvares-Sabin J, Huertas R, Quintana M, Rubeira M, Delgado P, Ribo M, Molina CA, Montaner J. Prior statin use may be associated with improved stroke outcome after tissue plasminogen activator. Stroke. 2007;38:1076–8.
28. Margulies S, HicksR, The Combination Therapies for Traumatic Brain Injury Workshop Leaders. Combination therapies for traumatic brain injury: prospective considerations. J Neurotrauma. 2009;26:925–39. https://doi.org/10.1089/neu.2008.0794.

29. Heart Protection Study Collaborative Group. MRC/BHF heart protection study of cholesterol-lowering with simvastatin in 20,536 high-risk individuals. A randomized placebo-controlled trial. Lancet. 2002;360:7–22.
30. Jonsson N, Asplund K. Does pretreatment with statins improve clinical outcome after stroke? A pilot case reference study. Stroke. 2002;32:1112–5.
31. Bellander BM, Cantais E, Enblad P, Hutchinson P, Nordstrom CH, Robertson C, Sahuquillo J, Smith M, Stocchetti N, Ungerstedt U, Unterberg A, Olsen NV. Consensus meeting on microdialysis in neurointensive care. Intensive Care Med. 2004;30:2166–9.
32. Hillered L, Persson L, Nilsson P, Ronne-Engstrom E, Enblad P. Continuous monitoring of cerebral metabolism in traumatic brain injury: a focus on cerebral microdialysis. Curr Opin Crit Care. 2006;12:112–8.
33. Vriesendorp TM, DeVries JH, Holleman F, Dzoljic M, Hoekstra JB. The use of two continuous glucose sensors during and after surgery. Diabetes Technol Ther. 2005;7:315–22.
34. Anogianakis G, Daios S, Topouzis N, Barmpagiannos K, Kaiafa G, Myrou A, Ztriva E, Tsankof A, Karlafti E, Anogeianaki A, et al. Current trends in stroke biomarkers: the prognostic role of S100 calcium-binding Protein B and glial fibrillary acidic protein. Life. 2024;14(10):1247.
35. Thelin EP, Nelson DW, Bellander BM. A review of the clinical utility of serum S100B protein levels in the assessment of traumatic brain injury. Acta Neurochir. 2017;159:209–25.
36. Abboud T, Rohde V, Mielke D. Mini review: current status and perspective of S100B protein as a biomarker in daily clinical practice for diagnosis and prognosticating of clinical outcome in patients with neurological diseases with focus on acute brain injury. BMC Neurosci. 2023;24:38.
37. Thelin EP, Jeppsson E, Frostell A, et al. Utility of neuron-specific enolase in traumatic brain injury; relations to S100B levels, outcome, and extracranial injury severity. Crit Care. 2016;20:285.
38. Kim YJ, Kim YH, Youn CS, et al. Different neuro prognostication thresholds of neuron-specific enolase in shockable and non-shockable out-of-hospital cardiac arrest: a prospective multicenter observational study in Korea (the KORHN-PRO registry). Crit Care. 2023;27:313.
39. Abboud T, Rohde V, Mielke D. Mini review: current status and perspective of S100B protein as a biomarker in daily clinical practice for diagnosis and prognosticating of clinical outcome in patients with neurological diseases with a focus on acute brain injury. BMC Neurosci. 2023;24:38.
40. Warner DS, sheng H. anesthetic neuroprotection? It's Complicated. Anesthesiology. 2017;126:579–81.
41. Tu Z, Zhang Y, Lv X, et al. Accurate machine learning-based monitoring of anesthesia depth with EEG recording. Neurosci Bull. 2024;41:449.
42. Zhang T, Deng D, Huang S, Fu D, Wang T, Xu F, MaL, Ding Y, Wang K, Wang Y, Zhao W, Chen X. A retrospect and outlook on the neuroprotective effects of anesthetics in the era of endovascular therapy. Front Neurosci. 2023;17:1140275.
43. Chen H, Cui Y, Li X, et al. Effect of remote ischemic conditioning vs usual care on neurologic function in patients with acute moderate ischemic stroke: the RICAMIS randomized clinical trial. JAMA. 2022;328(7):627–36.
44. Saccaro LF, Aimo A, Emdin M, Pico F. Remote ischemic conditioning in ischemic stroke and myocardial infarction: similarities and differences. Front Neurol. 2021;12:716316.
45. Purroy F, García C, Mauri G, et al. Induced neuroprotection by remote ischemic perconditioning as a new paradigm in ischemic stroke at the acute phase, a systematic review. BMC Neurol. 2020;20:266.

Controversies in Neurorehabilitation 18

Kaustuv Dutta, R. P. Sangeetha, and Deepak Ganjigere

Abstract

Neurorehabilitation is a multidisciplinary, goal-oriented intervention aimed at enhancing recovery and quality of life in patients with neurological impairments. This chapter critically explores ongoing controversies in neurorehabilitation, focusing on the timing and intensity of interventions, physical versus cognitive prioritisation, outcome assessment metrics, and management strategies in severe brain injury. While early rehabilitation is associated with improved neuroplasticity and functional outcomes, concerns remain regarding safety and individual readiness. Similarly, the superiority of high-intensity protocols is debated, with evidence suggesting benefits while also cautioning against overexertion. The chapter also addresses disparities in access and implementation between high- and low-resource settings, the appropriateness of intracranial pressure (ICP)–focused care in acute traumatic brain injury (TBI), and the limitations of current outcome measurement tools. A patient-centred, multidisciplinary, and phased strategy is advocated to enhance functional independence and long-term recovery.

Keywords

Neurorehabilitation · Traumatic brain injury · Cognitive–motor integration Early mobilisation · Functional outcome metrics · Rehabilitation intensity

K. Dutta (✉)
Neuroanaesthesia & Neurocritical Care, Dr PKSH, Cooch Behar, West Bengal, India

R. P. Sangeetha · D. Ganjigere
Neuroanaesthesia & Neurocritical Care, National Institute of Mental Health and Neurosciences, Bangalore, Karnataka, India

P. U. Bidkar, M. Krishnakumar (eds.), *Controversies in Neurocritical Care*,
https://doi.org/10.1007/978-981-95-4419-6_18

18.1 Introduction to Neurorehabilitation

Neurorehabilitation is a multidisciplinary approach that aims to enhance recovery and improve the quality of life for individuals with sequelae of neurological injuries. It involves multiple therapeutic interventions that aim to enhance functional proficiency and alleviate disability to lead an independent life and fulfil social responsibilities. To put it simply, rehabilitation requires overcoming the disability and assisting the person to be independent, as far as possible, to achieve personal, societal, and professional well-being. The importance of neurorehabilitation is emphasised by the growing incidence of neurological disorders, including stroke, traumatic brain injury (TBI), and neurodegenerative diseases [1].

Effective neurorehabilitation encompasses a holistic approach to enhance physical, cognitive, emotional, and psychological health [2]. It essentially assists the individual with a disability to set targets for functional recovery with professional guidance [3].

18.2 Controversies in Neurorehabilitation

There are several controversies and challenges in the field of neurorehabilitation for head injuries, strokes, and other neurological disorders (Fig. 18.1). In traumatic brain injury (TBI), while neurorehabilitation efforts are emerging, there is a lack of consensus regarding rehabilitation following TBI of any severity. Another widely debated aspect of neurorehabilitation is the timing of intervention, followed by other aspects like the intensity of rehabilitation (high-intensity versus low-intensity) and physical versus cognitive focus in rehabilitation, to reach a consensus on a successful rehabilitation outcome measure. This chapter will discuss some of these common controversies in neurorehabilitation in detail.

18.2.1 Timing of Rehabilitation

One of the most widely debated aspects of neurorehabilitation is the timing of intervention. Timing of neurorehabilitation is a critical aspect of patient recovery following neurological injuries such as stroke, traumatic brain injury (TBI), or spinal cord injury (SCI). The debate on when to initiate rehabilitation as early as possible or after a certain recovery period depends upon balancing the potential benefits of early mobilisation against the risks of exacerbating the injury.

The rehabilitation should begin as soon as the patient is haemodynamically stable and medically fit to tolerate mobilisation. Early mobilisation may be associated with improved outcomes and functional gains [4].

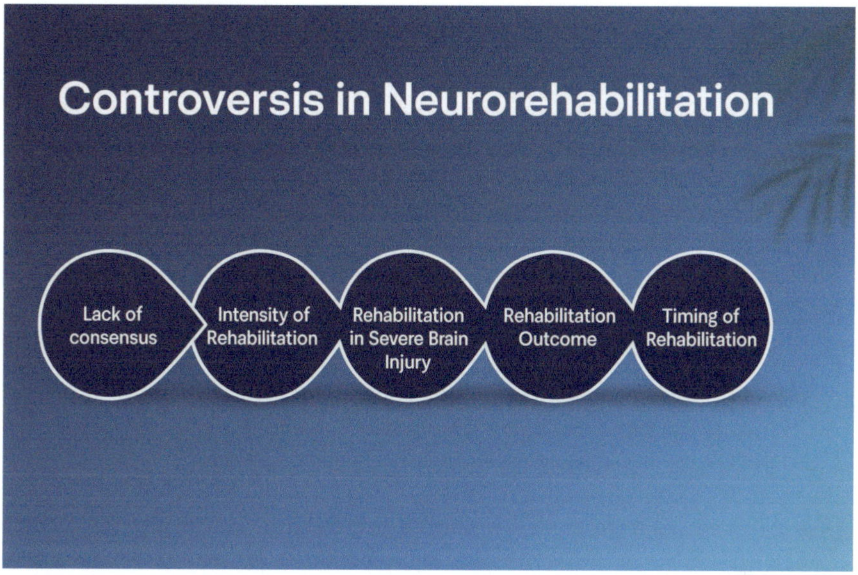

Fig. 18.1 Areas of controversy in neurorehabilitation

18.2.1.1 Early Rehabilitation

Benefits

1. *Neuroplasticity*: The injured brain is able to reorganise itself, and early rehabilitation can enhance neuroplasticity and recovery [5].
2. *Functional Mobility*: Initiating rehabilitation early can promote functional mobility, helping patients regain movement and independence sooner. This can improve muscle strength and coordination [6, 7].
3. *Preventing Complications*: Early mobilisation can reduce the risk of complications associated with immobility, such as pressure ulcers, deep vein thrombosis, and pulmonary complications [8].
4. *Psychological Benefits*: Early engagement in rehabilitation can foster motivation, reduce anxiety, and improve overall psychological well-being, as patients see the progress and regain control over their bodies [9, 10].

Risks of Early Rehabilitation

1. *Exacerbation of Injuries*: There is a concern that without appropriate assessment, early mobilisation might result in further damage to fragile tissues, particularly in cases of traumatic brain injury or spinal cord injuries [11, 12].
2. *Increased Pain and Discomfort*: Early rehabilitation might lead to increased pain if patients are pushed to move before they are sufficiently ready, resulting in a negative experience and decreased compliance.
3. *Fatigue and Overexertion*: Patients, especially those with neurological deficits, can fatigue quickly. Overexertion during early rehabilitation could be counterproductive and lead to setbacks.

18.2.2 Intensity of Rehabilitation: Are High-Intensity Rehabilitation Protocols Superior to Moderate- or Low-Intensity Approaches for Long-Term Recovery?

Before we draw the lines between high- and low-intensity rehabilitation protocols, we must understand specific terminologies. In simple words, intensity is the time the patient spends each day on a particular intervention. An accurate way to define it is the amount of physical or mental work put forth by the patient during a specific movement or series of movements, exercises, or activities during a therapy session [13]. Hence, intensity is not limited to the time spent; it can be defined in muscular capacity, cardiovascular reserve, movement counts, and task performance. A total dose is the total activity performed during the training period. The time-based definition is helpful for better understanding and analysis of the evidence available. There is no clear definition for high and low intensities based on the patient's dose. In their systematic review, Emma V et al. found that patients who received exercise-based training in the intensity group received 13.8–91.8 h [14]. The control or low-intensity group received 9.2–27.7 h. Marsh et al., in their meta-analyses, described 20 h a week under a high-intensity group [15]. To further simplify it, low-intensity or usual care involves 30–100 min daily for 4–5 days a week. An intense protocol involves 2–5 h daily for 4–7 days a week. Intensity protocols (5 h/day) in a retrospective analysis showed better results than low-intensity protocols [16].

The Spanish Society of Neurorehabilitation recommends typically 3 h a day, at a frequency of 5 days a week, to achieve their rehabilitation objectives. Hence, a more intensive protocol should be suggested, and the patient's needs should be adapted [17]. It is essential to individualise specific therapies for patients before increasing the dosage. Also, patient tolerance should be considered while implementing high-intensity protocols. Any increase or decrease in intensity can be done based on patient feedback. Table 18.1 highlights the key features of moderate-/low-intensity and high-intensity rehabilitation.

Table 18.1 Key features of moderate–/low-intensity and high-intensity rehabilitation

Key features	Moderate–/low-intensity	High-intensity
Advantages	Safer for early stages, joint protection, gradual mobility, psychological benefits, lower risk of overuse	Faster strength and endurance gains, improved functional capacity, stimulated neuroplasticity, reduced risk of re-injury
Risks	Slower progress may lack sufficient challenge for advanced recovery	Overuse injuries, fatigue, risk of re-injury if not managed well
Best for	Early-to-mid-recovery stages, joint mobility, pain management, low fitness levels, general fitness recovery	Advanced recovery stages, building strength, neurorehabilitation (e.g. stroke), improving athletic performance

18.2.3 Physical Versus Cognitive Focus in Rehabilitation: Should Rehabilitation Prioritise Motor Recovery over Cognitive and Emotional Rehabilitation, or Is an Integrated Approach Better?

The primary goal of motor rehabilitation is to help individuals regain physical functioning, mobility, and independence. This is especially important for patients recovering from injuries like stroke, traumatic brain injury, and spinal cord injury. Physical recovery, such as regaining the ability to walk or use a hand, is often seen as the most immediate and visible improvement. Hence, clinicians and families keep up their expectations of physical recovery. Motor rehabilitation usually takes the front seat in these patients. It involves physical therapy and occupational therapy to train muscles, joints, and limbs for mobility. However, focusing solely on motor recovery may overlook other aspects of an individual's well-being, particularly cognitive and emotional health, closely linked to the overall quality of life.

Conversely, cognitive rehabilitation focuses on improving memory, attention, problem-solving, and executive functions, which are essential for daily life. Emotional rehabilitation addresses issues such as anxiety, depression, and emotional regulation. For individuals who have suffered brain injuries or neurological disorders, cognitive and emotional functions can be just as impaired as physical abilities and often require specific intervention. Cognitive rehabilitation therapies (e.g. neuropsychological rehabilitation and cognitive training) and emotional support therapies (e.g. psychotherapy and counselling) are designed to help patients regain their cognitive and emotional stability.

That brings us to an integrated approach where a rehabilitation team focuses on individuals' motor, cognitive, and emotional deficits. For example, cognitive impairments like attention deficits or memory problems can impede motor learning and recovery. Similarly, emotional states such as depression can reduce motivation for physical therapy and affect motor recovery. Treating one aspect in isolation may decrease the overall progress. Every individual's rehabilitation needs are unique. An integrated, individualised approach allows for tailored care that considers the person as a whole rather than in isolated domains. Treating emotional and cognitive aspects alongside physical rehabilitation can improve psychological outcomes. Many patients struggle with feelings of frustration, helplessness, or anxiety, especially when physical progress is slow. Addressing these emotions can improve patient engagement and resilience, facilitating better adherence to the rehabilitation process. There is strong evidence from clinical studies that combining physical and cognitive therapies leads to superior outcomes [18–22].

While the immediate focus of rehabilitation may depend on the specific condition (e.g. if the patient is recovering from a stroke, motor recovery may take precedence initially), long-term success is most likely to come from an integrated approach that addresses the whole person. This involves treating both motor functions and the cognitive–emotional components that influence recovery. Table 18.2 summarises the key features of physical, cognitive, and integrated approaches to rehabilitation.

Table 18.2 Key features of physical, cognitive, and integrated approaches to rehabilitation

Aspect of rehabilitation	Physical focus (motor recovery)	Cognitive/emotional focus	Integrated approach
Key features	Focus on restoring physical abilities (strength, mobility, and coordination)	Focus on cognitive functions (memory and attention) and emotional health (mood and resilience)	Simultaneous focus on physical, cognitive, and emotional recovery
Advantages	Faster improvement in functional independence. Immediate physical quality-of-life gains	Improves cognitive functions like memory, planning, and attention. Enhances emotional Well-being and resilience	Optimises overall recovery by addressing body and mind. Supports neuroplasticity and brain–body connection
Risks	May overlook emotional and cognitive challenges. Can impede progress if emotional/ cognitive issues persist	Risk of neglecting physical recovery needs. It may hinder functional independence if not balanced	Requires careful coordination to prevent overloading in one area. Needs an individualised approach for best results
Best for	Early recovery from physical injuries. Restoring functional independence (e.g. stroke and musculoskeletal injuries)	Addressing cognitive impairments or emotional disorders (e.g. depression and anxiety after injury). Neurological conditions affecting brain function	Comprehensive recovery for complex conditions (e.g. stroke and TBI). Long-term functional, cognitive, and emotional health
Type of injury	Musculoskeletal injuries. Stroke recovery (physical rehabilitation focus)	Brain injury with cognitive deficits. Mental health conditions post-injury (e.g. depression after surgery)	Stroke recovery (addressing both physical and cognitive impairments). Traumatic brain injury (TBI) and spinal cord injury (SCI)

18.2.4 Rehabilitation in Severe Brain Injury: How Effective Is Rehabilitation in Patients with Severe Neurological Injury, and When Is It Futile?

Severe brain injury, either traumatic or non-traumatic, has a profound negative impact on the survivors' cognitive and functional recovery and the quality of life that is directly linked to the primary aetiology and severity of brain injury, the time lag between the injury and the institution of therapeutic management, and a multitude of other factors, such as pre-morbid status, response to therapy, and so on. TBI has adverse cognitive, physical, and functional consequences, which makes rehabilitation interventions an integral part of its management—the potential beneficiaries of rehabilitation range across different severity grades, from mild to severe.

Neurorehabilitation in the context of brain injury ranges from early rehabilitation of patients with impaired physical, cognitive, communicative, and sensory functions to reintegrating patients into their pre-morbid social and work environments. These are accomplished through inpatient and outpatient rehabilitation, nursing home care, and community-based services.

The controversies involved in the neurorehabilitation of TBI patients revolve around the geographic location that determines access to technological support, the feasibility of different rehabilitative interventions, the timing of institution, applicability across different severity grades, consistency of expected outcomes, and phasing of targeted interventions to suit the various illness stages.

18.2.4.1 Neurorehabilitation in Developed Versus Developing Countries

The beneficial role of neurorehabilitation has been consistently demonstrated across various studies, especially in developed countries [23]. The consistent clinical translation of these therapies has improved cognitive function, productivity, and early return to professional life, as well as better efficiency in daily activities and retained language and speech faculties. However, extrapolating these manoeuvres to improve outcomes has remained a challenge in developing countries, as reported by a study conducted among African survivors of TBI [24]. The challenges faced were limited resources, difficulty setting up multidisciplinary teams, and, hence, disparities in patient care. Low-resource countries often face additional barriers to accessing comprehensive inpatient rehabilitation secondary to the need for insurance pre-authorisation, insufficient beds available in rehabilitation facilities, and, hence, the inconsistent quality of rehabilitation services. This inadequacy could be circumvented by a trans-disciplinary model proposed as the gold standard for more integrated and patient-oriented care [25, 26].

18.2.4.2 Severity-Based Approach Versus Tailored Neurorehabilitation for All

Unlike the general belief that only moderate and severe TBI grades are predisposed to poor cognitive and functional recovery, there is evolving awareness about the consequences of concussive head injury, such as post-traumatic stress disorder, fatigue, and headaches [27]. However, the non-admission or early hospital discharge–related restricted access to these mild TBI patients precludes the opportunity to administer rehabilitative sessions [28].

18.2.4.3 ICP Control Over Early Rehabilitation

Another controversy concerning neurorehabilitation in TBI patients is prioritising intracranial pressure (ICP) stabilisation during the acute phase versus the early initiation of neurorehabilitation. Early rehabilitation has been demonstrated to contribute to shorter critical phases, shorter duration of hospital/ICU stays, and improved outcomes at hospital discharge in both adult and paediatric patients [29, 30]. This is supported by a systematic review and meta-analysis [31] and a Cochrane Review [15] of bread-earning, young adult TBI survivors, in whom intensive rehabilitation led to earlier gains. Despite this, studies have consistently emphasised ICP stabilisation as a prerequisite for neurorehabilitation initiation. The possible recommendation is that interventions such as intensive chest physiotherapy; regular posture management to avert thrombosis, deformity, and contractures; and neuromuscular electrical stimulation (NMES) to avoid muscle atrophy may be adopted when ICP is unstable. At the same time, other modalities like mobilisations can be delayed until the ICP normalises.

18.2.4.4 Multi-phased Versus Single-Phase Neurorehabilitation in TBI

Multi-phased targeted neurorehabilitation has undoubtedly phased out the single-phase rehabilitation technique that focuses on the post-acute phase alone. Hyper-acute, sub-acute, and post-acute phases of neurorehabilitation target distinct aspects of patient recovery [32].

18.2.4.5 Patient-Centred Versus a More Comprehensive Cover to Involve the Patient's Family

Families are rightfully entitled to culturally competent information on their loved one's injury and their likely recovery course. TBI rehabilitation interventions need to prioritise patient-centred outcomes and consider not only the person with injury but also the person's family and caregiver(s) [33].

18.2.5 Rehabilitation Outcome Metrics: Is There a Consensus on a Successful Rehabilitation Outcome (e.g. Return to Work, Mobility, and Cognitive Function)?

The translation of the rehabilitation outcome metrics objectively evaluates the clinical utility of rehabilitative interventions to clinically useful patient outcomes. The definition of a successful rehabilitation outcome varies across different centres, interventions, illness severity grades, and the course of illness.

A huge database of rehabilitation outcome metrics exists, spanning various primary disease processes. The most extensively studied and validated rehabilitation outcome measure used in inpatient rehabilitation facilities is the Functional Independence Measure (FIM) [34]. According to most meta-analyses, the Functional Independence Measure (FIM) is considered the most widely used and well-validated rehabilitation outcome measurement tool, particularly in inpatient rehabilitation settings, as it comprehensively assesses both motor and cognitive functions across various activities of daily living [35]. Its key advantages are that it measures a broad spectrum of functional abilities, including self-care, mobility, communication, and cognitive skills, with broad applicability, including inpatient facilities, skilled nursing homes, and clinical trials. Other commonly used rehabilitation outcome measures are the Barthel Index (BI) [36] and the Modified Rankin Scale (MRS) [37].

The currently used functional measurement scales are developed for Western countries, considering specific functional requirements and the overall healthcare systems in these countries. These scales are of limited utility for low- and middle-income countries (LMICs) due to differences in social structure, accessibility, and healthcare systems [38, 39]. The International Classification of Functioning, Disability and Health (ICF) is another recent tool that provides a comprehensive framework for directly examining the relevance and comprehensiveness of activity and function [40].

A Comprehensive Rehabilitation Outcome Measurement (CROM) scale has been recently developed to evaluate the functional independence of patients with predominantly neurological dysfunction. This 32-item comprehensive tool compares well to similar items on FIM; however, it remains to be validated across more extensive and diverse populations [41].

An important point is that return to work, mobility, and cognitive function are critical components of these scales. However, the routine application of these fixed parameters may be irrelevant to patients with a more severe primary injury. Hence, restoring the pre-injury or close-to-pre-morbid functional, cognitive, and physical status in all patients is essential.

18.3 Conclusion

Neurorehabilitation should begin as early as possible in individuals with neurological impairments. The controversial areas involve the timing and intensity of initial rehabilitation, primary areas of focus like cognitive and physical rehabilitation, and the factors that define a successful rehabilitation outcome. Neurorehabilitation involves enabling individuals with disability to lead their lives independently, guided by trained professionals, with the support of family members. As discussed, early mobilisation can tap the brain's potential for neuroplasticity, enabling early recovery, with inherent risks of exacerbating injury, haemodynamic instability, and pain. The rehabilitation team should consider the merits of early rehabilitation to design approaches that are best suited for each individual's clinical condition and possibility for recovery. Increased intensity of rehabilitation may improve outcome, but defining the optimal dose and duration of therapy involves finding a fine balance between intense rehabilitation measures and the risk of over-straining. A multidimensional approach that addresses physical, cognitive, and psychological dimensions is best suited for individuals to yield optimal recovery. However, the implementation of a holistic approach may be challenging, especially in healthcare systems with constrained resources.

Finally, standardised metric systems should be used to measure rehabilitation outcomes and guide clinical work and research. The lack of a uniform metric system across all domains of neurorehabilitation can impair effective evaluation of the progress of patients. There is a scope for developing robust metric systems to improve the understanding of rehabilitation success.

The road ahead in neurorehabilitation should focus on research involving an interdisciplinary collaboration to develop evidence-based protocols. Emphasis should be on patient-centric, individualised care to optimise recovery and overcome disability. Effective rehabilitation strategies can enhance affected individuals' quality of life and help them achieve functional independence.

References

1. Langhorne P, Bernhardt J, Kwakkel G. Stroke rehabilitation. Lancet. 2011;377(9778):1693–702. https://doi.org/10.1016/S0140-6736(11)60325-5. PMID: 21571152.
2. Baker C, Worrall L, Rose M, Hudson K, Ryan B, O'Byrne L. A systematic review of rehabilitation interventions to prevent and treat depression in post-stroke aphasia. Disabil Rehabil. 2018;40(16):1870–92. https://doi.org/10.1080/09638288.2017.1315181. Epub 2017 Apr 19. PMID: 28420284.
3. Barnes MP. Principles of neurological rehabilitation. J Neurol Neurosurg Psychiatry. 2003;74(Suppl 4(Suppl 4)):iv3–7. https://doi.org/10.1136/jnnp.74.suppl_4.iv3. PMID: 14645459; PMCID: PMC1765644.
4. Rodgers H, Price C. Stroke unit care, inpatient rehabilitation and early supported discharge. Clin Med. 2017;17(2):173–7. https://doi.org/10.7861/clinmedicine.17-2-173.
5. Zotey V, Andhale A, Shegekar T, Juganavar A. Adaptive neuroplasticity in brain injury recovery: strategies and insights. Cureus. 2023;15(9):e45873. https://doi.org/10.7759/cureus.45873. PMID: 37885532; PMCID: PMC10598326.
6. Pollock A, Baer G, Campbell P, Choo PL, Forster A, Morris J, et al. Physical rehabilitation approaches for the recovery of function and mobility following stroke. Cochrane Database Syst Rev. 2014;2014(4):CD001920. https://doi.org/10.1002/14651858.CD001920.pub3. PMID: 24756870; PMCID: PMC6465059.
7. Bai Y, Hu Y, Wu Y, Zhu Y, He Q, Jiang C, et al. A prospective, randomized, single-blinded trial on the effect of early rehabilitation on daily activities and motor function of patients with hemorrhagic stroke. J Clin Neurosci. 2012;19(10):1376–9. https://doi.org/10.1016/j.jocn.2011.10.021. Epub 2012 Jul 18. PMID: 22819061.
8. Alaparthi GK, Gatty A, Samuel SR, Amaravadi SK. Effectiveness, safety, and barriers to early mobilization in the intensive care unit. Crit Care Res Prac. 2020;2020:7840743. https://doi.org/10.1155/2020/7840743. PMID: 33294221; PMCID: PMC7714600.
9. Van Dongen L, Hafsteinsdóttir TB, Parker E, Bjartmarz I, Hjaltadóttir I, Jónsdóttir H. Stroke survivors' experiences with rebuilding life in the community and exercising at home: a qualitative study. Nurs Open. 2021;8(5):2567–77. https://doi.org/10.1002/nop2.788. Epub 2021 Mar 10. PMID: 33690972; PMCID: PMC8363348.
10. Rapolienė J, Endzelytė E, Jasevičienė I, Savickas R. Stroke patients motivation influence on the effectiveness of occupational therapy. Rehabil Res Pract. 2018;2018:9367942. https://doi.org/10.1155/2018/9367942. PMID: 30155309; PMCID: PMC6091285.

11. Young B, Moyer M, Pino W, Kung D, Zager E, Kumar MA. Safety and feasibility of early mobilization in patients with subarachnoid hemorrhage and external ventricular drain. Neurocrit Care. 2019;31(1):88–96. https://doi.org/10.1007/s12028-019-00670-2. PMID: 30659467.
12. Sommers J, Engelbert RH, Dettling-Ihnenfeldt D, Gosselink R, Spronk PE, Nollet F, et al. Physiotherapy in the intensive care unit: an evidence-based, expert driven, practical statement and rehabilitation recommendations. Clin Rehabil. 2015;29(11):1051–63. https://doi.org/10.1177/0269215514567156. Epub 2015 Feb 13. PMID: 25681407; PMCID: PMC4607892.
13. Goikoetxea-Sotelo G, van Hedel HJA. Defining, quantifying, and reporting intensity, dose, and dosage of neurorehabilitative interventions focusing on motor outcomes. Front Rehabil Sci. 2023;4:1139251.
14. Cooke EV, Mares K, Clark A, Tallis RC, Pomeroy VM. The effects of increased dose of exercise-based therapies to enhance motor recovery after stroke: a systematic review and meta-analysis. BMC Med. 2010;8(1):60.
15. Königs M, Beurskens EA, Snoep L, Scherder EJ, Oosterlaan J. Effects of timing and intensity of Neurorehabilitation on functional outcome after traumatic brain injury: a systematic review and meta-analysis. Arch Phys Med Rehabil. 2018;99(6):1149–1159.e1.
16. Ballester BR, Ward NS, Brander F, Maier M, Kelly K, Verschure PFMJ. Relationship between intensity and recovery in post-stroke rehabilitation: a retrospective analysis. J Neurol Neurosurg Psychiatry. 2022;93(2):226–8.
17. Noé E, Gómez A, Bernabeu M, Quemada I, Rodríguez R, Pérez T, et al. Guidelines: basic principles of neurorehabilitation for patients with acquired brain injury. Recommendations of the Spanish Society of Neurorehabilitation. Neurol Engl Ed. 2024;39(3):261–81.
18. Hagovska M, Nagyova I. The transfer of skills from cognitive and physical training to activities of daily living: a randomised controlled study. Eur J Ageing. 2017;14(2):133–42.
19. Hagovská M, Olekszyová Z. Impact of the combination of cognitive and balance training on gait, fear and risk of falling and quality of life in seniors with mild cognitive impairment. Geriatr Gerontol Int. 2016;16(9):1043–50.
20. Lipardo DS, Tsang WW. Effects of combined physical and cognitive training on fall prevention and risk reduction in older persons with mild cognitive impairment: a randomized controlled study. Clin Rehabil. 2020;34(6):773–82.
21. Hagovská M, Takáč P, Dzvoník O. Effect of a combining cognitive and balanced training on the cognitive, postural and functional status of seniors with a mild cognitive deficit in a randomized, controlled trial. Eur J Phys Rehabil Med. 2016;52(1):101–9.
22. Combourieu Donnezan L, Perrot A, Belleville S, Bloch F, Kemoun G. Effects of simultaneous aerobic and cognitive training on executive functions, cardiovascular fitness and functional abilities in older adults with mild cognitive impairment. Ment Health Phys Act. 2018;15:78–87.
23. Min JH, Shin YI. Treatment and rehabilitation for traumatic brain injury: current update. Brain Neurorehabil. 2022;15(2):e14. https://doi.org/10.12786/bn.2022.15.e14. PMID: 36743200; PMCID: PMC9833473.
24. Buh FC, Hutchinson PJA, Anwar F. Early neuro-rehabilitation in traumatic brain injury: the need for an African perspective. BMC Med. 2023;21:290. https://doi.org/10.1186/s12916-023-03009-z.
25. Ramaswamy S, Seshadri S, Bunders-Aelen J. Shifting landscapes of global child mental health: imperatives for transdisciplinary approaches. Asian J Psychiatr. 2022;69:103002. https://doi.org/10.1016/j.ajp.2021.103002.
26. Karol RL. Team models in neurorehabilitation: structure, function, and culture change. NeuroRehabilitation. 2014;34(4):655–69. https://doi.org/10.3233/NRE-141080.
27. Dean PJ, Sterr A. Long-term effects of mild traumatic brain injury on cognitive performance. Front Hum Neurosci. 2013;12(7):30. https://doi.org/10.3389/fnhum.2013.00030.
28. McInnes K, Friesen CL, MacKenzie DE, Westwood DA, Boe SG. Mild traumatic brain injury (mTBI) and chronic cognitive impairment: a scoping review. PLoS One. 2017;12(4):e0174847. https://doi.org/10.1371/journal.pone.0174847.

29. Eghbali M, Khankeh H, Ebadi A. The importance of early rehabilitation in traumatic brain injury. Nurs Pract Today. 2020;7(2):84–6.
30. Kreitzer N, Rath K, Kurowski BG, Bakas T, Hart K, Lindsell CJ, Adeoye O. Rehabilitation practices in patients with moderate and severe traumatic brain injury. J Head Trauma Rehabil. 2019;34(5):E66–72.
31. Turner-Stokes L, Pick A, Nair A, Disler PB, Wade DT. Multi-disciplinary rehabilitation for acquired brain injury in adults of working age. Cochrane Database Syst Rev. 2015;2015(12):CD004170.
32. Lalwani SS, Dadgal R, Harjpal P, Saifee SS, Lakkadsha TM. Perks of early physical therapy rehabilitation for a patient with diffuse axonal injury. Cureus. 2022;14(10):e30886. https://doi.org/10.7759/cureus.30886.
33. National Academies of Sciences, Engineering, and Medicine; Health and Medicine Division; Board on Health Care Services; Board on Health Sciences Policy; Committee on Accelerating Progress in Traumatic Brain Injury Research and Care; Matney C, Bowman K, Berwick D, editors. Traumatic brain injury: a roadmap for accelerating progress. Washington (DC): National Academies Press (US); 2022. Rehabilitation and Long-Term Care Needs After Traumatic Brain Injury. Available from: https://www.ncbi.nlm.nih.gov/books/NBK580075/.
34. Granger CV, Hamilton BB, Linacre JM, Heinemann AW, Wright BD. Performance profiles of the functional independence measure. Am J Phys Med Rehabil. 1993;72(2):84–9.
35. Shultz S, Olszewski A, Ramsey O, Schmitz M, Wyatt V, Cook C. A systematic review of outcome tools used to measure lower leg conditions. Int J Sports Phys Ther. 2013;8(6):838–48. PMID: 24377070; PMCID: PMC3867077.
36. Hsueh IP, Lin JH, Jeng JS, Hsieh CL. Comparison of the psychometric characteristics of the functional independence measure, 5 item barthel index, and 10 item Barthel index in patients with stroke. J Neurol Neurosurg Psychiatry. 2002;73(2):188–90.
37. Quinn TJ, Dawson J, Walters MR, Lees KR. Reliability of the modified Rankin scale: a systematic review. Stroke. 2009;40(10):3393–5.
38. Jette AM, Haley SM, Ni P. Comparison of functional status tools used in post-acute care. Health Care Financ Rev. 2003;24(3):13–24.
39. Rogers JC, Green Gwinn SM, Holm MB. Comparing activities of daily living assessment instruments: FIM™, MDS, OASIS, MDS-PAC. Phys Occup Ther Geriatr. 2001;18(3):1–25.
40. Organization, W. H. International classification of functioning, disability, and health: children & youth version: ICF-CY, World Health Organization; 2007.
41. Rashid M, Harish SP, Mathew J, et al. Comprehensive rehabilitation outcome measurement scale (CROMS): development and preliminary validation of an interdisciplinary measure for rehabilitation outcomes. Health Qual Life Outcomes. 2022;20:160. https://doi.org/10.1186/s12955-022-02048-z.

Controversies in Neuroprognostication in Neurocritical Illness

19

Kanchan V. Bilgi and Seham Syeda

Abstract

Healthcare providers of severely neurological ill and critical patients are faced with the difficult task of communicating neurological prognosis to the families of patients who are often incapacitated or comatose during the acute phase. Withdrawal of life-sustaining treatments (WLST) accounts for more than a third of deaths in neurocritical care, and there is a lot of heterogeneity in the data about possibly avoidable mortality. Guidelines are now available for neuroprognostication in the survivors of cardiac arrest, severe acute brain injury (SABI), spinal cord injury (SCI), and Guillain–Barré syndrome (GBS), but the current evidence is mostly of moderate-to-low quality. Certain well-validated prognostic models, rather than individual clinical variables, seem to be moderately reliable in predicting defined outcomes. There is a lot of scope for the improvement of the quality of evidence and the formulation of decision aids for clinicians to communicate neurological prognosis with more certainty and enable surrogates to make informed decisions, along with healthcare teams.

Keywords

Neuroprognostication · Disorders of consciousness · Cardiac arrest · Prognostic biomarkers · Diffusion tensor imaging · Quantitative EEG

K. V. Bilgi (✉)
Neuroanesthesia, Chinmaya Mission Hospital, Bengaluru, Karnataka, India

S. Syeda
Department of Anesthesiology, M S Ramaiah Institute of Neurosciences, Ramaiah Medical College and Hospitals|, Bengaluru, Karnataka, India

P. U. Bidkar, M. Krishnakumar (eds.), *Controversies in Neurocritical Care*,
https://doi.org/10.1007/978-981-95-4419-6_19

Controversies in Neuroprognostication

- Can we cope with the uncertainties in neuroprognostication?
- Self-fulfilling prophecies and clinical nihilism in neurocritical care: Can we make better clinical and ethical decisions?
- Shared decision-making and effective communication: What does the evidence say?
- What is the quality of evidence for neuroprognostication at present? Do we have guidelines to conduct better studies and improve upon the existing evidence and recommendations?

19.1 Introduction

Prognostication in neurocritical care appears to be distinct, given its enormous uncertainty due to various medical, ethical, and legal factors. Neurologically critically ill patients often survive the first 7–10 days and then remain incapacitated for long durations or even for life. Goals of care decisions are often made by the patient's kin or surrogates based on the information provided by the healthcare providers, who may often not be accurate in their prognostication, largely due to the lack of evidence and concrete guidelines and the bias due to nonmedical factors. Healthcare teams and families are often faced with several challenges when a patient suffers severe acute brain damage (Fig. 19.1). Several questions arise about when

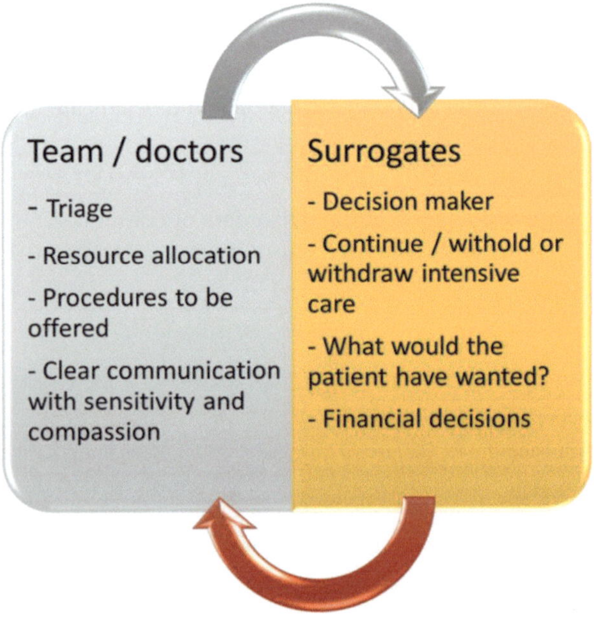

Fig. 19.1 Challenges faced by the healthcare team and the surrogate decision-makers (SDMs) of neurocritically ill patients

the patient will awaken, what constitutes a "good outcome," and the resources needed in the process.

Physician decisions should primarily be determined by the four ethical principles of beneficence, non-maleficence, justice, and patient autonomy [1]. Evidence must be gathered using all components of prognostic models and effects of intervention, and decisions must be made after applying clinical expertise and considering the preferences of the patient and their surrogates [2]. In India, forgoing life-sustaining therapy is defined under a medicolegal framework by the Honorable Supreme Court of India. The Indian Society of Critical Care Medicine and the Indian Association of Palliative Care have published their consensus and position statement and elaborated on the evidence, ethical considerations, and the legal framework available for decision support by the bedside in Indian intensive care units (ICUs) [3].

Neuroprognostication has long been an art that clinicians have practiced, which has remained so due to heterogeneous historical data and poor quality of evidence in studies. Studies such as the Clinician JUdgment vs Risk Score to predict Stroke outComes (JURaSSiC) study have shown that even experienced clinicians often underperform in prognostication after stroke and prediction scores perform better [4]. With the introduction of electronic clinical data and machine learning technologies, it is now feasible to accumulate extensive and large clinical datasets. These innovations facilitate the development of prognostic models that combine variables from clinical, physiological, and radiological fields. Outcomes are measured using time-tested and validated outcome scores, such as the Glasgow Outcome Score (GOS) or GOS-Extended (GOS-E), the modified Rankin Scale (mRS), the Coma Recovery Scale–Revised (CRS-R), and the Cerebral Performance Category Scale (CPC), among many others. Despite ongoing efforts in this regard, there is great variability in the withdrawal of life-sustaining treatment (WLST) and consequently a high variability in morbidity and mortality, as seen across various centers [5]. The contributors to such variability are several. A heuristic approach oversimplifies assumptions and takes mental shortcuts to neuroprognostication. Biases often lead clinicians to make predictions based on little evidence, potentially putting patients at risk of death due to a premature WLST. Prognosticating too early in the clinical course (for example, within 72 h post-resuscitation after cardiac arrest) is often the most common reason for WLST, contributing to variability in outcomes after cardiac arrest [6].

The process of prognostication consists of the formulation of the prognosis, as well as the proper communication of the possible outcomes to the next of kin. A 2019 scientific statement from the American Heart Association (AHA) gave an overview of the specific challenges researchers face with the conduct of studies in this population and the recommended standards for studies to follow in the future. One of the most challenging factors identified was the self-fulfilling prophecy. WLST continues to be the most common reason for in-hospital death of patients resuscitated from in-hospital cardiac arrest (IHCA) as well as out-of-hospital cardiac arrest (OHCA) [7]. A *self-fulfilling prophecy* is a conjecture one makes that comes true, at least in part, due to a person's belief or anticipation that the prediction would come true. The outcomes due to this may be positive or negative. Apart from clinician-associated factors, such as internal biases leading to self-fulfilling prophecies, prognostic nihilism, the clinician's affirmation of substituted judgment, and varying levels of experience and personal comfort, environmental factors, family dynamics, and preferences of the patient's surrogates may play a role as well [8].

The following sections describe various common neurological conditions that present prognostication challenges, along with up-to-date evidence and the controversies surrounding them. The Neurocritical Care Society has published several guidelines for different neurological conditions that call for careful neuroprognostication. The most clinically relevant predictors and prediction models were listed, and the Grading of Recommendations Assessment, Development, and Evaluation (GRADE) methodology was used to make recommendations and good practice statements.

19.2 Pathophysiology of Brain Injury Following Cardiac Arrest: *The Two-Hit Model*

The onset of primary brain injury, marked by an ischemic cascade, takes place within seconds after cardiac arrest due to the cessation of cerebral blood flow (CBF). Neuronal tissue, which lacks energy reserves, is critically dependent on a continuous supply of oxygen and glucose provided by CBF. When CBF abruptly stops following cardiac arrest, there is a rapid depletion of these critical resources, leading to significant impairment of neuronal integrity and function [9]. This cessation of aerobic metabolism results in a decrease in adenosine triphosphate (ATP), disrupting the Na-K ATPase pump. As a result, sodium and water accumulate within the cells, leading to cytotoxic edema. Additionally, the efflux of potassium leads to membrane depolarization and the activation of voltage-gated calcium channels, causing an increase in intracellular calcium levels (Fig 19.2).

Secondary brain injury (Reperfusion injury) begins once the return of spontaneous circulation (ROSC) is achieved. Increased intracellular calcium following primary injury increases the excitatory neurotransmitter glutamate, which further increases calcium levels via the mGlu and NMDA receptors. Increased calcium stores cause cleavage of the cell membrane, cell death, and apoptosis by releasing lytic enzymes (proteases, caspases, and phospholipases). There is associated mitochondrial dysfunction with failure of the electron transport chain and further reduction in ATP production, leading to a vicious cycle.

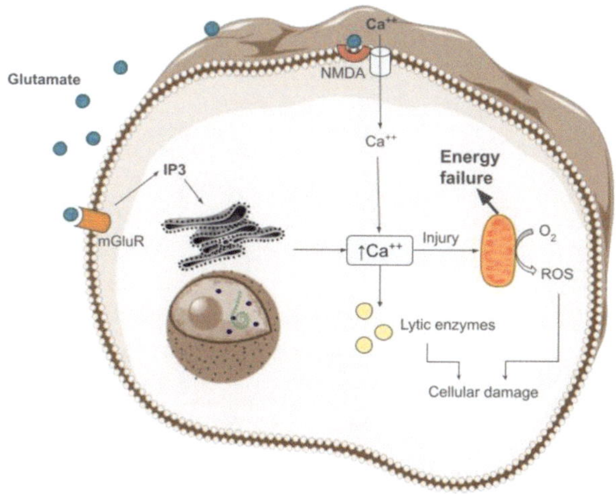

Fig. 19.2 Cellular events in primary brain injury. In the aftermath of ischemic injury, cells release glutamate, a neurotransmitter that binds to two key receptors on the cell membrane. The mGlu receptor (illustrated on the left) activates an intracellular mediator, IP3, which triggers the release of calcium from the endoplasmic reticulum. Concurrently, the N-methyl-d-aspartic acid (NMDA) receptor (positioned at the top) opens a channel that allows calcium to enter the cell. The resulting rise in intracellular calcium levels activates various calcium-dependent lytic enzymes, such as caspases, proteases, and phospholipases, leading to cellular structural damage. Additionally, the influx of calcium into the mitochondria disrupts the electron transport chain, resulting in the generation of reactive oxygen species (ROS) from oxygen. This cascade of events further aggravates intracellular damage and leads to energy failure, creating a vicious cycle that ultimately culminates in cell injury and death [10]

Role of neuroinflammation in secondary brain injury As a result of a hypoxic–ischemic event affecting the brain, resident innate immune cells, specifically microglia, become activated. This is followed by the migration of peripheral macrophages, monocytes, and neutrophils, which release various cytokines and chemokines [10]. Furthermore, the permeability of the blood-brain barrier (BBB) is heightened, leading to the development of vasogenic edema (Fig. 19.3).

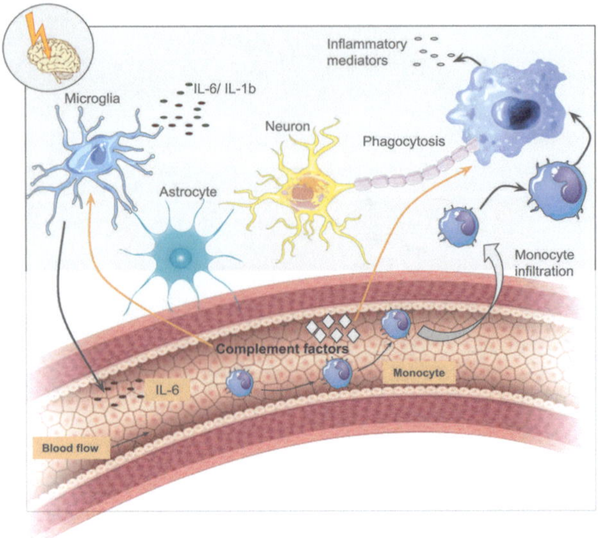

Fig. 19.3 Neuroinflammation in secondary brain injury. When blood flow is restored to the cerebrovascular area after tissue ischemia, the innate immune system initiates an inflammatory response characterized by the activation of astroglial cells due to hypoxia or ischemia in the brain. The resident macrophages (microglia) are primarily activated and produce pro-inflammatory cytokines (interleukin 6 and interleukin 1–beta) as well as chemokines that attract circulating mononuclear cells from the bloodstream. In response, the endothelium enhances the expression of leukocyte adhesion molecules, which allows monocytes to infiltrate the tissue. This infiltration further amplifies the release of pro-inflammatory cytokines, resulting in damage to the neurovascular unit's cellular components. Furthermore, the activation of the complement cascade contributes to the inflammatory injury and creates a pro-thrombotic environment within the cerebral microvasculature. (Adapted from Sandroni et al. [10])

19.3 Functional Markers of Neuroprognostication

Because no prognostic marker has perfect accuracy, markers are likely to have greater predictive value when combined (Fig. 19.4) [11].

Importantly, levels of consciousness in disorders of consciousness (DoC) commonly fluctuate, particularly in the ICU. The "mesocircuit" hypothesis considers the susceptibility of the frontal/prefrontal cortical–striatopallidal– thalamocortical loop systems to extensive deafferentation or loss of neurons after severe brain injury. The central thalamus projects connections to the cortex, which plays an important role in the reduction in cerebral metabolism that is observed following cerebral injury [12].

Standardized clinical evaluation, electroencephalogram (EEG)-based parameters, and functional neuroradiological studies should be used in combination for the multimodal evaluation of patients with DoC. The state of consciousness can be classified based on the highest level revealed by any of these three methods of evaluation [13].

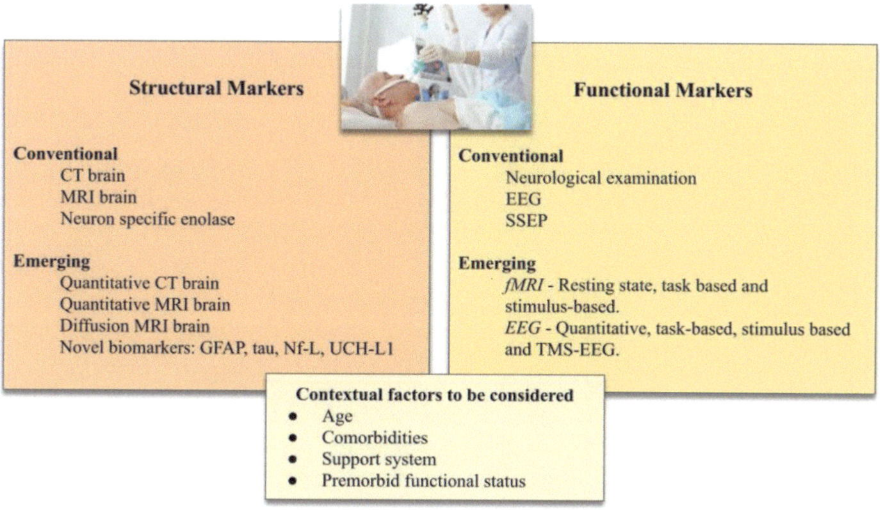

Fig. 19.4 The various markers of neuroprognostication. CT computed tomography, EEG electroencephalogram, fMRI functional magnetic resonance imaging, GFAP glial fibrillary acidic protein, MRI magnetic resonance imaging, Nf-L neurofilament light chain, SSEP somatosensory evoked potential, TMS transcranial magnetic stimulation, and UCH-L1 ubiquitin carboxy-terminal hydrolase L1

19.3.1 Conventional Markers

1. Clinical examination:
   (a) *Mental status or the type of DoC*: The JFK Coma Recovery Scale–Revised (CRS-R) is popular and distinguishes patients between vegetative state, minimally conscious state (MCS), and MCS+ or emerging from MCS, based on a bedside clinical assessment and scoring system [14] (Table 19.1). The Cerebral Performance Category (CPC) score is another outcome measure scoring method often used [15]. Abbreviated scores that can be administered with relative ease are coma recovery scale–revised: functional assessment of self-care tasks (CRSR-FAST), Simplified Evaluation of CONsciousness Disorders (SECONDs), Glasgow Coma Scale (GCS), and the full outline of unresponsiveness (FOUR) score [16–18]. Importantly, levels of consciousness in DoC commonly fluctuate, particularly in the ICU, and therefore, serial assessments may be necessary to sensitively detect periods of consciousness [19].
   (b) *Brain stem reflexes*: Absent pupillary reflexes for 72 h post-hypoxic-ischemic brain injury (HIBI) indicate a poor prognosis. A sub-study of the Blood Pressure and Oxygenation Targets After Out-of-Hospital Cardiac Arrest (BOX) trial concluded that automated pupillometry with a Neurological Pupil index [NPi] of ≤ 2 and a quantitatively assessed pupillary light reflex [qPLR] <4% correlated with a poor neurological outcome measured 90 days after ROSC, defined as a Cerebral Performance Category (CPC) score ≥ 3, with a 0% false positive rate (FPR). This also increased the sensitivity of a marker of brain injury, the neuron-specific enolase (NSE) >60 μg/L [20].

Table 19.1 The JFK Coma Recovery Scale–Revised

Auditory function scale	Visual function scale	Motor function scale	Oromotor/verbal function scale	Communication scale	Arousal scale
4-consistent movement to command[a]	5-object recognition[a]	6-functional object use[b]	3-intelligible verbalization[a]	2-functional: accurate[b]	3-attention[a]
3-reproducible movement to command[a]	4-object localization: reaching[a]	5-automatic motor response[a]	2-vocalization/oral movement	1-nonfunctional: intentional[a]	2-eye opening without stimulation
2-localization to sound	3-visual pursuit[a]	4-object manipulation[a]	1-Oral reflexive movement	0-none	1-eye opening with stimulation
1-auditory startle	2-Fixation[a]	3-localization to noxious stimulation[a]	0-none		0-unarousable
0-none	1-visual startle	2-flexion withdrawal			
1-auditory startle	0-none	1-abnormal posturing			
0-none		0-none/flaccid			

Adapted from Giacino et al. [14]
[a]Denotes MCS
[b]Denotes emergence from MCS

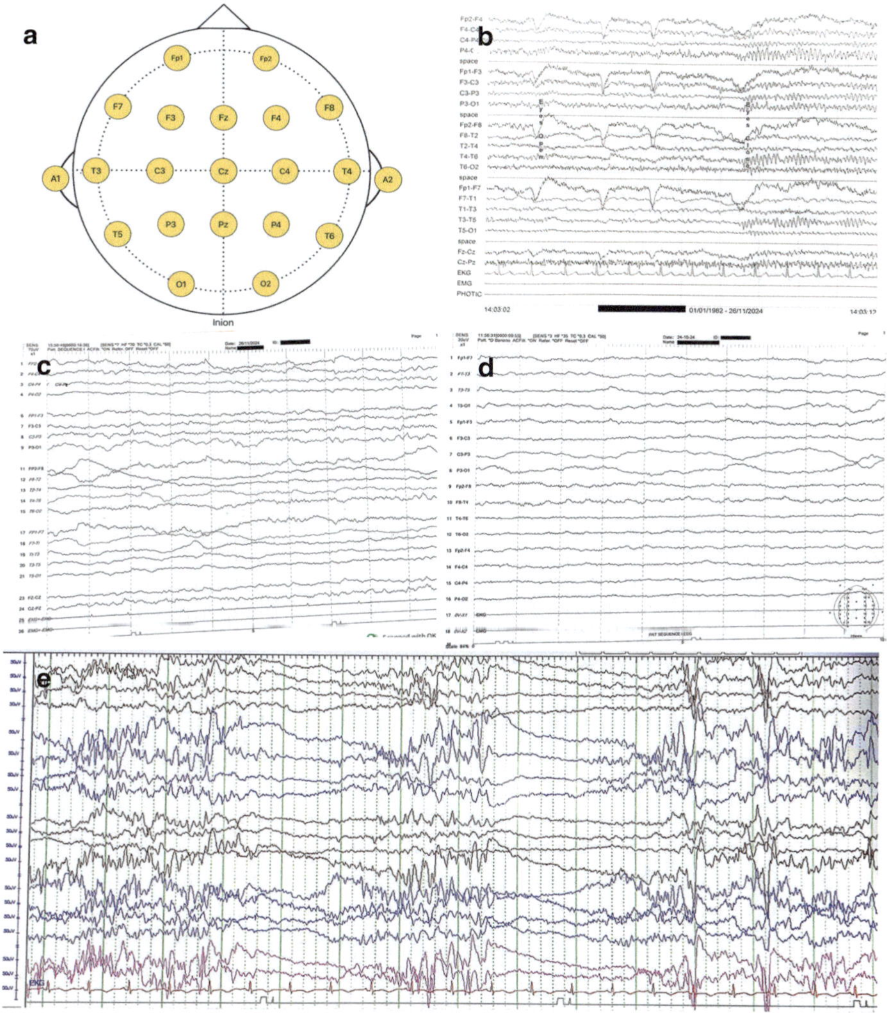

Fig. 19.5 EEG patterns. (**a**) The standard 10–20 system for electroencephalography. (**b**) Normal background activity with alpha reactivity, eyes open and closed. (**c**) EEG slowing, with mainly delta and theta frequencies seen. (**d**) EEG suppression. (**e**) Burst suppression

2. EEG patterns: Suppressed background or burst suppression (termed highly malignant features) reliably predicts poor functional recovery [21] (Fig. 19.5). The *mesocortical hypothesis* suggests that resting-state EEG patterns reflect levels of thalamocortical network functioning that correlate with the outcome in comatose survivors of cardiac arrest. These patterns have been classified by the ABCD framework. EEG power spectra have been classified based on spectral

peaks within predefined frequency bands: "A" (complete thalamocortical disruption) = no peaks above delta (<4 Hz) range, "B" (severe thalamocortical disruption) = theta (4–8 Hz) peak, "C" (moderate thalamocortical disruption) = theta and beta (13–24 Hz) peaks, or "D" (normal thalamocortical function) = alpha (8–13 Hz) and beta peaks. This classification demonstrates a longitudinal improvement of patients from better to worse EEG patterns ($p < 0.05$) and helped differentiate between patients with and without command following in the sub-acute-to-chronic phase of recovery. It is possible to characterize channel-level EEG dynamics and identify fluctuations in the integrity of the functional thalamocortical network in spatial detail [22].

3. Absent somatosensory evoked potential (SSEP) (N20 response): A cortical electrical response following stimulation of the upper-limb nerve indicates preserved somatosensory pathway integrity. Sensitivity in detecting cortical damage and predicting poor prognosis in HIBI is increased when a preserved N9 response is elicited at the brachial plexus with absent cortical N20 for a median nerve SSEP stimulation [23]. Guidelines endorse this modality for HIBI, but it seems to carry prognostic significance in other severe acute brain injuries like traumatic brain injury (TBI) as well.

19.3.2 Emerging Functional Markers

Functional magnetic resonance imaging (fMRI) and studies of emerging EEG applications have shown prognostic relevance across both traumatic and nontraumatic etiologies of DoC.

1. *EEG: Task-Based, Stimulus-Based, Quantitative, Resting-State, and TMS-EEG*
   Interpretation of conventional EEG is subjective as opposed to emerging techniques that use quantitative interpretation under task-based, stimulus-based, or resting-state conditions. Identifying cognitive motor dissociation (CMD) seems key when patients show no motor response to stimuli. The category of cognitive motor dissociation (CMD) sets apart a subset of patients with DoC, in whom there exists neuroimaging evidence of consciousness but no command-following behaviors. Major improvements in CMD patients have been observed 3 months after the injury when treatment is continued, with up to a quarter of patients achieving recovery to a GOS-E of 4 or better when compared with 3% of patients without CMD (odds ratio (OR): 11.3, 95% CI, 3.3–41.4, $P = 0.001$) [24]. CMD detected with task-based EEG has prognostic significance, predicting greater neurological function at 3 months and 1 year (odds ratio: 4.6; 95% CI, 1.2–17.1) following injury, along with a more rapid recovery compared to patients without CMD [25, 26]. In the months following severe acute brain injury (SABI), greater recovery of neurological function was noted in patients who showed EEG cortical responses, particularly to more complex, syntactical features of language [27]. A fairly easy-to-perform and passive auditory EEG protocol has been shown to improve prognostic accuracy during a critical period of clinical deci-

sion-making, as it discriminates well between good and poor prognosis of patients with DoC [28].

2. *fMRI: Task-Based, Stimulus-Based, Resting-State, and Positron Emission Tomography (PET).*
   - Task-based fMRI helped identify CMD in 2006, which was followed by increasing research in this domain. Clinical guidelines released by the American Academy of Neurology, the American Congress of Rehabilitation Medicine, and the National Institute on Disability, Independent Living, and Rehabilitation Research have endorsed stimulus-based fMRI for clinical neuroprognostication, albeit with low confidence, given the early stages of these technologies [29].
   - Resting-state fMRI assesses functional brain integrity by measuring the synchronization of spontaneous activity between brain network regions. Evaluation of average functional connectivity across the set of region-to-region pairs for the resting-state networks, namely, the default mode, fronto-parietal, sensorimotor, visual, auditory, and salience networks, indicates superior functional network integrity with greater synchronization [11].
   - MCS*: Patients with hypometabolism of the frontoparietal network were classified as "vegetative state/unresponsive wakefulness syndrome (VS/UWS)." The reservation of metabolism in this circuit either confirmed the behavioral diagnosis of "MCS" or, in the nonexistence of behavioral signs of consciousness, may point to a diagnosis of "MCS*."
   - Patients with DoC but preserved cortical metabolism on PET are more likely to achieve a robust functional recovery at 1 year following injury than patients without a similarly preserved metabolism [30].

19.4 Structural Markers of Neuroprognostication

19.4.1 Conventional Structural Markers

Conventional structural markers include neuroimaging and serum biomarkers.

(a) Neuroimaging: To assess the structural integrity of the brain, structural markers are used, most of which are contributed by neuroradiological studies.

Non-contrast computed tomography (NCCT) of the brain: Hypoxic–ischemic brain injury (HIBI) during cardiac arrest leads to cytotoxic edema, which is characterized by a loss of gray–white matter differentiation, accompanied by basal cistern and sulcal effacement (Fig. 19.6). The average gray–white matter radiodensity ratio (avGWR) is measured at three levels in a CT scan: (1) at the level of basal ganglia (putamen and caudate nucleus for gray matter and internal capsule for white matter), (2) at the level of centrum semiovale, and (3) at the high-convexity level—axial cut 5 mm above the centrum semiovale [31, 32].

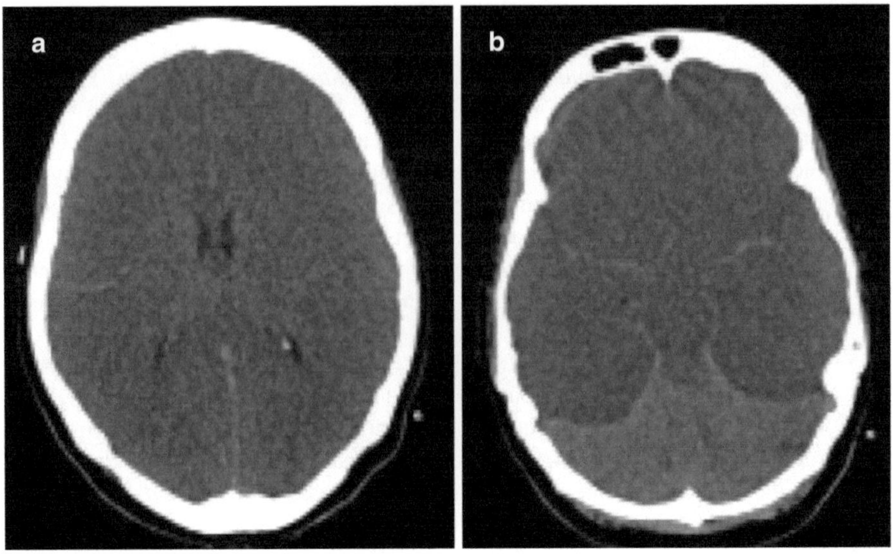

Fig. 19.6 Non-contrast computed tomography of the brain following hypoxic–ischemic brain injury. (**a**) Showing diffuse loss of gray–white matter differentiation. (**b**) Effacement of basal cisterns

CT, being a moderately reliable predictor, should ideally be used with a combination of functional predictors like SSEP or EEG for neuroprognostication. Various pitfalls for the use of CT as a reliable predictor are as follows: (1) To quantify avGWR accurately, one must possess specialized skills and access to specific software, resources that are often limited. (2) The assessment of CT has to be performed in the absence of artifacts like motion or metal artifacts. (3) A misdiagnosis of acute ischemic stroke can be overcome by looking for diffuse involvement across vascular distribution, including the cerebral cortex, supplied by the bilateral anterior and posterior circulation, and deep gray matter. The suggested timing to perform a CT scan for neuroprognostication is >48 h following ROSC, after which the ischemic changes become evident. Any scan performed earlier is referred to as an "etiology scan," which can be used to rule out the possibility of a neurological cause for cardiac arrest.

Magnetic Resonance Imaging (MRI) of the brain MRI is the most specific and sensitive predictor of neuroprognostication at days 3–5 following ROSC [33]. HIBI results in the restriction of water molecules across the brain cell. The diffusion-weighted imaging (DWI) sequence shows the characteristic diffuse restriction pattern involving bilateral anterior and posterior circulation territories, including the cerebral cortex and deep gray matter like the caudate nucleus and putamen. The timing observed in MRI scans corresponds to the sequential injury pattern identified on a structural level. Within the first 24–48 h following ROSC, diffusion-weighted

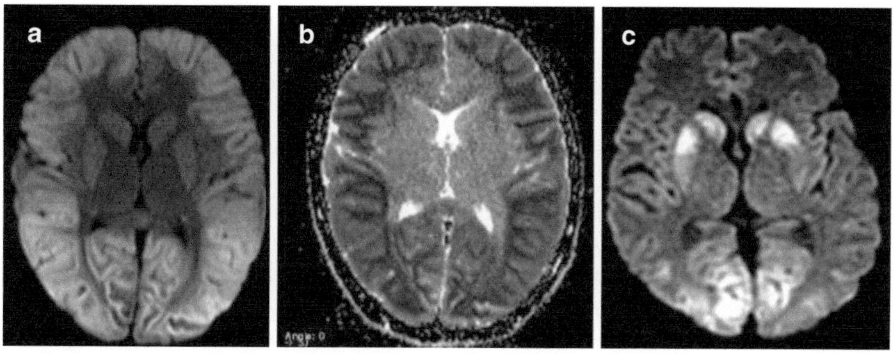

Fig. 19.7 Magnetic resonance imaging with diffusion restriction pattern in cortical and subcortical structures. (**a**) Diffuse restriction involving the DWI sequence's anterior and posterior circulation territories. (**b**) Corresponding restriction changes in apparent diffusion coefficient (ADC) scan. (**c**) Diffusion restriction in the subcortex and white matter

changes indicative of acute ischemia are most evident in regions with high metabolic activity, such as the basal ganglia and cerebellum (specifically the Purkinje cells). Between days 3 and 5 after ROSC, the involvement of the cerebral cortex increases, particularly affecting the parietal and occipital lobes. By 10–14 days after the event, diffusion-weighted changes may be noted in the white matter, while earlier changes become more pronounced on fluid-attenuated inversion recovery sequences, indicating potential permanent injury (Fig. 19.7) [34, 35]. Quantitative assessment of diffusion restriction can be done by calculating the apparent diffusion coefficient (ADC) value in each image voxel. The two thresholds validated in higher-quality studies for the prediction of long-term outcomes are as follows: >10% of voxels with ADC <650 × 10–6 mm^2/s and >2.5% of voxels with ADC <400 × 10–6 mm^2/s [36, 37].

The limitations of using MRI for neuroprognostication are as follows: (a) lengthy duration of imaging as compared to CT scan, with limited monitoring options in patients with hemodynamic instability; (b) subjective analysis of DWI sequence is done more commonly owing to the inaccessibility of expertise and specialized software required for the quantitative evaluation of ADC to many clinicians; and (c) false positive results in the presence of pathologies like status epilepticus and hyperammonemic encephalopathy; hence, MRI-DWI is not a reliable predictor for outcome assessment in the presence of seizures [38, 39].

The absence of diffusion restriction or the presence of isolated restriction lesions on MRI-DWI performed >72 h following ROSC is associated with good long-term functional outcomes, with a sensitivity of 92–100% and a specificity of 93% [40].

Positron emission tomography (PET) and single-photon emission computed tomography are of limited use and are not feasible as prognostic predictors in acute settings.

(b) Serum Biomarkers.

Biomarkers indicative of neurovascular unit injury encompass neuron-specific enolase (NSE; associated with neuron cell bodies), S100 calcium-binding protein β (S100β; related to glial cells), glial fibrillary acidic protein (GFAP; found in astrocytes), neurofilament light (Nf-L; present in axons), tau protein (also in axons), and ubiquitin carboxyl hydrolase L1 (UCH-L1; linked to neuron cell bodies). Among these, NSE is the most frequently investigated prognostic marker for outcomes in comatose patients. Enolase functions as a glycolytic enzyme and exists in three isoforms: enolase α, which is widely distributed; enolase β, which is specific to muscles; and enolase γ, which is specific to neurons. NSE serves as a highly specific indicator for neurons and peripheral neuroendocrine cells [41]. Following HIBI, there is increased anaerobic glycolysis metabolism in the neurons, leading to increased levels of NSE in the bloodstream [42]. In a multicenter observational study conducted prospectively by Kim et al., NSE levels were found to be different among cardiac arrest survivors of shockable and non-shockable rhythms. The NSE cutoff values that maintained a false positive rate (FPR) below 1% were 69.3 ng/mL (sensitivity of 76.0%) for the non-shockable group and 102.7 ng/mL (sensitivity of 42.1%) for the shockable group [43]. The evidence to suggest that NSE is a reliable predictor of neurological outcome following ROSC is less robust due to differing sensitivity and specificity based on the threshold value; hence, it should always be combined with other reliable markers for prognostication.

Limitations The cost and availability of the testing in low- and middle-income countries, the lack of a standardized technique to measure the NSE levels, and the absence of a consistent validated threshold value for NSE restrict their routine use. Studies have shown that for NSE >60 μg/L, False positive rate (FPR) was 7%, and it was 2% for a threshold >80 μg/L, with large variability. Extra-cerebral causes such as neuroendocrine tumors, small-cell lung cancer, gastroenteropancreatic tumors, neuroblastoma, and hemolysis of blood samples can lead to spurious values.

A recent systematic review by Sandorini et al. suggested that the presence of a normal serum NSE level (<17–18 μg/L), measured 24–72 h following ROSC, predicted a good long-term functional outcome, with a specificity of >80% and a sensitivity of >40% [44].

19.4.2 Emerging Structural Markers

19.4.2.1 Quantitative Whole-Brain White Matter Fractional Anisotropy (WWM-FA)

There has been an emerging body of evidence to demonstrate the prognostic promise of axonal integrity/neural integrity in patients after ROSC. Diffusion measures the movement of water molecules across the neural cell membrane. Loss of uniformity in this movement results in fractional anisotropy in diffusion tensor imaging (DTI) and has been implicated in poor prognosis. The quantitative measurement of whole-brain white matter fractional anisotropy (WWM-FA) through diffusion tensor imaging (DTI) in comatose patients after ROSC between days 7 and 28 can serve as a dependable predictor of neurological outcomes (area under the receiver operating characteristic curve: 0.95, 95% CI, 0.91–0.98) [45]. Notably, the absence of fractional anisotropy has been linked to favorable neurological and cognitive recovery [46].

19.4.3 Novel Brain Injury Biomarkers

Axonal injury markers (Nf-L, followed by tau) have higher diagnostic accuracy in predicting favorable and unfavorable outcomes following ROSC. A systematic review and meta-analysis involving 10,000 comatose patients after ROSC demonstrated that neurofilament light chain (Nf-L), a marker of white matter injury, had the highest prognostic accuracy, with an AUC of 0.92 (95% CI, 0.84–0.97), followed by tau protein with an AUC of 0.89 (95% CI, 0.71–0.97), when measured within 48 hours after ROSC [47]. The difference between the levels of serum Nf-L and tau in patients with HIBI vs healthy volunteers is much higher when compared to classic biomarkers such as NSE. Nevertheless, the absence of prospective randomized controlled trials and standardized measurement criteria results in inadequate data to incorporate novel biomarkers as prognostic indicators within current guidelines.

19.5 Approaches to the Communication of Prognosis in Neurocritical Care

Communication of the risk in neurocritical care is heavily influenced by prognostication. As seen in the preceding sections of this chapter, the timing and objectivity of the assessment of factors predicting the outcomes will influence the decisions regarding the continuation or withdrawal of life-sustaining treatments. Early neuroprognostication and nihilism in the acute stages are the most common causes of the probable underestimation of a good outcome [48].

Communication with patient surrogates could be informational, authoritative, responsive, or, more commonly, advisory in nature. Long-term outcomes discussed with families focus on cognitive, physical, functional, and survival outcomes [49]. Shared decision-making is characterized as a cooperative approach where both the physician and the patient, or their representative, engage in making significant healthcare choices. This process integrates the values, preferences, and objectives of patients and their families with the physician's expertise and evidence-based medical practices to arrive at optimal healthcare decisions tailored to the individual patient (Fig. 19.8) [50].

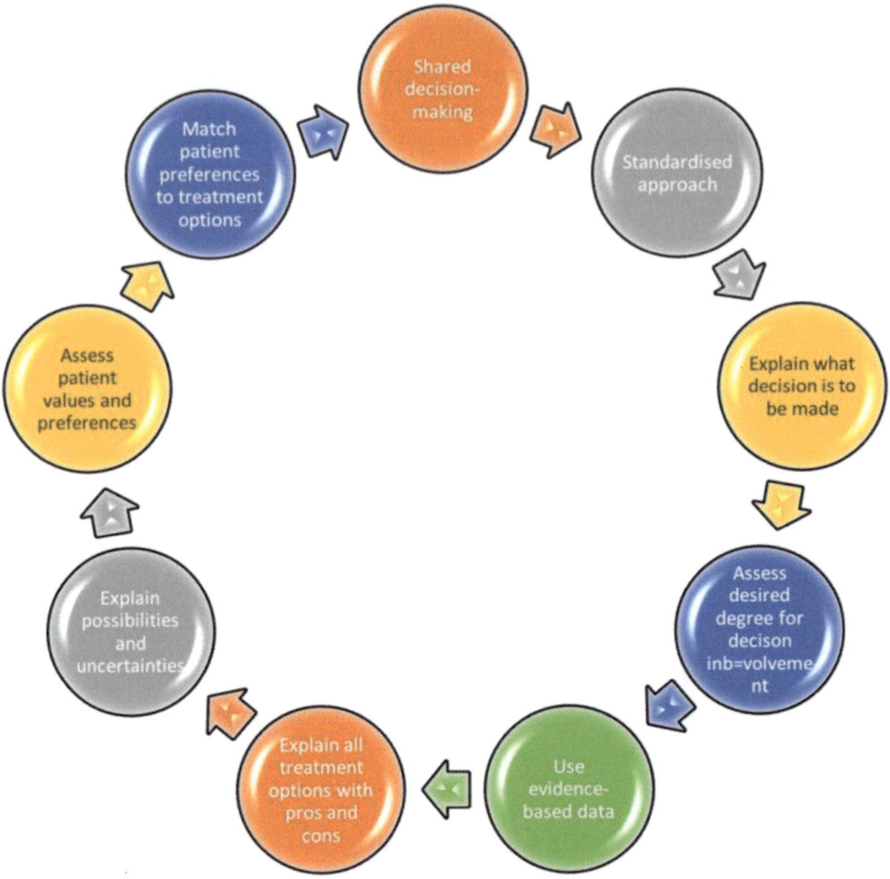
Shared decision-making
Standardised approach
Explain what decision is to be made
Assess desired degree for decison inb=volveme nt
Use evidence-based data
Explain all treatment options with pros and cons
Explain possibilities and uncertainties
Assess patient values and preferences
Match patient preferences to treatment options

Fig. 19.8 The process of shared decision-making. (Adapted from Khan et al. [50])

19.6 Guidelines for Neuroprognostication

Clinical questions that could not be answered by using the GRADE criteria were given as *good practice statements*. These guidelines, based on the evidence gathered from eligible studies, provide recommendations and indicate the degree of reliability of each predictor of certain defined outcomes for each condition. Clinicians are suggested to use the appropriate language to convey the degree of uncertainty of the prognosis arrived at after considering all recommended predictors, composite models, and the overall clinical picture while counseling the surrogates of any neurocritically ill patient (Table 19.2).

Table 19.2 Grading of reliability of predictors, the quality of the body of evidence available, and the suggested language to be used for the communication of prognosis

Category of prediction	Body of evidence	Suggested language during counseling of the outcome	Degree of uncertainty
Reliable	High: well-defined threshold values or valid clinical/ radiological definition	"Very likely"	Present but low
Moderately reliable	High: well-defined threshold values or valid clinical/ radiological definition	"Likely"	Substantial
Not reliable	Low	–	–

19.7 Neuroprognostication After ROSC

The outcomes considered critical were functional outcomes assessed at or beyond 3 months from ROSC, mortality assessed at or beyond discharge, and cognitive outcomes assessed at or beyond 3 months from ROSC [21].

Good practice statements Evaluation of the neurological prognosis of patients who are comatose after surviving a cardiac arrest must be deferred for at least 72 h following the return of spontaneous circulation without inducing therapeutic hypothermia (goal temperature <36.5 °C) and at least 72 h after rewarming in those treated with targeted temperature management (TTM). In addition, a coma that persists beyond 72 h in the ICU should not be assumed to be equal to a poor neurological prognosis. Sedation or other confounders must be stopped and abnormalities corrected prior to assessment for neuroprognostication (Figs. 19.9 and 19.10). Factors such as a premorbid poor baseline functional status, a preexisting illness known to limit life expectancy, and multi-organ failure must be considered before and independent of neurological prognosis in post–cardiac arrest comatose survivors. Prognostication must never be based on a single clinical variable and should be based on a multimodal assessment of the complete clinical scenario. It is strongly recommended to counsel the surrogates of such patients, emphasizing that the possibility of, extent of, and time taken for any degree of recovery are uncertain. Any neurologically significant improvement in functional outcome may take several days to months. Discussion with surrogates of patients with indeterminate prognosis should establish goals of care, and an extended period of observation for clinical signs of neurological recovery is recommended in such patients.

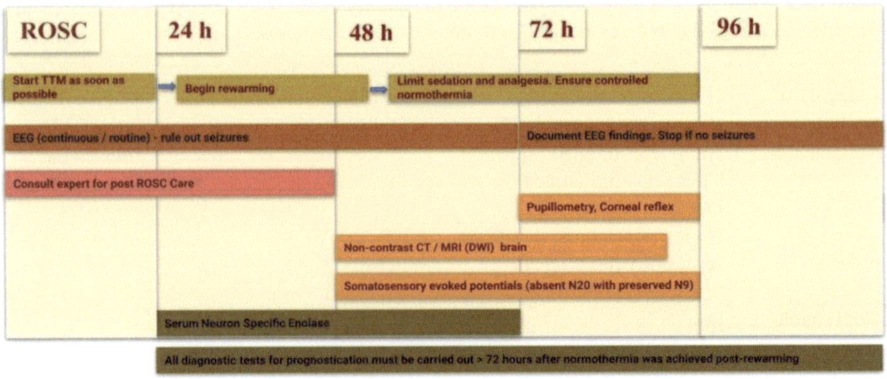

Fig. 19.9 Bedside tests for prognostic studies to evaluate the neurological status in cardiac arrest survivors in the first 72–96 h

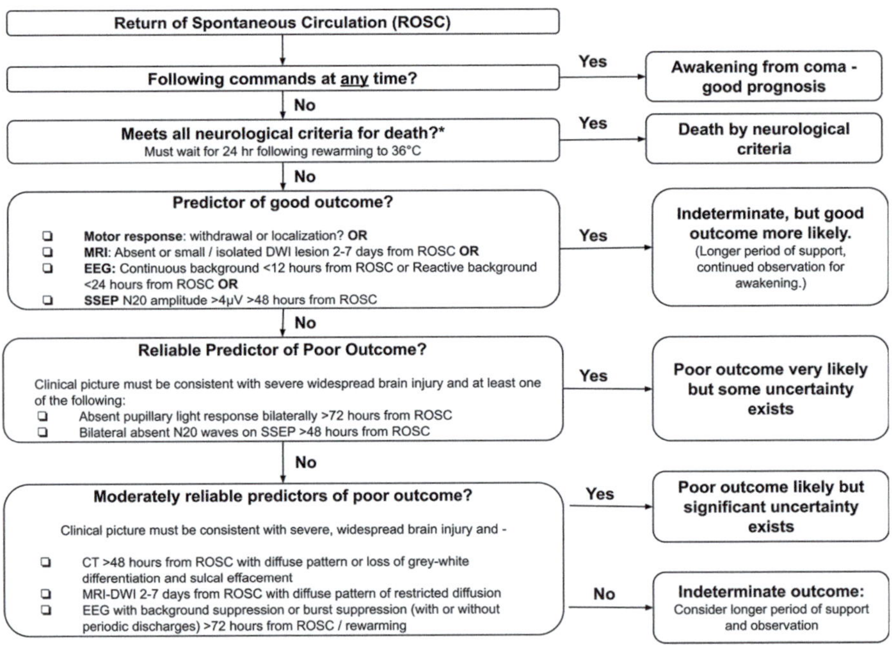

Fig. 19.10 Interpretation of clinical, radiological, and neurophysiological predictors and tests in cardiac arrest survivors. (Adapted from Rajajee et al. [21])

*Pediatric and Adult Brain Death/Death by Neurologic Criteria Consensus Guideline. Report of the American Academy of Neurology (AAN) Guidelines Subcommittee, American Academy of Pediatrics (AAP), Congress of Neurological Surgeons (CNS), and Society of Critical Care Medicine (SCCM) [34]

19.7.1 Functional Outcomes Assessed at or Beyond 3 Months from ROSC

Clinical variables Age, initial cardiac rhythm (shockable vs non-shockable), the time to ROSC, bilateral absent corneal reflex, bilaterally absent or extensor motor response to stimulus, and the occurrence of myoclonus <48 h after ROSC (without concomitant EEG recording) *cannot be considered alone to predict poor outcomes at 3 months or beyond.* On the condition that pupillary assessment is carried out accurately and in the setting of severe, widespread neurological injury and absent confounding factors like medication, hypothermia, or prior surgery, it is suggested that the absence of a pupillary light response bilaterally, checked at least 72 h from ROSC, should be considered a reliable predictor of poor functional outcome evaluated at 3 months or later.

Brain imaging Non-contrast CT of the brain performed at least 48 h from ROSC that demonstrates a diffuse pattern of loss of gray–white matter differentiation (in the distributions of bilateral anterior and posterior circulation, involving the cerebral cortex and deep gray matter), with effacement of sulci, or diffusion restriction on magnetic resonance imaging (MRI) of the brain performed between 2 and 7 days from ROSC in the above areas is suggested to be a moderately reliable predictor of poor functional outcome.

Electrodiagnostics Suppressed or burst suppression background, with or without periodic discharges, on EEG performed at least 72 h from ROSC or after rewarming after TTM is considered a moderately reliable predictor. Absent N20 response on somatosensory evoked potential, with preserved N9 response at the Erb's point, and ensuring the absence of confounders when evaluated at least 48 h from ROSC, is considered a reliable predictor of poor functional outcome.

Biomarkers A consistent threshold for serum NSE level is yet to be validated for this purpose and is unreliable when measured <72 h after ROSC as a predictor.

Prediction models Insufficient evidence in support of the out-of-hospital cardiac arrest (OHCA), Cardiac Arrest Hospital Prognosis (CAHP), and Good Outcome Following Attempted Resuscitation (GOFAR) models precludes their utility for functional outcome prediction at present.

19.8 Neuroprognostication in Intracerebral Hemorrhage (ICH)

Six candidate clinical variables (age, clinical presentation, ICH volume on admission scan, infratentorial location, intraventricular blood on admission CT scan, and anticoagulant intake history at ICH onset) and two clinical grading scales (the original ICH score and maximally treated (max-) ICH score) were selected for recommendation creation [51–53]. These guidelines offer dependable recommendations for addressing unfavorable outcomes following intracerebral hemorrhage (ICH) when counseling patients or their surrogates.

Good practice statements: Neurological prognostication in patients with ICH should ideally be deferred until 48–72 h unless severe clinical deterioration is noted. Preexisting cognitive impairment, a poor baseline level of functioning, a preexisting illness associated with limited life expectancy, and multi-organ failure are considered at the time of prognostication. Long-term cognitive and psychological impairment is common in patients surviving ICH. Patients and surrogates need to be counseled that neurological recovery following ICH would take a long duration of time, ranging from days to months.

Poor functional outcome prediction at 3 months (defined as a modified Rankin Scale (mRS) score of $\geq$3, an mRS score of $\geq$4, or a Glasgow Outcome Score $\leq$ 3): Clinical variables (age, clinical exam on admission, volume of ICH on admission, infratentorial location of ICH, intraventricular hemorrhage, and anticoagulant use at the time of ICH) alone cannot be considered as reliable predictors of poor functional outcome assessed at 3 months or later. Clinical grading scales such as the original ICH score and max-ICH score cannot be considered reliable predictors.

Prediction of 30-day mortality: The clinical grading scale, the original ICH score, cannot be considered a reliable predictor of 30-day mortality following ICH. There is insufficient evidence to utilize the max-ICH score as a predictor of 30-day mortality to make a formal recommendation.

19.9 Neuroprognostication in Subarachnoid Hemorrhage (SAH)

Survivors of SAH often suffer from poor quality of life, failure to achieve functional independence, and neurocognitive decline. To evaluate functional outcomes, a range of clinical models has been created and externally validated for prognostic purposes. In addition to established scoring systems like the Hunt–Hess score (HHS) and the World Federation of Neurosurgical Societies (WFNS) score, several composite scoring systems have been formulated, a selection of which is listed below:

Prognosis on Admission of Aneurysmal Subarachnoid Hemorrhage (PAASH) and the Glasgow Coma Scale (GCS) [54].

Functional Recovery Expected after Subarachnoid Hemorrhage (FRESH) score: A comprehensive tool designed to forecast long-term functional, cognitive, and quality-of-life outcomes following spontaneous subarachnoid hemorrhage [55]. This tool incorporates the HHS and the acute physiology and chronic health evaluation II (APACHE II) scores recorded at admission, along with the patient's age and the occurrence of aneurysmal rebleeding within 48 h. FRESH comprises two distinct scores aimed at predicting cognitive function (FRESH cog) and quality of life (FRESH quol) after 1 year [56].

Subarachnoid Hemorrhage International Trialists (SAHIT): This included the development of three prediction models: (1) a core model comprising age, hypertension, and WFNS grade; (2) a neuroimaging model that incorporates the Fischer grade, aneurysm size, and site; and (3) a final model that combines the core and neuroimaging models [57].

VASOGRADE scale: Patients were classified into green, yellow, and red categories based on a combination of the modified Fischer and WFNS grading systems. This model, initially designed to assess the risk of delayed cerebral ischemia (DCI), has also proven to be highly effective in forecasting functional outcomes [58].

HATCH score: The key components of this score are Hemorrhage, Age, Treatment, Clinical State, and the presence or absence of Hydrocephalus, which are used to predict functional outcomes following aneurysmal SAH [59].

Serum biomarkers: In addition to conventional biomarkers, including NSE, S100B, and GFAP, there has been an increasing interest in novel biomarkers such as tau protein and the ratio of arginine to ornithine in cerebrospinal fluid as markers to predict functional outcomes [60, 61].

19.10 Neuroprognostication in Ischemic Stroke

The introduction of intravascular thrombolysis and endovascular thrombectomy has led to notable improvements in the outcomes of ischemic stroke; however, considerable morbidity and poor functional outcomes continue to be prevalent. Numerous point-based prediction scores and modules have been established to estimate clinical outcomes, a few of which are listed below:

Preadmission comorbidities, Level of consciousness, Age, and Neurological deficit (PLAN) score [62].
Ischemic stroke predictive risk score (IScore) [63].
Acute Stroke Registry and Analysis of Lausanne (ASTRAL) score [64].
Houston intra-arterial recanalization therapy (HIAT) score [65].
Totaled Health Risks in Vascular Events (THRIVE) score [66].
Stroke Prognostication using Age and National Institutes of Health Stroke Scale (SPAN score 100) [67].

19.11 Neuroprognostication After Moderate-to-Severe Traumatic Brain Injury

Withdrawal of life-sustaining treatments (WLSTs) by surrogate decision-makers (SDMs) is the leading cause of death after moderate-to-severe TBI (msTBI, defined as a Glasgow Coma Scale (GCS) score of 3–12 on admission). In more than 50%, deaths related to msTBI have been observed to occur as early as 72 h [5, 68]. Apprehensions about predicted long-term disability and poor quality of life often prompt SDMs to permit WLST. This may vary considerably between countries and communities, influenced by the severity of TBI, age, race and ethnicity, religious beliefs, socioeconomic status, availability of resources, geography, and preexisting conditions such as functionally dependent status, dementia, and disseminated cancer [69].

Individual predictors, when considered alone, are not reliable predictors of mortality at discharge or beyond [70]. The following variables have been identified: age, pupillary reactivity on admission, admission GCS score or motor GCS sub-score following adequate resuscitation, hypotension (systolic blood pressure [SBP] <90 mm Hg on admission, hypoxia (oxygen saturation) <90%, or arterial partial pressure of oxygen (PaO_2) <110 mm Hg before or after admission), major extracranial injury, alcohol intoxication, hypernatremia, prolonged elevated intracranial pressure (ICP) >20 mm Hg for >60 min/day, acute kidney injury during ICU treatment, and post-traumatic cerebral infarction.

Bilateral absent pupillary reactivity was found to be a moderately reliable predictor of poor functional outcome (measured using the Glasgow Outcome Scale or the Glasgow Outcome Scale–Extended, disability-free outcome, Functional Independence Measure, Ranchos Los Amigos Score, and others).

19.12 Prediction Models in TBI

The corticosteroid randomisation after significant head injury (CRASH)-basic and corticosteroid randomisation after significant head Injury-computed tomography model (CRASH-CT) clinical prediction models are considered moderately reliable predictors of short-term (14-day) mortality. The IMPACT-core, IMPACT-extended (core + CT), and IMPACT-core + CT + lab clinical prediction models are moderately reliable predictors of 6-month mortality. Scoring systems based on imaging findings alone, such as the Marshall, Rotterdam, Helsinki, or Stockholm scores, are not reliable predictors of mortality after msTBI. Poor functional outcome at 6 months and beyond can be predicted with moderate reliability by the CRASH-basic and CRASH-CT (https://crash.lshtm.ac.uk/Risk%20calculator/index.html), the IMPACT-core, the IMPACT-extended (core + CT), and the IMPACT-core + CT + lab (http://www.tbi-impact.org/?p=impact/calc) [71] models. In the TrackTBI study with 1-year follow-up, one-fifth of patients on 12-month follow-up had zero disability [72].

19.13 Neuroprognostication in Spinal Cord Injuries

Guidelines for neuroprognostication after spinal cord injuries (SCIs) are crucial since, oftentimes, in these cases, patients are conscious and are not only capable of participating in the decision-making process but are also susceptible to the effects of depression, anxiety, and post-traumatic stress disorder [73, 74].

Good practice statements: One must consider the patient's complete clinical condition and not individual variables alone while formulating and communicating the prognosis to the patient or their kin. Communication of significant challenges of probable functional deficits, as well as the potential for improvement and for long-term quality of life with SCI-related deficits, is essential.

The outcomes in SCI have been defined as follows:

1. Mortality: Acute, in-hospital, and measured at discharge.
2. Functional outcome: Assessed by the Functional Independence Measure (FIM) or the Spinal Cord Independence Measure (SCIM) scores at 1 year.
3. AIS grade conversion: American Spine Injury Association (ASIA) Impairment Scale.
4. Independent ambulation: Broadly defined as the ability to walk for short distances with or without assistive devices.
5. Bowel and bladder control: Broadly defined as the ability to maintain continence with or without the use of adjuncts, an outcome that impacts quality of life.

Variables and predictors: Although the body of evidence is of low quality, guidelines recommend that age, comorbidities, concomitant injuries, magnetic resonance imaging findings, the neurological level of injury (NLI), and the severity of the spinal cord injury (ASIA impairment scale) each considered alone not be considered reliable predictors of acute inpatient mortality or mortality measured after discharge or even the functional outcome at 1 year [75]. However, incomplete motor injury can be associated with a greater probability of functional recovery, and the severity of injury, as assessed by the initial ASIA impairment score, can be considered a moderately reliable predictor of AIS conversion on follow-up at 6–12 months. NLI can be considered a moderately reliable predictor of AIS conversion at 6–12 months. The probability of an improvement in AIS is more after a lumbar and thoracolumbar injury than with a cervical or dorsal spine injury (weak recommendation; moderate quality evidence). The Dutch Clinical Prediction Rule (DCPR) is a composite model that has proven to be a useful tool for predicting independent ambulation at 1 year after traumatic Spinal Cord Injury (tSCI) with moderate reliability [76] (Table 19.3).

Table 19.3 The Dutch Clinical Prediction Rule (DCPR)

Variable	Range of test scores	Weighted coefficients	Minimum score	Maximum score
Age >65 years	0–1	−10	−10	0
Motor score L3	0–5	2	0	10
Motor score S1	0–5	2	0	10
Light touch score L3	0–2	5	0	10
Light touch score S1	0–2	5	0	10
Total			−10	40

Adapted from van Middendorp et al. [76]

19.14 Neuroprognostication in Guillain–Barré Syndrome

Guillain–Barré syndrome is a dynamic illness, especially in the acute stages, and may take weeks to months for partial or complete recovery. Guidelines to help clinicians prognosticate these cases offer the clinicians some tools for shared decision-making with patients and their families [77].

19.15 Good Practice Statements (Strong Recommendation; Evidence Cannot Be Graded)

Two phases of the illness should simultaneously be focused upon during the assessment of the neurological prognosis for patients with GBS: the acute course of hospitalization and long-term recovery. It is a very dynamic illness in its acute stages; hence, the possible need for mechanical ventilation and the need for direct enteral feeding and bypassing oral feeds and swallowing must be communicated to the patient and their surrogates. Prognostication in GBS must always be based on the complete clinical picture and never on a single variable alone.

19.16 Outcomes and Predictors

Need for mechanical ventilation within 14 days of disease onset: The presence of bulbar weakness and motor weakness (less than antigravity strength in arms and legs), assessed on admission or during the early course of hospitalization, is considered a moderately reliable predictor of the need for mechanical ventilation within 14 days of disease onset. Bulbar function assessment is done by examination of the cranial nerves IX, X, XI, and XII bilaterally on admission and daily for the first few days after onset until stabilized. The degree of motor weakness is assessed reliably by the Medical Research Council–Sum Score (MRC-SS) [78]. “Rapid” progression of motor weakness, neck weakness, dysautonomia, and the axonal electrophysiological subtype, although found to be good predictors in many studies, were found to be unreliable predictors when considered in isolation. Among the prediction models, the Erasmus Guillain–Barré Syndrome Respiratory Insufficiency Score (EGRIS) is moderately reliable [79].

Independent ambulation at $\geq$3 months: The Erasmus GBS Outcome Score (EGOS) within 2 weeks of admission and the modified EGOS at hospital admission and at 1 week may be considered moderately reliable predictors [80].

Functional outcome at 6 months: It is most commonly assessed using the GBS disability scale (GBSDS, or the Hughes Scale), which ranges from mild signs and symptoms of neuropathy to the grading of the ability of the patient to walk or, finally, being dependent on mechanical ventilation. In some studies, the outcomes are dichotomized as good (GBSDS: 0–2) and poor (GBSDS: 3–6). The mRS has also been used. The predictors studied were the need for mechanical ventilation, an axonal electrophysiological subtype, the patient's age, and the disability grade at disease nadir. No reliable predictors or composite scales measured in the acute stages could predict the functional outcome at 6 months.

19.17 Conclusion

Neuroprognostication, with its uncertainties, be it for the survivors of cardiac arrest, severe acute brain injury, spinal cord injury, GBS, or any other condition in neurocritical care, must be carried out using multiple predictors, and shared decisions regarding WLST or continuation must be taken by giving adequate time to eliminate confounding factors. Avoidance of nihilism and the use of objective assessment tools help in making better prognostications. Effective communication of the prevailing uncertainty using appropriate language during the counseling of surrogates will aid a joint decision-making process. Methodological discrepancies, inadequately powered studies, and variability in definitions and assessment have contributed to the low quality of evidence and failure to establish several predictors as objectively applicable, reliable predictors. Currently, there is a high variability in the measurement of the functional outcome, uncovering a growing need to use standardized scoring systems and appropriate dichotomization or ordinal classification to identify various outcomes [70]. Several studies were associated with a risk of bias due to self-fulfilling prophecy, inadequate statistical analysis, confounding, study attrition, and participation issues. Future studies in neuroprognostication should adhere to specific guidelines to improve the quality of evidence necessary for the development of index tests aimed at predicting functional outcomes and quality of life [7].

Acknowledgments We extend our sincere gratitude to Mr. Suhas, an electrophysicist, and Dr. Vinay Prabhu, a radiologist, for their valuable contributions to this chapter.

References

1. Varkey B. Principles of clinical ethics and their application to practice. Med Princ Pract. 2021;30(1):17–28.
2. Creutzfeldt CJ, Holloway RG. Treatment decisions after severe stroke: uncertainty and biases. Stroke. 2012;43(12):3405–8.
3. Gupta S, Kumar A, Mathur R, Gursahani R, Bhatnagar S, Deodhar J, et al. Indian society of critical care medicine and Indian association of palliative care expert consensus and position statements for end-of-life and palliative care in the intensive care unit. Indian J Crit Care Med. 2024;28(3):200–50.
4. Saposnik G, Cote R, Mamdani M, Raptis S, Thorpe KE, Fang J, et al. JURaSSiC. Neurology. 2013;81(5):448–55.
5. Turgeon AF, Lauzier F, Simard JF, Scales DC, Burns KEA, Moore L, et al. Mortality associated with withdrawal of life-sustaining therapy for patients with severe traumatic brain injury: a Canadian multicentre cohort study. Can Med Assoc J. 2011;183(14):1581–8.

6. May TL, Ruthazer R, Riker RR, Friberg H, Patel N, Soreide E, et al. Early withdrawal of life support after resuscitation from cardiac arrest is common and may result in additional deaths. Resuscitation. 2019;139:308–13.
7. Geocadin RG, Callaway CW, Fink EL, Golan E, Greer DM, Ko NU, et al. Standards for studies of neurological prognostication in comatose survivors of cardiac arrest: a scientific statement from the American Heart Association. Circulation. 2019;140(9):e517.
8. Ge C, Goss AL, Crawford S, Goostrey K, Buddadhumaruk P, Shields AM, et al. Variability of prognostic communication in critically ill neurologic patients: a pilot multicenter mixed-methods study. Crit Care Explor. 2022;4(2):e0640.
9. Sekhon MS, Ainslie PN, Griesdale DE. Clinical pathophysiology of hypoxic ischemic brain injury after cardiac arrest: a "two-hit" model. Crit Care. 2017;21(1):90.
10. Sandroni C, Cronberg T, Sekhon M. Brain injury after cardiac arrest: pathophysiology, treatment, and prognosis. Intensive Care Med. 2021;47(12):1393–414.
11. Amiri M, Raimondo F, Fisher PM, Cacic Hribljan M, Sidaros A, Othman MH, et al. Multimodal prediction of 3- and 12-month outcomes in ICU patients with acute disorders of consciousness. Neurocrit Care. 2024;40(2):718–33.
12. Schiff ND. Recovery of consciousness after brain injury: a mesocircuit hypothesis. Trends Neurosci. 2010;33(1):1–9.
13. Kondziella D, Bender A, Diserens K, van Erp W, Estraneo A, Formisano R, et al. European academy of neurology guideline on the diagnosis of coma and other disorders of consciousness. Eur J Neurol. 2020;27(5):741–56.
14. Giacino JT, Kalmar K, Whyte J. The JFK coma recovery scale-revised: measurement characteristics and diagnostic utility. Arch Phys Med Rehabil. 2004;85(12):2020–9.
15. Grossestreuer AV, Abella BS, Sheak KR, Cinousis MJ, Perman SM, Leary M, et al. Inter-rater reliability of post-arrest cerebral performance category (CPC) scores. Resuscitation. 2016;109:21–4.
16. Bodien Y, Vora I, Barra A, Chiang K, Chatelle C, Goostrey K, et al. Feasibility and validity of the coma recovery scale-revised for accelerated standardized testing (CRSR-FAST): a practical assessment scale for detecting consciousness in the intensive care unit. Arch Phys Med Rehabil. 2024;105(4):e117.
17. Aubinet C, Cassol H, Bodart O, Sanz LRD, Wannez S, Martial C, et al. Simplified evaluation of CONsciousness disorders (SECONDs) in individuals with severe brain injury: a validation study. Ann Phys Rehabil Med. 2021;64(5):101432.
18. Wijdicks EFM, Bamlet WR, Maramattom BV, Manno EM, McClelland RL. Validation of a new coma scale: the FOUR score. Ann Neurol. 2005;58(4):585–93.
19. Wannez S, Heine L, Thonnard M, Gosseries O, Laureys S, Coma Science Group Collaborators. The repetition of behavioral assessments in diagnosis of disorders of consciousness. Ann Neurol. 2017;81(6):883–9.
20. Nyholm B, Grand J, Obling LER, Hassager C, Møller JE, Schmidt H, et al. Validating quantitative pupillometry thresholds for neuroprognostication after out-of-hospital cardiac arrest. A predefined substudy of the blood pressure and oxygenations targets after cardiac arrest (BOX)-trial. Intensive Care Med. 2024;50(9):1484–95.
21. Rajajee V, Muehlschlegel S, Wartenberg KE, Alexander SA, Busl KM, Chou SHY, et al. Guidelines for Neuroprognostication in comatose adult survivors of cardiac arrest. Neurocrit Care. 2023;38(3):533–63.
22. Curley WH, Bodien YG, Zhou DW, Conte MM, Foulkes AS, Giacino JT, et al. Electrophysiological correlates of thalamocortical function in acute severe traumatic brain injury. Cortex J Devoted Study Nerv Syst Behav. 2022;152:136–52.
23. Comanducci A, Boly M, Claassen J, De Lucia M, Gibson RM, Juan E, et al. Clinical and advanced neurophysiology in the prognostic and diagnostic evaluation of disorders of consciousness: review of an IFCN-endorsed expert group. Clin Neurophysiol. 2020;131(11):2736–65.
24. Egbebike J, Shen Q, Doyle K, Der-Nigoghossian CA, Panicker L, Gonzales IJ, et al. Cognitive-motor dissociation and time to functional recovery in patients with acute brain injury in the USA: a prospective observational cohort study. Lancet Neurol. 2022;21(8):704–13.

25. Pan J, Xie Q, Qin P, Chen Y, He Y, Huang H, et al. Prognosis for patients with cognitive motor dissociation identified by brain-computer interface. Brain. 2020;143(4):1177–89.
26. Claassen J, Doyle K, Matory A, Couch C, Burger KM, Velazquez A, et al. Detection of brain activation in unresponsive patients with acute brain injury. N Engl J Med. 2019;380(26):2497–505.
27. Sokoliuk R, Degano G, Banellis L, Melloni L, Hayton T, Sturman S, et al. Covert speech comprehension predicts recovery from acute unresponsive states. Ann Neurol. 2021;89(4):646–56.
28. Ling Y, Xu C, Wen X, Li J, Gao J, Luo B. Cortical responses to auditory stimulation predict the prognosis of patients with disorders of consciousness. Clin Neurophysiol. 2023;153:11–20.
29. Giacino JT, Katz DI, Schiff ND, Whyte J, Ashman EJ, Ashwal S, et al. Practice guideline update recommendations summary: disorders of consciousness: report of the guideline development, dissemination, and implementation subcommittee of the American academy of neurology; the American congress of rehabilitation medicine; and the National institute on disability, independent living, and rehabilitation research. Neurology. 2018;91(10):450–60.
30. Thibaut A, Panda R, Annen J, Sanz LRD, Naccache L, Martial C, et al. Preservation of brain activity in unresponsive patients identifies MCS star. Ann Neurol. 2021;90(1):89–100.
31. Torbey MT, Selim M, Knorr J, Bigelow C, Recht L. Quantitative analysis of the loss of distinction between gray and white matter in comatose patients after cardiac arrest. Stroke. 2000;31(9):2163–7.
32. Kirsch K, Heymel S, Günther A, Vahl K, Schmidt T, Michalski D, et al. Prognostication of neurologic outcome using gray-white-matter-ratio in comatose patients after cardiac arrest. BMC Neurol. 2021;21(1):456.
33. Wijman CAC, Mlynash M, Finley Caulfield A, Hsia AW, Eyngorn I, Bammer R, et al. Prognostic value of brain diffusion-weighted imaging after cardiac arrest. Ann Neurol. 2009;65(4):394–402.
34. Greer D, Scripko P, Bartscher J, Sims J, Camargo E, Singhal A, et al. Serial MRI changes in comatose cardiac arrest patients. Neurocrit Care. 2011;14(1):61–7.
35. Mlynash M, Campbell DM, Leproust EM, Fischbein NJ, Bammer R, Eyngorn I, Hsia AW, Moseley M, Wijman CA. Temporal and spatial profile of brain diffusion-weighted MRI after cardiac arrest. Stroke. 2010;41(8):1665–72.
36. Hirsch KG, Fischbein N, Mlynash M, Kemp S, Bammer R, Eyngorn I, et al. Prognostic value of diffusion-weighted MRI for post-cardiac arrest coma. Neurology. 2020;94(16):e1684.
37. Moon HK, Jang J, Park KN, Kim SH, Lee BK, Oh SH, et al. Quantitative analysis of relative volume of low apparent diffusion coefficient value can predict neurologic outcome after cardiac arrest. Resuscitation. 2018;126:36–42.
38. Rennebaum F, Kassubek J, Pinkhardt E, Hübers A, Ludolph AC, Schocke M, et al. Status epilepticus: clinical characteristics and EEG patterns associated with and without MRI diffusion restriction in 69 patients. Epilepsy Res. 2016;120:55–64.
39. Rosario M, McMahon K, Finelli PF. Diffusion-weighted imaging in acute hyperammonemic encephalopathy. The Neurohospitalist. 2013;3(3):125–30.
40. Park JS, In YN, You YH, Min JH, Ahn HJ, Yoo IS, et al. Ultra-early neurologic outcome prediction of out-of-hospital cardiac arrest survivors using combined diffusion-weighted imaging findings and quantitative analysis of apparent diffusion coefficient. Resuscitation. 2020;148:39–48.
41. Isgrò MA, Bottoni P, Scatena R. Neuron-specific enolase as a biomarker: biochemical and clinical aspects. In: Scatena R, editor. Advances in cancer biomarkers. Advances in experimental medicine and biology, vol. 867. Dordrecht: Springer; 2015.
42. Haque A, Polcyn R, Matzelle D, Banik NL. New insights into the role of neuron-specific enolase in neuro-inflammation, neurodegeneration, and neuroprotection. Brain Sci. 2018;8(2):33.
43. Kim YJ, Kim YH, Youn CS, Cho IS, Kim SJ, Wee JH, et al. Different neuroprognostication thresholds of neuron-specific enolase in shockable and non-shockable out-of-hospital cardiac arrest: a prospective multicenter observational study in Korea (the KORHN-PRO registry). Crit Care. 2023;27:313.

44. Sandroni C, D'Arrigo S, Cacciola S, Hoedemaekers CWE, Westhall E, Kamps MJA, et al. Prediction of good neurological outcome in comatose survivors of cardiac arrest: a systematic review. Intensive Care Med. 2022;48(4):389–413.
45. Velly L, Perlbarg V, Boulier T, Adam N, Delphine S, Luyt CE, et al. Use of brain diffusion tensor imaging for the prediction of long-term neurological outcomes in patients after cardiac arrest: a multicentre, international, prospective, observational, cohort study. Lancet Neurol. 2018;17(4):317–26.
46. Wang JY, Bakhadirov K, Abdi H, Devous MD, Marquez De La Plata CD, Moore C, et al. Longitudinal changes of structural connectivity in traumatic axonal injury. Neurology. 2011;77(9):818–26.
47. Hoiland RL, Rikhraj KJK, Thiara S, Fordyce C, Kramer AH, Skrifvars MB, et al. Neurologic prognostication after cardiac arrest using brain biomarkers: a systematic review and meta-analysis. JAMA Neurol. 2022;79(4):390.
48. Hemphill JC, White DB. Clinical nihilism in neuro-emergencies. Emerg Med Clin North Am. 2009;27(1):27–viii.
49. Goss A, Ge C, Crawford S, Goostrey K, Buddadhumaruk P, Hough CL, et al. Prognostic language in critical neurologic illness. Neurology. 2023;101(5):e558–69.
50. Khan MW, Muehlschlegel S. Shared decision making in neurocritical care. Neurol Clin. 2017;35(4):825–34.
51. Hwang DY, Kim KS, Muehlschlegel S, Wartenberg KE, Rajajee V, Alexander SA, et al. Guidelines for neuroprognostication in critically ill adults with intracerebral hemorrhage. Neurocrit Care. 2024;40(2):395–414.
52. Hemphill JC 3rd, Farrant M, TA N Jr. Prospective validation of the ICH score for 12-month functional outcome. Neurology. 2009;73(14):1088–94.
53. Sembill JA, Castello JP, Sprügel MI, Gerner ST, Hoelter P, Lücking H, et al. Multicenter validation of the max-ICH score in intracerebral hemorrhage. Ann Neurol. 2021;89(3):474–84.
54. Jaja BNR, Cusimano MD, Etminan N, Hanggi D, Hasan D, Ilodigwe D, et al. Clinical prediction models for aneurysmal subarachnoid hemorrhage: a systematic review. Neurocrit Care. 2013;18(1):143–53.
55. Witsch J, Frey HP, Patel S, Park S, Lahiri S, Schmidt JM, et al. Prognostication of long-term outcomes after subarachnoid hemorrhage: the FRESH score. Ann Neurol. 2016;80(1):46–58.
56. Witsch J, Kuohn L, Hebert R, Cord B, Sansing L, Gilmore EJ, et al. Early prognostication of 1-year outcome after subarachnoid hemorrhage: the FRESH score validation. J Stroke Cerebrovasc Dis Off J Natl Stroke Assoc. 2019;28(10):104280.
57. Macdonald RL, Cusimano MD, Etminan N, Hanggi D, Hasan D, Ilodigwe D, et al. Subarachnoid hemorrhage international trialists data repository (SAHIT). World Neurosurg. 2013;79(3):418–22.
58. Oliveira Souza NV, Rouanet C, Solla DJF, Barroso de Lima CV, d Souza CA, Rezende F., et al. The role of VASOGRADE as a simple grading scale to predict delayed cerebral ischemia and functional outcome after aneurysmal subarachnoid hemorrhage. Neurocrit Care. 2023;38:96–104.
59. Maldaner N, Visser V, Hostettler IC, Bijlenga P, Haemmerli J, Roethlisberger M, et al. External validation of the HATCH (hemorrhage, age, treatment, clinical state, hydrocephalus) score for prediction of functional outcome after subarachnoid hemorrhage. Neurosurgery. 2022;91(6):906.
60. Heilig M, Rass V, Lindner A, Kofler M, Ianosi BA, Gaasch M, et al. Brain microdialysate tau dynamics predict functional and neurocognitive recovery after poor-grade subarachnoid haemorrhage. Brain Commun. 2022;5(1):fcac342.
61. Weller J, Lampmann T, Asoglu H, Schneider M, Ehrentraut SF, Lehmann F, et al. Additive prognostic impact of the cerebrospinal fluid arginine/ornithine ratio to established clinical scores in aneurysmal subarachnoid hemorrhage. Front Neurol. 2023;14:1156505.
62. O'Donnell MJ, Fang J, D'Uva C, Saposnik G, Gould L, McGrath E, et al. The PLAN score: a bedside prediction rule for death and severe disability following acute ischemic stroke. Arch Intern Med. 2012;172(20):1548–56.

63. Saposnik G, Kapral MK, Liu Y, Hall R, O'Donnell M, Raptis S, et al. IScore: a risk score to predict death early after hospitalization for an acute ischemic stroke. Circulation. 2011;123(7):739–49.
64. Ntaios G, Faouzi M, Ferrari J, Lang W, Vemmos K, Michel P. An integer-based score to predict functional outcome in acute ischemic stroke: the ASTRAL score. Neurology. 2012;78(24):1916–22.
65. Hallevi H, Barreto AD, Liebeskind DS, Morales MM, Martin-Schild SB, Abraham AT, et al. UCLA intra-arterial therapy investigators; identifying patients at high risk for poor outcome after intra-arterial therapy for acute ischemic stroke. Stroke. 2009;40(5):1780–5.
66. Flint AC, Xiang B, Gupta R, Nogueira RG, Lutsep HL, Jovin TG, et al. Thrive score predicts outcomes with a third-generation endovascular stroke treatment device in the trevo-2 trial. Stroke. 2013;44(12):3370–5.
67. Saposnik G, Guzik AK, Reeves M, Ovbiagele B, Johnston SC. Stroke prognostication using age and NIH stroke scale: SPAN-100. Neurology. 2013;80(1):21–8.
68. Van Veen E, Van Der Jagt M, Citerio G, Stocchetti N, Gommers D, Burdorf A, et al. Occurrence and timing of withdrawal of life-sustaining measures in traumatic brain injury patients: a CENTER-TBI study. Intensive Care Med. 2021;47(10):1115–29.
69. Williamson T, Ryser MD, Ubel PA, Abdelgadir J, Spears CA, Liu B, et al. Withdrawal of life-supporting treatment in severe traumatic brain injury. JAMA Surg. 2020;155(8):723–31.
70. Muehlschlegel S, Rajajee V, Wartenberg KE, Alexander SA, Busl KM, Creutzfeldt CJ, et al. Guidelines for neuroprognostication in critically ill adults with moderate–severe traumatic brain injury. Neurocrit Care. 2024;40(2):448–76.
71. Prognostic calculator | TBI-IMPACT.org [Internet]. [cited 2025 Jan 7]. Available from: http://www.tbi-impact.org/?p=impact/calc.
72. MA MC, Giacino JT, Barber J, Temkin NR, Nelson LD, Levin HS, et al. Functional outcomes over the first year after moderate to severe traumatic brain injury in the prospective, longitudinal TRACK-TBI study. JAMA Neurol. 2021;78(8):982–92.
73. Mahanes D, Muehlschlegel S, Wartenberg KE, Rajajee V, Alexander SA, Busl KM, et al. Guidelines for neuroprognostication in adults with traumatic spinal cord injury. Neurocrit Care. 2024;40(2):415–37.
74. Budd MA, Gater DR, Channell I. Psychosocial consequences of spinal cord injury: a narrative review. J Pers Med. 2022;12(7):1178.
75. Roberts TT, Leonard GR, Cepela DJ. Classifications In brief: American spinal injury association (ASIA) impairment scale. Clin Orthop. 2017;475(5):1499–504.
76. Van Middendorp JJ, Hosman AJ, ART D, Pouw MH, Ditunno JF, Curt A, et al. A clinical prediction rule for ambulation outcomes after traumatic spinal cord injury: a longitudinal cohort study. Lancet. 2011;377(9770):1004–10.
77. Busl KM, Fried H, Muehlschlegel S, Wartenberg KE, Rajajee V, Alexander SA, et al. Guidelines for neuroprognostication in adults with Guillain–Barré syndrome. Neurocrit Care. 2023;38(3):564–83.
78. Kleyweg RP, Van Der Meché FGA, Schmitz PIM. Interobserver agreement in the assessment of muscle strength and functional abilities in Guillain-Barré syndrome. Muscle Nerve. 1991;14(11):1103–9.
79. Walgaard C, Lingsma HF, Ruts L, Drenthen J, van Koningsveld R, Garssen MJP, et al. Prediction of respiratory insufficiency in Guillain-Barré syndrome. Ann Neurol. 2010;67(6):781–7.
80. Walgaard C, Lingsma HF, Ruts L, van Doorn PA, Steyerberg EW, Jacobs BC. Early recognition of poor prognosis in Guillain-Barré syndrome. Neurology. 2011;76(11):968–75.

Controversies in Brain Death

20

Ankita Dey and Prasanna Udupi Bidkar

Abstract

Despite the availability of national and international guidelines and protocols for the determination of brain death, there are several areas of contention, including but not limited to pregnancy, primary posterior fossa injury, the number of examinations required, and so on. This chapter attempts to elucidate these gray areas pertaining to the determination of brain death or death by neurologic criteria (BD/DNC).

Keywords

Brain death · Uniform Determination of Death Act · Death by neurologic criteria Apnea testing · Pediatric brain death · Organ donation

20.1 Introduction

Mollaret et al. first introduced the concept of brain death/death by neurologic criteria (BD/DNC) in 1959, terming it "coma depasse" [1]. The term "brain death" appeared in publication for the first time in 1968, as part of the Harvard Brain Death Criteria [2]. The Uniform Determination of Death Act (UDDA), established in 1981, provides two ways to determine death: irreversible loss of circulatory and respiratory function or irreversible loss of all brain function, including the brain stem [3]. The American Academy of Neurology (AAN) defines BD/DNC as the

A. Dey (✉)
Department of Anaesthesiology, AIIMS, Bathinda, Punjab, India

P. U. Bidkar
Department of Anaesthesiology and Critical Care, JIPMER, Pondicherry, India

P. U. Bidkar, M. Krishnakumar (eds.), *Controversies in Neurocritical Care*,
https://doi.org/10.1007/978-981-95-4419-6_20

irreversible cessation of all brain function, including the brain stem, leading to coma, the absence of brain stem reflexes, and apnea [4]. However, despite the availability of guidelines and protocols to guide the determination of BD/DNC, controversies and dilemmas abound pertaining to BD. The World Brain Death Project (WBDP) was undertaken to mitigate, if not resolve, these controversies surrounding BD/DNC [5].

20.2 Controversies Around Brain Death

20.2.1 Brain Death During Pregnancy

Brain death during pregnancy is an exceedingly rare event, with approximately 30 cases reported in the literature [6]. Therefore, the physician dealing with a brain-dead pregnant woman is confronted with ethical, legal, and medical challenges pertaining to whether life-sustaining therapies should be discontinued, leading to fetal demise, or if organ-preservative support should continue with the aim of sustaining fetal viability. These challenges have to be navigated with extreme caution. According to the 2023 updated guidelines for the declaration of BD/DNC by the AAN, pregnancy is not a contraindication to brain death declaration [7]. However, whether or not the pregnancy should be continued following BD/DNC declaration is shrouded in controversy. A retrospective study revealed that very few health institutions in the United States have policies and protocols to manage brain death in pregnant women [8]. A 2019 position statement from the American Academy of Neurology (AAN) emphasizes that when brain death occurs in a pregnant woman, ethical considerations should prioritize the well-being of the fetus [9]. The AAN further advises that the family and legal representatives of the deceased pregnant woman should be informed about relevant laws and the potential outcomes for the fetus, acknowledging that these outcomes can be uncertain. In addition, the AAN also endorses requests for prolonged life-sustaining therapies in these patients, regardless of the gestational age, with the following caveats:

1. The relatives should be completely cognizant of the deleterious effects of prolonged life-sustaining therapies on the fetal outcome.
2. The intention to withdraw life-sustaining therapies following the completion of pregnancy should be informed to the lawful surrogates.
3. The decision of the lawful surrogates to withdraw life-sustaining therapies if the fetus has not reached a viable gestational age should also be honored.

If a legally valid advance medical directive exists that outlines the pregnant woman's wishes regarding the care of her unborn child in the event of her death, it should be taken into account while remaining subject to legal interpretation [10]. A multidisciplinary team comprising obstetricians, neonatologists, neurologists, anesthesiologists, transplant surgeons, and medical ethicists should discuss the risks and benefits of continuing life-sustaining therapies for the fetus with the lawful surrogates and help them make an informed choice [5, 7].

20.2.2 Brain Death Declaration in Patients with Primary Posterior Fossa Injury

The incidence of primary infratentorial injury leading to brain death is to the tune of 6% [11]. The declaration of brain death in these patients remains an area of contention because of the differences in the definition of brain death employed in different countries and even within different states of the same country [12]. A systematic review and meta-analysis of 3602 brain death declarations revealed 38 cases of isolated brain stem injury. Of those, 28 patients later experienced a loss of cerebral blood flow or electrical activity, supporting the concept of "whole-brain" death [11]. In a small case series of four patients with catastrophic primary posterior fossa injury, the authors observed the eventual evolution of the complete absence of intracranial blood flow despite initial evidence of preserved supratentorial blood flow. The authors concluded that, should this natural history be confirmed in larger studies, ancillary testing may not be required in these patients if clinical examination and apnea test are indicative of BD/DNC [13]. Furthermore, in an editorial published in a reputed journal, the author notes that recovery in patients with isolated primary brain stem injury fulfilling the brain stem death criteria has not been reported so far [14]. The WBDP recommends that when isolated brain stem damage is suspected, ancillary tests should be used to verify the absence of cerebral blood flow. Even if clinical examination and apnea testing align with the brain death criteria, BD/DNC should not be diagnosed in the presence of supratentorial blood flow [5]. Similarly, the AAN's updated 2023 guidelines recommend that before initiating a BD/DNC evaluation, clinicians should confirm that a primary infratentorial injury has also caused catastrophic damage to the supratentorial region, as evidenced by conventional neuroimaging [7].

20.2.3 Preserved Neuroendocrine Function and BD/DNC Determination

The UDDA mandates the cessation of all brain functions, including those of the brain stem, for BD/DNC declaration [3]. However, it has been argued that preserved neuroendocrine function, which can be simplified to mean the absence of diabetes insipidus, does not translate to the "loss of all functions of the entire brain" [15, 16].

It may be pertinent to discuss the unique circulation of the hypothalamic–pituitary axis here. The inferior hypophyseal artery follows an extradural course until it reaches the posterior pituitary, where it penetrates the dura mater. The fact that it remains outside the dura for most of its course likely provides added protection to the hypothalamus and pituitary perfusion, shielding them from the effects of elevated intracranial pressure [17]. This may account for preserved neuroendocrine function in some patients who otherwise fulfill the criteria for BD/DNC. As such, the updated 2023 AAN guideline advises that clinicians may proceed with initiating and declaring BD/DNC even in the presence of evidence of neuroendocrine function [7]. This is also endorsed by the WBDP [5].

20.2.4 Number of Examinations Required to Establish BD/DNC

The literature provides limited guidance on the number of neurologic examinations necessary to declare BD/DNC. The updated AAN guidelines, published in 2023, recommend at least one neurologic exam for the declaration of BD/DNC in adults. The latest guidelines aim to minimize the risk of incorrectly diagnosing brain death. To achieve this, they recommend a separate, independent examination by a second clinician [7, 18]. A large study on adult and pediatric patients who were declared brain dead demonstrated that the second examination did not add anything to the first in adult patients. Additionally, it resulted in a significant delay in the declaration of death, resulting in significant intensive care costs, and also reduced the viability of organs for transplantation [19]. These findings were reciprocated in another study conducted by Varelas et al., in which the authors found that the second examination was not useful and resulted in a significant delay in the procurement of organs [20]. A single brain death examination was found to be faster and easier to perform and was not associated with the recovery of brain function. It also resulted in a lower financial burden and an equivalent or better organ function status [21]. However, it is important to note that the priority while conducting a BD/DNC determination should be preserving the integrity of the examination. It may be preferable to err on the side of caution, given the finality and the implications of this process [7]. Further research is warranted to help us discern whether a single neurologic examination should suffice in adults for the declaration of BD/DNC.

20.2.5 Consent Before the Declaration of BD/DNC

According to the 2023 AAN guideline, clinicians are not required to obtain consent before conducting an evaluation for BD/DNC unless mandated by the institution's policy or state laws and regulations [7]. Similarly, the WBDP and the AAN's 2019 position statement emphasize that while clinicians should make reasonable efforts to inform the patient's family of the intent to perform a BD/DNC evaluation, obtaining informed consent is not required [5, 9]. Death by neurologic criteria and cardiopulmonary death are treated equally under the law [3]. Therefore, it follows that since informed consent is not required for the determination of cardiopulmonary death, there should be no need for informed consent before determining death by neurologic criteria. Determination of death should not represent a choice. Respect for the patient's autonomy should be balanced against the implications of delaying the declaration of death with respect to the triaging of allocation of hospital resources, as well as prolonging the agony of the family members [22]. Therefore, unless mandated by institutional policy or state laws, there should be no obligation to obtain consent for the determination of BD/DNC.

20.2.6 Considerations in the Pediatric Population

A child is defined as someone who is at least 37 weeks corrected gestational age and less than 18 years of age for the purpose of BD/DNC determination [7]. Some of the recommendations for the determination of BD/DNC are different in children on account of the unique anatomical and physiological considerations in children, along with the varied age-dependent pathophysiological responses to brain injury. Children suspected of brain death require two separate neurologic exams, including apnea testing, with an observation period between exams, which varies depending on the child's age. The recommended observation period is 24 h in neonates (from 37 weeks corrected gestational age to term infants 30 days of age) and 12 h in infants and children (>30 days of age to 18 years of age) [23]. The two examinations must be performed by two independent examiners. The apnea tests can be conducted by the same physician, ideally the one responsible for the care of the ventilated child [7, 18, 23]. A waiting period of at least 48 h after a catastrophic brain injury allows for a more accurate assessment of BD/DNC in children [7].

20.3 Conclusions

The various controversies pertaining to BD/DNC determination need to be navigated with caution, keeping in mind the updated guidelines of well-established medical associations and regulatory bodies. When in doubt, it is always advisable to err on the side of caution.

References

1. Mollaret P, Goulon M. The depassed coma (preliminary memoir). Rev Neurol (Paris). 1959;101:3–15.
2. A definition of irreversible coma. Report of the Ad Hoc Committee of the Harvard Medical School to examine the definition of brain death. JAMA. 1968;205(6):337–340.
3. Guidelines for the determination of death. Report of the medical consultants on the diagnosis of death to the president's Commission for the Study of ethical problems in medicine and biomedical and behavioral research. JAMA. 1981;246(19):2184–6.
4. Wijdicks EFM, Varelas PN, Gronseth GS, Greer DM, American Academy of Neurology. Evidence-based guideline update: determining brain death in adults: report of the quality standards Subcommittee of the American Academy of neurology. Neurology. 2010;74(23):1911–8.
5. Greer DM, Shemie SD, Lewis A, Torrance S, Varelas P, Goldenberg FD, et al. Determination of brain death/death by neurologic criteria: the world brain death project. JAMA. 2020;324(11):1078–97.

6. Esmaeilzadeh M, Dictus C, Kayvanpour E, Sedaghat-Hamedani F, Eichbaum M, Hofer S, et al. One life ends, another begins: management of a brain-dead pregnant mother – a systematic review. BMC Med. 2010;8(8):74.
7. Kirschen MP, Lewis A, Greer DM. The 2023 American academy of neurology, American academy of pediatrics, child neurology society, and society of critical care medicine pediatric and adult brain death/death by neurologic criteria determination consensus guidelines: what the critical care team needs to know. Crit Care Med. 2024;52(3):376–86.
8. Lewis A, Varelas P, Greer D. Pregnancy and brain death: lack of guidance in U.S. Hospital policies. Am J Perinatol. 2016;33(14):1382–7.
9. Russell JA, Epstein LG, Greer DM, Kirschen M, Rubin MA, Lewis A. Brain death, the determination of brain death, and member guidance for brain death accommodation requests: AAN position statement. Neurology. 2019;92(5):228–32.
10. Lewis A. Contemporary legal updates to the definition of brain death in Nevada. JAMA Neurol. 2017;74(9):1031–2.
11. Neves Briard J, Plourde G, Nitulescu R, Boyd JG, Carrier FM, Couillard P, et al. Infratentorial brain injury among patients suspected of death by neurologic criteria: a systematic review and meta-analysis. Neurology. 2023;100(4):e443–53.
12. Wijdicks EFM. The transatlantic divide over brain death determination and the debate. Brain J Neurol. 2012;135(Pt 4):1321–31.
13. Varelas PN, Brady P, Rehman M, Afshinnik A, Mehta C, Abdelhak T, et al. Primary posterior fossa lesions and preserved supratentorial cerebral blood flow: implications for brain death determination. Neurocrit Care. 2017;27(3):407–14.
14. Varelas PN. Brainstem or entire brain-based declaration of death: is there a difference? Pract Neurol. 2016;16(2):85–6.
15. Nair-Collins M, Joffe AR. Hypothalamic function in patients diagnosed as brain dead and its practical consequences. Handb Clin Neurol. 2021;182:433–46.
16. Nair-Collins M, Joffe AR. Frequent preservation of neurologic function in brain death and brainstem death entails false-positive misdiagnosis and cerebral perfusion. AJOB Neurosci. 2023;14(3):255–68.
17. Nair-Collins M, Northrup J, Olcese J. Hypothalamic-pituitary function in brain death: a review. J Intensive Care Med. 2016;31(1):41–50.
18. Lewis A, Kirschen MP, Greer D. The 2023 AAN/AAP/CNS/SCCM pediatric and adult brain death/death by neurologic criteria consensus practice guideline: a comparison with the 2010 and 2011 guidelines. Neurol Clin Pract. 2023;13(6):e200189.
19. Lustbader D, O'Hara D, Wijdicks EFM, MacLean L, Tajik W, Ying A, et al. Second brain death examination may negatively affect organ donation. Neurology. 2011;76(2):119–24.
20. Varelas PN, Rehman M, Mehta C, Louchart L, Schultz L, Brady P, et al. Comparison of 1 vs 2 brain death examinations on time to death pronouncement and organ donation: a 12-year single center experience. Neurology. 2021;96(10):e1453–61.
21. Varelas PN, Rehman M, Abdelhak T, Patel A, Rai V, Barber A, et al. Single brain death examination is equivalent to dual brain death examinations. Neurocrit Care. 2011;15(3):547–53.
22. Lewis A, Greer D. POINT: should informed consent be required for apnea testing in patients with suspected brain death? No. Chest. 2017;152(4):700–2.
23. Nakagawa TA, Ashwal S, Mathur M, Mysore M, Society of Critical Care Medicine, Section on Critical Care and Section on Neurology of American Academy of Pediatrics, Child Neurology Society. Clinical report—guidelines for the determination of brain death in infants and children: an update of the 1987 task force recommendations. Pediatrics. 2011;128(3):e720–40.

Controversies in Glycemic Control in Neurocritical Care

21

R. P. Sangeetha, Shweta S. Naik, and K. R. Shwethashri

Abstract

Controversies concerning clinical management practices have prevailed from time immemorial. The management of glycemic status is one such management arm. This requires a physiological range to be individually defined and targeted for each patient during each phase of the critical illness. Ongoing research continues attempts to gain knowledge in this aspect to provide the best possible management guidelines, especially for the neurocritically ill. Despite the ongoing extensive research in these areas to provide the best possible practice guidelines, ambiguity still needs to be addressed concerning the intensity of treatment, target thresholds, and duration of therapies. A "personalized" approach to glycemic control in the critically ill, with recognition of preadmission glycemia, is supported by an emerging literature. This chapter will review the different sources of evidence available in the literature concerning this critical intervention. We suggest the best practices for this commonly faced controversy and elaborate on what needs to be researched further.

Keywords

Hypoglycemia · Hyperglycemia · Insulin therapy · Neurointensive care unit

R. P. Sangeetha (✉) · S. S. Naik · K. R. Shwethashri
Neuroanaesthesia and Neurocritical care, National Institute of Mental Health and Neurosciences, Bangalore, Karnataka, India

P. U. Bidkar, M. Krishnakumar (eds.), *Controversies in Neurocritical Care*,
https://doi.org/10.1007/978-981-95-4419-6_21

21.1 Introduction

An ongoing controversy concerning the care of neurocritically ill patients prevails in the face of continuing research to dictate optimal management practices. This includes the management of glycemic status during the acute and chronic phases of the disease course in the neurointensive care unit (NICU). A single target is difficult to define for uniform application to all patients across different diagnoses. A physiological range should be individually determined and targeted for each patient during each phase of the critical illness. Despite the ongoing extensive research in these areas to provide the best possible practice guidelines, ambiguity still needs to be addressed concerning the intensity of treatment, target thresholds, and duration of therapies. This chapter will review the different sources of evidence available in the literature concerning this critical intervention. We suggest the best practices for this commonly faced controversy and elaborate on what needs to be researched further.

Glycemic control in the neuro-ICU is key in patients' routine critical care management involving normoglycemia maintenance. The goal of glycemic monitoring is to avoid hyperglycemia (and its attendant complications, such as multisystemic inflammation and infections) and hypoglycemia-induced neurological and cardiac insults. Extreme surges at either end of the spectrum, hyper- and hypoglycemia, strongly influence outcomes in critically ill patients. Patients admitted to neurocritical care (NCC) are a unique population whose optimal glycemic targets may differ across heterogeneous diagnoses.

21.1.1 Evidence for Glycemic Control

The traditional glycemic targets have varied over the past several decades. Earlier, the Leuven trials led by Greet Van Den Berghe were instrumental in implementing a strict glucose control regimen that was in vogue for a reasonable period until the NICE-SUGAR trial challenged this. The Leuven trials: The landmark study of the 2001 Leuven Surgical Trial conducted by Greet Van Den Berghe signaled the trend of intensive glucose control in the ICU. This study showed a decrease in ICU mortality from 8% to 4.6% with tight control (blood glucose = 4.5–6.5 mmol/L) [1]. The Leuven Medical Trial 2006 found improved morbidity but not mortality in ICU patients with medical disorders receiving intensive insulin therapy (IIT) [2]. The 2008 Efficacy of Volume Substitution and Insulin Therapy in Severe Sepsis (VISEP) study in severe sepsis raised concerns about severe hypoglycemia and adverse events due to intensive insulin therapy (IIT) [3].

The subsequent Normoglycemia in Intensive Care Evaluation-Survival Using Glucose Algorithm Regulation (NICE-SUGAR) trial contradicted and superseded the Leuven trials. This was a definitive multicenter randomized clinical trial (RCT) of over 6000 ICU patients, where increased mortality and more severe hypoglycemia were found in the intensive control group (glucose 4.6–6 mM) [4]. They also found that intensive glucose control increased mortality among adults in the ICU. A blood glucose concentration (BGC) ≤180 mg/dL leads to lower mortality than a target of 81–108 mg/dL [5].

21.1.2 Extrapolations to Neurocritical Care

Neurocritical patients have unique attributes, with differences owing to their primary neurological and neurosurgical diagnoses. In patients with acute brain injury (ABI) admitted to NCC, careful BGC management is a priority. Blood glucose concentration (BGC) management among neurocritical patients is challenging [6–9]. Hypoglycemia (BGC <80 mg/dL)-induced neuroglycopenia and cerebral dysfunction occur through sympathetic stimulation, altered cerebral flow, and metabolism by use of non-glucose substrates, such as pyruvate, glycogen, ketone bodies, glutamate, glutamine, and aspartate [7]. Hyperglycemia and high BGC variability have been established to denote adverse outcomes in patients with acute brain injury (ABI) secondary to different causes, such as traumatic brain injury (TBI), acute ischemic stroke (AIS), intracranial hemorrhage (ICH), and subarachnoid hemorrhage (SAH) [7, 8]. The exacerbation of hyperglycemia occurs primarily through the hypothalamus–hypophyseal–adrenal axis activation, elevated cortisol secretion, and induction of gluconeogenesis. Optimal BGC target range and BGC management in neurocritical care (NCC) patients have significantly evolved in the past decades [8, 10].

21.1.3 Glycemic Control in Critical Neurosurgical Patients

Hyperglycemia can occur in 30–70% of neurosurgical patients in the postoperative phase, especially among patients with a Glasgow Coma Scale (GCS) score below 13 and in those with intracranial hematoma or traumatic brain injury (TBI) [11].

21.1.4 Glycemic Control in TBI

An RCT conducted in 97 patients with severe TBI showed that the maintenance of glycemia at 80–120 mg/dL (4.44–6.66 mmol/L) significantly increased the risk of hypoglycemic episodes. Though patients receiving intensive insulin therapy (IIT) had shorter ICU stays and infection rates like those who received conventional insulin therapy, both groups had similar follow-up mortality and neurological outcomes [12].

21.1.5 Glycemic Control in Patients with Subarachnoid Hemorrhage (SAH)

In patients with SAH, acute hyperglycemia at presentation may mirror the severity of brain injury and may not be a modifiable target for the prevention of secondary brain injury. Hyperglycemia after SAH is associated with prolonged intensive care unit stay, increased mortality, and severe disability [13]. A recent randomized clinical trial of 78 patients with subarachnoid hemorrhage (SAH) reported a significantly reduced infection rate among patients receiving intensive insulin therapy targeting glycemic values of 80–120 mg/dL. However, this regimen failed to demonstrate any benefit over the conventional vasospasm prevention treatment and improve neurological outcomes [14]. The recent 2023 guidelines on managing SAH do not provide any definitive consensus on the intensity of glycemic control in these patients [15]. The mean hospital glucose (MHG), minimum (MinG), maximum (MaxG), and variability are clinically significant. The MHG has been demonstrated as independently associated with ($p < 0.001$) mortality, MaxG ($p = 0.017$) with complications, and lower MinG ($p = 0.015$) with vasospasm. While inpatient insulin appears to be associated with increased complications, with no mortality benefit, among those with MHG ≥140 mg/dL, insulin therapy resulted in lower mortality (OR = 0.3; 95% CI 0.1–0.9; $p = 0.0358$) but no increased complication risk [16].

21.1.6 Glycemic Control in Intracerebral Hemorrhage (ICH)

Stress hyperglycemia ratio (SHR), measured as admission glucose–to–glycated hemoglobin (HbA1c) ratio, correlates with unfavorable clinical outcomes during hospital discharge and at 90 days among the survivors of ICH [17]. In the face of such conflicting data, the relevance of systemic hypoglycemia–induced neuroglycopenia and, hence, cerebral metabolic crisis and worse neurological outcomes needs further evaluation [18].

21.1.7 Glycemic Control in Stroke

Stress hyperglycemia predisposes to adverse outcomes and mortality among patients with acute ischemic stroke (AIS). A recent meta-analysis of 13 studies encompassing 184,179 patients with AIS showed that a higher SHR correlates with a 2.64 times increased risk of poor functional outcomes, a 3.11-fold increased risk of mortality at 3 months, a 2.80-fold increased risk of 1-year mortality, a 3.90-fold increased risk of intracerebral hemorrhage (ICH), a 4.57 times increased risk of symptomatic ICH, a 1.73-fold increased risk of neurological deficits, and a 2.84-fold increased risk of stroke recurrence [19].

21.1.8 Intensive Versus Conventional Glycemic Control and Optimal Glycemic Range

A systematic review and meta-analysis of 16 randomized controlled trials (RCTs) involving 1248 neurocritical care patients compared intensive insulin therapy (IIT) with conventional techniques of glycemic control among patients with traumatic brain injury, ischemic or hemorrhagic stroke, anoxic encephalopathy, central nervous system infections, or spinal cord injury. Glycemic targets with IIT ranged from 70 to 140 mg/dL (3.9–7.8 mmol/L), while conventional protocols aimed to keep glucose levels below 144–300 mg/dL (8.0–16.7 mmol/L). These studies indicate that IIT carries a significant hypoglycemic risk and does influence mortality among neurocritical care patients. Liberal glucose control was associated with worse neurological recovery and was preferred to be avoided. These results suggest that intermediate glycemic goals [threshold for insulin administration: 140–180 mg/dL (7.8–10.0 mmol/L)] may be the most appropriate target [20]. The currently available clinical evidence supports the use of IIT therapy among patients in the NCC. In this subset, a target BGC range of 90–140 mg/dL helps reduce the incidence of iatrogenic-induced hypoglycemia.

Among the NCC patients, insulin infusion therapy should be initiated at a BGC ≥180 mg/dL. This should be titrated and stopped at a BGC ≤140 mg/dL. Few studies recommend IIT to manage BGC in NCC patients [10, 14, 21].

21.1.9 Nutrition [Enteral Nutrition (EN) and Parenteral Nutrition (PN)]

The timely institution of adequate nutrition is warranted in NCC. Therefore, EN or PN should be started when indicated, particularly as continuous EN/PN if IIT is instituted. The recent Brain Trauma Foundation guidelines recommend initiating appropriate nutritional support no later than the fifth day and at least by the seventh day after injury in patients with severe TBI to reduce mortality [22].

21.1.10 Clinical Pitfalls

The current debate focuses on whether to implement strict glycemic control or not. Instead, the focus must shift to a more individual, patient-targeted management approach. The focus should change from a systemic perspective to a more clinical, target organ–based assessment through advanced neuromonitoring systems, such as cerebral microdialysis, in neurocritical patients. The management approaches may significantly vary for diabetic hyperglycemia and stress-induced hyperglycemia, and both should be managed through different techniques in the critically ill. A targeted, value-driven approach should be replaced by glucose variability control, whose relevance over existing targets remains to be elucidated and is a potential area for future research. The key take-home points for consideration are as follows.

1. A history of diabetes and hemoglobin A1C levels (when available) may help guide management.
2. Measuring glucose from drawn blood may be more accurate than a fingerstick glucose. More frequent monitoring may be warranted in those with higher glycemic variability.
3. Avoid being dogmatic about specific glucose targets. In the current scenario, there cannot be a single number-based target.
4. Efforts to reduce glucose should be gentle and cautious. Avoid overdosing of insulin.
5. Run intensive insulin therapy when an effective nutrition supplementation is established.
6. Stop insulin infusion when BGC is lowering and reaches values <140 mg/dL to prevent iatrogenic-induced hypoglycemic episodes [23].
7. To reduce BGC variability, continuous PN or EN with continuous glucose monitoring should be used.
8. Short-acting insulin formulation has a quicker onset and offset time than regular insulin formulation and is, hence, preferred.
9. Insulin infusions require mandatory continuous hourly glucose monitoring.
10. Careful insulin titration is essential when patients are made nil per oral and during steroid discontinuation to avoid hypoglycemia.

21.2 Conclusion

A "personalized" approach to glycemic control in the critically ill, with recognition of preadmission glycemia, is supported by an emerging literature. The evidence in NCC supports BGC values <146 mg/dL with IIT and concurrent, appropriate, ongoing nutrition therapies. Future evaluation of "closed-loop systems" that regulate caloric supply and insulin infusion titrated by a "real-time," continuous BGC monitor might further contribute to optimizing clinical management.

References

1. Van den Berghe G, Wouters P, Weekers F, et al. Intensive insulin therapy in critically ill patients. N Engl J Med. 2001;345(19):1359–67.
2. van den Berghe G, Wilmer A, Milants I, et al. Intensive insulin therapy in mixed medical/surgical intensive care units: benefit versus harm. Diabetes. 2006;55(11):3151–9.
3. Brunkhorst FM, Engel C, Bloos F, et al. Intensive insulin therapy and pentastarch resuscitation in severe sepsis. N Engl J Med. 2008;358(2):125–39. https://doi.org/10.1056/NEJMoa070716.
4. NICE-SUGAR Study Investigators, Finfer S, Chittock DR, et al. Intensive versus conventional glucose control in critically ill patients. N Engl J Med. 2009;360(13):1283–97. https://doi.org/10.1056/NEJMoa0810625.

5. NICE-SUGAR Study Investigators, Finfer S, Liu B, et al. Hypoglycemia and risk of death in critically ill patients. N Engl J Med. 2012;367(12):1108–18. https://doi.org/10.1056/NEJMoa1204942.
6. Bilotta F, Rosa G. Glucose management in the neurosurgical patient: are we yet any closer? Curr Opin Anaesthesiol. 2010;23(5):539–43.
7. Amaral AI. Effects of hypoglycaemia on neuronal metabolism in the adult brain: role of alternative substrates to glucose. J Inherit Metab Dis. 2013;36(4):621–34.
8. Bilotta F, Giovannini F, Caramia R, Rosa G. Glycemia management in neurocritical care patients: a review. J Neurosurg Anesthesiol. 2009;21(1):2–9.
9. Jauch-Chara K, Oltmanns KM. Glycemic control after brain injury: boon and bane for the brain. Neuroscience. 2014;283:202–9.
10. Bilotta F, Rosa G. Glycemia management in critical care patients. World J Diabetes. 2012;3(7):130–4.
11. Bilotta F, Caramia R, Cernak I, et al. Intensive insulin therapy after severe traumatic brain injury: a randomized clinical trial. Neurocrit Care. 2008;9(2):159–66. https://doi.org/10.1007/s12028-008-9084-9.
12. Yuksel S, Altun Ugras G, Sirin K, Turan Y, Kurucu S. Stress hyperglycemia and glycemic control in critical neurosurgical patients: a retrospective study. Annals of Medical Research. 2020;27(9):2298–2305.
13. Kruyt ND, Biessels GJ, DeVries JH, et al. Hyperglycemia in aneurysmal subarachnoid hemorrhage: a potentially modifiable risk factor for poor outcome. J Cereb Blood Flow Metab. 2010;30(9):1577–87. https://doi.org/10.1038/jcbfm.2010.102.
14. Bilotta F, Spinelli A, Giovannini F, Doronzio A, Delfini R, Rosa G. The effect of intensive insulin therapy on infection rate, vasospasm, neurologic outcome, and mortality in neuroin tensive care unit after intracranial aneurysm clipping in patients with acute subarachnoid hemorrhage: a randomized prospective pilot trial. J Neurosurg Anesthesiol. 2007;19(3):156–60. https://doi.org/10.1097/ANA.0b013e3180338e69.
15. Hoh BL, Ko NU, Amin-Hanjani S, et al. 2023 guideline for the management of patients with aneurysmal subarachnoid hemorrhage: a guideline from the American Heart Association/American Stroke Association [published correction appears in Stroke. 2023;54(12):e516. https://doi.org/10.1161/STR.0000000000000449]. Stroke. 2023;54(7):e314–70. https://doi.org/10.1161/STR.0000000000000436.
16. MK MI, Halabi M, Li B, et al. Glycemic indices predict outcomes after aneurysmal subarachnoid hemorrhage: a retrospective single center comparative analysis. Sci Rep. 2021;11(1):158. Published 2021 Jan 8. https://doi.org/10.1038/s41598-020-80513-9.
17. Li S, Wang Y, Wang W, et al. Stress hyperglycemia is predictive of clinical outcomes in patients with spontaneous intracerebral hemorrhage. BMC Neurol. 2022;22:236. https://doi.org/10.1186/s12883-022-02760-9.
18. Huang YW, Li ZP, Yin XS. Stress hyperglycemia and risk of adverse outcomes in patients with acute ischemic stroke: a systematic review and dose-response meta-analysis of cohort studies. Front Neurol. 2023;14:1219863. https://doi.org/10.3389/fneur.2023.1219863.
19. Kramer AH, Roberts DJ, Zygun DA. Optimal glycemic control in neurocritical care patients: a systematic review and meta-analysis. Crit Care. 2012;16(5):R203. Published 2012 Oct 22. https://doi.org/10.1186/cc11812.
20. Bilotta F, Badenes R, Lolli S, Belda FJ, Einav S, Rosa G. Insulin infusion therapy in critical care patients: regular insulin vs short-acting insulin. A prospective, crossover, randomized, multicenter blind study. J Crit Care. 2015;30(2):437.e1–6.
21. Carney N, Totten AM, O'Reilly C, et al. Guidelines for the management of severe traumatic brain injury. Neurosurgery. 2017;80(1):6–15.
22. Bilotta F, Qeva E, Prete A, Pugliese F. Clinical relevance of blood glucose concentration and hyperglycemia management in Neurocritical Care Patients. J Neuroanaesth Crit Care. 2019;06:087–95. https://doi.org/10.1055/s-0039-1689069.
23. McDonnell ME, Umpierrez GE. Insulin therapy for the management of hyperglycemia in hospitalized patients. Endocrinol Metab Clin N Am. 2012;41(1):175–201. https://doi.org/10.1016/j.ecl.2012.01.001.

Controversies in Thromboprophylaxis in Neurocritical Care

22

Ajay Prasad Hrishi, R. P. Sangeetha, and S. Rakul Prasath

Abstract

Controversies around critical care practices have prevailed since time unknown. This includes the management of coagulation status and the administration of thromboprophylaxis (TP). Extensive research remains ongoing in these areas to provide the best possible practice guidelines, especially for the neurocritically ill. Here, this chapter will take you through the different phases of evidence available in the literature concerning this clinically important preventive and therapeutic intervention. The prevention of venous thromboembolism (VTE) in susceptible populations is crucial to improve patient morbidity and mortality. However, TP-induced benefits need careful balancing with its potential complications, which are, in turn, contributory to life-threatening haemorrhage. The evidence-based guideline provided by the Neurocritical Care Society (NCS) provides useful insights to safely reduce the burden of VTE, with the avoidance of its associated complications. We try to provide the best possible solutions to this commonly faced controversy and focus on the possible areas of future research prospects. In this chapter, we delve deep into the controversies of this aspect of patient management and attempt to inform the best approach to patient care in each scenario.

Keywords

Thromboprophylaxis · Neurocritical care · Heparin · Thromboembolism Haemorrhage

A. P. Hrishi
Department of Anaesthesiology, Sree Chitra Tirunal Institute for Medical Sciences and Technology, Trivandrum, Kerala, India

R. P. Sangeetha (✉) · S. Rakul Prasath
Neuroanaesthesia and Neurocritical Care, National Institute of Mental Health and Neurosciences, Bangalore, Karnataka, India

P. U. Bidkar, M. Krishnakumar (eds.), *Controversies in Neurocritical Care*,
https://doi.org/10.1007/978-981-95-4419-6_22

22.1 Introduction

Controversies in neurocritical care (NCC) prevail in the face of ongoing research that supports and challenges the current management practices in various patient care arenas. The management of coagulation status in the backdrop of thromboprophylaxis (TP) is one such controversy, which requires a case-based approach. Ideal beneficiaries are difficult to define for the uniform application of different thromboprophylaxis techniques across different diagnoses and time points of care. A combination of the definitive indication, the phase of illness, the haematological and coagulation status, the need for imminent invasive intervention, and time since previous intervention, such as surgery, epidural catheter, or central vascular access, all have the potential to impact the decision to either consider or delay the institution of pharmacological thromboprophylaxis. The treatment decision revolves around patient-centred and disease-targeted factors for each patient during each phase of the critical illness. Despite the ongoing extensive research in this arena to provide the best possible practice guidelines, ambiguity persists concerning the modality and intensity of treatment, frequency and thresholds for coagulation monitoring, and the duration of therapies. This chapter will explore the different sources of evidence available in the literature concerning this potentially life-saving intervention. We suggest the best possible practices for this routinely encountered controversy and focus on the potential areas of future research prospects.

Thromboprophylaxis (TP) in neurocritical care (NCC) remains an extensively debated grey area in managing acute post-neurosurgical and chronic neurological patients. The decision to administer TP, the modality, and the dose depend on the patient's predisposition to thrombotic and thromboembolic complications. A systematic, case-based approach ensures a maximum benefit versus risk ratio to ensure therapeutic gain with minimal clinical side effects.

A recent cross-sectional survey that evaluated the current practices among neurointensivists informs that nearly 53% of respondents practise thromboprophylaxis with a lesser zeal in NCC compared to the general critical care setting. A wide variation in its execution exists across different diagnoses [1].

22.1.1 Risk Stratification for Thromboembolism (TE)

Two different approaches are recognised for TE risk stratification. The first approach is the default administration of standardised thromboprophylaxis to the entire cohort of patients, such as neurosurgery, after ruling out the contraindications. The key deciding parameter is the patient's primary reason for hospitalisation. However, there exists extreme variability in VTE incidence based on several patient-specific factors. This calls for a second approach that assesses the individual VTE risk of patients and their risk factors, in addition to their morbidity level at presentation or the definitive interventions planned. Diagnosis-based guidelines provided by the Neurocritical Care Society (NCS) in 2016 remain the most recent reckoners to refer for TP in NCC, lacking further updates [2].

22.1.2 Low-Dose Heparin (LDH) Versus Low-Molecular-Weight Heparin (LMWH)

LDH has remained the default thromboprophylaxis of choice, with an effective reduction of VTE in a varied spectrum of patients for more than three decades [3]. Although the efficacy and safety profiles of LDH and LMWH are similar among NCC patients, LMWH is more efficacious than LDH after significant trauma [4]. LMWH fares better than LDH owing to the requirement of fewer doses in a day and a lesser risk of heparin-induced thrombocytopenia [5].

22.1.3 Decision on the Duration of TP

This aspect remains unknown for most hospitalised patients, exposing the need for more research in this area. Post-discharge thromboprophylaxis, especially for those with relatively brief hospital stays (hence shorter prophylaxis), requires consideration [6]. For most neurosurgical diagnoses, the NCS recommends thromboprophylaxis for the entire duration of hospitalization during the acute phase of brain injury [2].

22.1.4 Combined Versus Single Modalities for TP

Mechanical TP modalities, such as graduated compression stockings (GCSs) and intermittent pneumatic compression (IPC) devices, do not fare better than anticoagulant prophylaxis owing to several limitations.

These devices lack pre-established standardisation in terms of their size or application pressure [6]. This mandates resources and attempts to ensure their use to the maximum benefit.

Their non-predisposition to bleeding per se and the feasibility of combining them with pharmacological prophylaxis have demonstrated their efficacy as an effective deep vein thrombosis (DVT) prevention strategy in clinical trials and scenarios [7, 8].

Among patients with significant trauma who have a significant bleeding risk at presentation, initial mechanical prophylaxis preceding LMWH-based anticoagulant prophylaxis, when deemed safe, appears to be an optimal strategy in postoperative conditions associated with a high risk of bleeding [9].

Dual-mode TP, combining pharmacological and non-pharmacological methods, has also been used [10].

22.1.5 New Oral Anticoagulants Versus Heparin and Heparinoids in Thromboprophylaxis

The advent of new oral anticoagulants, such as factor Xa inhibitors like rivaroxaban and thrombin inhibitors like dabigatran, that do not need laboratory monitoring represents a significant advantage for thromboprophylaxis. These have similar or greater efficacy than standard LMWH, with comparable safety [11, 12]. These agents have a simplified regimen in terms of once-daily dosing, a lack of daily injections, and an absent requirement for international normalized ratio (INR) monitoring. This is especially advantageous among hospital-discharged patients [13].

22.1.6 Neurocritical Care Society Guidelines, 2016 [2]

In post-craniotomy patients, a strong recommendation is for mechanical thromboprophylaxis using intermittent pneumatic compression (IPC) or graduated compression stockings (GCS) in the perioperative period. Pharmacological thromboprophylaxis should be considered following the elapse of at least 24 h postoperatively, especially among high-risk populations, only after confirming haemostasis. Thromboprophylaxis needs to be continued till hospital discharge.

In patients with aneurysmal rupture–induced subarachnoid hemorrhage (SAH), for surgery, unfractionated heparin (UFH) is found to supersede LDH. Strong recommendations advocate the use of IPC-based mechanical thromboprophylaxis at hospital admission. UFH is weakly recommended 24 h after clipping and immediately after coiling among patients undergoing clipping or coiling of ruptured aneurysm, respectively.

In all patients with ischaemic stroke, early mobilisation and good hydration are strongly recommended. In stroke patients with restricted or no mobility (strong recommendation), pharmacological prophylaxis, LMWH/LDH, is started immediately (unless there is a contraindication to anticoagulants). LMWH is preferred to UFH. Pharmacological prophylaxis should be started within 48 h of stroke and continued for 2 weeks. Watch for haemorrhagic transformation in CT scan—an indication to stop anticoagulation. Aspirin can be used concurrently with other pharmacological thromboprophylaxis but is not used as sole therapy in stroke patients undergoing decompressive procedures. UFH/LMWH with/without IPC is preferred immediately post-surgery, except when a patient has received recombinant tissue plasminogen activator (TPA). If TPA is started, delay pharmacological methods for 24 h. Here is a strong recommendation for mechanical thromboprophylaxis in patients with stroke as a stand-alone therapy, using IPC and GCS only when pharmacological prophylaxis (PP) is contraindicated.

In patients with traumatic brain injury (TBI), pharmacological thromboprophylaxis using LMWH/LDH is to be used 24–48 h after TBI or 24 h after craniotomy only in a stable brain injury if its benefits outweigh the possibility of intracranial haemorrhage (ICH).

In patients with ICH, in addition to IPC and GCS, prophylactic UFH/LMWH is administered only for a stable haematoma or normal coagulation status.

22.2 Conclusion

The prevention of VTE in vulnerable populations is crucial to improve patient morbidity and mortality. However, TPP-induced benefits need careful balancing with its potential complications, which are, in turn, contributory to life-threatening haemorrhage. The evidence-based guideline using the grading of recommendations assessment, development and evaluation (GRADE) provided by the Neurocritical Care Society provides useful insights to safely reduce the burden of VTE, with the avoidance of its associated complications.

References

1. Sinha S, Ahuja B, Pandit R, Mishra R, Chatterjee R, Choudhuri AH. Thromboprophylaxis practices in neurocritical care-a cross-sectional survey among neurocritical care practitioners. Indian J Anaesth. 2023;67(8):703–7. https://doi.org/10.4103/ija.ija_862_22.
2. Nyquist P, Bautista C, Jichici D, et al. Prophylaxis of venous thrombosis in neurocritical care patients: an evidence-based guideline: a statement for healthcare professionals from the neurocritical Care Society. Neurocrit Care. 2016;24(1):47–60.
3. Collins R, Scrimgeour A, Yusuf S. Reduction in fatal pulmonary embolism and venous thrombosis by perioperative administration of subcutaneous heparin: overview of results of randomized trials in general, orthopedic, and urologic surgery. N Engl J Med. 1988;318:1162–73.
4. Geerts WH, Bergqvist D, Pineo GF, et al. Prevention of venous thromboembolism: American college of chest physicians evidence-based clinical practice guidelines (8th Edition). Chest. 2008;133:381S–443S.
5. Martel N, Lee J, Wells PS. Risk for heparin-induced thrombocytopenia with unfractionated and low molecular-weight heparin thromboprophylaxis: a metaanalysis. Blood. 2005;106:2710–5.
6. Selby R, Geerts W. Prevention of venous thromboembolism: consensus, controversies, and challenges. Hematology Am Soc Hematol Educ Program. 2009:286–92. https://doi.org/10.1182/asheducation-2009.1.286.
7. Best AJ, Williams S, Crozier A, Bhatt R, Gregg PJ, Hui AC. Graded compression stockings in elective orthopaedic surgery. An assessment of the in vivo performance of commercially available stockings in patients having hip and knee arthroplasty. J Bone Joint Surg Br. 2000;82:116–8.
8. Wille-Jørgensen P, Rasmussen MS, Andersen BR, Borly L. Heparins and mechanical methods for thromboprophylaxis in colorectal surgery. Cochrane Database Syst Rev. 2003;(4):CD001217.
9. Turpie AG, Bauer KA, Caprini JA, Comp PC, Gent M, Muntz JE, Apollo Investigators. Fondaparinux combined with intermittent pneumatic compression vs. intermittent pneumatic compression alone for prevention of venous thromboembolism after abdominal surgery: a randomized, double-blind comparison. J Thromb Haemost. 2007;5:1854–61.
10. Khan NR, Patel PG, Sharpe JP, Lee SL, Sorenson J. Chemical venous thromboembolism prophylaxis in neurosurgical patients: an updated systematic review and meta-analysis. J Neurosurg. 2018;129(4):906–15.
11. Henwood PC, Kennedy TM, Thomson L, et al. The incidence of deep vein thrombosis detected by routine surveillance ultrasound in neurosurgery patients receiving dual modality prophylaxis. J Thromb Thrombolysis. 2011;32(2):209–14.
12. Abrams PJ, Emerson CR. Rivaroxaban: a novel, oral, direct factor Xa inhibitor. Pharmacotherapy. 2009;29:167–81.
13. Eriksson BI, Quinlan DJ, Weitz JI. Comparative pharmacodynamics and pharmacokinetics of oral direct thrombin and factor Xa inhibitors in development. Clin Pharmacokinet. 2009;48:1–22.

Scoring Systems in the Neuro ICU

23

Shweta S. Naik, R. P. Sangeetha, and Amruta Nirale

Abstract

Scoring systems play a pivotal role in neurocritical care by providing structured methodologies to assess disease severity, guide therapeutic interventions, and predict patient outcomes. This chapter delves into the evolution, applications, and limitations of widely used scoring systems in the neuro ICU, such as the Glasgow Coma Scale (GCS), FOUR) Score, and the Hunt and Hess Scale, among others. It critically examines key controversies, including the reliability and predictive accuracy of these tools, their applicability across diverse clinical scenarios, and the challenges of incorporating biomarkers and advanced technologies like machine learning. Furthermore, the chapter explores the debate surrounding the need for neuro-specific scoring systems versus adaptations of general ICU tools and discusses future directions, such as real-time integration with electronic health records and personalized scoring models. These discussions aim to refine the clinical utility of scoring systems and enhance patient outcomes in neurocritical care.

Keywords

Scoring system · FOUR · GCS · Traumatic brain injury · Neuro ICU

S. S. Naik (✉) · R. P. Sangeetha
Department of Neuroanaesthesia and Neurocritical care, NIMHANS, Bengaluru, Karnataka, India

A. Nirale
Neuroanaesthesia, Trustwell Hospital, Bengaluru, Karnataka, India

P. U. Bidkar, M. Krishnakumar (eds.), *Controversies in Neurocritical Care*,
https://doi.org/10.1007/978-981-95-4419-6_23

Controversies in Scoring Systems in Neurocritical Care

1. *Predictive Accuracy*: Limited long-term outcome prediction and a lack of biomarkers.
2. *Generalizability*: Challenges in diverse settings and limited neuro-specific tools.
3. *Inter-rater Variability*: Subjectivity and inconsistency in scoring.
4. *Tool Complexity*: Barriers to use in emergencies and resource-limited settings.
5. *Stroke-Specific Tools*: National Institutes of Health Stroke Scale (NIHSS) bias toward anterior strokes and imaging variability in Alberta Stroke Program Early CT Score (ASPECTS).
6. *Static Nature*: Inability to reflect evolving patient conditions.
7. *Biomarker Integration*: High costs, poor standardization, and limited accessibility.
8. *Imaging Reliance*: Subjectivity and a lack of clinical severity incorporation.

23.1 Introduction to Scoring Systems

Scoring systems are integral tools in the neuro intensive care unit (neuro ICU), providing structured methods for evaluating the severity of neurological injuries, guiding clinical decisions, and predicting patient outcomes. Historically, these systems have evolved from simple observational scales to complex models incorporating various physiological and clinical parameters. Their role in neurocritical care has expanded as our understanding of neurological pathophysiology and critical care management has deepened.

The development of scoring systems dates back to the introduction of the Glasgow Coma Scale (GCS) in the 1970s, which provided a standardized method to assess consciousness in traumatic brain injury (TBI) patients [1]. Since then, numerous scoring systems have been developed, each aiming to address specific clinical needs and improve prognostic accuracy. Despite their utility, these systems are not without controversies, particularly concerning their predictive accuracy, applicability across diverse clinical scenarios, and the need for neuro-specific adaptations.

23.2 Commonly Used Scoring Systems

23.2.1 Traumatic Brain Injury (TBI)

23.2.1.1 Glasgow Coma Scale (GCS)

The GCS, widely used for assessing consciousness levels in TBI patients, evaluates eye, verbal, and motor responses, providing a score ranging from 3 to 15. However, there is significant variability in inter-rater reliability, especially in nonspecialist settings, which can affect the consistency of patient assessment [2]. The GCS is also insufficient for intubated or sedated patients, as it does not account for brain stem function and lacks a detailed neurological assessment [3]. Consequently, there is ongoing debate about whether the Full Outline of UnResponsiveness (FOUR) Score should replace GCS in certain scenarios due to its comprehensive nature, which includes brain stem reflexes and respiratory patterns [4].

23.2.1.2 Glasgow Coma Scale–Pupils (GCS-P)

The GCS-P is a modification of the GCS that includes pupil reactivity to enhance prognostic accuracy. Despite its potential, the GCS-P has limited validation in diverse clinical settings, raising concerns about its generalizability [5]. Additionally, the inclusion of pupil reactivity adds complexity, and reliable assessment may not always be feasible in emergency situations [6]. While GCS-P has the potential to improve predictive accuracy over GCS, further research is needed to confirm its effectiveness and facilitate widespread acceptance [7].

23.2.2 Full Outline of UnResponsiveness (FOUR) Score

The FOUR Score was developed to provide a more detailed neurological assessment, including brain stem reflexes and respiratory patterns. However, it is less familiar to many clinicians compared to the GCS, and there are concerns about the consistency and training required for its use [8]. Furthermore, the FOUR Score is more complex and time-consuming, which may hinder its adoption in emergency settings [9]. Despite these challenges, the FOUR Score provides a comprehensive neurological assessment, making it potentially superior to the GCS in certain TBI cases [10].

23.2.3 Subarachnoid Hemorrhage (SAH)

23.2.3.1 Hunt and Hess Scale

The Hunt and Hess Scale categorizes SAH patients into five grades based on clinical presentation, ranging from mild headache to deep coma and decerebrate posturing. However, the subjectivity in assessment leads to significant interobserver variability [11]. Additionally, the scale has poor correlation with long-term outcomes [12]. There are calls for developing a more objective and reproducible scoring system to improve the consistency of SAH severity assessment [13].

23.2.3.2 The World Federation of Neurosurgical Societies (WFNS) Scoring System

This scoring system incorporates both the Glasgow Coma Scale (GCS) score and the presence of focal neurological deficits to categorize patients into five grades. One major issue is the variability in inter-rater reliability, particularly concerning the assessment of focal neurological deficits. This can lead to inconsistent grading and potentially impact clinical decision-making and outcomes. Additionally, the WFNS scale has been criticized for its limited predictive value in long-term outcomes, as it primarily focuses on the initial neurological status without incorporating other critical factors such as patient age, comorbidities, and the extent of the hemorrhage. Some studies have suggested that combining the WFNS scale with other scoring systems or biomarkers may improve its prognostic accuracy, but this approach has yet to be universally accepted and standardized in clinical practice [14].

23.2.3.3 Modified Fisher Scale

The Modified Fisher Scale is an improvement over the original Fisher Scale, incorporating the presence of intraventricular hemorrhage. Despite its advancements, the scale still relies heavily on imaging findings, which can vary in interpretation [15]. While it includes the assessment of intraventricular hemorrhage, it may not fully capture the clinical severity of SAH [16]. The Modified Fisher Scale is an improvement over its predecessor, but further refinement and clinical correlation are needed to enhance its utility [17].

23.2.4 Stroke (Ischemic and Hemorrhagic)

23.2.4.1 National Institutes of Health Stroke Scale (NIHSS)

The NIHSS is a comprehensive tool for assessing the severity of stroke based on neurological deficits. However, the scale emphasizes anterior circulation strokes and is less sensitive to posterior circulation strokes [18]. The complex and time-consuming nature of the NIHSS can be a hindrance in acute settings [19]. There is an ongoing debate about simplifying the NIHSS or developing separate scales for different types of strokes to improve its applicability [20].

23.2.5 Alberta Stroke Program Early CT Score (ASPECTS)

ASPECTS is used to quantify early ischemic changes on CT scans in patients with acute ischemic stroke. Its reliance on imaging interpretations can lead to variability in scoring [21]. Moreover, ASPECTS is not universally applicable to all stroke patients, particularly those with posterior circulation involvement [22]. ASPECTS is valuable for early stroke assessment but needs further validation across diverse populations and stroke types [23].

23.2.6 Intracerebral Hemorrhage (ICH)

23.2.6.1 ICH Score

The ICH Score is a widely used tool for assessing the severity of intracerebral hemorrhage based on clinical and radiological findings. However, the score's limited scope does not account for evolving clinical and radiological changes, making it less dynamic [24]. As a static measure, the ICH Score may not reflect the dynamic nature of patient status over time [25]. There are arguments for developing a dynamic or serial assessment approach to better predict outcomes and guide management in ICH patients [26].

23.2.7 General Neurocritical Care

23.2.7.1 APACHE II and SAPS II

Both acute physiology and chronic health evaluation II (APACHE II) and simplified acute physiology score II (SAPS II) are general ICU scoring systems that have been applied to neurocritical care. These scores may not accurately reflect neuro-specific morbidity and mortality due to the lack of neuro-specific variables [27]. Their poor predictive power in neuro ICU settings limits their utility for neurocritical patients [28]. There is an ongoing debate about developing neuro-specific severity scores versus adapting existing ones to better suit the needs of neuro ICU patients [29].

23.2.8 SOFA Score

The sequential organ failure assessment (SOFA) Score is used to track a patient's status during their ICU stay and determine the extent of organ function or rate of failure. However, the underrepresentation of neurological dysfunction in the SOFA scoring criteria is a significant limitation [30]. The SOFA Score primarily focuses on multi-organ failure, without adequate emphasis on the neurological status [31]. Suggestions have been made to modify the SOFA Score to better accommodate neuro ICU patients and accurately reflect their neurological status [9]. Another point of contention is the broad focus of these scoring systems, which are not tailored to the specific pathophysiological nuances of neurocritical patients. For instance, APACHE II and SOFA are designed for general ICU populations, which may not capture the intricacies of neurological deterioration. This lack of specificity can lead to misclassification and inappropriate management decisions.

23.2.9 Integration of Biomarkers

The integration of biomarkers into scoring systems presents both an opportunity and a challenge. Biomarkers such as neuron-specific enolase (NSE), glial fibrillary acidic protein (GFAP), and S100 calcium-binding protein B (S100B) have shown promise in enhancing the prognostic accuracy of traditional scores [32]. However, the standardization of these biomarkers and their routine incorporation into clinical practice remain contentious issues. The reliability, cost-effectiveness, and accessibility of these biomarkers are critical factors that need to be addressed before they can be widely adopted in clinical settings [33]. A summary of the various neuro-specific scoring systems, with their sensitivity and specificity (Fig. 23.1) and their pros and cons (Table 23.1), is provided at the end of the chapter.

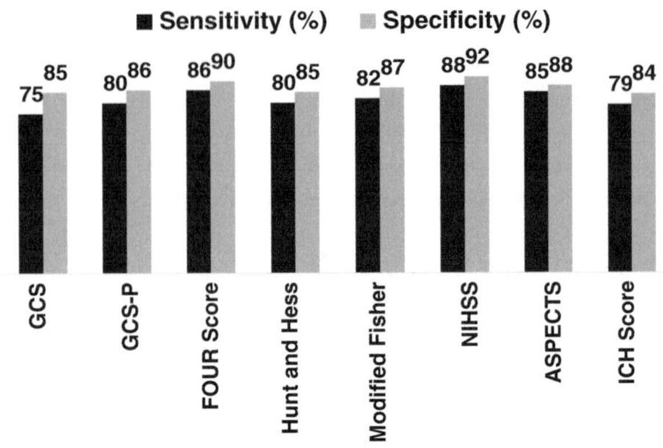

Fig. 23.1 Sensitivity and specificity of neuro-specific scoring systems

Table 23.1 Advantages and disadvantages of neuro-specific scoring systems

Scoring system	Advantages	Disadvantages
GCS	Widely used and understood; simple and quick to apply	Variability in inter-rater reliability; insufficient for intubated or sedated patients; lacks detailed brain stem assessment
GCS-P	Includes pupil reactivity, enhancing prognostic accuracy	Limited validation in diverse clinical settings; adds complexity; pupil reactivity may not always be reliably assessed
FOUR score	Comprehensive neurological assessment; includes brain stem reflexes and respiratory patterns	Less familiar to clinicians; requires more training; more complex and time-consuming
WFNS	Combines GCS and focal neurological deficits; widely used for SAH	Variability in inter-rater reliability; limited predictive value for long-term outcomes
Hunt and Hess scale	Simple and easy to use; commonly used for SAH severity	Subjectivity in assessment; significant interobserver variability; poor correlation with long-term outcomes
Modified fisher scale	Incorporates intraventricular hemorrhage; improved over the original fisher scale	Relies heavily on imaging findings, which can vary in interpretation; may not fully capture clinical severity
NIHSS	Comprehensive tool for stroke severity; highly predictive for outcomes	Emphasizes anterior circulation strokes; less sensitive to posterior circulation strokes; complex and time-consuming
ASPECTS	Quantifies early ischemic changes on CT; valuable for early stroke assessment	Relies on imaging interpretations, leading to variability; not applicable to all stroke patients, particularly those with posterior circulation involvement
ICH score	Widely used for assessing ICH severity; combines clinical and radiological findings	Limited scope; does not account for evolving clinical and radiological changes; static measure may not reflect dynamic patient status

23.3 Future Directions

23.3.1 Emerging Trends and New Developments

The future of scoring systems in neurocritical care lies in the integration of advanced technologies such as machine learning (ML) and the inclusion of emerging biomarkers. ML models can analyze vast amounts of data, identify patterns, and provide personalized prognostic insights that surpass traditional scoring methods. For instance, ML algorithms can incorporate a multitude of variables, including clinical parameters, imaging data, and biomarkers, to predict outcomes with higher accuracy and granularity [34].

23.3.2 Personalized Scoring Systems

Personalized scoring systems, driven by ML, have the potential to revolutionize neurocritical care. These systems can adapt to the unique characteristics of individual patients, providing tailored risk assessments and treatment recommendations. However, the implementation of these systems requires rigorous validation and integration into clinical workflows to ensure their efficacy and safety [35].

23.3.3 Integration with Electronic Health Records (EHRs)

Utilizing EHRs to automatically calculate and update scores in real time offers significant advantages for accurate, efficient, and comprehensive patient monitoring. The integration of EHRs with scoring systems can streamline the assessment process and ensure that up-to-date information is readily available to clinicians [36].

23.3.4 Validation and Standardization

The need for ongoing validation and standardization of scoring systems across different neurocritical care populations is crucial. Establishing universally accepted guidelines and protocols for the implementation of scoring systems will help ensure their reliability and comparability across various clinical settings [37].

23.4 Conclusion

Scoring systems are indispensable in neurocritical care, offering valuable tools for prognosis and clinical decision-making. However, the controversies surrounding their predictive accuracy, specificity, and integration with emerging biomarkers underscore the need for ongoing research and refinement. Neuro-specific scores such as the FOUR Score, NIHSS, and the Hunt and Hess Scale provide more tailored assessments for neurological conditions, addressing some of the limitations of traditional scoring systems. The future integration of machine learning holds promise for developing personalized, dynamic scoring models that enhance patient outcomes and optimize resource allocation in neurocritical care.

References

1. Jennett B, Teasdale G. Assessment of coma and impaired consciousness: a practical scale. Lancet. 1974;2(7872):81–4.
2. Reith FC, Van den Brande R, Synnot A, Gruen R, Maas AI. The reliability of the Glasgow coma scale: a systematic review. Intensive Care Med. 2016;42(1):3–15.
3. Fearnside MR, Cook RJ, McDougall P, RJ MN. The Westmead head injury project outcome in severe head injury. A comparative analysis of pre-hospital, clinical and CT variables. Br J Neurosurg. 1993;7(3):267–79.
4. Wijdicks EF, Bamlet WR, Maramattom BV, Manno EM, McClelland RL. Validation of a new coma scale: the FOUR score. Ann Neurol. 2005;58(4):585–93.
5. Fischer J, Mathieson C. The history of the Glasgow coma scale: implications for practice. Crit Care Nurs Q. 2001;23(4):52–8.
6. Kelly CA, Upex A, Bateman DN. Comparison of consciousness level assessment in the poisoned patient using the Glasgow coma scale and the alert/verbal/painful/unresponsive scale. Resuscitation. 2004;61(1):117–20.
7. Brennan PM, Murray GD, Teasdale GM. Simplifying the use of prognostic information in traumatic brain injury. Part 1: the GCS-pupils score: an extended Glasgow coma scale. J Neurosurg. 2018;129(4):945–54.
8. Stead LG, Wijdicks EF, Bhagra A, Kashyap RS, Bellolio MF, Nash DL, Enduri S, Schears G. Validation of a new coma scale, the FOUR score, in the emergency department. Neurocrit Care. 2009;10(1):50–4.
9. Iyer VN, Mandrekar JN, Danielson RD, Zubkov AY, Elmer JL, Wijdicks EF. Validity of the FOUR score coma scale in the medical intensive care unit. Mayo Clin Proc. 2009;84(8):694–701.
10. Fugate JE, Rabinstein AA, Claassen DO, White RD, Wijdicks EF. The FOUR score predicts outcome in patients after traumatic brain injury. Neurocrit Care. 2010;12(1):44–9.
11. Hunt WE, Hess RM. Surgical risk as related to time of intervention in the repair of intracranial aneurysms. J Neurosurg. 1968;28(1):14–20.
12. Gruber A, Reinprecht A, Illievich UM, Fitzgerald R, Dietrich W, Czech T, Richling B. Evaluation of cerebral vasospasm after early surgical and endovascular treatment of ruptured intracranial aneurysms. Neurosurgery. 1998;42(2):258–68.
13. Van Gijn J, Kerr RS, Rinkel GJ. Subarachnoid haemorrhage. Lancet. 2007;369(9558):306–18.
14. Rosen DS, Macdonald RL. Subarachnoid hemorrhage grading scales: a systematic review. Neurocrit Care. 2005;2(2):110–8.
15. Frontera JA, Claassen J, Schmidt JM, Wartenberg KE, Temes R, Connolly ES Jr, MacDonald RL, Mayer SA. Prediction of symptomatic vasospasm after subarachnoid hemorrhage: the modified fisher scale. Neurosurgery. 2006;59(1):21–7.
16. Connolly ES Jr, Rabinstein AA, Carhuapoma JR, Derdeyn CP, Dion J, Higashida RT, Hoh BL, Kirkness CJ, Naidech AM, Ogilvy CS, Patel AB, Thompson BG, Vespa P, American Heart Association Stroke Council, Council on Cardiovascular Radiology and Intervention; Council on Cardiovascular Nursing; Council on Cardiovascular Surgery and Anesthesia; and Council on Clinical Cardiology. Guidelines for the management of aneurysmal subarachnoid hemorrhage: a guideline for healthcare professionals from the American heart association/American stroke association. Stroke. 2012;43(6):1711–37.
17. Lovelock CE, Molyneux AJ, Rothwell PM. Early complications of subarachnoid hemorrhage and outcome. Lancet Neurol. 2010;9(3):311–24.

18. Brott T, Adams HP Jr, Olinger CP, Marler JR, Barsan WG, Biller J, Spilker J, Holleran R, Eberle R, Hertzberg V. Measurements of acute cerebral infarction: a clinical examination scale. Stroke. 1989;20(7):864–70.
19. Lyden P, Brott T, Tilley B, Welch KM, Mascha EJ, Levine S, Haley EC, Grotta J, Marler J. Improved reliability of the NIH stroke scale using video training. NINDS TPA Stroke Study Group. Stroke. 1994;25(11):2220–6.
20. Kasner SE. Clinical interpretation and use of stroke scales. Lancet Neurol. 2006;5(7):603–12.
21. Barber PA, Demchuk AM, Zhang J, Buchan AM. Validity and reliability of a quantitative computed tomography score in predicting outcome of hyperacute stroke before thrombolytic therapy. Lancet. 2000;355(9216):1670–4.
22. Grotta JC, Chiu D, Lu M, Patel S, Levine SR, Tilley BC, Brott TG, Haley EC Jr, Lyden PD, Kothari R. Agreement and variability in the interpretation of early CT changes in stroke patients qualifying for intravenous rtPA therapy. Stroke. 1999;30(8):1528–33.
23. Hill MD, Demchuk AM, Goyal M, Jovin TG, Foster LD, Tomsick TA, von Kummer R, Yeatts SD, Palesch YY. Alberta stroke program early CT score (ASPECTS) in acute ischemic stroke: outcomes from the INTERRSeCT study. Am J Neuroradiol. 2016;37(3):504–9.
24. Hemphill JC 3rd, Bonovich DC, Besmertis L, Manley GT, Johnston SC. The ICH score: a simple, reliable grading scale for intracerebral hemorrhage. Stroke. 2001;32(4):891–7.
25. Becker KJ, Baxter AB, Cohen WA, Bybee HM, Tirschwell DL, Newell DW, Winn HR, Longstreth WT Jr. Withdrawal of support in intracerebral hemorrhage may lead to self-fulfilling prophecies. Neurology. 2001;56(6):766–72.
26. Qureshi AI, Tuhrim S, Broderick JP, Batjer HH, Hondo H, Hanley DF. Spontaneous intracerebral hemorrhage. N Engl J Med. 2001;344(19):1450–60.
27. Vincent JL, Moreno R. Clinical review: scoring systems in the critically ill. Crit Care. 2010;14(2):207.
28. Metnitz PG, Moreno RP, Almeida E, Jordan B, Bauer P, Campos RA, Iapichino G, Edbrooke D, Capuzzo M, Le Gall JR. SAPS 3—from evaluation of the patient to evaluation of the intensive care unit. Part 2: development of a prognostic model for hospital mortality at ICU admission. Intensive Care Med. 2005;31(10):1345–55.
29. Vincent JL, de Mendonça A, Cantraine F, Moreno R, Takala J, Suter PM, Sprung CL, Colardyn F, Blecher S. Use of the SOFA score to assess the incidence of organ dysfunction/failure in intensive care units: results of a multicenter, prospective study. Crit Care Med. 1998;26(11):1793–800.
30. Mikkelsen ME, Miltiades AN, Gaieski DF, Goyal M, Fuchs BD, Shah CV, Bellamy SL, Christie JD. Serum lactate is associated with mortality in severe sepsis independent of organ failure and shock. Crit Care Med. 2009;37(5):1670–7.
31. Ferreira FL, Bota DP, Bross A, Mélot C, Vincent JL. Serial evaluation of the SOFA score to predict outcome in critically ill patients. JAMA. 2001;286(14):1754–8.
32. Vos PE, Jacobs B, Andriessen TM, Lamers KJ, Borm GF, Beems T, et al. GFAP and S100B are biomarkers of traumatic brain injury: an observational cohort study. Neurology. 2010;75(20):1786–93.
33. Zetterberg H, Smith DH, Blennow K. Biomarkers of mild traumatic brain injury in cerebrospinal fluid and blood. Nat Rev Neurol. 2013;9(4):201–10.
34. Fischer M, Ansari S, De Georgia M. Four score and Glasgow coma scale in predictive modeling for traumatic brain injury. Surg Neurol Int. 2010;1:78.
35. Nasrallah F, Sengupta S, Schreiber S, et al. PREdiction and Diagnosis using Imaging and Clinical data for traumatic brain injury: a machine-learning model study. BMJ Open. 2023;13(4):e067740.
36. Yang S, Varghese P, Stephenson E, Tu K, Gronsbell J. Machine learning approaches for electronic health records phenotyping: a methodical review. J Am Med Inform Assoc. 2023;30(2):367–81.
37. Chaudhry F, Srei PKL, Ganatra A, et al. Machine learning applications in the neuro ICU: current status and future directions. Frontiers in Neurology. 2020;11:554633.

24 End-of-Life Care in the Neuro ICU

Shweta S. Naik, Mathangi Krishnakumar,
and Amruta Nirale

Abstract

End-of-life (EOL) care in the neurocritical care unit (neuro ICU) is fraught with ethical, medical, and logistical challenges. Prognostic uncertainty, family dynamics, cultural and religious considerations, and resource limitations add layers of complexity to EOL decision-making.

This chapter explores the key controversies in EOL care, including the timing and accuracy of prognostic assessments, the role of advance directives, the influence of surrogate decision-making, and the ethical principle of medical futility. It also addresses challenges in implementing do-not-resuscitate (DNR) orders, managing conflicts between family wishes and medical recommendations, and integrating palliative care in neurocritical settings.

Controversial topics such as sedation and analgesia use, artificial nutrition and hydration, and the ethical dilemmas of withdrawing life support are analyzed. The chapter emphasizes the need for effective communication strategies and multidisciplinary collaboration to align treatment goals with patient and family values. By understanding and addressing these controversies, healthcare professionals can navigate the complexities of EOL care with compassion and sensitivity, ultimately enhancing patient-centered outcomes in the neuro ICU.

S. S. Naik (✉)
Department of Neuroanaesthesia and Neurocritical Care, NIMHANS, Bengaluru, Karnataka, India

M. Krishnakumar
Surgical and Neuro Intensive Care Unit, Department of Anaesthesia, St John's Medical College Hospital, Bengaluru, Karnataka, India

A. Nirale
Neuroanaesthesia, Trustwell Hospital, Bengaluru, Karnataka, India

P. U. Bidkar, M. Krishnakumar (eds.), *Controversies in Neurocritical Care*,
https://doi.org/10.1007/978-981-95-4419-6_24

Keywords

End-of-life care · Neurocritical care · Prognostic uncertainty · Medical futility · Palliative care, Ethical dilemmas

Controversies

1. *Prognostic Uncertainty*: Limitations of scoring systems and biomarkers in predicting outcomes
2. *Family Communication*: Balancing patient autonomy, family wishes, and medical recommendation
3. *Medical Futility*: Lack of consensus on when treatments are futile.
4. *Do-Not-Resuscitate (DNR) Orders:* Misinterpretations and conflicts during implementation
5. *Palliative Care Integration*: Resistance due to misconceptions and ethical concerns about symptom management
6. *Resource Allocation*: Ethical dilemmas in prioritizing ICU resources for patients with poor prognoses

24.1 Introduction

End-of-life (EOL) care in neurocritical care presents unique challenges and ethical dilemmas due to the complex and often uncertain prognoses of patients with severe neurological conditions. As medical technology advances, the capacity to sustain life artificially has increased, leading to difficult decisions regarding the prolongation of life versus the quality of life. The ethical dilemma revolves around determining when continued aggressive treatment is futile and when to initiate palliative care [1].

24.2 The EOL Decision Process

The process of making end-of-life decisions in neurocritical care involves several stages, each with potential controversies (Fig. 24.1).

Fig. 24.1 End-of-life decision process

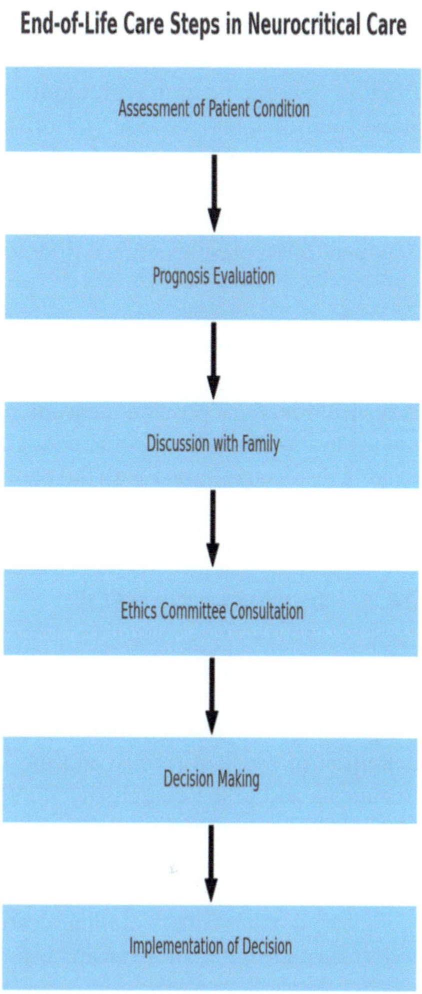

24.3 Assessment and Prognosis

Accurate prognostication in neurocritical care is inherently difficult due to the variability in neurological injuries. Scoring systems like the Glasgow Coma Scale (GCS) and the Full Outline of UnResponsiveness (FOUR) score help guide clinical decisions but are often uncertain. Controversies arise regarding the timing of prognostic assessments, potential biases in clinical judgment, and the limitations of current diagnostic tools. Studies suggest a need for improved prognostic models and biomarkers to better predict outcomes [2–5]. There is a significant difference in decision-making between acute and chronic conditions, requiring multiple assessments to proceed to the next step.

24.4 Family Discussions

Effective communication with families is critical yet challenging due to emotional stress and complex medical information. Misunderstandings about the patient's prognosis can lead to conflicts. The Setting, Perception, Invitation, Knowledge, Emotions, and Summary (SPIKES) protocol is one approach to structure these discussions. However, balancing patient autonomy with family wishes and medical judgment often presents ethical dilemmas [6].

24.5 Decision-Making

Advance directives provide clear instructions about a patient's preferences but are not always available or specific enough. Surrogate decision-makers are tasked with making decisions aligned with the patient's values, which can be contentious if family members disagree or if the patient's wishes are not well-documented [7].

24.6 Implementing EOL

Deciding when to withdraw or withhold treatments is ethically and emotionally charged. The concept of medical futility, where interventions are unlikely to benefit the patient, is a significant source of controversy. The lack of a universally accepted definition of medical futility and the extent of physician authority to cease futile treatments add to the complexity [8, 9]. Do-not-resuscitate (DNR) orders are challenging to obtain, especially when there are conflicts between patient or family preferences and medical recommendations. Miscommunications and fears that DNR implies the cessation of all care complicate the process. Thorough documentation and clear, compassionate communication are essential to ensure that DNR orders reflect the patient's wishes and are respected by all healthcare team members [10, 11].

24.7 Decision-Making and Care Planning

Despite the availability of various scoring systems, both neuro-specific (Glasgow Coma Scale [GCS] and Full Outline of UnResponsiveness [FOUR] score) and non-neuro-specific acute physiology and chronic health evaluation II (APACHE II) and sequential organ failure assessment (SOFA), the accuracy in predicting prognosis for guiding clinical decisions, especially on end-of-life care, is uncertain due to the variable nature of neurological injuries and illnesses [2–5]. Other controversies in assessment and planning include the limitations of current diagnostic tools and biomarkers in providing definitive prognoses; the optimal timing for prognostic assessments, given that early predictions may change with time and treatment; and potential biases and variability in clinicians' assessments influenced by personal experience and institutional practices.

Balancing patient autonomy and family wishes with medical judgment and ethical considerations is a recurring challenge in EOL care. Conflicts often arise from differing opinions on appropriate care pathways. Advance directives and surrogate decision-makers play a crucial role in guiding these decisions [6]. Advance directives provide clear instructions about a patient's preferences for EOL care, while surrogate decision-makers are tasked with making decisions that align with the patient's values and wishes. Clinicians must navigate these dynamics with sensitivity, ensuring that the patient's autonomy is respected while also considering the emotional and ethical concerns of the family [5].

Prognostic uncertainty is a significant challenge in neurocritical care. Predicting outcomes in neurocritical care patients is notoriously difficult, leading to challenges in making EOL decisions [11]. The need for better prognostic tools and strategies to manage uncertainty is evident. Current prognostic models often rely on clinical judgment, which can be subject to bias and variability. Efforts to develop more accurate and reliable prognostic tools, such as biomarkers and advanced imaging techniques, are ongoing [12]. In the meantime, clinicians must communicate the inherent uncertainties to families and involve them in shared decision-making processes, emphasizing the importance of aligning treatment goals with the patient's values and preferences [13].

Determining the right time to shift from aggressive curative treatments to palliative care can be controversial, often leading to disputes between medical teams and families. The ethical principle of double effect, where an action (like administering high-dose opioids) can have two effects (relieving pain and potentially hastening death), is often at the center of these debates [14]. Misconceptions that palliative care is synonymous with giving up can lead to resistance from patients, families, and some healthcare providers. Timing the introduction of palliative care, particularly in conjunction with aggressive treatment efforts, requires careful consideration and communication [15].

24.8 Symptom Management and Palliative Care

Integrating palliative care into neurocritical care can address many of the controversies surrounding EOL care. Palliative care focuses on symptom management, psychological support, and the improvement of quality of life for patients with serious illnesses [16]. Early involvement of palliative care teams can facilitate better communication, support decision-making, and align treatment goals with patient and family wishes [17].

In neurocritical care, symptom management is paramount, especially for patients nearing the end of life. Pain, agitation, and respiratory distress are common and require careful management to ensure comfort [18]. Palliative care principles emphasize the importance of comfort care, even when life-sustaining treatments are being considered or withdrawn [19]. Resistance to integrating palliative care into neurocritical care persists due to perceptions that it is synonymous with giving up. However, highlighting the role of palliative care in improving the quality of life and supporting both patients and families can help shift perceptions and facilitate its integration [20].

Symptom management in neurocritical care is aimed at alleviating suffering with the right use of appropriate medications. The use of opioids in the management of severe pain raises concerns about respiratory depression, excessive sedation, and their impact on neurological assessment and prognostication. Patients often develop a tolerance, necessitating higher doses for the same relief, which can lead to concerns about oversedation and hastening death [21]. Clinicians must carefully balance the need for pain relief with potential side effects that can complicate the assessment of neurological function.

The use of sedatives in neurocritical care has the potential to mask neurological symptoms, complicate prognosis, and contribute to prolonged ventilation and ICU stays. Critics argue that it may hasten death, blurring the lines between palliative care and euthanasia. Decisions about when and how to initiate sedation involve complex ethical considerations, balancing relief from suffering with the potential for reducing consciousness and life expectancy. The development of sedation protocols that involve light sedation with sedation interruption is debated for their effectiveness and impact on patient outcomes [22].

While oxygen therapy can relieve dyspnea, its use in patients with limited life expectancy must be balanced against the potential for increased discomfort and the prolongation of the dying process [23]. The use of artificial nutrition and hydration (ANH) in patients nearing the end of life is contentious, particularly in patients with neurological illness, due to impaired consciousness, swallowing, and gastrointestinal function. Decisions regarding ANH involve ethical dilemmas about prolonging life versus ensuring comfort, with varying practices based on cultural, religious, and personal beliefs [13].

24.9 Ethical and Legal Considerations

Withdrawal of life support is a profound ethical dilemma in neurocritical care (Table 24.1). Clinicians must balance the potential benefits of continued treatment against the possibility of prolonged suffering and diminished quality of life. Institutional protocols for withdrawing life support vary widely, influenced by cultural, religious, and personal beliefs. For instance, in some cultures, withdrawal of life support may be seen as morally unacceptable, whereas in others, it may be viewed as a way to alleviate suffering [1, 7].

The variability in legal frameworks across jurisdictions further complicates the decision-making process, necessitating that clinicians are well-versed in the legal standards and ethical guidelines that govern their practice [24]. The Indian Council of Medical Research (ICMR) National Ethical Guidelines for Biomedical and Health Research Involving Human Participants emphasize the importance of respecting patient autonomy, ensuring informed consent, and considering the ethical principles of beneficence, non-maleficence, and justice [25].

Table 24.1 Ethical and legal considerations in end-of-life care

Consideration	Description
Patient autonomy	Respecting the patient's right to make their own healthcare decisions
Informed consent	Ensuring that patients and families understand the illness and treatment options
Advance directives	Legal documents specifying patients' preferences for end-of-life care
Surrogate decision-making	Designated individuals making decisions for incapacitated patients
Role of ethics committees	Committees providing oversight in complex ethical cases
Legal frameworks	Laws and regulations guiding end-of-life care decisions
Cultural and religious beliefs	Influence of cultural and religious values on end-of-life choices
Resource allocation	Ethical distribution of limited healthcare resources

DNR orders present another layer of complexity. Obtaining DNR orders can be challenging, particularly when patient or family preferences conflict with medical recommendations. These conflicts often arise from misunderstandings about the patient's prognosis or differing values regarding the sanctity of life versus quality of life [9, 10]. Miscommunications are common, with some families fearing that a DNR order implies a cessation of all care, rather than just refraining from invasive resuscitation measures. Clear, compassionate communication and thorough documentation are essential to ensure that DNR orders accurately reflect the patient's wishes and are respected by all members of the healthcare team [26].

Controversial aspects include establishing clear and consistent criteria for when it is appropriate to withdraw or withhold treatments, balancing respect for patient and family wishes with medical recommendations and ethical considerations, and navigating varying legal frameworks and institutional policies regarding withdrawal of life-sustaining therapy (WLST) [2]. The concept of medical futility, where interventions are unlikely to benefit the patient, is a significant source of controversy. Key issues include the lack of a universally accepted definition of medical futility, the extent of physicians' authority to unilaterally decide to cease futile treatments, and strategies for resolving conflicts between healthcare providers and families regarding futile treatments [8].

24.10 Communication Strategies

Effective communication is critical in navigating EOL care decisions in neurocritical care. Discussing prognosis and EOL options with families is particularly challenging due to the emotional stress and complexity of medical conditions. The involvement of multidisciplinary teams, including social workers, chaplains, and palliative care specialists, can provide additional support, helping families understand the medical situation and make informed decisions [27].

Coordination among multidisciplinary team members is essential to avoid inconsistent messaging and decision-making. Regular team meetings and case conferences can help align treatment goals and care plans [11]. A unified approach ensures coherent communication with families, reducing confusion and fostering trust. Multidisciplinary teams, including neurologists, intensivists, nurses, palliative care specialists, and ethicists, should collaborate to develop a consensus on the best course of action, considering both the medical aspects and the patient's and family's values and preferences [12].

24.11 Emerging Controversies

Ethical dilemmas in allocating limited resources, such as ICU beds and staff, to patients with poor prognoses are particularly acute in neurocritical care [7]. Criteria for resource allocation and prioritization must be developed transparently and equitably. These criteria should consider factors such as the likelihood of meaningful recovery, the patient's wishes and values, and broader public health considerations. The impact on patient care and outcomes can be significant, and efforts to ensure fair and just allocation of resources are essential to maintaining trust and integrity in the healthcare system [28]. Some examples encountered in the neurocritical care unit are given in Table 24.2.

Table 24.2 Examples of clinical conditions and controversies in EOL care

Neurocritical care condition	Controversies in implementing EOL care
Traumatic brain injury (TBI)	Prognostic uncertainty and the potential for recovery, leading to difficulty in making EOL decisions
Subarachnoid hemorrhage (SAH)	High mortality and morbidity rates create ethical dilemmas about the extent of aggressive treatment versus comfort care
Stroke	Variability in recovery potential and differing views on the quality of life post-stroke complicate EOL decision-making
Intracerebral hemorrhage (ICH)	High rates of poor outcomes lead to complex decisions about continuing aggressive treatment versus palliation
Coma	Challenges in determining the irreversibility of the condition and the potential for misdiagnosis affecting EOL decisions
Severe meningitis/encephalitis	Uncertain recovery potential and the impact of severe neurological deficits
Spinal cord injury	Balancing aggressive treatment with the potential for significant disability and the patient's quality of life
Brain tumors	Ethical dilemmas regarding the aggressiveness of treatment in the context of a terminal illness
Neuromuscular diseases (e.g., amyotrophic lateral sclerosis (ALS) and Guillain–Barré syndrome)	Difficulty in assessing the long-term prognosis and balancing life-sustaining treatments with quality-of-life considerations

24.12 Conclusion

End-of-life care in neurocritical care involves navigating numerous controversies and ethical challenges. From withdrawal of life support and DNR orders to communication strategies, decision-making processes, and symptom management, each aspect requires careful consideration and a nuanced approach. By understanding and addressing these controversies through ethical frameworks, legal guidelines, and cultural sensitivity, healthcare professionals can provide compassionate, patient-centered care that honors the wishes and values of neurocritical patients and their families.

References

1. Beauchamp TL, Childress JF. Principles of biomedical ethics. 7th ed. Oxford University Press; 2013.
2. Sternbach GL. The Glasgow coma scale. J Emerg Med. 2000;19(1):67–71.
3. Marion DW, Carlier PM, Viña-Ribes R. The use of barbiturates in the treatment of head injury. Neurochirurgie. 1991;37(2):81–5.
4. Wijdicks EF, Bamlet WR, Maramattom BV, Manno EM, McClelland RL. Validation of a new coma scale: the FOUR score. Ann Neurol. 2005;58(4):585–93.
5. Quill TE, Arnold RM, Back AL. Discussing treatment preferences with patients who want "everything". Ann Intern Med. 2009;151(5):345–9.
6. Bosslet GT, Pope TM, Rubenfeld GD, et al. An official ATS/AACN/ACCP/ESICM/SCCM policy statement: responding to requests for potentially inappropriate treatments in intensive care units. Am J Respir Crit Care Med. 2016;193(11):1318–30.
7. Truog RD, Campbell ML, Curtis JR, et al. Recommendations for end-of-life care in the intensive care unit: a consensus statement by the American college of critical care medicine. Crit Care Med. 2008;36(3):953–63.
8. Bosslet GT, Kesecioglu J, White DB, et al. Critical care societies collaborative statement on the use of intensive care unit beds for patients with little or no expected benefit. Crit Care Med. 2017;45(1):110–5.
9. Lautrette A, Darmon M, Megarbane B, et al. A communication strategy and brochure for relatives of patients dying in the ICU. N Engl J Med. 2007;356(5):469–78.
10. Smith TJ, Temin S, Alesi ER, et al. American society of clinical oncology provisional clinical opinion: the integration of palliative care into standard oncology care. J Clin Oncol. 2012;30(8):880–7.
11. Nelson JE, Bassett R, Boss RD, et al. Models for structuring a clinical initiative to enhance palliative care in the intensive care unit: a report from the improving palliative care in the ICU (IPAL-ICU) project. Crit Care Med. 2010;38(9):1765–72.
12. Curtis JR, Vincent JL. Ethics and end-of-life care for adults in the intensive care unit. Lancet. 2010;376(9749):1347–53.
13. Teno JM, Gozalo PL, Bynum JP, et al. Change in end-of-life care for medicare beneficiaries: site of death, place of care, and health care transitions in 2000, 2005, and 2009. JAMA. 2013;309(5):470–7.
14. Sulmasy DP. The rule of double effect: clearing up the double talk. Arch Intern Med. 1999;159(6):545–50.
15. Quill TE, Abernethy AP. Generalist plus specialist palliative care — creating a more sustainable model. N Engl J Med. 2013;368(13):1173–5.
16. Gade G, Venohr I, Conner D, et al. Impact of an inpatient palliative care team: a randomized controlled trial. J Palliat Med. 2008;11(2):180–90.

17. Grady C. End-of-life care for critically ill patients in the United States: the intensive care unit and beyond. Curr Opin Crit Care. 2014;20(6):656–63.
18. Azoulay E, Pochard F, Chevret S, et al. Meeting the needs of intensive care unit patient families: a multicenter study. Am J Respir Crit Care Med. 2001;163(1):135–9.
19. Meier DE, Beresford L. Palliative care in the intensive care unit. Intensive Care Med. 2008;34(4):616–7.
20. Wunsch H, Wagner J, Herlim M, et al. ICU occupancy and mechanical ventilator use in the United States. Crit Care Med. 2013;41(12):2712–9.
21. Devlin JW, et al. Clinical practice guidelines for the prevention and management of pain, agitation/sedation, delirium, immobility, and sleep disruption in adult patients in the ICU. Crit Care Med. 2018;46(9):e825.
22. Shehabi Y, et al. Sedation depth and long-term mortality in mechanically ventilated critically ill adults: a prospective longitudinal multicentre cohort study. Intensive Care Med. 2013;39:910–8.
23. Rocker GM, Simpson AC. Dyspnea at the end of life: how to recognize, assess, and manage. J Palliat Med. 2016;19(6):567–73.
24. Luce JM. End-of-life decision making in the intensive care unit. Am J Respir Crit Care Med. 2010;182(1):6–11.
25. Indian Council of Medical Research. National Ethical Guidelines for biomedical and Health Research involving human participants. New Delhi: ICMR; 2017.
26. Fins JJ. A palliative ethic of care: clinical wisdom at life's end. Jones & Bartlett Learning; 2006.
27. Halpern SD, Hansen-Flaschen J, Brennan TA. Allocation of intensive care resources during an influenza pandemic. N Engl J Med. 2008;358(14):1379–80.
28. Cook D, Rocker G. Dying with dignity in the intensive care unit. N Engl J Med. 2014;370(26):2506–14.

MIX
Papier aus verantwortungsvollen Quellen
Paper from responsible sources
FSC® C105338

If you have any concerns about our products,
you can contact us on
ProductSafety@springernature.com

In case Publisher is established outside the EU,
the EU authorized representative is:
Springer Nature Customer Service Center GmbH
Europaplatz 3, 69115 Heidelberg, Germany

Printed by Libri Plureos GmbH
in Hamburg, Germany